E. Molinari   A. Compare   G. Parati

Clinical Psychology and Heart Disease

E. Molinari ▪ A. Compare ▪ G. Parati

Clinical Psychology
and
Heart Disease

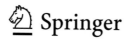 Springer

ENRICO MOLINARI
Faculty of Psychology
Catholic University of Milan
Italian Auxologic Institute
Milan, Italy

GIANFRANCO PARATI
University of Milano-Bicocca
Cardiology II - St. Luca Hospital
Italian Auxologic Institute
Milan, Italy

ANGELO COMPARE
Faculty of Psychology
Catholic University of Milan
Italian Auxologic Institute
Milan, Italy

Cover: figure reproduced from the brochure
"Lo stress in ambiente di lavoro" (with permission)

Library of Congress Control Number: 2006926658

ISBN-10   88-470-0377-6 Springer Milan Berlin Heidelberg New York
ISBN-13   978-88-470-0377-4 Springer Milan Berlin Heidelberg New York

Springer is a part of Springer Science+Business Media
springer.com
© Springer-Verlag Italia 2006
Printed in Italy

Cover design: Simona Colombo, Milan, Italy
Typesetting: Graficando, Milan, Italy
Printing: Grafiche Porpora, Cernusco s/N (MI), Italy

Foreword

Among the various areas of interest studied in the Laboratory of Clinical Psychology of the Faculty of Psychology at the Catholic University in Milan and in the Psychology Laboratory of the Italian Auxologic Institute, the study and care of the psychological aspects of cardiac illness constitute a particularly interesting challenge.

The decline in infectious diseases, brought about by important medical discoveries over the past hundred years, has witnessed the emergence of other, more evident causes of pathology. Today in Italy, as in the United States and the United Kingdom, cardiac illness constitutes the principal cause of death. In Italy, cardiovascular pathologies cause 27% of the deaths (this datum can be compared to a mortality rate of 21% of deaths caused by tumours). In the United States over the past twenty years, deaths caused by cardiac illness have remained high: about 5 million people are affected by cardiac illness and 400,000 new cases are registered every year. In Italy there is a yearly incidence of 130,000 new cases of heart attacks, of which 80,000 represent new episodes and 50,000 recurrences.

An international survey of contemporary research and clinical comparisons outlines how cardiac illness is often associated with psychological stress, which represents an important risk factor both in the onset of the disease and in its progression. This demonstrates the importance of developing care and rehabilitation programs within a bio-psycho-social perspective, in which biological, social and psychological factors, both individually and relationally, are viewed as a collection of interdependent or systemic variables that interact either in keeping individuals healthy or in causing illness.

As reflected in the international guidelines on cardiac rehabilitation, the scientific world acknowledges the importance of multidisciplinary, integrated models in the clinical area, in which the competences of cardiologists and the psychologists operate in an integrated way.

We are very proud to present this volume on "Clinical Psychology and Heart Disease," by Enrico Molinari, Angelo Compare and Gianfranco Parati. In our view, the study and care of cardiac illness and the psychological symptomatology connected to it deserve a privileged space in the medical literature, one in which both medical and psychological competences can be integrated within a bio-psycho-social framework.

This volume tackles psychological suffering in cardiac patients and is the result of the collaboration of the most important international researchers in the fields of clinical and health psychology, as applied to cardiac illness. The focus encompasses: a) the most up-to-date information available on the link between psychological variables and cardiac functionality; b) clinical indications for the diagnosis and treatment of psychological factors connected to cardiac risk; and c) possible directions future research might take.

In addition to discussing and illustrating the theoretical and technical aspects of the complex psychological variables associated with cardiac illness, this book presents a proposal to give a "heart to cardiology," in keeping with our belief, as affirmed by Bernard Lown (Nobel Peace Prize 1985), that: *"Medicine is based both on taking care of people and on science. If one takes care of others without science, there might be good intention, but it is certainly not medicine. On the other hand, if there is science, but one does not take care of patients, medicine is emptied of its thaumaturgical aspect, making it similar to other sciences, such as physics, engineering…these two aspects, taking care of others, and science, complement one another and are essential in medicine. I would like to add that taking care of people is different from healing them; in the first case, one has to do with organs that don't function well, and in the second case with a human being who suffers. I believe that medicine should orient itself towards healing."*

Among the more salient points presented in the first part of the book is the connection between personality factors (the so called Type A and Type D personality traits) and the relational aspects of cardiac illness. Another noteworthy area of research we present contextualizes cardiac illness within an interpersonal perspective, placing particular emphasis on the relationship of couples.

The second part of the book focuses on the various psychological interventions used in cardiac rehabilitation and emphasizes the therapeutic value of the psychologist's understanding of the psychological suffering involved in cardiac disease. Other psychological approaches examined include interpersonal psychotherapy in the treatment of depression, the treatment of anxious symptomatology with the use of "couples therapy" and relaxation techniques and the application of new computer technology in the integrated psychological-cardiac treatment of the psychological symptomatology of cardiac insufficiency.

We believe that this volume can be a useful reference for clinicians, medical and psychological researchers as well as others who want to understand and explore the link between cardiac pathology and its psychological components.

Eugenia Scabini
Director of the Laboratory of Psychological Research
Italian Auxologic Institute
Dean Faculty of Psychology
Catholic University of Milan, Italy

Alberto Zanchetti
Scientific Director
Italian Auxologic Institute
Milan, Italy

Foreword

It is a propitious time for a volume examining the range of ways that clinical psychology can inform and influence the understanding of the development and treatment of heart disease. Although the possible relationships between heart disease and psychological factors such as personality type have been discussed for several decades, it is only recently that theory and research have begun to fully explicate the bio-psycho-social influences on heart disease and the ways that psychological treatments can be brought to bear to increase the quality of life of those with heart disease and perhaps even decrease the prevalence of disease.

Enrico Molinari, Angelo Compare and Gianfranco Parati in this wonderful edited volume provide a valuable guide to the study of clinical psychology in the cardiological field, covering the key areas of investigation and intervention. There are sections describing the physiological basis of the mind-heart link, the relationships between heart disease and depression and anxiety, the relationship of heart disease to personality types, statistical methods that enable the study of psychological risks, and psychological treatments. Much of this book is on the cutting edge of the investigations into these phenomena; for example, the chapters by Coyne, Compare, and Ruiz (on the quality of the couple relationship as protective and risk factors) and by Johnson, Lee, and DiGuilio (on the application of emotion-focused couple therapy in this population) provide unique insights about interpersonal processes related to heart disease and how interpersonal systems can be helpful in treatment.

Molinari, Compare and Parati bring a much needed systemic vision to the psychological aspects of heart disease. In their introductory chapter, they point to the complex interrelationships between the psychological and somatic aspects of heart disease, how each can influence the other, and how treatments need to account for these complex mutual influences.

Humans are bio-psycho-social entities, affected by a range of internal subsystems and external social systems, which influence one another in endless loops of causality. It therefore behooves us to fully understand the effects of each system on the other systems and to carefully consider how to utilize our understanding to improve the welfare of patients. This volume reflects the advances in recent theory and research that allows us to make significant progress in that direction. This is an area where there are many reasonable sounding ideas, but in which volumes of this kind are needed to help understand the breadth of thought and what the evidence says about these thoughts.

Such understandings can serve as the underpinning for what truly would be an evidence-based practice for treating heart disease. Incorporating the evidence reviewed in this book, such an evidence-based practice needs to include consideration of the psychological intervention, as well as the biological. With the powerful impact of the various heart diseases themselves and the heroic developments in surgery, technology, medicine, and other disciplines, it becomes easy to focus exclusively on biological factors and biological solutions. Yet, biology remains only part of the story, even though an important part. Engaging in health-promoting behaviors over a lifetime makes a considerable impact on heart disease, as does the presence of family support. Additionally, certain psychological patterns seem clearly related to a greater likelihood of the development of heart disease. Treatments that engage family support, promote individual coping, and change behaviors that promote heart disease have considerable impact. Additionally, as the chapters in section 2 of this book clearly indicate, understanding and treating the psychological co-morbidities of anxiety and depression is of great importance in treating heart disease patients. Hopefully, this volume will help call attention to the now well-established relationships between psychological factors and heart disease, and the important role for clinical psychology in both understanding heart disease and in treating patients suffering from the resulting set of disorders.

Jay Lebow, PhD, ABPP
Clinical Professor
Family Institute at Northwestern
and Northwestern University
Evanston, IL, USA

Contents

List of Contributors XIII

About the Editors XVII

Introduction 1
S. Mendis

Chapter 1: Clinical Psychology for Cardiac Disease 5
E. Molinari, L. Bellardita, A. Compare

▌**Part I**
▌**Psychological Risk Factors for Cardiac Disease**

Chapter 2: Psychological Risk Factors for Cardiac Disease
and Pathophysiological Mechanisms: An Overview 21
A. Compare, L. Gondoni, E. Molinari

Physiological Basis of Mind-Heart Link

Chapter 3: Psychophysiology of Heart Disease 35
G. Parati, M. Valentini, G. Mancia

Chapter 4: Mental Stress Ischemia: Characteristics, Pathophysiology,
Prognosis and Treatment 71
M.M. Burg

Depression and Anxiety

Chapter 5: Depression and CHD: Prevalence, Prognosis,
Pathophysiology and Treatment 85
K. Maier, D. Chatkoff, M.M. Burg

Chapter 6: Prevalence of Depression in Chronic Heart Failure 99
E.P. Havranek

Chapter 7: Depression in Coronary Artery Disease:
Assessment and Treatment 109
W.J. Kop, D.N. Ader

Chapter 8: Anxiety and Heart Disease 121
D.K. Moser, M.J. De Jong

Chapter 9: Anxiety, Depressive Symptoms and Heart
Transplantation 149
S. Zipfel, A. Schneider, J. Jünger, W. Herzog

Chapter 10: Psychological Factors in Hypertension
Development and Treatment 165
T. Rutledge

Personality and Relational Aspects

Chapter 11: Type A, Type D, Anger-Prone Behavior
and Risk of Relapse in CHD Patients 187
A. Compare, G.M. Manzoni, E. Molinari

Chapter 12: Defensive Hostility and Cardiovascular Disease:
Theoretical and Empirical Bases for an Interpersonal
Approach-Avoidance Conflict Perspective 217
R.S. Jorgensen, R. Thibodeau

Chapter 13: In Sickness and In Health: Interpersonal Risk
and Resilience in Cardiovascular Disease 233
J.M. Ruiz, H.A. Hamann, J.C. Coyne, A. Compare

Chapter 14: Psychological Stress in Women:
the Stockholm Female Coronary Risk Study 273
K. Orth-Gomèr

Advanced Statistical Tools for the Study of Psychological Risks Aspects

Chapter 15: Application of Neural Networks and Other
Artificial Adaptive Systems in Prediction and Data
Mining of Risk Psychological Profile for CHD 281
E. Grossi, A. Compare

Chapter 16: Person Measurement and Rehabilitation Outcome:
the New Perspective of Rasch Analysis 319
L. Tesio

Interlude

The "Heart" of Cardiology:
an Imaginary Conversation with Bernard Lown 339
E. Molinari

Part II
Psychological Treatments in Cardiac Rehabilitation

Chapter 17: *The Art* of Listening to Cardiac Patient and his Family:
the Meanings of Suffering Along Temporal Dimension 349
A. Compare, M. Simioni

Chapter 18: Interpersonal Psychotherapy for Depression
in Patients with Coronary Heart Disease 369
D. Koszycki

Chapter 19: Hanging onto a Heartbeat: Emotionally
Focused Therapy for Couples Dealing with the Trauma
of Coronary Heart Disease 391
H.B. MacIntosh, S.M. Johnson, A. Lee

Chapter 20: Type A Behavior Pattern and Its Treatment 413
A.T. Möller

Chapter 21: Relaxation Techniques and Hypnosis
in the Treatment of CHD Patients 435
L. Bellardita, M. Cigada, E. Molinari

Chapter 22: Cardiological and Psychological Mobile Care
through Telematic Technologies for Heart Failure Patients:
ICAROS Project 451
A. Compare, E. Molinari, L. Bellardita, A. Villani, G. Branzi,
G. Malfatto, S. Boarin, M. Cassi, A. Gnisci, G. Parati

Chapter 23: Functioning and Disability in Patients with
Cardiovascular Disease within the ICF Classification Framework:
Proposals for Using ICF to Classify Functioning
and Disability in Patients with Cardiovascular Disease 471
M. Leonardi, A. Raggi

Chapter 24: Coherence-Building Techniques and Heart
Rhythm Coherence Feedback: New Tools for Stress
Reduction, Disease Prevention and Rehabilitation 487
R. McCraty, D. Tomasino

Subject Index 511

List of Contributors

Dr. D.N. Ader, PhD
National Institutes of Health, NIAMS
Bethesda, MD, USA

Dr. L. Bellardita, PsyD, MS
University of Bergamo
Catholic University of Milan, Italy

Dr. S. Boarin, MD
Cardiologist, Cardiology II
St. Luca Hospital
Italian Auxologic Institute
Milan, Italy

Dr. G. Branzi, MD
Cardiologist, Cardiology II
St. Luca Hospital
Italian Auxologic Institute
Milan, Italy

Prof. M.M. Burg, PhD
Associate Clinical Professor of Medicine
Behavioral Cardiovascular Health and
Hypertension Program Department of Medicine
Columbia University School of Medicine
New York, USA
and Associate Clinical Professor of Medicine
Section of Cardiovascular Medicine
Yale University School of Medicine
New Haven, CT, USA

Ing. M. Cassi
ICAROS FIRB
Project Manager, Senior Partner
Mobile Medical Technologies
Genoa, Italy

Prof. D. Chatkoff, PhD
Assistant Professor
Department of Behavioral Sciences Psychology
University of Michigan–Dearborn
Dearborn, Michigan, USA

Dr. M. Cigada, MD
European School of Hypnotic Psychotherapy
Milan, Italy

Prof. J.C. Coyne, PhD
Co-Director Cancer Control and Outcomes
Amramson Cancer Center
Professor of Psychology, Department of Psychiatry
Professor, Department of Family Practice
and Community Medicine
University of Pennsylvania, Philadelphia
USA

Dr. M.J. De Jong, PhD, CCNS, CCRN, Lt Col
Director, Nursing Research
Flight Commander, Support Flight
59th Clinical Research Squadron
Wilford Hall Medical Center
Lackland AFB, TX, USA

Prof. A. Gnisci, PhD
Associate Professor in Psychometry
II University
Naples, Italy

Dr. L.A. Gondoni, MD
Unit of Cardiac Rehabilitation
Ospedale San Giuseppe, IRCCS
Italian Auxologic Institute
Verbania, Italy

Dr. E. Grossi, MD
Director Medical Affairs
Pharma Department, Bracco SpA
Milan, Italy

Dr. J. Jünger, MD
Department of General Internal
and Psychosomatic Medicine
University Medical Hospital
Heidelberg, Germany

Prof. H.A. Hamann, PhD
Assistant Professor
Department of Psychology
Washington State University
Pullman, WA, USA

Prof. E.P. Havranek, MD
Denver Health Medical Center
University of Colorado at Denver
and Health Sciences Center
Denver, CO, USA

Prof. W. Herzog, MD
Professor of Medicine and Head, Department of
General Internal and Psychosomatic Medicine
University Medical Hospital
Heidelberg, Germany

Prof. S. Johnson, EdD
Professor of Clinical Psychology
Ottawa University
Director of the Ottawa Couple and Family Institute
and Center for Emotionally Focused Therapy
Ottawa, Canada
Research Professor at Alliant U, San Diego, CA, USA

Prof. R.S. Jorgensen, PhD
Associate Professor
Director of the Psychophysiology Laboratory
Center for Health and Behavior
and Department of Psychology
Syracuse University
New York, NY, USA

Dr. J. Jünger, MD
Department of General Internal
and Psychosomatic Medicine
University Medical Hospital
Heidelberg, Germany

Dr. W.J. Kop, PhD
Department of Medical and Clinical Psychology
Uniformed Services
University of the Health Sciences, Bethesda
Division of Cardiology, Department of Medicine
University of Maryland
Baltimore, MD, USA

Prof. D. Koszycki, PhD, C Psych
Research Director
Stress and Anxiety, Clinical Research Unit
University of Ottawa
Institute of Mental Health Research
Royal Ottawa Hospital
Associate Professor of Psychiatry
University of Ottawa, Canada

Prof. J. Lebow, PhD, ABPP
Clinical Professor
Family Institute at Northwestern
and Northwestern University
Evanston, IL, USA

Dr. A. Lee, PhD
Ottawa Couple & Family Institute
Ottawa, Canada

Dr. M. Leonardi, MD
Responsible Headnet Research Group:
Public Health, Disability, ICF
Scientific Direction
Italian National Neurological Institute Carlo Besta
Milan, Italy

Prof. K. Maier, PhD
Assistant Professor
Psychology Department, Salisbury University
Salisbury, MD, USA

Dr. G. Malfatto, MD
Cardiologist, Cardiology II
St. Luca Hospital
Italian Auxologic Institute
Milan, Italy

Prof. G. Mancia, MD
Full Professor of Medicine
Past President of European Society of Hypertension
Deputy Editor of the Journal of Hypertension
Chief, Department of Medicine
University of Milano-Bicocca, Italy

Dr. G.M. Manzoni, PsyD Candidate
Clinical Psychology Service and Laboratory
St. Giuseppe Hospital
Italian Auxologic Institute
Verbania, Italy

Prof. H.B. MacIntosh, PhD
Assistant Professor
Faculty of Human Sciences
St. Paul University
Ottawa, Canada

Dr. R. McCraty, PhD
Director of Research
HeartMath Research Center
Institute of HeartMath
Boulder Creek, California, USA

Dr. S. Mendis, MD, FRCP, FACC
Senior Adviser
Cardiovascular Diseases
World Health Organization
Geneva, Switzerland

Prof. A.T. Möller, Dphil
Professor of Clinical Psychology
Head, Department of Psychology
Stellenbosch University
South Africa

Prof. D.K. Moser, DNSc, RN, FAAN
Professor and Gill Endowed Chair of Nursing
Editor, The Journal of Cardiovascular Nursing
University of Kentucky, College of Nursing
Lexington, KY, USA

Prof. K. Orth-Gomèr, MD, PhD
Professor in Community Medicine
Karolinska Institutet
Stockholm, Sweden

Dr. A. Raggi, PsyD
Junior Researcher
Italian National Neurological Institute Carlo Besta
Scientific Direction
Italian National Neurological Institute Carlo Besta
Milan, Italy

Prof. J.M. Ruiz, PhD
Assistant Professor
Department of Psychology
Washington State University
Pullman, WA, USA

Prof. T. Rutledge, PhD
Assistant Professor
Department of Psychiatry
University of California - San Diego
San Diego, USA

Prof. E. Scabini, PsyD, MS
Dean, Faculty of Psychology
Full Professor of Social Psychology of Family
Faculty of Psychology
Director, Centre for Family Studies and Research
Catholic University of Milan
Director of the Laboratory of Psychological Research
Italian Auxologic Institute
Milan, Italy

Dr. A. Schneider, MD
Department of General Practice
and Health Service Research
University Medical Hospital
Heidelberg, Germany

Dr. M. Simioni, PsyD, MS
Legnano Hospital, Italy

Prof. L. Tesio, MD
Chair of Rehabilitation Medicine
University of Milan
Head, Clinical Unit and Laboratory
of Research of Neuromotor Rehabilitation
Italian Auxologic Institute
Milan, Italy

Dr. R. Thibodeau, MS
Doctoral Candidate
Department of Psychology
Syracuse University
Syracuse, NY, USA

Dr. D. Tomasino, BA
HeartMath Research Center
Institute of HeartMath
Boulder Creek, CA, USA

Dr. C. Valentini, MD
University of Milano-Bicocca
Cardiology II, St. Luca Hospital
Italian Auxologic Institute
Milan, Italy

Dr. A.A. Villani, MD
Cardiologist, Cardiology II
St. Luca Hospital
Italian Auxologic Institute
Milan, Italy

Prof. A. Zanchetti, MD
Editor in Chief of Journal of Hypertension
Scientific Director
Italian Auxologic Institute
Milan, Italy

Prof. S. Zipfel, MD
Prof. of Medicine and Head
Department Internal Medicine VI
Psychosomatic Medicine and Psychotherapy
University Medical Hospital
Tübingen, Germany

About the Editors

■ **Enrico Molinari,** MS, PsyD in Clinical Psychology

Full Professor of Clinical Psychology at the Faculty of Clinical Psychology, Catholic University, Milan, Italy and Head of the Clinical Psychology Service at St. Joseph Hospital, Italian Auxologic Institute, Milan. His scientific activity in the field of cardiac psychology includes the participation in Italian and European research projects involving the use of telematic technologies. He is a member of several international and national scientific societies such as the Italian Society of Systemic Therapy and Research (SIRTS) and the Society of Psychotherapy Research (SPR). Since 2002, he has been the Scientific Secretary of the Board of Professors of Clinical Psychology of Italian Universities. Since 2003 he has been the coordinator of the PhD Program in Clinical Psychology at the University of Milano-Bicocca. He is a member of the Commission for the recognition of Psychotherapy schools in Italy, Italian Ministry of Research & University and of the Committee for Eating Disorders, Italian Ministry of Health. He has been the President of the Regional (Lombardy) Professional Board of Psychologists in Italy since 2006.

■ **Angelo Compare,** PhD, MS, PsyD in Clinical Psychology

Researcher in Clinical Psychology, Department of Psychology, Catholic University of Milan, and Clinical Psychologist for the Cardiology Unit of Clinical Psychology Service Laboratory, St. Joseph Hospital, Italian Auxologic Institute, Milan. He was a visiting scientist at the Boston University School of Medicine, the Department of Psychological Medicine of Gartnavel Hospital, University of Glasgow, and at the London Institute of Family Therapy. He is a member of several international and national scientific societies, such as the International Society for Psychotherapy Research (SPR), the European Society of Health Psychology (ESHP) and the Italian Society of Health Psychology. His scientific activity in the field of cardiac psychology includes the following Italian and European research projects: Home Managed Care through Telematic Technologies for the cardiological and psychological integrated assistance to patient with Congestive Heart Failure (FIRB-MIUR 2001), Universal Service for Managing and Monitoring Cardiac and Psychological Health of European Cardiac Patients (European Commission - Information Society).

◼ Gianfranco Parati, MD

Associate Professor of Medicine, Department of Clinical Medicine, Prevention and Applied Biotechnology, University of Milano-Bicocca, and Head of II Department of Cardiology, St. Luca Hospital, Italian Auxologic Institute, Milan. He was a visiting Scientist at the Massachusetts Institute of Technology and at Children's Hospital, Harvard Medical School. His editorial activity includes the following: member of the Editorial Board of Blood Pressure Monitoring Journal, Executive Editor of the Journal of Hypertension, official Journal of the European and of the International Society of Hypertension, and member of the Editorial Board of the American Journal of Physiology. He is member of a number of important international and national scientific societies, such as International Society of Hypertension, European Society of Hypertension, European Society of Cardiology, Italian Society of Cardiology and Italian Society of Hypertension. He is an International Fellow of the High Blood Pressure Council of the American Heart Association. Since 1998 he has been a member of the Scientific Committee of the Italian Society of Cardiology, and since 2002 he has been a Fellow of the European Society of Cardiology.

Introduction:

Heart Disease and Psychosocial Factors*

S. MENDIS

There are approximately 35 million deaths attributable to chronic diseases annually. Approximately one third of these deaths are due to cardiovascular disease alone. Cardiovascular disease also accounts for 10% of the global disease burden, of which 80% is borne by low and middle-income countries [1].

The main causes of the cardiovascular disease epidemic are tobacco use, unhealthy diets and physical inactivity [2]. Social, economic, cultural, political and environmental factors promote and support the adoption of these unhealthy behaviors. Ageing of populations, globalisation and rapid urbanization are important driving forces of the epidemic, particularly in low and middle-income countries. According to the first ever global analysis of the impact of risk factors on global health conducted by the World Health Organization, the major cardiovascular risk factors are high blood pressure, tobacco use and elevated cholesterol, and these are among the top 10 risks to global health [2]. Overall, rised blood pressure causes 7 million premature deaths each year, tobacco use causes almost 5 million and rised cholesterol more than 4 million deaths.

Many recent studies provide epidemiological evidence for causal links between coronary heart disease incidence among healthy populations, and prognosis among coronary heart disease patients and psychosocial factors [3, 4]. Psychosocial factors for which such an association has been reported include depression, anxiety, personality traits, social isolation and chronic stress [5]. Further, in a recent case control study of myocardial infarction conducted in 52 countries, psychosocial stress was reported to account for approximately 30% of the risk of acute myocardial infarction [6].

There are several plausible behavioral and biological pathways by which psychosocial factors can be linked to the incidence and prognosis of coronary heart

---

* Disclaimer: The opinions expressed in this paper are solely those of the author and do not represent those of the affiliate institution.

disease. First, psychosocial factors may influence health related behaviors such as tobacco use, unhealthy diet and physical inactivity, which in turn lead to the development of major cardiovascular risk factors (obesity and elevated blood pressure, blood sugar and blood cholesterol) [7]. Second, psychosocial factors may produce pathophysiological changes that increase the risk of coronay heart disease [8]. These include autonomic disturbances, hormonal imbalance, metabolic abnormalities, inflammation, insulin resistance, and endothelial dysfunction. These changes may promote atherogenesis or the progression of subclinical disease. Thirdly, psychosocial factors such as depression may act as a barrier to adherence and to the assessment of the need for medical care, resulting in a more rapid progression of clinical disease [9]. Lastly, some medications used in the treatment of depression , in particular tricyclic antidepressants, may be a risk factor for coronary heart disease [10].

The key test of whether psychosocial factors are aetiological for coronary heart disease lies on proof of reversibility; might clinical or social interventions aimed at reducing psychosocial factors such as anxiety and depression be effective in preventing coronary heart disease and reducing recurrent attacks and mortality? Randomized control trials have examined the effects of a variety of interventions including relaxation, stress management and counselling, in patients with coronary heart disease. A meta-analysis combining the results of 23 trials reported reductions in overall mortality (41%, 95%, CI 8 to 62%) and in non-fatal cardiovascular events (46%, 95%, CI 11 to 67%) at 2-years follow-up [11]. However, the trials on which these estimates were based were generally small and of short follow-up duration; and in some cases the trials were based on systematic rather than random allocation and widely different interventions. Large individual trials have provided little evidence of benefit in this context. A large multicenter trial showed no impact on event-free survival in those treated with cognitive behavioral therapy plus serotonin reuptake inhibitors if depressive symptoms were sufficiently severe [12].

Whether psychotherapeutic and psychopharmacological interventions will prevent coronary heart disease or alter mortality in patients with coronary heart disease still remain to be clarified. Future research need to focus less on the observational demonstration of associations, and more on identifying the critical components of depression and other psychosocial conditions, and the mechanism by which these critical components operate. Research also needs to focus on reversibility.

However, there is enough scientific knowledge to take action to prevent coronary heart disease now. Factors that increase the risk of coronary heart disease are known and are similar worldwide in men and women. Therefore, public health approaches to prevention can be based on similar principles globally. They need to target tobacco use, physical inactivity, unhealthy diet, obesity, elevated blood pressure, diabetes and psychosocial factors. A combination of population-wide prevention strategies and strategies aimed at early detection and treatment of those at high cardiovascular risk are required for this purpose [1, 2].

Based on available evidence, action can be taken to minimize the impact of psychosocial risk factors. Simple screening questions are available for a reliably detecting inappropriate levels of psychosocial stress. Physicians need to use them and to emphasize the role of psychosocial risk factors in counselling their patients. When physicians engage patients in the identification of psychosocial issues in this manner, alteration in the psychosocial risk factors are more likely. Patients can also be helped to reduce psychosocial stress levels through psychosocial support, regular exercise and stress reduction training [13, 14].

Based on current evidence, anxiety and depression are contributors to the course and severity of coronary heart disease. Patients with coronary heart disease should be assessed and treated for symptoms of anxiety or depression. Comprehensive cardiac rehabilitation programmes should include patient education, counselling, cognitive behavioral techniques and family and social support [15].

◼ References

1. WHO (2003) Preventing chronic diseases a vital investment
2. WHO (2002) The world health report. Reducing risks, promoting healthy life. World Health Organization, Geneva
3. Kuper H, Marmot M, Hemingway H (2002) Systematic review of prospective cohort studies of psychosocial factors in the etiology and prognosis of coronary heart disease. Semin Vasc Med 2:267-314
4. Hemingway H, Whitty CJ, Shipley M et al (2001) Psychosocial risk factors for coronary disease in White, South Asian and Afro-Caribbean civil servants: the Whitehall II study. Ethn Dis 11:391-400
5. Bunker SJ, Colquhoun DM, Esler MD et al (2003) "Stress" and coronary heart disease: psychosocial risk factors. Med J Aust 178:272-276.
6. Rosengren A, Hawken S, Ounpuu S et al; INTERHEART investigators (2004) Association of psychosocial risk factors with risk of acute myocardial infarction in 11119 cases and 13648 controls from 52 countries (the INTERHEART study):case-control study. Lancet 364:953-962
7. Rozanski A, Blumenthal JA, Kaplan J (1999) Impact of psychological factors on the pathogenesis of cardiovascular disease and implications for therapy. Circulation 99:2192-2217
8. Bairey Merz CN, Dwyer J, Nordstrom CK (2002) Psychosocial stress and cardiovascular disease: pathophysiological links. Behav Med 27:141-147
9. Brunner E (1997) Stress and the biology of inequality. Br Med J 314:1472-1476
10. Roose SP, Glassman AH (1994) Antidepressant choice in the patient with cardiac disease: lessons from Cardiac Arrhythmia Suppression Trial (CAST) studies. J Clin Psychiatry 55[Suppl A]:83-100
11. Jones DA, West RR (1996) Psychological rehabilitation after myocardial infarction; multicenter randomized controlled trial. Br Med J 313:1517-1521
12. Berkman LF, Blumenthal J, Burg M et al (2003) Effects of treating depression and low perceived social support on clinical events after myocardial infarction: the

Enhancing Recovery in Coronary Heart Disease Patients Randomized trial. JAMA 89:3106-3116

13. Walton KG, Schneider RH, Nidich SI et al (2002) Psychosocial stress and cardiovascular disease Part 2: effectiveness of the Transcendental Meditation program in treatment and prevention. Behav Med 28:106-123

14. Blumenthal JA, Sherwood A, Babyak MA et al (2005) Effects of exercise and stress management training on markers of cardiovascular risk in patients with ischemic heart disease: a randomized controlled trial. JAMA 293:1626-1634

15. WHO (2003) Prevention of recurrent heart attacks and strokes in low and middle income populations. Evidence-based recommendations for policy makers and health professionals. World Health Organization, Geneva

Chapter 1

Clinical Psychology for Cardiac Disease

E. MOLINARI ▪ L. BELLARDITA ▪ A. COMPARE

> *"When we try to pick out anything by itself, we find it hitched to everything else in the Universe."*
>
> J. Muir [1]

From its very beginning, modern scientific psychology has dealt with issues regarding mind-body, health-disease relationships; in particular, clinical psychology, in its various applications, has tried to provide a structure to psychological concepts tied to organic disease. Clinical psychology is described as the "area of psychology whose objectives are the explanation, understanding, interpretation and reorganization of dysfunctional or pathological mental processes, both individual and interpersonal, together with their behavioral and psychobiological correlates" [2]. Clinical psychology is characterized by a variety of models, methods, theories and techniques, each of which has its own historical reason. Its core and indispensable common denominator is clinical practice, be it intended for individuals, groups or collectives [3]. Among its areas of application we can include psychosomatics, health psychology and hospital psychology, where clinical psychology offers a relevant and coherent scientific, professional and training frame through contributions aimed at health maintenance and promotion, identification of etiological and diagnostic correlates, analysis and improvement of health care, and enhancement of public health [4].

The applications of clinical psychology to medicine have obviously been influenced by the historical, epistemological and operational changes in psychological paradigms (behavioral, cognitive-behavioral, psychodynamic, systemic, phenomenological and so forth). It can be argued that the common element of different approaches is the idea that we deal with an "environmental" subject, whose identity is built through and inside the relationships with other persons. As such, the care process cannot be restricted to organic dysfunction, but should be extended to anything that is or could be related to disease itself. From this perspective, the concept of disease that begins to emerge is the result of complex interactions of individual characteristics, developmental dynamics, genetically determined biological processes and significant social experiences.

We believe that the systemic approach, among the others, has particularly promoted the shift from a mechanistic, linear-causality perspective to a relational one [5], where each part of a system (familial, social, biological) influences the others and is influenced in turn. If we assume that in a systemic circuit each element that is inserted interacts with the entirety, the organic-mental dichotomy loses its significance, as well as its pragmatic value, in the care process. Along this line of thought, Engel proposed the biopsychosocial model [6], according to which disease results from the interaction of a variety of factors that can be approached and investigated at different levels (from subcellular to environmental). Psychological constructivism also has provided an important contribution toward the capsizing of linear causal models [7]. Constructivism is particularly interesting as far as illness perception and cognitive beliefs and emotions related to illness are concerned. As a matter of fact, according to constructivist theory, individual knowledge does not represent objective reality but is the result of the observer's process of construction and specification, and, consequently, limited by the observer. Piaget [8] argued that cognitive development occurs through the process of assimilation and accommodation: each new object or event is subject to a person's attempt to assign meaning based on available perceptive and mental schema (assimilation); at the same time, new experiences modify, to a certain extent, the cognitive organization based upon the requirements set by the experiences themselves (accommodation).

According to constructivist psychology, health practitioners can intervene on how patients and their families perceive disease using an "illness and disability" model that is constructed by both the practitioner and patient.

A consequence of the constructivist approach is the reorganization of patient expectations regarding the clinician's "omnipotence," and a more symmetric relationship between physician and patient [9]. This enables the patient to experience a stronger sense of control and autonomy, in contrast to the sense of impotence typically resulting from having a disease. Moreover, several studies [10-13] have reported that an increase in self-efficacy and internal locus of control have a positive impact on adherence to therapy. This effect is particularly relevant for patients with cardiac disease, since most cardiovascular problems are of a chronic nature and usually require complex pharmacological programs.

The application of psychological theories and interventions to particular classes of patients has led to the emergence of specific research and clinical fields such as psycho-oncology, psycho-neuro-endocrinology, psychosomatic dermatology, psycho-neuro-immunology, psycho-cardiology and so forth. There is much debate on whether we should consider such applications as parts of clinical psychology or as new, autonomous disciplines. We believe that the relationship of the various applications of clinical psychology to the different forms of disease have their own specific theoretical, methodological and operational characteristics. At the same time, we argue that they should constantly refer back to basic assumptions of clinical psychology, such as those previously presented.

It is important to emphasize that, rather than creating a definition for a presumably new discipline - psycho-cardiology (or cardio-psychology, according to which aspects one is stressing) - we should try to find out how clinical psychology can contribute to prevention, treatment and rehabilitation of patients with cardiac disease. As such, the term *psycho-cardiology* will be used for practical purposes, but the following distinctions should be made:

a. The association of psychological, social and emotional factors with cardiac disease has long been acknowledged by both common sense and clinical tradition. In 1628, William Harvey stated that "mental agitation" that induces either pleasure or emotional pain influences the heart's functioning [14]. In 1910, Sir William Osler described cardiac patients as extremely ambitious and prone to push their bodies to the limit [15]. Alexander [16] postulated that high blood pressure of unknown etiology (primary or essential hypertension) was prevalent in individuals strongly focused on achieving high social goals, who also tend to defensively inhibit emotional and cognitive aspects of anger in order to avoid interpersonal conflict.

b. As far as so-called "psycho-cardiology" is concerned, rather than considering psychological and cardiological components as a single unit, we prefer to emphasize the need for professionals with different competencies to communicate on the same level and to integrate specific and complementary skills and knowledge in order to achieve common objectives in the areas of improving prevention, and in the treatment and rehabilitation for the escalating problem of cardiac disease.

c. As far as psychological intervention is concerned, it is necessary to reflect upon the knowledge and skills deriving from training in clinical psychology, and how this knowledge and these skills should to tailored to the cardiac patient, based on "needs analysis," specific features of cardiac disease, and typical characteristics deriving from life experiences.

"Psycho-Cardiology" Activities

For patients with established cardiac disease, as well as individuals at risk for developing cardiovascular dysfunction, the focus of psycho-cardiology is prevention, diagnosis, treatment and rehabilitation, both within and outside the hospital setting. Psychologists in this field deal with the behavioral, emotional and relational problems associated with chronic or acute cardiac dysfunction. Psychological interventions often also involve family members and medical staff.

In order to implement an ad-hoc intervention, one should consider some fundamental issues, such as:

a. understanding specific characteristics and needs of cardiac patients, as reported in relevant scientific literature;

b. taking into account patient attitudes toward disease, medical and para-medical staff, and the psychologist (patient self-expectations and family expectations should be considered as well);

c. understanding the type of relationship established between psychologist and patient.

The development of psycho-cardiology. The studies that tended to promote the growth of psycho-cardiology focused on personality factors and cardiac disease. In the fifties, Friedman and Rosenman started to investigate possible associations and found that cardiac patients generally exhibited a complex sequence of behaviors and affects falling into the category "type A behavior pattern" (TABP) [17, 18]. TABP is described as an action-emotion complex characterized by impatience, exaggerated competitiveness, a chronic sense of time urgency, aggressive drive and hostility. Friedman provided a psychodynamic explanation of the underlying mechanisms of TABP. He argued that poor self-esteem was the basis of hostility and time-urgency (which are believed to be the most "toxic" components of coronary prone behavior) - in other words, individuals trying to confront their sense of inadequacy by continuously striving for the achievement of more and more ambitious goals.

Despite some interesting results, subsequent studies failed to generate a unanimous conclusion on the relationship between TABP and cardiac disease, mainly because of methodological issues related to the investigation of TABP subcomponents. Nevertheless, the studies represented a noteworthy turning point, since they demonstrated how specific personality traits may negatively influence cardiac health.

More recent studies on personality traits associated with cardiac disease conducted by Denollet and colleagues [19-22] identify a new personality pattern potentially associated with cardiac disease – namely, Type D personality or "Distressed personality." The taxonomy is based on two traits, negative affectivity and social inhibition [23]. Specifically, negative affectivity indicates the tendency to experience general, diffuse distress and a pervasive pessimism. Social inhibition refers specifically to a difficulty in expressing one's emotions and ideas, and to a general difficulty in social interactions. Type D individuals, according to Denollet [19] and other authors [24], are often worried without specific reasons, have a pessimistic perspective, often feel depressed and irritated, and rarely experience positive feelings. Between 1996 and 2000, studies of psychological risk factors and cardiac disease tended to focus on correlations between psychological risk factors (stress, depression, vital exhaustion) and Type D personality. Despite the fact that Type A and Type D patterns are usually considered to be opposite, we argue that they may present a common underlying feature, that being *social desirability*. In Type D patients this characteristic leads to inhibition of the expression of feelings that may be negatively judged or not accepted within the usual social contexts; and in Type A individuals it leads to compulsive overachievement in an attempt to bring about social acknowledgement.

Other types of research focused on behavioral risk factors. Beginning in the sixties, a great number of studies emerged on addictive behaviors (particularly, smoking and alcoholism), and on health-related lifestyle (exercise and diet). Results showed that smoking was the main cause of premature death [25], but that the solution was also the easiest to implement [26-28]. Based on these findings, cognitive-behavioral programs that were focused on modifying risk factors began to develop. Another research current in the field of psycho-cardiology focused on the identification of associations between cardiac disease and psychopathology. Anxiety, depression, excessive workload, stress and social isolation have been the most investigated variables. Rozanski's extensive meta-analysis [29] reveals the relevance and plausibility of the association between psycho-social factors and the occurrence and course of cardiac disease.

Illness behavior. One important aspect to consider is the patient's attitude toward illness. The idea of "illness behavior" derives from Parson's concept of "sick role" [30-33]. *Illness behavior* refers to how individuals interpret their symptoms and react to them, and also to how they search for medical advice and cure.

Mechanic [34] argues that illness behavior is more a function of social and cultural factors than illness itself. The basic sociological concepts of "sick role" and "illness behavior" were later integrated by Pilowsky [35-39], who suggested a psychological mechanism.

Pilowsky [38] defines illness behavior as the manner in which people react to their psychological and biological functioning and how they define it in terms of health and disease. The author also talks about "abnormal illness behavior" (AIB), defined as an inappropriate and/or dysfunctional perspective on one's health condition, which persists even when disconfirmed by a physician or another health practitioner, based upon a complete and appropriate medical examination [38].

Quite often, AIB is associated with an inappropriate sick role. It is also connected to the patient's denial of the influence of psychological factors on actual health status [35]. There are a variety of health-related dysfunctional behaviors, such as lying in bed most of the time or having inappropriate health-related feelings. For example, the patient may think that the physician has not offered an adequate explanation of reported symptoms and that alternative explanations as well as treatments should be explored. AIB is often associated with a secondary gain, such as being dependent upon significant others or one's physician, or not complying with responsibilities deriving from one's social role [40]. The introduction of the concept of illness behavior represents a significant step forward in understanding patients' relationship with their own disease. An evaluation for illness behavior provides the opportunity to recognize somatic symptoms that cannot be connected with physical disease but can be connected with psychopathological conditions. When patients complain of poorly defined, anatomically localized, time-related symptoms that cannot be associated with specific events or activities, it is appropriate to conduct a thorough evaluation of psychological functioning. Moreover, it is important to collect information on a patient's psychological distress as it relates to physical pathology, since the patient's psychological stress is often not sufficiently evident. Only by getting to know the patient can psycho-physiological symptoms be seen as the expression of a painful and constant search for help that, if not met, may dramatically increase disability or compromise compliance [41].

Relationship between patient and psychologist. The therapeutic relationship requires a lively and active interaction between patient and psychologist. Each session should yield a concrete achievement or provide an innovative direction (in the form, e.g., of new information, or homework designed to improve quality of life or reduce risk of relapse). A more passive approach seems inappropriate with cardiac patients, who may find it difficult to adapt to the demands of lengthy psychotherapy [14]. Moreover, although most psychotherapies focus on achieving insight, the interventions with cardiac patients must also necessarily obtain behavioral changes able to reduce disease-associated risk factors.

Family context. Much attention should be given to family dynamics. The research [42] emphasizes how both emotional and practical social support perception influences mental health and treatment adherence. Couple and family relationships are characterized by the connection with a significant other that represents the main source of satisfaction of tangible and emotional needs, and this becomes particularly evident at the onset of physical pathology. For example, the research shows that marital conflict increases cardiac reactivity [43].

In the field of psycho-cardiology, many investigations conducted within a relational paradigm have focused on:
a. the impact of cardiac disease on the couple relationship;
b. the influence of the couple relationship on the progression of cardiac disease;
c. the influence of the couple relationship on psycho-social adaptation to cardiac disease.

The quality of a relationship in which one partner suffers from a cardiac pathology may gradually deteriorate. Marital satisfaction, emotion communication and involvement, conflicts and changes in lifestyle and marital roles are usually considered to be reliable indicators of relationship quality. The adoption of proper coping strategies is also considered a marker of a good marital relationship [44]. In this manual, relational and familial issues will be broadly treated (especially in the Coyne, Compare et al. and Johnson et al. chapters).

In conclusion, many of the problems that emerge when physicians try to work with cardiac patients – e.g., lack of compliance – can generate conflicts and even lead to treatment drop-out. Patients, families, and medical staff may have different, and sometimes conflicting, priorities, making therapy a frustrating and expensive challenge. How can we facilitate the development of common objectives? The act of listening itself fosters the development of positive interactions, thereby establishing the basis for a systemic clinical and therapeutic intervention, where physical, individual and familial components reciprocally influence each other [45].

International and Italian Guidelines

Developments in knowledge, experience and technical and scientific skills have resulted in a series of guidelines for practitioners who work with cardiologists in the treatment and rehabilitation of cardiac patients. In some cases, ad-hoc guidelines have been created for the implementation of psychological intervention in preventive and rehabilitative cardiology. According to American Heart Association [46], the term *cardiac rehabilitation* refers to a multi-component and coordinated intervention aimed at optimizing the cardiac patient's physical, psychological and social functioning and reducing morbidity and mortality. Some studies report controversial results regarding the efficacy of psychosocial interventions on cardiac patient prognosis. Nonetheless, the American Heart Association guidelines consider psychological intervention to be an important part of the rehabilitation process and recommend it as a tool for improving psychological well-being and quality of life in cardiac patients.

In 1999, the Italian Group of Preventive and Rehabilitative Cardiology (Gruppo Italiano di Cardiologia Riabilitativa e Preventiva - GICR), together with the National Association of Hospital Cardiologists (Associazione Nazionale dei Medici Cardiologi Ospedalieri - ANMCO) and the Italian Society of Cardiology (Società Italiana di Cardiologia - SIC) assembled comprehensive guidelines on rehabilitative cardiology [47]. The GICR has identified different phases in which the *client* (primarily the patient but also family members, cardiologists and general practitioners) should have contact with psychologists. The GICR also describes main activities, emphasizing that professional interventions need to be appropriate and accurate both from a clinical and organizational point of view. In particular, the following elements in the relationship-building process between patient and psychologist have been identified:

- *Selection*: starts care process and is characterized by patient's or professional's choice of health center. Psychologist should guide patient's requests toward the most appropriate care process.
- *Entry:* patient establishes first contact with psychologist.
- *Assessment*: identification of patient's care needs.
- *Intervention*: implementation of a series of actions that meet patient's needs previously identified.
- *Follow-up*: evaluation of patient's satisfaction regarding expressed needs and of conditions that may suggest continuity of care.

For each of these phases, the GICR has identified proper assessment and intervention instruments, including the clinical interview and administration of self-report questionnaires.

Psychologists in "Psycho-Cardiology"

Since World War II, the number of psychologists in medical settings has progressively increased in North America, resulting in the development of clinical psychology as a profession. Between 1950 and 1990, for example, the number of psychologists rose from 255 to 3000 [48]. Physicians collaborate with psychologists primarily in the management of psychological problems related to medical problems, and in order to assess psychological change in patients with chronic diseases. In Italy, about 136 psychologists work in community health centers [48]. In the area of psycho-cardiology, the GICR conducted a study to define the current status of psychological intervention in rehabilitative cardiology programs [49]. This study, called YSIDE-Y (Italian SurveY on CarDiac REhabilitation - Psychology), evaluated the extent to which rehabilitative cardiology guidelines are followed, and identified training needs for health operators. Clearly, practitioners and institutions are becoming more and more interested and involved in trying to delineate the psychological interventions that can improve prevention and rehabilitation outcomes in cardiac disease.

In a multi-disciplinary setting, psychologists represent a crucial link. Research shows that they play a critical role in helping cardiologists in a variety of ways [14]:

- Offering in-hospital and out-hospital support to patients in the areas of therapy adherence, life-style modification, and processing trauma deriving from being a "victim" of a cardiac "insult" (as patients often refer to cardiac disease).
- Tailoring therapy: medical therapy optimization, understanding of interpersonal and work stress, and anticipation of emotional distress and its physiological consequences seem to play a significant role in facilitating patient compliance and in decreasing hospitalization rates due to relapse.
- Improving communication with patients: psychologists may be an important resource in managing patients who, due to repeated hospitalization, assume a recalcitrant role. It is fundamental for cardiologists to be aware of patient attitudes and consult with psychologists in managing possible self-injuring behaviors.
- Conducting differential diagnosis: for example, panic disorder presents a relevant somatic symptomatology, primarily assuming the form of chest pain and dyspnea. It is necessary to distinguish when such symptoms are due to cardiac dysfunctions and when they might be related to panic attack. A recent meta-analysis conducted on 1364 subjects that reported chest pain showed that among the subjects who received a diagnosis of panic disorder (i.e., 30% of the total sample, n = 411), 74% had no cardiac problems. 7.7% of the subjects received a diagnosis of both cardiac disease and panic attack. In conclusion, early recognition of panic disorder in the ER setting may avoid invasive and expensive coronary artery disease tests, such as cardiac catheterization, and may also improve the prognosis in cardiac patients affected by cardiac disease and panic disorder.

Clinical interview. The clinical interview is perhaps the psychologist's favorite instrument, both for psychodiagnostic purposes [47] and in counseling. In the psychodiagnostic phase, the purpose of the interview is to investigate current psychological problems and how they interfere with rehabilitation outcomes.

Italian guidelines for psychological activity in preventive and rehabilitative cardiology list dysfunctional and functional areas that should be considered:

1) Symptomatology
2) Physical functionality
3) Psychological functionality
4) Disease history
5) Disease perception/processing
6) Resources, coping, self-efficacy
7) Familiar and social support

8) Motivation toward therapy and attitude with respect to adherence
9) Expectations

Characteristics of psychological intervention. Based upon Italian guidelines [47], the goal of psychological intervention is identified as supporting patients and their families in:
- recognizing and expressing disease-related emotions;
- identifying and using strategies to control risk factors and modify life-style;
- implementing proper self-management of rehabilitation treatments;
- regaining satisfying quality of life.

Existing literature shows the efficacy of multi-component, multi-disciplinary disease management programs that target a variety of risk factors through the use of different intervention techniques, including relaxation procedures, psycho-educational activities, cognitive-behavioral therapy, counseling and so forth.

Psychologist's training. The psychologist's emotional, cognitive and relational system represents the elective intervention instrument in the field of clinical psychology. This system is the product of specific training and clinical practice [50]. Despite the fact that an explicit, ad-hoc training for psychologists that work in the field of psycho-cardiology does not exist yet, it is possible to identify some basic elements that, among theoretical and methodological approaches typical of clinical psychology, are particularly suitable in psycho-cardiology:

a. The idea concept behind Carl Roger's therapeutic approach. Rogers was committed to researching and explaining characteristics of the "patient-focused therapist" [51]. He had an optimistic view of the patient, whom he considered the protagonist. Another characteristic of Roger's therapy is its non-directivity: the therapist allows the client to lead the therapeutic process. Therapists, according to Rogers, should merely function as facilitators in the process of achieving awareness, since the main focus is the achievement of autonomous individual development, i.e., "self-realization." Rogers believed that therapists should always maintain a positive attitude and an emphatic understanding in their relationship toward patients and their resources, in the hope that this attitude and understanding would motivate patients to engage in a self-knowledge process, learn to value themselves and develop stronger self-esteem.

b. Contributions of positive psychology. During the past decade, the medical and social sciences have been characterized by a growing attention to the study of well-being and quality of life. Initially, these aspects were evaluated through objective markers such as housing conditions, annual income and social role. But several studies have demonstrated that objective indicators do not offer a valid examination of individual well-being and quality of life, which turn out to be relative and subjective concepts. In psychological research, the study of subjective well-being has given rise to the broad and multi-faced current of positive psychology [52], which emphasizes the fundamental role of individual resources and abilities. This approach represents a change in perspective in the design of a rehabilitation program, where personal resources and activities, rather than limits-compensatory interventions, are the central and preferred mechanisms of therapy [53]. The positive psychology perspective, in summary, can bring about important contributions in the field of psycho-cardiology, particularly as far as activities aimed at promoting the quality of life in the care process are concerned, for both patients and family members.

c. Cognitive-behavioral therapy [54, 55]. The cognitive-behavioral approach focuses on the "hic-et-nunc" changes of dysfunctional behavior. Therapists seek to activate patients' skills and propose valid strategies in overcoming problems. The main elements of therapeutic process are:
   * Defining how and when dysfunctional behavior is acted out;
   * Defining ineffective strategies used to face the problematic situation; and
   * Finding and using problem- or emotion-oriented effective strategies (coping skills) [56].

Cognitive-behavioral therapy is particularly indicated for cardiac patients since it is usually a brief intervention, where both therapist and patient play an active role in goal setting and in the identification of specific cognitive patterns that may generate problems. One of the goals is to encourage an increase in self-efficacy, self-esteem[10], and the internal locus of control. The cognitive-behavioral approach is highly advisable for the reduction of risk factors such as smoking and unbalanced diet. It is important to understand that a patient's lack of co-operation may be due to the fact that the therapist adopts a "psycho-educational" position, focusing on what he or she knows about the problem and about solutions. The patient may not always share the therapist's ideas; establishing a constructive working alliance that also incorporates the patient's perspective is critical.

d. Systemic family therapy [9]: after the occurrence of a cardiac event (or any serious disease), a "crisis" occurs: the existing balance structure, involving all members of the family system, breaks down, and role re-negotiation becomes necessary, above all, to settle on "who takes care of whom." If family members cannot re-establish a new "homeostasis" - characterized by a functional assignment of responsibilities - emotional difficulties and conflicts may emerge and be expressed through closure, hostility, and aggressiveness and guilt, with direct and/or indirect consequence on the whole family's quality of life and on the patient's medical and psychological condition [57, 58].

The training of psychologists should include the acquisition of basic cardiovascular knowledge, such as cardiovascular system anatomy and functioning, development and symptomatology of cardiac disease, and behavioral risk factors. Being familiar with these aspects becomes fundamental in order to properly communicate, not only with cardiologists, but also with the patients themselves, who are often very knowledgeable in the field of cardiac disease. It is also important to have a good knowledge of the psychophysiological mechanisms underlying psychopathology (above all depression, stress and anxiety), since they may contribute to cardiac disease onset and/or exacerbation.

Finally, psychologists should develop the ability to work inside a team of professionals with different competencies and backgrounds in order to ensure the implementation of a multi-disciplinary intervention.

Conclusion

It well recognized that clinical psychology can significantly contribute to preventive and rehabilitative cardiology. This book has the ambitious intent of revealing the links between psychological factors and cardiac disease and providing current hypotheses and explanations on mechanisms underlying these linkages. The general agreement on the usefulness of biopsychosocial model [6] should lead researchers and practitioners to further investigate the most effective diagnostic and psychotherapeutic solutions for addressing the complex interactional patterns that link somatic, emotional and psycho-social factors. In the second part of the book some therapeutic approaches are presented, illustrating how clinical psychology practice can be employed in the treatment of cardiac patients.

In addition to investigating effective treatments for cardiology patients, it also important to evaluate the processes and outcomes of psychological interventions in the field of preventive and rehabilitative cardiology by conducting expressly designed program evaluations [59] that offer focused, professional support to patients and their families, thereby contributing to their health status, as described by the accepted WHO definition.

References

1. Muir J (1911) My first summer in the Sierra. Houghton Mifflin, Boston, MA
2. Collegio dei professori e ricercatori di Psicologia Clinica delle Università italiane (2003) Definizione della Psicologia Clinica. Available from: *http://www.collegiopsiclinicauniv.it/eng_ambiti.htm*
3. Statuto del Collegio dei professori e ricercatori di Psicologia Clinica delle Università italiane. Available from: *http://www.collegiopsiclinicauniv.it/eng_statuto.htm*
4. Imbasciati A (2000) Medical psychology through institutions. Psichiatria e Psicoterapia Analitica 19:38-48
5. Ricci C, Selvini-Palazzoli M (1984) Interactional complexity and communication. Family Process 23:169-176
6. Engel GL (1977) The need for a new medical model. Science 196:129-136
7. Maturana HR, Varela FJ (1987) The tree of knowledge: biological roots of human understanding, pp 263. New Science Library/Shambhala Publications, Boston
8. Piaget J, Inhelder R (1987) The construction of reality. In: Oats J, Sheldon S (Eds) Cognitive development in infancy, pp 165-169. Lawrence Erlbaum Associates, Inc., England, NJ
9. Boscolo L, Bertrando P, Novick C (1996) Systemic therapy with individuals. Karnac Books, England

10. Bandura A (1992) Self-efficacy mechanism in psychobiologic functioning. In: Schwarzer R (Ed) Self-efficacy: thought control of action, pp 355-394. Hemisphere Publishing Corp, Washington, DC
11. Bandura A (2005) The primacy of self-regulation in health promotion. Applied Psychology: an International Review 54:245-254
12. Bandura A (2004) Health promotion by social cognitive means. Health Education & Behavior 31:143-164
13. Bandura A (2000) Health promotion from the perspective of social cognitive theory. In: Norman P, Abraham C, Conner M (Eds) Understanding and changing health behavior: from health beliefs to self-regulation, pp 299-339. Harwood Academic Publishers, Netherlands
14. Allan R, Scheidt SS (1996) Heart & mind: the practice of cardiac psychology. American Psychological Association, US
15. Williams R Jr, Barefoot JC (1988) Coronary-prone behavior: the emerging role of the hostility complex. In: Houston B Kent, Snyder CR (Eds) Type A behavior pattern: research, theory, and intervention. John Wiley & Sons., Oxford, UK
16. Alexander F (1984) Psychological aspects of medicine. Advances 1:53-60
17. Friedman M, Rosenman RH (1959) Association of specific overt behavior pattern with blood and cardiovascular findings: blood cholesterol level, blood clotting time, incidence of arcus senilis, and clinical coronary artery disease. JAMA 169:1286-1296
18. Friedman M, Rosenman RH (1974) Type A behavior and your heart. Knopf, New York
19. Denollet J (2000) Type D personality: a potential risk factor refined. J Psychosom Res 49:255-266
20. Denollet J (1997) Personality, emotional distress and coronary heart disease. Eur J Personal 11:343-357
21. Denollet J (1994) Health complaints and outcome assessment in coronary heart disease. Psychosom Med 56:463-474
22. Denollet J (1991) Negative affectivity and repressive coping: pervasive influence on self-reported mood, health and coronary-prone behavior. Psychosom Med 53:538-556
23. Denollet J (1998) Personality and risk of cancer in men with coronary heart disease. Psycholog Med 28:991-995
24. Lesperance F, Frasure-Smith N, Talajic M (1996) Major depression before and after myocardial infarction: its nature and consequences. Psychosom Med 58:99-110
25. Ezzati M, Lopez AD (2003) Estimates of global mortality attributable to smoking in 2000. Lancet 362:847-852
26. Sebregts E, Falger P, Bar F (2000) Risk factor modification through nonpharmacological interventions in patients with coronary heart disease. J Psychosom Res 48:425-441
27. Fitzgerald TE, Prochaska JO, Pransky GS (2000) Health risk reduction and functional restoration following coronary revascularization: a prospective investigation using dynamic stage typology clustering. Int J Rehab Health 5:99-116
28. Scherwitz L, Ornish D (1994) The impact of major lifestyle changes on coronary stenosis, CHD risk factors, and psychological status: results from the San Francisco Lifestyle Heart Trial. Homeostasis in Health and Disease 35:190-197
29. Rozanski A et al (2005) The epidemiology, pathophysiology, and management of

psychosocial risk factors in cardiac practice: the emerging field of behavioral cardiology. J Am Coll Cardiol 45:637-51

30. Mechanic D (1986) The concept of illness behavior: culture, situation and personal predisposition. Psycholog Med 16:1-7

31. Mechanic D (1995) Sociological dimensions of illness behavior. Soc Sci Med 41:1207-1216

32. Mechanic D (1992) Health and illness behavior and patient-practitioner relationships. Soc Sci Med 34:1345-1350

33. Hansell S, Mechanic D (1986) The socialization of introspection and illness behavior. In: McHugh S, Vallis T (Eds) Illness behavior: a multidisciplinary model, pp 253-260. Plenum Press, New York

34. Mechanic D (1986) Illness behavior: an overview. In: McHugh S, Vallis TM (Eds) Illness behavior: a multidisciplinary model, pp 101-109. Plenum Press, New York

35. Pilowsky I (1990) The concept of abnormal illness behavior. Psychosom J Consult Liaison Psychiat 31:207-213

36. Pilowsky I, Murrell T, Gordon A (1979) The development of a screening method for abnormal illness behavior. J Psychosom Res 23:203-207

37. Pilowsky I, Spence N, Waddy J (1979) Illness behavior and coronary artery by-pass surgery. J Psychosom Res 23:39-44

38. Pilowsky I (1978) A general classification of abnormal illness behaviors. Bri J Med Psychol 51:131-137

39. Pilowsky I (1969) Abnormal illness behavior. Bri J Med Psychol 42:347-351

40. Winefield HR (1991) Health psychology for medical students. In: Jansen MA, Weinman J (Eds) The international development of health psychology, pp 135-143. Harwood Academic Publishers, Netherlands

41. Strepparava MG (2003) La qualità della vita nel malato in dialisi. Giornale di tecniche nefrologiche e dialitiche 14:11-17

42. House JS, Landis KR, Umberson D (2003) Social relationships and health. Salovey, In: Rothman P, Alexander J (Eds) Social psychology of health, pp 218-226. Psychology Press, New York

43. Broadwell SD, Light KC (1999) Family support and cardiovascular responses in married couples during conflict and other interactions. Int J Behav Med 6:40-63

44. Bunzel B et al (1992) Does changing the heart mean changing personality? A retrospective inquiry on 47 heart transplant patients. Quality of life research: an International Journal of Quality of Life Aspects of Treatment, Care & Rehabilitation 1:251-256

45. Molinari E, Valtolina G (1996) L'approccio integrato medico psicologico nel trattamento dell'obesità: un modello di intervento. Ricerche di Psicologia, FrancoAngeli, Milano

46. Leon AS, Franklin BA, Costa F et al (2005) Cardiac rehabilitation and secondary prevention of coronary heart disease. An American Heart Association scientific statement from the Council on Clinical Cardiology and the Council on Nutrition, Physical Activity, and Metabolism, in Collaboration with the American Association of Cardiovascular and Pulmonary Rehabilitation. Circulation 111:369-376

47. Task Force per le Attività di Psicologia in Cardiologia Riabilitativa e Preventiva Gruppo Italiano di Cardiologia Riabilitativa e Preventiva GICR (2003) Linee guida per le attività di psicologia in cardiologia riabilitativa e preventiva. Monaldi Archives for Chest Disease 60:184-234

48. Speed L (1999) Ruolo degli psicologi nei setting medici. Società Italiana di Psicologia dei Servizi Ospedalieri e Territoriali *http://www.sipsot.it/html/ricercafolder/ric_settori.particolari/documenti/serviziautonomi/prinsetmed2.html*

49. Sommaruga M, Tramarin R, Balestroni G et al (2005) ISYDE- Prima fase dell'implementazione delle linee guida per le attività di psicologia in cardiologia riabilitativa e preventiva. Italian survey on cardiac rehabilitation - Psychology. Monaldi Archives for Chest Disease 64:53-58

50. Collegio dei professori e ricercatori di Psicologia Clinica delle Università italiane (2003) Available from: *http://www.collegiopsiclinicauniv.it/ita_ambiti.htm*

51. Raskin NJ, Rogers CR (1989) Person-centered therapy. In: Corsini RJ, Wedding D (Eds) Current psychotherapies, 4th ed., pp 155-194. FE Peacock Publishers Inc., Chicago, IL

52. Seligman ME, Csikszentmihalyi M (2000) Positive psychology: an introduction. Am Psychologist 55:5-14

53. Delle Fave A (2004) Editorial: positive psychology and the pursuit of complexity. Ricerche di psicologia. Special Issue on Positive Psychology 27:7-12

54. Emmelkamp PM, Oppen PV (1998) Cognitive interventions in behavioral medicine. In: Fava GA, Freyberger H (Eds) Handbook of psychosomatic medicine. International Universities Press, Inc., Connecticut, US

55. Hollon SD, Beck AT (1994) Cognitive and cognitive-behavioral therapies. In: Bergin AE, Garfield SL (Eds) Handbook of psychotherapy and behavior change, 4th ed., pp 428-466. John Wiley & Sons, London

56. Meichenbaum D (1997) The evolution of a cognitive-behavior therapist. In: Zeig JK (Ed) The evolution of psychotherapy: the third conference, pp 95-104. Brunner/Mazel, Inc., Philadelphia

57. Invernizzi G et al (1991) Emotional profiles of families with a heart-operated patient: a pilot study. Psychother Psychosom 55:1-8

58. Invernizzi G et al (1990) Emotional and relational state of the family of the cancer patient. Psychologie Medicale 22:208-212

59. Posavac EJ, Carey RG (1997) Program evaluation: methods and case studies. Prentice-Hall, Englewood Cliffs, NJ

Part I
Psychological Risk Factors for Cardiac Disease

Chapter 2

Psychological Risk Factors for Cardiac Disease and Pathophysiological Mechanisms: An Overview

A. COMPARE ▪ L. GONDONI ▪ E. MOLINARI

Psychological Risk Factors for Coronary Heart Disease

Coronary heart disease (CHD) is a classical psychosomatic disease within the framework of reference of the so-called biopsychosocial model.[1] More than any other disease, it reflects the realities of living in modern society, such as stress, lack of time, competitiveness and excessive ambition, which are all part of the dynamic of success in contemporary cultures.

We do not have a complete knowledge of the etiology of CHD, which is multifactorial. We have therefore to concentrate our efforts on risk factors rather than on causes. Most material published prior to 1930 consists of empirical accounts by recognised experts. During the 1930s or thereabout, the earliest clinically impressive studies describing the psychodynamics of the disease process began to emerge [1, 2]. 1950 marks the beginning of systematic scientific research using larger samples and control groups [3, 4]. The marked increase in cardiovascular disease in industrial nations during the second half of the 20th century further accelerated the research effort. The aim was to use epidemiological methods to ascertain the factors associated with the disease etiology. By modifying these factors, it was hoped that a reduction in the incidence of cardiovascular disease and premature mortality could be achieved. This approach was bound up from the start with the principle of intervention. The first and most famous research project was the Framingham study. Launched in 1948 in the small town of Framingham, Massachusetts, by 1952 the study already had more than 5000 healthy people on its books. It was one of the earliest of Kannel's group publications in 1961 to use the term *risk factor*. A whole series of long-term

---

[1] The mechanistic conceptual model of medicine (the so-called mechanical paradigm), dating back to the 17th and 18th centuries, is based on a body-soul dualism, which is responsible for the psychosocial aspects of disease. This model has been largely disregarded in standard medical practice. The biopsychosocial model incorporates modern epistemological thinking [4] and gives greater prominence to psychosocial aspects.

prospective[2] studies followed, which together built up the canonical list of so-called classical risk factors for CHD [5-7].

The actual number of risk factors cannot be definitively established, as costs and the enormous demands on the subjects' time render it impossible for a single prospective study to follow up on all known variables. It is not possible to derive results by an additive process using a number of separate studies, because a risk factor, if it is to be regarded as existing in its own right (rather than as an indicator variable), must not correlate with any other factor. The only way to test for this would be to cover all known risk factors in a single study. Additionally, the terms *predictor variable* and *risk factor* were ill defined and imprecisely used from the outset, although this leads to premature conclusions.

If a predictor variable is to become a risk factor in the proper sense of the term, then – in addition to the confirmed and independent prediction of the disease – the following requirements must be satisfied [8]:

a. It must be established that an increased risk rating increases the probability of disease occurring.	**Dose/effect relationship**
b. The dose/effect relationship must be confirmed in studies involving different population groups within a single culture, or in various groups in different countries or on different continents.	**Generalisation**
c. The pathway through which the risk factor operates must be established with both basic and clinical research.	**Pathomechanisms**
d. It must be demonstrated in prospective, controlled, randomized studies that the population's mortality and/or morbidity is reduced when the risk factor is reduced.	**Results confirmation by means of intervention studies**

In addition to increasing age, the established risk factors for CHD include male gender and genetic predisposition (i.e. the non-modifiable risk factors), as well as conditions that favor the occurrence of CHD: diabetes and insulin resistance, hypertension and dyslipidemia (high LDL cholesterol) [9]. Other risk factors currently under investigation include homocysteine, fibrinogen, fibrinolysis markers (such as PAI-1, t-PA, D-dimer) and inflammatory markers (such as hs-CRP, ICAM-1, IL-6). In this continuously evolving framework, the role of psychosocial components – including behaviors or life-styles such as smoking, lack of exercise and poor diet – is not altogether clear, although they appear to be involved indirectly. Depression, vital exhaustion and socio-economic status also appear to be relevant, but do not fulfill the criteria for being considered risk factors. Despite these reservations, recent recommendations of the European Society of Cardiology include systematic screening for psychosocial risk factors [10].

---

[2] Prospective studies are large-scale, fully representative studies carried out on healthy persons (subjects) who subsequently are re-examined repeatedly over a period of many decades. This permits identification of variables noted at the outset as present in healthy subjects (e.g. lack of exercise) that, in time, lead to increased risk of disease (e.g. diabetes, heart disease, high blood pressure).

◼ Brief Overview of the Biological Mechanisms Underlying the Pathogenesis of Ischemic Heart Disease

It is useful to define a framework within which to understand the complex inter-actions between body and mind in the pathogenesis of ischemic heart disease. CHD is almost always secondary to an obstruction of the flow in the coronary arteries due to atherosclerosis. We still do not have a satisfactory knowledge-base of the early phases of atherosclerosis, but they are probably characterised by the accumulation of lipids in the internal layer of the artery called intima. This is likely followed by an increase of oxidative stress in the region of lipid accu-mulation, although this is still partly speculative. The second macroscopic event in the formation of the atheroma is the adhesion of lymphocytes to the endothe-lium with subsequent diapedesis and intima penetration guided by cytokines. These cells transform subsequently into foamy cells, i.e. cells that are full of lipids. Moreover, they express several molecules that increase adhesion of other cells (namely, T lymphocytes and monocytes) to the endothelium. This early phase of atherogenesis, involving the formation of the so-called *lipid stripes,* is most likely reversible. The evolution of the atheroma involves muscular cells that are generally located in the intermediate layer of the artery (called the media). It is believed that, under the action of chemotactic factors such as PGDF (platelet derived growth factor), the muscular cells of the media migrate towards the intima where they may possibly divide and multiply, although some of the muscular cells probably die as a result of apoptosis. The extracellular matrix also increases in volume under the action of several factors produced locally, while other stimuli tend to reduce the matrix. The overall result is an increase in size of the involved vessel, usually secondary to intima and media thickening, that results in a reduction in the internal diameter of the vessel itself - i.e. the stenosis that begins to reduce blood flow. Thickness of intima-media, measured in the carotid artery by means of echodoppler technique, is currently considered a marker of future cardiovascular events in healthy subjects. Two other process-es are fundamental in the development of the atherosclerotic plaque: angio-genesis and mineralization. The creation of new small vessels inside the plaque facilitates the passage of nutrients and allows further growing of the plaque itself, while mineralization consists mainly in the accumulation of calcium, which is secondary to the increased secretion of cytokines by the muscular cells.

After a period of time, usually several years, a stenosis develops, reducing blood flow through the vessel. A reduction of about 60% of the internal lumen is necessary to determine ischemia in stressful conditions such as physical effort and/or strong emotions. Angina is often symptomatic of ischemia. CHD behaves generally as a chronic disease. However, periods of instability that may lead to myocardial infarction (MI) or unstable angina may occur at anytime. MI may be the first episode of CHD without preceding anginal symptoms; indeed, it has been shown that MI is often secondary to obstruction in lesions that are non-obstructive, i.e. in lesions that, even though often large, reduce the lumen of the coronary artery by less than 60% and, therefore, do not determine significant ischemia. The mechanism more frequently involved in the genesis of an MI is thrombosis of a ruptured plaque.

But why does a plaque rupture? This process involves either the fibrous external layer of the atheroma or an erosion of the intima surface, and it reflects complex interactions between various factors such as mechanical stress, collagen metabolism, catabolism of the extracellular matrix, inflammatory status and loss of muscular cells. The so-called vulnerable plaque is characterized by an accumulation of macrophages and a large amount of lipids, both of which play a role in the mechanical compression that facilitates the rupture. The complete occlusion of the vessel that precedes myocardial necrosis (i.e. the infarction) is the final event in the cascade and is determined by the formation of a thrombus in the lumen.

How Does the Psyche Interact with Physical Health in CHD?

Rozanski and Kubzansky [11] provided a very interesting answer to this question. Our physical well being is maintained by a complex interaction of regulatory influences that respond with a non-linear dynamic – i.e. parameters such as blood pressure are to be kept in a narrow range (the less blood pressure varies during the day, the better for our health status) while other parameters have a different behavior: heart rate variability, for instance, is directly related to survival after a MI; therefore, a high heart rate variability is a sign of physiological health, while blood pressure variability is not. Homeostatic efficacy "controls" parameters such as blood pressure and "responds" to various stimuli in the regulation of heart rate. This mechanism progressively loses its efficacy as a result of increasing age and various medical illnesses. Psychological aspects not only interact in complex ways, they exhibit a non-linear functionality with respect to homeostatic control. Vitality (a positive state associated with enthusiasm and energy) is a reservoir for our mind. Chronic stress and chronic negative emotion negatively affect vitality, thus initiating a destructive cycle, while emotional competence and effective coping skills positively affect our vital energy and initiate a health-promoting cycle. When "psychological flexibility" is lost, we no longer are capable of facing everyday psychological tasks, particularly if they are very demanding. Reduced flexibility may be looked at as the basis of pathological reactions to environmental stressors. Although the specific mechanisms underlying this process are under investigation, we can describe the general framework of the physiological pathway. Various states potentially determine hyperarousal. Examples are pessimism, emotional or job distress, lack of rest, caregiver strain, etc. These and other conditions can result in continuous stimulation of the sympathetic nervous system and hypothalamic-pituitary-adrenal axis, which, in turn, can cause a series of dysregulations that negatively affect clinical status. The most relevant issues seem to be altered cortisol levels, elevated resting heart rate and reduced heart rate variability and baroreceptor control.

A thorough analysis of all the mechanisms linking psychosocial aspects to CHD is beyond the scope of this review. On no other psychosomatic issue have there been so many empirical studies distinguished by excellent methodology published worldwide, or so many reviews or meta-analyses. Understandably, the heart has always been regarded as a highly emotional organ. At one time it was even believed to be the location of emotions, pain, love and generosity. The stock of established knowledge is vast: on the topic of psychological factors in high blood pressure alone, some 4000 publications have appeared; on the psychosocial aspects of angiography and coronary angioplasty there are 145 publications; and on heart transplants there are about 200. The following sections summarise the most prominent associations thought to exist between psychosocial variables with CHD.

Type A Behavior Pattern

Type A behavior pattern, characterised by hard driving and competitive behavior, a potential for hostility, pronounced impatience and abrupt speech, has been shown to result in a two-fold occurrence of CHD compared to controls. Long-term mental stress and negative emotions such as anger, hostility, excessively competitive attitudes, and undue ambition in conjunction with social timidity increase the probability of CHD and adversely affect prognosis in patients with established CHD [12]. Anger and hostility are among the main characteristics of type A behavior pattern. These psychological constructs encompass a broad range of negative orientations toward interpersonal relationships, and include traits such as mistrust and cynicism. The underlying mechanisms have a detrimental influence on the cardiovascular system not only through unfavorable lifestyle, but biological mechanisms as well (examples are endothelial damage and increased heart rate and blood pressure). People with hostile behavior also have increased plasma homocysteine [13]. Homocysteine is an amino acid derived from dietary methionine. Its levels are regulated through a complex interaction of genetic, dietary and hormonal factors, and it plays a role in the process or atherogenesis. Increased plasma homocysteine is therefore a possible risk factor, through endothelial toxicity, LDL oxidation and reduced flow-mediated arterial vasodilation.

Depression

After the onset of CHD, persistent clinical depression increases morbidity and mortality [14]. This is secondary to a cluster of unfavorable behaviors that are directly related to depression itself – e.g. poor diet, excessive alcohol use, non-compliance to medications etc. It is likely that the presence of so-called vital exhaustion (which includes a variety of the depressive cluster of symptoms characterised by fatigue, severe chronic exhaustion, irritability and demoralized feelings, with various concomitant physical symptoms) is a prodromal syndrome (early-warning syndrome) for CHD and cardiac infarction [15-18]. There is also a direct biological action associated with depression: depressed patients exhibit an increase in cortisolemia in sympathetic tone, with reduced heart rate variability. This may explain the high incidence of sudden cardiac death in subjects affected with CHD and depression: an increase in free fatty acid level and platelet aggregation. In and of itself, however, depression seems to be a weak risk factor for the development of CHD.

Anxiety

Anxiety is weakly associated with the development of CHD: panic disorder and worry (i.e. a subcategory of generalized anxiety disorder) seem to be the most significant aspects of anxiety that relate to CHD. Anxiety also reduces vagal activity, however, and a direct association with sudden cardiac death has been documented. The pathway, once again, is a reduction in heart rate variability. Like depression, anxiety also favors unhealthy lifestyle behaviors.

Post-Traumatic Stress Disorder (PTSD)

Post-traumatic stress disorder (PTSD), i.e. "an event that is outside the range of usual human experience and that would be markedly distressing to almost anyone," has been examined both as a factor that influences the pathogenesis and progression of CHD, and also as a possible consequence of CHD itself, since, in the last revision of DSM, medical illness and subjective perception of the event were added as qualifying events for PTSD, thus rendering cardiac problems more likely to fulfill the stressor criterion. Indeed, a recently published review that addresses this issue [19] documented that a subgroup of patients are at high risk of PTSD after a cardiac event. MI, life-threatening arrhythmias, congestive heart failure, cardiac surgery and heart transplantation were all associated with an increased incidence of PTSD. This observation underscores the need for prospective studies addressing the issue of whether PTSD should be regarded as a causative agent in CHD or only as a consequence of established CHD. In many cases, heart surgery is also associated with significant psychological distress.

Mental Stress

Beyond platelet aggregation, blood coagulation and fibrinolysis have been studied as possible links between psychological stress and CHD [20], with findings that seem to support this hypothesis. Job stress has long been acknowledged as a cause of accelerated blood coagulation. More recently it has been associated with an increase in fibrinogen and a decrease in fibrinolytic capacity. Low socioeconomic status, as defined using a wide range of measures such as education, income, and work environment, has also been shown to be related to fibrinogen levels, while fibrinolysis seems to be less affected.

In the recently published INTERHEART study [21], subjects with MI reported a higher prevalence of all the stressors identified as markers of psychosocial risk, compared with controls. The markers, including episodic and permanent work stress, stress at home, financial stress and stressful events, were all found to be independent risk factors for the occurrence of MI. Although this was an epidemiological survey and did not provide a detailed interpretation of the findings, it is interesting that the findings were consistent across regional, ethnicity and gender demographics.

Acute stressors may also favor sudden cardiac death. Approximately 20% of patients that survive a potentially fatal arrhythmia experienced a stressful situation in the preceding period of time.

Stress cardiomyopathy syndrome is of particular interest in the setting we are exploring. It has been defined as profound myocardial stunning precipitated by acute emotional stress [22]. The onset of symptoms rapidly follows emotional stress: within a couple of days all patients have ECG abnormalities, including a marked prolongation of the QTc interval (i.e. ventricular repolarization time), with T wave inversion sometimes accompanied by pathological Q waves (classical ECG markers of myocardial necrosis). Interestingly, all these ECG abnormalities resolve within few days, in contrast to classical MI alterations, which persist over time. Patients show little (if any) increase in cardiac enzymes, while MI patients always have a significant release of intracellular enzymes. Myocardial function is severely depressed: the mean ejection fraction (a widely used descriptor of systolic function in the work of Wittstein and coworkers) is 0.20, compared with normal values above 0.50. In particular, akynesis or dyskinesis of left ventricular apex is present, with recovery of normal function occurring in less than one month, while once again patients with MI rarely fully recover contractile function. Coronary arteries are normal in almost every patient, without evidence of ruptured plaques or significant stenosis. Plasma catecholamines are much higher than normal controls and even patients with a classical picture of MI. Brain natriuretic peptide, which is regarded as a biomarker of right atrial pressure and, therefore, of hemodynamic status, is also markedly elevated during the acute phase. Even if the pathogenetic mechanism underlying this condition is not fully understood, the marked increase in sympathetic activity is the main feature in this syndrome. Myocardial stunning can occur as a result of coronary spasm or direct myocytic injury by calcium overload and the subsequent increase of free radicals. Interestingly, women are by far more often affected with stress cardiomyopathy, but, again, the reason remains to be explored.

Mental stress induced in the laboratory has been shown to be a highly significant predictor of cardiac major events in patients already affected with CHD. Patients who had a reduction in contractility (documented as a reduction in radionuclide measured ejection fraction) experienced a three-fold higher incidence of events at four-year follow-up [23].

A correlation between stress – particularly long-term familial stress (marital tension, caregiving strain) and job stress – and CHD [24] has been documented. Moreover, social isolation – i.e. an insufficiently supportive social network or lack of friends and leisure activities (such as hobbies, sports, playing with children, conversations, etc.) – impairs compensatory resources that have health-promoting properties, increases susceptibility to disease [25-27], and results in an unfavorable prognosis in those with established CHD. Although several researchers have questioned the direct effect of social variables on CHD, suggesting that they act through covariates rather than directly, some interesting animal models support the direct effect hypothesis [28]. While the biological mechanism is not fully understood, the most likely candidate is the role of hypercortisolemia and exaggerated stress response, i.e. pronounced elevations in heart rate and blood pressure in response to stressful stimuli.

■ Syndrome X: A Conceptual Framework for Discussing the Interaction Between Heart and Mind

Syndrome X(SX), a pathological condition characterised by anginal chest pain, ECG and/or scintigraphic signs of ischemia, but normal epicardial coronary arteries, represents a useful conceptual framework for discussing the interaction between heart and mind. Since 1973, when the syndrome was first described by Kemp [29], a number of hypotheses have been proposed to account for the physiopathological mechanisms underlying this disease. Ischemia was at first thought to reduce flow in the distal branches of the coronary arteries; however, recently noninvasive techniques of flow measurement such as positron emission tomography (PET) have disproved this hypothesis. Ischemia itself was questioned when preservation of contractile function during stress was demonstrated. An alternative hypothesis considered autonomic deregulation as a causative factor. Indeed, several indices of increased sympathetic activity (namely, excessive heart rate and blood pressure increase during stress, shortening of exercise diastolic time, and metabolic responses to stress) were present in affected patients. However, coronary vasoconstriction, the purported link between enhanced sympathetic activity and chest pain, has never been demonstrated. Moreover, recent studies have found normal concentrations of catecholamines in the myocardial tissue of SX patients.

Heart rate variability is another marker of autonomic balance. The majority of patients affected with SX exhibit reduced vagal tone. This observation served as a bridge to another major finding relative to SX patients: frequently they have abnormal pain perception. In particular, these patients often experience painful stimuli coming from the heart during catheterization of the ventricle or injection of a contrast media in the coronary arteries, procedures that are usually painless. Also, while the intracoronary injection of adenosine, which can provoke chest pain in many patients, is at least as painful in SX patients as in those with evidence of coronary stenosis, dipyridamole-induced ischemia, documented through wall motion abnormality in the latter, has no effect on SX patients. The hypothesis that chest pain in SX is a sympathetic-maintained pain of neurologic origin due to dysregulation in the cardiac nervous system was formulated, and, in fact, abnormalities in the perception of visceral pain have been demonstrated in SX patients.

Shifting the paradigm away from ischemia led to the formulation of a new hypothesis. Because PET studies of the brain during chest pain documented extensive cortical activation (greater than in coronary patients) in the absence of myocardial pathology, it was proposed that SX might be thought of as a cortical pain syndrome (the stimulus arises in the brain and goes towards the heart, rather than arising in the heart and ascending to brain as in angina due to coronary artery disease). Indirect support for this hypothesis is the lower level of classical risk factors (excepted smoking) in SX patients, compared with established CHD patients.

SX represents a very interesting model of interaction between heart and mind. The psychological factors that characterize affected patients have been studied by comparing SX to established CHD and normal controls. The main finding includes an anxiety level that is higher than healthy controls and CHD patients. Family and social difficulties are often increased, as is an inhibited emotion expression. There is a high prevalence of panic disorder, depression and somatization of symptoms. Type A behavior pattern is infrequent in SX patients, who usually have low levels of irritability and hostility.

Conclusion

In conclusion, risk factors can be systematically influenced by means of psychological techniques. For example, when standard cardiological therapy is supplemented by professional psychological intervention of sufficient intensity and duration, there is a noticeable improvement in lifestyle (i.e. risk-linked behavior) and quality of life, and a consequent reduction in morbidity and mortality [25, 30]. In about 20-30% of patients with recent heart surgery, supportive psychological intervention is relevant and helpful [29-35]. Intervention studies deal mainly with depression in patients with prior MI. Theoretically, a significant reduction in the prevalence of depression, regardless of the method that one uses, could lead to a 30% reduction in cardiovascular morbidity and mortality through life style improvement and direct effect on blood pressure, cholesterol and autonomic balance. Studies of antidepressant treatment are currently underway, and include the use of sertraline, one of the selective serotonin reuptake inhibitors (SSRI). Sertraline is safe to use in patients with heart disease, in contrast to tricyclic antidepressants, which may worsen cardiac function and cause arrhythmias. Potentially, SSRI may increase heart rate variability and reduce platelet activity. However, at present there is no evidence that treating depression with SSRI reduces cardiac events or mortality in patients with established CHD.

This rather complex scenario, which is peculiar to psychosocial risk factors, is further complicated by the fact that psychosocial factors can aggregate in clusters and exert different effects during different stages of life. Also, access to medical care might be influenced by psychosocial constructs even if we lack a straightforward demonstration. As a consequence, one can state that any life situation that has the capacity to evoke chronic negative emotional responses may promote heart disease.

Although a great amount of work remains to be done, it is possible to conclude that psychosocial status is a relevant issue in the development of CHD and its prognosis in patients who already have CHD. Recognized psychosocial risk factors include low socio-economic status, social isolation, chronic family conflict, chronic job stress, acute stress, negative emotional states (i.e. depression, anxiety, vital exhaustion, PTSD) and negative behavior patterns (hostility). These act either indirectly, by affecting behavior and favoring unhealthy lifestyles (smoking, diet, alcohol consumption, physical inactivity) or directly, through biological pathways that are not at present fully understood, although blood coagulation, autonomic balance, catecholamine release and inflammation seem to be the most affected. Prospective, controlled interventional studies are needed to determine whether the amelioration of psychological problems is effective in improving the prognosis of CHD patients.

Finally, it is important to mention a potential confusion that exists relative to the roles of cardiologists, who, generally, are not eager to serve as mental health professionals, and psychologists, who should be contacted when a psychological issue emerges during patient evaluation. The failure to do so has probably both slowed research, on the one hand, and clinical and therapeutic approaches on the other. A new, highly integrated pattern of cooperation between different health providers is necessary and should be pursued.

■ References

1. Menninger KA, Menninger WC (1936) Psychoanalytic observations in cardiac disorders. Am Heart J 11:10-22
2. Arlow JA (1945) Identification mechanisms in coronary occlusion. Psychosom Med 7:195-209
3. Dunbar F (1954) Emotions and bodily changes, 4th ed. New York: Columbia University Press
4. Dunbar F (1950) Psychosomatic medicine. In: Lorand S (Ed) Psychoanalysis today, 4th edition, New York: International University Press, pp 23-42
5. Kannel WB, Castelli WP, Gordon T, McNamara PM (1971) Serum cholesterol, lipoproteins, and the risk of coronary heart disease. The Framingham Study. Ann Intern Med 74:1-12
6. Haynes SG, Feinleib M, Kannel WB (1980) The relationship of psychosocial factors to coronary heart disease in the Framingham study: III. Eight-year incidence of coronary heart disease. Am J Epidemiol 111:37-58

7. Kannel WB, Gordon T (1968) The Framingham Study. Washington, D.C.
8. Stamler J, Epstein FH (1972) Coronary heart disease: risk factors as guides to preventive action. Preventive Med 1:27-48
9. Abholz HH, Borgers D, Karmaus W, Korporal J (1982) Risikofaktorenmedizin Konzept und Kontroverse. Berlin: de Gruyter
10. Albus C, Jordan J, Herrmann-Lingen C (2004) Screening for psychosocial risk factors in patients with coronary heart disease. Recommendations for clinical practice. Eur J Cardiovasc Prev Rehabil 11: 75-79
11. Rozanski A, Kubzansky LD (2005) Psychologic functioning and physical health: a paradigm of flexibility. Psychosom Med 67, Suppl 1: S47-S53
12. Denollet J (2000) Type D personality. A potential risk factor refined. J Psychosom Res 49:255-66
13. Panagiotakos DB, Pitsavos C, Chrysohoou C et al (2004) Increased plasma homocysteine in healthy people with hostile behavior: the ATTICA study. Med Sci Monit 10:CR457-462
14. Herrmann-Lingen C, Buss U (2002) Angst und Depressivität im Verlauf der koronaren Herzerkrankung. Frankfurt: VAS
15. Appels A, Schouten E (1993) Erschoepftes Erwachen als Risikofaktor der koronaren Herzkrankheit. Psychotherapie 43:166-170
16. Appels A (1980) Psychological prodromata of myocardial infarction and sudden death. Psychotherapy and Psychosomatics 34:187-195
17. Kop WJ, Appels A-PWM, Mendes-de-Leon CF, Baer FW (1996) The relationship between severity of coronary artery disease and vital exhaustion. J Psychosom Res 40:397-405
18. Appels A, Siegrist J, De-Vos Y (1997) "Chronic workload," "need for control," and "vital exhaustion" in patients with myocardial infarction and controls: A comparative test of cardiovascular risk profiles. Stress Medicine 13:117-121
19. Spindler H, Pedersen SS (2005) Posttraumatic stress disorder in the wake of heart disease: prevalence, risk factors, and future research directions. Psychosom Med 67: 715-723
20. von Känel R, Mills PJ, Fainman C, Dimsdale JE (2001) Effects of psychological stress and psychiatric disorders on blood coagulation and fibrinolysis: a biobehavioral pathway to coronary artery disease. Psychosom Med 63: 531-544
21. Rosengren A, Hawkin S, Öunpuu S et al (2004) Association of psychosocial risk factors with risk of acute myocardial infarction in 11119 cases and 13648 controls from 52 counties (the INTERHEART study): case-control study. Lancet 364:953-962
22. Wittstein IS, Thiemann DR, Lima JAC et al (2005) Neurohormonal features of myocardial stunning due to sudden emotional stress. N Engl J Med 352: 539-548
23. Jiang W, Babyak M, Krantz SD et al (1996) Mental stress induced myocardial ischemia and cardiac events. JAMA 275: 1651-1656
24. Siegrist J (1996) Soziale Krisen und Gesundheit. Göttingen: Hogrefe
25. Jones DA, West RR (1996) Psychological rehabilitation after myocardial infarction: multicentre randomised controlled trial. Brit Med J 313: 1517-1521
26. Badura B, Kaufhold G, Lehmann H (1988) Soziale Unterstützung und Krankheitsbewältigung - Neue Ergebnisse aus der Oldenburger Longitudinalstudie 4 1/2 Jahre nach Erstinfarkt. Psychotherapie und medizinische Psychologie 38:48-58

27. Badura B, Schott T (1989) The significance of psychosocial factors for coping with chronic illness. Zeitschrift fuer Gerontopsychologie und Psychiatrie 2:149-154
28. Lown B, Verrier RL, Corbalan R (1973) Psychologic stress and threshold for repetitive ventricular response. Science 182:834-836
29. Kempt HG Jr (1973) Left ventricular function in patients with the anginal syndrome and normal coronary arteriograms. Am J Cardiol 32:375-376
30. Linden W, Stossel C, Maurice J (1996) Psychosocial interventions for patients with coronary artery disease. A meta-analysis. Arch Intern Med 156:745-752
31. Bunzel B (1995) Heart transplantation: psychosocial correlations in the postoperative period. Schweiz Rundsch Med Prax 84:866-871
32. Riedel-Keil B, Strenge H (1994) Practical experiences in the psychological care of heart transplant patients. Seiten 125:111-125
33. Zipfel S, Lowe B, Paschke T et al (1998) Psychological distress in patients awaiting heart transplantation. J Psychosom Res 45:465-470
34. Zipfel S, Loewe B, Schneider A et al (1999) Quality of life, depression and coping in patients awaiting heart transplantation. Psychotherapie, Psychosomatik, medizinische Psychologie 99 A.D.
35. Zipfel S, Lowe B, Schneider A et al (1999) Quality of life, depression and coping behavior in patients awaiting heart transplant. Psychother Psychosom Med Psychol 49:187-194

Physiological Basis of Mind-Heart Link

Chapter 3

Psychophysiology of Heart Disease

G. Parati ▪ M. Valentini ▪ G. Mancia

The link between heart and mind has represented for centuries an intriguing topic for researchers; it is interesting and at the same time difficult to explore [1]. A number of pathophysiological, epidemiological and clinical studies have emphasized the complex interactions that exist between neural influences and cardiovascular function, both physiologically and in the context of neural or cardiovascular diseases [1].

Among the neural factors reported to affect cardiovascular parameters, influences stemming from the central nervous system in response to environmental stress have repeatedly been suggested to be important determinants of changes in cardiovascular function and structure [2]. Indeed, acute and chronic stress, as well as psychological disorders, have been shown to play a role in the genesis of a number of cardiovascular diseases. Research has focussed primarily on the mechanisms underlying the association between stress on one hand and hypertension or coronary artery disease on the other. This association this has resulted in discrepant conclusions over the years, mainly due to methodological problems [3, 4].

This chapter provides a brief critical review on results of studies focusing on cardiovascular reactivity to stress, as well as on important methodological issues involved. In particular, we address the assessment of blood pressure and heart rate responses evoked in the laboratory by a wide range of physical and psychological stressors, as well as the hemodynamic effects of real-life stress, ranging from sudden natural disasters to sustained psychosocial influences. Proposed mechanisms and pathways potentially responsible for the deleterious effects of stress on the cardiovascular system are outlined, with particular attention on the role of sympathetic nervous system activation.

Finally, the clinical relevance of enhanced blood pressure and heart rate reactivity to stress is discussed in relation to the complex interaction between genetic factors and psychosocial stressors in predisposing individuals to various manifestations of cardiovascular disease, ranging from sustained hypertension to coronary and carotid atherosclerosis and left ventricular hypertrophy.

■ Introduction

Although behavioral and psychological factors have been repeatedly related to cardiovascular disease in the context of epidemiological, clinical and laboratory studies, the mechanisms by which either intermittent or sustained stress, as well as psychological illness, may lead to hypertension and coronary artery disease are not yet fully understood.

Historically, Hines and Brown [5, 6], back in early 30s, reported their first observations on cardiovascular reactivity. Subjects showing "exaggerated heart rate and blood pressure responses when encountering behavioral stimuli experienced as engaging, challenging or aversive" were defined as hyper-reactors [7]. By recording blood pressure changes following hand immersion in ice-cold water, Hines and Brown tried to devise a simple test capable of identifying subjects prone to future hypertension. These authors were the first to report that hypertensive patients exhibit a greater blood pressure response to cold, and a longer recovery time, than normotensive controls. They concluded that enhanced reactivity to physical stress could be regarded as a predictor of future hypertension, and suggested that normotensive subjects showing pronounced hemodynamic responses to stress are at increased risk for developing hypertension later in life.

Although a number of studies [8-11] replicated and confirmed these original findings, better controlled investigations [12-17], including studies from our own group [18], failed to corroborate such results.

Wolff and Wolf [19], almost two decades later, introduced a mental stressor (stressful interview) instead of a physical stressor to test cardiovascular reactivity. Behaviorally induced cardiovascular reactivity was still viewed simply as a marker of future hypertension rather than being causally related to it. Again, there were conflicting results on the occurrence of more pronounced hemodynamic responses to mental stressors in essential hypertensive subjects than in normotensive subjects. Although in some investigations a difference in reactivity was demonstrated in essential hypertensive subjects undergoing a wide array of psychological stimulations - including stressful interviews, mental arithmetic tests as well as the induction of fear or anger [20-24] - a number of other studies revealed that essential hypertensive patients showed similar blood pressure and heart rate increases to mental stressors compared to normotensive subjects [25-29]. In particular, the classic study by Brod et al. [26] revealed that mental aritmetics induced similar effects in hypertensives and normotensives, including cardiac output increase, vasoconstriction of the systemic, renal and splanchnic circulation, and vasodilation in the skeletal muscles.

Since then, several additional investigations have been conducted, trying to control for possible confounders, in an attempt to better elucidate the various mechanisms linking emotional, cognitive and physical stress with cardiovascular disease. In contrast to previous investigations, these studies recognized the difficulties and limitations involved in reproducing the effects of real-life stress in the laboratory. This chapter presents these issues, in an attempt to acquaint the reader with the available epidemiological evidence, with respect to the link between various forms of psychological stress and cardiovascular disease, and with respect to the proposed mechanisms possibly underlying this link.

▦ Assessing the Response to Stress in the Laboratory

A number of tests have been developed to assess cardiovascular reactivity (CVR) to stress in the laboratory environment. These tests are aimed at qualitatively and quantitatively assessing blood pressure and heart rate responses to discrete stressors. Some of these tests have been introduced in the attempt to reproduce, under controlled experimental conditions, what people experience in real life as stressful from the psycho-emotional or physical standpoint. They roughly belong to the broad categories of mental (or cognitive) and physical stressors [18]. The latter involve essentially the subjects emotionally by requesting them to solve mathematical, technical or organizational problems. The former involve essentially a physical stimulus or a physical performance [18].

▦ Mental Stressors

The most widely recognized mental stressor is the mental arithmetic test in which subjects are asked to compute subtractions of increasing complexity under a time constraint. Additionally, subjects can be mentally challenged by memory tasks, by items of the IQ test, or by complex psychomotor tasks. These include the mirror drawing test (during which subjects are asked to replicate a geometrical drawing looking at their writing hand only as reflected by a mirror (Fig. 1), the Stroop-color-word test (in which subjects are asked to select a colored object while under the influence of conflicting visual and auscultatory inputs), video-game tests of increasing complexity, and public speaking. Finally, cardiovascular changes that may occur in anticipation of physical exercise similarly fall into the category of psychologically challenging stressors. As in

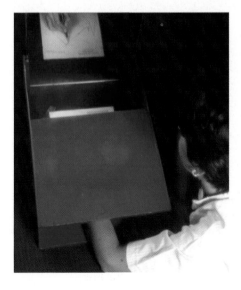

Fig. 1. Mirror drawing test

the effects of mental tests that do not involve a motor component, the anticipatory responses are mostly driven by descending cortical efferent neural influences, and not by peripheral neural afferent influences signalling the exercise-induced increase in metabolic demands. Similarly to traditional mental stressors, the anticipation of exercise can trigger substantial blood pressure elevations [4]. In longitudinal studies, there is evidence that enhanced blood pressure responses to these stressors are associated with left ventricular hypertrophy [30], carotid wall lesions [31] and subsequent development of chronic blood pressure increase [32]. The public speaking test, introduced more recently, has strong social features as it involves interpersonal relationships. This test elicits strong β-adrenergic stimulation and larger cardiovascular responses than the traditionally structured mental stress tests used in the laboratory [33].

■ Physical Stressors

The physical stressors most commonly used in the laboratory are the cold pressure test [5] (which usually involves hand immersion in ice cold water for 60 seconds) and the hand-grip test [9] (which involves the application of a hand isometric exercise usually for 90 seconds at 30% of the subject's maximal strength) (Fig. 2). Sometimes dynamic exercise on a treadmill or on a cycloergometer is also used.

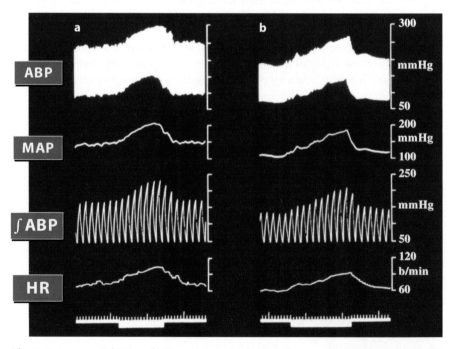

Fig. 2. Intra-arterial BP and HR responses to isometric exercise in two patients. BP, blood pressure; HR, heart rate. From [40]

In the cold pressure test, hand or foot immersion in iced cold water triggers a brisk blood pressure rise that is thought to be generated by peripheral vaso con-striction triggered by pain and temperature afferent signals [34]. When cold is applied to the forehead, vasoconstriction couples with bradycardia as is observed in the diving reflex (where stimulation of skin receptors is associated with chemoreflex activation by breath holding) [4].

In the case of aerobic exercise, increased peripheral metabolic activity is a major determinant of the observed cardiovascular responses. This may account for the weak correspondence between responses elicited by aerobic exercise and those elicited by mental tests [4]. Overall, during the application of physical stressors, the main responses assessed in cardiovascular reactivity studies con-sist of changes in blood pressure and heart rate. These changes are thought to be secondary to central activation of the sympathetic nervous system coupled with skin noci- and thermo-receptor stimulation as well as ergoceptor stimulation [18]. Less commonly, changes in other parameters, such as cardiac output, total peripheral resistance, regional blood flow, as well as plasma adrenaline and noradrenaline, have also been evaluated.

▣ Limitations of Laboratory Stress Tests

The laboratory assessment of cardiovascular reactivity to stress has the advan-tages of allowing the investigator to control the features of the stressor applied (quality, duration, intensity), as well of the environmental conditions (tem-perature, humidity, noise, etc.). This is done while collecting data on both the hemodynamic and neurohormonal changes occurring before, during and fol-lowing the administration of the stressful stimulation. In spite of these advan-tages, laboratory assessment of cardiovascular reactivity has its limitations [3, 35] (Table 1).

Major drawbacks relate both to the nature of the stressor (which has to be strong enough to elicit a detectable response in all subjects) and to the need for standardized test protocols, aimed at ensuring similar conditions in different laboratories. Even with meticulous attention on the methodological aspects of

Table 1. Limitations of laboratory methods for assessing cardiovascular reactivity to stress in humans

• Artificial laboratory environement
• Limited reproducibility of the responses
• Only spot quantifications of response to stress
• No information on daily-life cardiovascular reactivity
• Most stimuli are not specific to real life conditions
• Different responses to different tests in the same subject
• Different mechanisms of stress reactivity explored by different tests

cardiovascular reactivity testing, within-subject reproducibility of blood pressure and heart rate responses remains rather poor, with variation coefficients in the 15-33% range [36]. In our own laboratory, twenty essential hypertensives (studied after 7-10 days of pharmacological wash-out) and nineteen normotensives underwent cold pressure and hand-grip testing six times in a row, with 15 minute intervals between standardized sessions. R-R interval was derived by analysis of the conventional electrocardiographic signal, and blood pressure was invasively recorded at the radial artery level on a beat-by-beat basis. Average blood pressure and heart rate responses to either test markedly differed among subjects as shown in Figure 3. Furthermore, these responses exhibited a wide within-subject variability on repeat testing. In the whole population, the variation coefficient (SD X 100/mean response) of the blood pressure response to hand-grip and cold pressure test was respectively 22.2% (12.8-32.3%) and 17.2% (8.2-34.7%), being the coefficient of variation of the heart rate response to the same tests being 24.6% (11.9-49.1%) and 44.2% (18.1-158.1%). Both blood pressure and heart rate responses were independent of baseline values and test sequence.

The question whether cardiovascular reactivity is consistent and stable over time within and among subjects has been addressed by a number of investigations in addition to ours [37-39] and, overall, the evidence supporting the probability of reproducible results is far from being satisfactory.

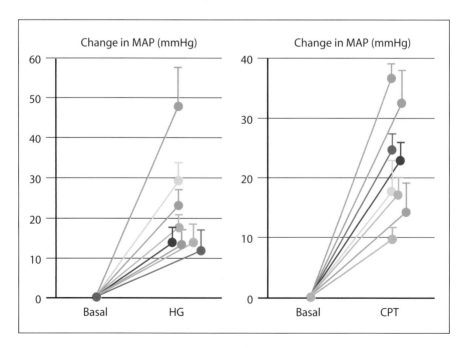

Fig. 3. Variability between and within subjects of the mean arterial pressure (MAP, intra-arterial recording) responses to hand-grip exercise (HG) and to cold pressure test (CPT). From [36]

Wide individual variation in hemodynamic responses to discrete stressors is not the only limitation faced while assessing cardiovascular reactivity in the laboratory environment. An additional problem lies in the limited correspondence of responses elicited by different tests [35]. In our laboratory [40], intra-arterial blood pressure and heart rate responses to mental challenges (mental arithmetic and mirror drawing test) and to physical stressors (hand-grip and cold pressure test) were compared in 22 subjects with untreated mild hypertension. As shown in Table 2, blood pressure responses to mental arithmetic and mirror drawing tests were significantly, although not highly, correlated; and the same was observed for blood pressure responses to hand-grip and cold pressure tests.

Table 2. Correlation coefficients between mean blood pressure responses to lab stressors and 24h mean blood pressure variability

MA	MI	HG	CPT
(n = 14)	(n = 15)	(n = 43)	(n = 31)
0.46	0.59*	0.28	0.01
0.10	0.14	0.10	0.07

*p<0.05; MA, mental arithmetic; MI, mirror drawing test; HG, hand-grip test; CPT, cold pressure test. From [40]

Of notice, blood pressure response to mental challenges showed little or no correlation with blood pressure response to physical stressors. Heart rate response to mental arithmetic significantly correlated with the heart rate response observed with the mirror drawing test. Heart rate responses to different physical stressors, however, did not correlate either between tests or with heart rate responses to mental challenges. In other words, subjects defined as hyper-, hypo- or normo-reactor to one test might be classified differently based on the results of another test (Fig. 4). Other researchers interested in the issue of the stability of cardiovascular responses across laboratory tests [25, 38, 41-44] have, overall, come to the same conclusion: although some correlation between responses to different tasks is apparent (more for blood pressure than for heart rate, and more among mental tests than between mental and physical tests), the evidence in favor of a consistent cardiovascular response pattern shared by both traditional mental and physical laboratory tests is not very strong.

Another limitation of the assessment of cardiovascular responses to discrete stressors in the laboratory environment is the fact that, in most tests, measures of heart rate and blood pressure response are taken at their peak, neglecting both the anticipation and the recovery phase. Assessment of peak response only may not adequately reflect the actual engagement of the cardiovascular system, in terms of both magnitude and time course. Because of these inadequacies, the use of discrete laboratory stressors to assess cardiovascular responses may significantly underestimate the overall hemodynamic load exerted in real life by the sustained and complex responses that characterize reactivity to stressful situations.

Indeed, a number of studies have confirmed the finding of Hines and Brown

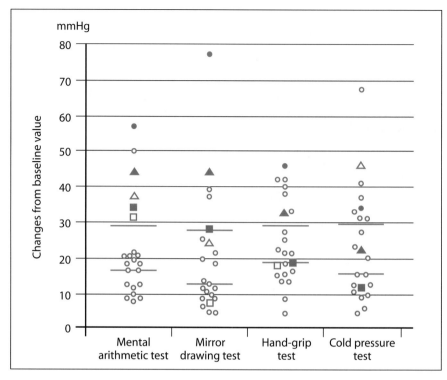

Fig. 4. Different classification of subject's cardiovascular reactivity to stress as a function of the type of stressor employed. From [40]

[22] that hypertensive patients are characterized not only by greater cardio-vascular reactivity but also by a slower recovery, compared with normotensive controls [45].

A possible way to better assess magnitude and time course of cardiovascular reactivity to stress, has been offered by new technology for the continuous, non-invasive beat-to-beat monitoring of blood pressure [46]. This technology is incor-porated in devices such as the Finapres (Ohmeda), the Finometer and the Por-tapres (Finapres Medical Systems, Arnhem, the Netherlands), as well as in the Task Force Monitor (CNSystems, Graz, Austria) (Fig. 5) [47]. These devices allow blood pressure and heart rate to be recorded on a beat-by-beat basis for pro-longed time periods without the need for intra-arterial catheters. This offers an obvious advantage in assessing dynamic blood pressure and heart rate respons-es to stimuli of short duration, a capability that is not allowed by conventional auto-mated blood pressure monitor, which are based on discontinuous readings (Fig. 5) [48]. Devices implementing the new technology use finger cuffs for assess-ment purposes; and their accuracy in detecting blood pressure changes in response to different laboratory tests, as well as real life simulations, has been shown to be quite good (this is treated elsewhere [47, 49] - see Figs. 6, 7).

Portapres model 2

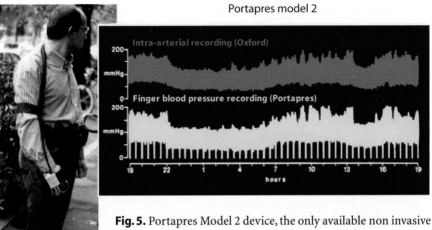

Fig. 5. Portapres Model 2 device, the only available non invasive device for continuous ambulatory blood pressure monitoring. Tracings obtained simultaneosuly by the Portapres device (lower panel) and by means of an intra-arterial cathereter (upper panel) are also shown

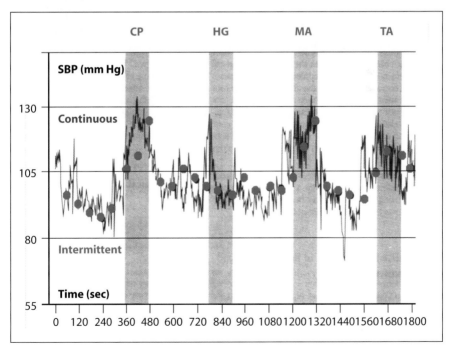

Fig. 6. Differences in the detection of systolic blood pressure peak respones to four laboratory stressors by using a continuous blood pressure recording (line) or discontinuous albeit frequent blood pressure measurements (dots). CP, cold pressure test; HG, hand-grip exercise; MA, mental arithmetics; TA, talking in public. From [49a]

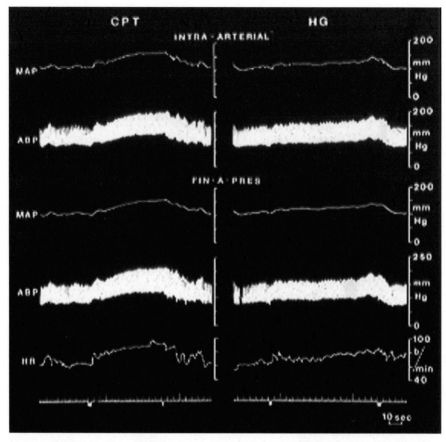

Fig. 7. Intra-arterial (upper panels) and non-invasive (Finapres, lower panels) blood pressure recordings simultaneously obtained during cold pressor tests (CPT) and hand-grip exercise (HG) in the same subject. MAP, mean arterial pressure; ABP, pulsatile blood pressure; HR, heart rate. From [47]

A final problem with laboratory stressors is related to their limited ability to truly reflect blood pressure and heart rate responses evoked by physical or emotional stress in real life. This limitation has been overcome by the introduction of techniques for ambulatory blood pressure monitoring. These techniques allow direct measurement of blood pressure and heart rate responses to the challenges related to daily activities, such as public speaking, undergoing job interviews, taking exams or driving a car. They also offer the possibility of obtaining information on the cardiovascular effects of occasional but highly stressful situations, such as flying a jetfighter plane or being exposed to an earthquake. An example of these possibilities is represented by the recording of ambulatory blood pressure obtained from a subject during the strong earthquake that hit central Italy a few years ago. In line with previous observations collected only before or after an earthquake, exposure to an earthquake acutely triggered an important sympathetically-mediated increase in both heart rate and blood pressure, which was maximal at the time of the strongest hit [50]. Heart rate returned to baseline values soon after the catastrophic event, whereas blood pressure levels remained elevated for over an hour and were followed by a sustained period of increased blood pressure variability. These hemodynamic changes may help in understanding the pathophysiological mechanisms responsible for the substantial increase in the rate of myocardial infarction and sudden death reported in major earthquakes such as those which occured in the United States and Japan [50] (Fig. 8). Other examples of blood pressure responses triggered by real life stressors and identifiable thanks to continuous ambulatory blood pressure monitoring techniques include the effects of a) a university interview (Fig. 9) [51], b) a lengthy poker game (Fig. 10) [51] and c) driving a bus in heavy city traffic (Fig. 11).

The information collected with the help of either continuous blood pressure monitoring or discontinuous ambulatory blood pressure recorders has clearly shown that the hemodynamic responses recorded following stress exposure in the laboratory bear little relationship with the responses evoked by daily-life stress. This is exemplified by the absence of a correlation between a typical response to stress in daily life, e.g., an increase in blood pressure and heart rate

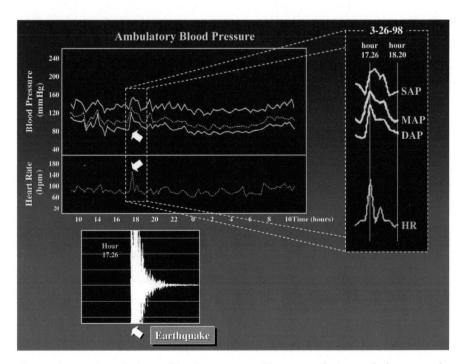

Fig. 8. Changes in ambulatory blood pressure and heart rate during and after an earthquake. From [50]

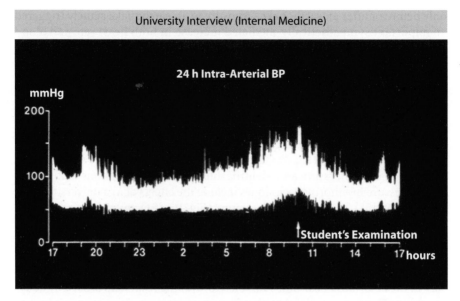

Fig. 9. Continuous intra-arterial ambulatory blood pressure monitoring during a stressful University interview. From [51]

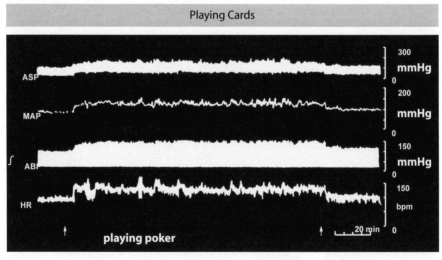

Fig. 10. Continuous intra-arterial ambulatory blood pressure monitoring during a poker game. From [51]

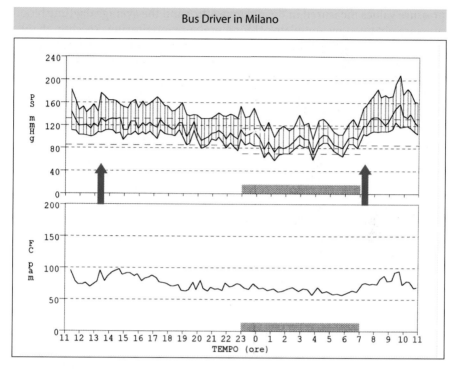

Fig. 11. Discontinuous non-invasive ambulatory blood pressure and heart rate monitoring of a bus driver (morning shift between 7 am and 13 pm)

induced by a doctor's visit (known as "white-coat effect"), and the response to most laboratory stressors. The first direct quantification of the white-coat effect was obtained by using techniques for ambulatory intra-arterial blood pressure monitoring over 24 hours. During the 24-hour recording, a visit by a physician was scheduled, and the increase in intra-arterial blood pressure triggered by consultation was recorded. As shown in Figure 12, the most pronounced blood pressure and heart rate increase was observed between two and four minutes after the visit began, and there was a tendency for blood pressure to slowly return towards baseline values thereafter [52]. This phenomenon, on average of significant magnitude, was characterized by pronounced between-subject variability, as shown in Figure 13, indicating a large between-subject difference in the reaction to this common stressful situation [53]. Given the invasiveness of this procedure, however, in clinical practice the magnitude of the white-coat effect is commonly and indirectly assessed as the difference between the blood pressure values measured in the doctor's office and the average daytime blood pressure obtained by ambulatory blood pressure monitoring. Recently, thanks to the application of methods for continuous noninvasive blood pressure monitoring in the assessment of blood pressure during a physician's visit [54], the surrogate quantification of white-coat effect, based on the difference between office and daytime average blood pressure, was clearly shown to be unrelated to the actual response in blood pressure triggered by the physician [54] (Fig. 14). In fact, the increase in blood pressure triggered by an unfamiliar physician was much greater than the difference between clinic and daytime average blood pressure. Lack of a significant correlation between these two measures of the white-coat effect has also been confirmed by other studies [33, 55]. In addition to the limited agreement between the different measures of the white-coat effect, the blood pressure and heart rate responses to this natural stressor resulted in either no or limited correlation with a number of stressful stimulations in the laboratory. In particular, blood pressure response to the doctor's visit showed no correlation with mental stressors applied in the laboratory [33, 40]. Another study, however, revealed that an exaggerated response in blood pressure to a doctor's visit *was* associated with a sustained reaction to other daily life stressors such as public speaking [33] (Fig. 15). Some correlation was conversely found between the response to a mental stressor such as the mirror drawing test and long term 24-hour blood pressure variability (Fig. 16), although no significant relationship was found between blood pressure variability over 24 hours and the responses to other laboratory stressors (Table 2), emphasizing discrepancies between laboratory and daily life conditions.

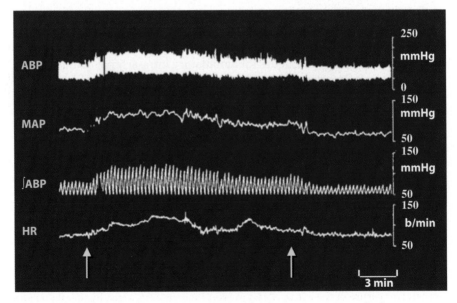

Fig. 12. Blood pressure and heart rate effects of a doctor's visit. From [52]

Maximal change in MAP and HR with doctor's visit (n = 88)

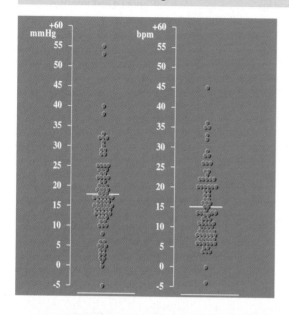

Fig. 13. Average and individual mean arterial pressure (MAP) and heart rate (HR) responses to the doctor's visit. Data refer to the acute effects, over the first few minutes of the visit. Modified from [54]

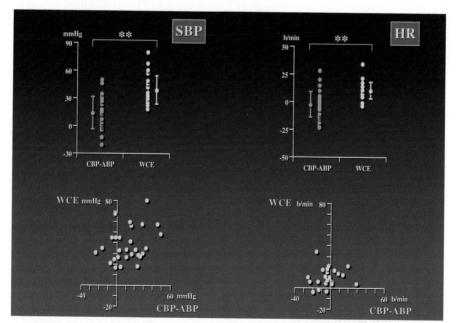

Fig. 14. Comparison between the surrogate measure of the white coat effect provided by the difference between clinic and ambulatory daytime blood pressure (CBP-ABP) and the direct measure of the actual blood pressure increase triggered by the physician's visit. Individual and average data from ***subjects are shown. From [55a]

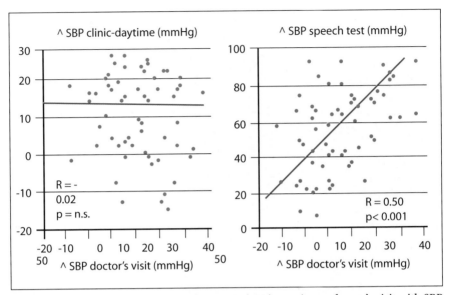

Fig. 15. Relationship of systolic blood pressure (SBP) reaction to doctor's visit with SBP response to speech test and clinic-daytime SBP difference. From [33]

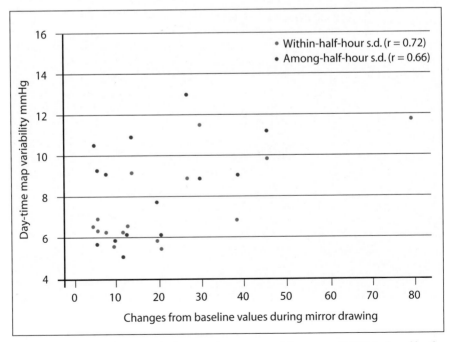

Fig. 16. Relationship between the increase in mean arterial pressure (MAP) induced by the mirror drawing test and the short- and long-term daytime MAP variabilities. From [40]

Daily life and laboratory stressors differ not only in the magnitude of the changes in blood pressure and heart rate that they induce, but also in the temporal characteristics of the stimulus applied. In fact, laboratory stressors elicit mostly acute reactions. Except for sudden natural disasters, naturally occurring forms of stress in most cases exert their action on a chronic and/or intermittent basis. The long lasting effect of chronic real-life stress is, indeed, one of the possible reasons for its adverse impact on cardiovascular outcome. This is exemplified by the features of some of recently acknowledged psychosocial risk factors, such as depression, anxiety, low socioeconomic status, lack of social support, work-related stress, poor quality of the marital relationship and caregiving strain [1, 7, 56-58].

Mechanisms

Acute and chronic stress - as well as psychological disorders - are thought to result in adverse cardiovascular consequences, such as arterial hypertension and coronary artery disease, through various pathophysiological mechanisms.

Studies conducted in selected human populations have yielded interesting insights on the link between stress and hypertension. A longitudinal follow-up of Italian nuns living in a secluded and unchanging environment did not demonstrate the expected rise in blood pressure with ageing, compared with that observed in a group of lay-women living in the same area. This difference was not accounted for by disparities in family history of hypertension, level of physical activity, baseline blood pressure or diet and body mass index, suggesting that the exposure to little or no stress and to little social conflict blunted the effects of a possible predisposition to develop hypertension [2, 10]. In keeping with this observation, several epidemiological studies of populations migrating from rural to urban environments demonstrated a substantial increase in blood pressure, as well as an increased incidence of new cases of hypertension, soon after migration [59-61]. Exposure to high levels of psychosocial stress or to new dietary habits have been thought to be responsible for this phenomenon, although it is notable that this was not universally observed in subjects migrating to areas at risk [2]. Overall, it is believed that important cardiovascular responses to stress lead to cardiovascular disease only after long-standing exposure to stressful events in subjects genetically or behaviorally predisposed [2, 34]. This was well exemplified by a study conducted on a group of male students [62] undergoing cold pressure and shock threat reactivity testing. The ability of laboratory cardiovascular reactivity to predict blood pressure levels ten years later emerged only in subjects who either self-reported high levels of daily stress or had a family history of hypertension, suggesting that cardiovascular responses to stress interact with both stress exposure and genetic predisposition in determining hypertension.

The results of other investigations have yielded the same conclusion: in a sample of Finnish men [31, 63], for example, it was discovered that a 4-year progression of carotid artery atherosclerosis was best predicted in subjects with the most pronounced cardiovascular responses in anticipation of an exercise stress test in association with either the hardest work demands or the worst socio-economic status.

The role of job stress in cardiovascular diseases has been suggested by several studies. In the London teachers study, job strain was associated with an increased blood pressure response to uncontrollable and not controllable tasks (this was a prospective study, including 162 school teachers) [64]. Blood pressure (systolic, mean and diastolic) decreased in the evening only in the low strain and not in the high strain group, probably because of a carryover effect. The prognostic role of these observations is supported by a report that a 3-fold higher risk for coronary disease was found in subjects who reported that they could not relax after work [65]. In another study, this time of fire-fighters, ambulatory blood pressure over 24 hours was elevated only during the working day and not during the non-working day [66] (Fig. 17). In women, the relation between ambulatory blood pressure and job strain is more controversial, due to conflicting data on the association between job strain and sustained hypertension in women [67]. The relationship between the menstrual cycle phase and blood pressure in working women is also controversial, with reports suggesting an increase in blood pressure during the luteal phase, along with increased sympathetic nerve activity [68]. Married working women (even more so if they have

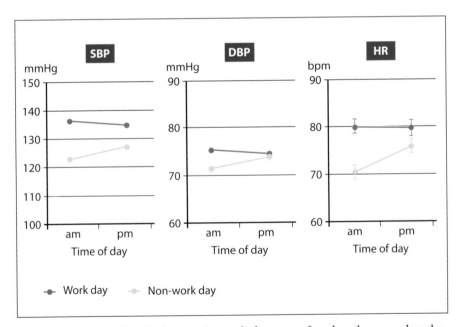

Fig. 17. SBP, DBP and HR in the morning and afternoon of work and non-work ambulatory monitoring days. SBP, systolic blood pressure; DBP, diastolic blood pressure; HR, heart rate. From [66]

children) are often found to have higher ambulatory blood pressure both during working hours and during the evening at home [68].

Finally, there is evidence that excessive workload (e.g., overtime work) can be particularly dangerous in terms of cardiovascular risk complications. Ambulatory blood pressure monitoring clearly shows that in a sleep-deficient day, followed by excessive work, 24 hour blood pressure is higher than in a normal work day [69].

Pathways

The activation of the sympathetic nervous system seems to be critical in mediating the stress-hypertension and coronary artery disease link. In fact, it has been seen that mental stress exerts a strong impact on the central nervous system leading to increased sympathetic nerve firing [1]. The sudden exposure to any form of stress prompts a sympathetically mediated increase in circulating catecholamines, heart rate and blood pressure [2]. This is the case when subjects are exposed to acute stress either in the laboratory environment or in real-life situations. The same response is seen even in the absence of a stressor when subjects feel under cognitive pressure [2, 70].

Whereas acute heart rate and blood pressure responses to stress are clearly attributable to enhanced sympathetic nervous system activity, the mechanisms by which chronic stressors lead to more sustained blood pressure elevation or to hypertension are not completely understood. Evidence suggests that essential hypertension is commonly neurogenic in nature, with the sympathetic nervous system, potentially under the influence of stress, playing a pivotal role [71]. This view is supported by observations that: a) in patients with essential hypertension, frequently the activity of the sympathetic nervous system is persistently elevated, as documented by increased cardiac and renal noradrenaline spillover [71, 72]; b) as in experimental models of stress, suprabulbar projections of noradrenergic neurons located in the brainstem are activated in hypertension [73-75]; and c) as can be seen in clinical models of sustained stress such as panic disorders, subjects with hypertension are releasing adrenaline as a co-transmitter, together with noradrenaline from the sympathetic endings. Under physiologic circumstances, adrenaline, the main hormone of the adrenal medulla, can be found in small amounts in the sympathetic nerve endings. According to the "adrenaline hypothesis" of the contribution of stress to the pathogenesis of hypertension [76], the exposure to stressful situations can increase the level of circulating plasma adrenaline and noradrenaline. As a consequence, the amount of adrenaline contained in the sympathetic nerve endings increases as well, and ends up being released in greater amounts, along with noradrenaline. The result is that adrenaline activates presynaptic β-adrenoceptors located on the sympathetic nerve endings, facilitating further release of noradrenaline and thus contributing to the hymodynamic perturbation. In support of the adrenaline hypothesis on the pathogenesis of hypertension, adrenaline co-transmission has been demonstrated both in cardiac [77] and in renal sympathetic nerves [78] of patients with hypertension, although it remains to be proven if it substantially contributes in these subjects to increased rates of cardiac and renal noradrenaline release [71]. In short, although the putative causal role of stress in the "adrenaline hypothesis" on the pathogenesis of hypertension is intriguing, to date, it remains presumptive, and adrenaline co-transmission can probably be regarded simply as a marker of chronic stress. In fact, although during a panic attack subjects exhibit evidence of stress-induced increases in the adrenaline content of cardiac sympathetic nerve endings and adrenaline co-transmission, as well as substantial increases in heart rate and blood pressure elevation, once the panic attack has resolved, they fail to show persistently elevated blood pressure.

The activation of the sympathetic nervous system by psychosocial stress is thought to be responsible for a number of other effects besides heart rate and blood pressure elevation. These effects, which include the promotion of arrhythmias, triggering of myocardial ischemia, pro-coagulation activity and, lastly, endothelial dysfunction, all contribute to creating conditions that are predisposing to sudden cardiac death and to various presentations of coronary artery disease.

Acute stress exposure can trigger potentially life-threatening arrhythmias, particularly in patients with coronary artery disease, by increasing myocardial electrical instability [7, 57, 79]. This has been clearly demonstrated, both in animal and human studies. The ventricular fibrillation threshold, defined as the amount of electrical stimulation needed to induce repetitive ventricular premature contractions, decreased by over 40% in dogs after they had spent three days in a stressful and harmful environment [80]. Treatment with β-adrenergic antagonists partially offsets the arrhythmogenic effect of acute stress, confirming the involvement of the sympathetic nervous system arousal in arrhythmia risk [81]. In humans with coronary occlusion, mental stress was found to induce ventricular tachycardia that was difficult to resolve and, in turn, lowered the threshold for ventricular fibrillation [82]. The beat-to-beat, exercise-induced variation of T-wave morphology (T-wave alternans = TWA) is a newly recognized marker of myocardial electrical instability and a potent predictor of major arrhythmias in susceptible patients [58]. Recently, the effects of mental stress (anger recall and mental arithmetic) on TWA have been compared with those of physical exercise in patients with known coronary artery disease and propensity to malignant arrhythmias [83]. Interestingly, compared to exercise, mental stress caused an impressive increase in electrical instability, as assessed by TWA, in spite of a relatively smaller heart rate increase (less than 15 beats/min). Furthermore, β-adrenergic blockade attenuated exercise-induced TWA increase, whereas it had no effect on mental stress-induced TWA increase, suggesting that mental activity can be a potent arrhythmogenic trigger in susceptible coronary artery disease patients, and that it acts via central and autonomic pathways that are different from those preferred by physical exercise. In summary, the role of stress in triggering malignant arrhythmias in the context of coronary artery disease is well documented, and recent evidence, as demonstrated in survivors of a cardiac arrest due to ventricular fibrillation [84], suggests that psychological stress can play such a causal role also in patients with apparently normal hearts.

It is well established that acute stress exposure precipitates myocardial ischemia in coronary artery disease patients [7, 57]. In the laboratory environment, patients with an established diagnosis of coronary artery disease undergoing (mostly) the mental arithmetic or public speaking test consistently develop myocardial ischemia as assessed via radionuclide ventriculography [85, 86], echocardiography [87], positron emission tomography (PET) [88], and 99mTc-sestamibi single photon emission computed tomography (SPECT) [89]. This is believed to depend, at least in part, on a sympathetically mediated increase in heart rate, blood pressure and oxygen demand. Despite the fact that heart rate elevations in response to laboratory mental stress are relatively small in magnitude, blood pressure elevations can be as substantial as the ones observed during physical exercise. Nevertheless, the double product threshold for myocardial ischemia during mental stress is much lower than the one observed during stress test [7], suggesting that other mechanisms, such as stress-induced endothelium-dependent coronary constriction, may come into play [90]. Interestingly, stress-induced episodes of myocardial ischemia are often silent, both in laboratory [7] and real-life settings [91] as assessed by Holter ECG 24-hour monitoring. It is even more interesting that laboratory stress-induced ischemia has the ability to predict cardiac events after adjustment for ejection fraction, history of myocardial infarction and age [86, 92].

Pro-coagulation effects and hemoconcentration are commonly seen in response to stress and are thought to be mostly secondary to sympathetic nervous system activation, although the possible causal role of stress-induced blood pressure elevation cannot be excluded [7, 57]. Both in the laboratory environment [93] and in real life [94], acute and sustained stress exposure induced a number of abnormalities, ranging from platelet activation, increased concentration of pro-coagulation substances (such as β-thromboglobulin and platelet factor 4) and hemoconcentration [95]. Interestingly, coagulation abnormalities were detected in human blood samples collected both within a couple of weeks from the Hanshin-Awaji earthquake [94] and several months after the occurrence of the natural disaster, suggesting that these abnormalities can persist for a considerable time after stress exposure.

There is recent evidence that psychological disturbances can interact with stress exposure to alter heart rate variability (HRV), which is known to be a measure of autonomic heart control and to predict selected heart diseases. In population studies, low HRV – reflecting reduced parasympathetic or increased sympathetic stimulation – has been shown to predict cardiovascular events [96], as well as cardiac and all-cause mortality [97]. Additionally, low HRV is an independent risk factor for mortality after acute myocardial infarction [98], owing, in part, to its ability to dispose individuals to arrhythmias. Depression, anxiety and hostility have all been associated with decreased HRV. Additionally, HRV is significantly lower in depressed than in non-depressed coronary artery disease patients, and there is some preliminary evidence that the depressed subjects show greater reductions in HRV in response to mental stress. Together, these data further support the view that autonomic nervous system involvement mediates the stress-cardiovascular disease link.

Baroreflex

An impaired baroreflex sensitivity (BRS) – i.e., blunted reflex heart rate changes secondary to either drug-induced or spontaneous systolic blood pressure variations – has been associated with adverse cardiovascular outcome [99]. Attempts to assess the effects of psychological stress on BRS variation, and to relate BRS and hemodynamic responses while under cognitive load, have led to inconsistent results [100-102]. In one study conducted on medical students, changes in BRS were assessed both during psychological and physical stress. An oral examination, considered a form of moderate psychological load, elicited a significant reduction in BRS. Of note, this effect was as sizable as the one elicited by light physical exercise, but it did not show any relation to stress-related blood pressure and heart rate responses. Similarly, in another study, resting BRS was not related to systolic blood pressure changes during the Stroop Color Word test [101].

In conclusion, although central modulation of BRS under psychological stress is thought to contribute to the development of hypertension, a relation between BRS and blood pressure responses to stress has never been demonstrated. In fact, very little correspondence between measures of baroreceptor functioning and cardiovascular reactivity has been found.

Endothelial Dysfunction

The endothelium controls the vascular tone and inhibits smooth muscle cell proliferation, platelet aggregation and leukocyte adhesion. All of these processes play a role in atherosclerosis, and a number of cardiovascular risk factors are known to cause vascular disease via endothelial dysfunction. A considerable body of evidence suggests that, in addition to traditional risk factors, acute and sub-acute psychological stress may be responsible for endothelial dysfunction both in animals and in humans. Borderline hypertensive rats exposed to air-jet stress in the face two hours a day for ten days exhibited impaired vasodilation in response to the endothelium-dependent vasodilator acetylcholine [103]. Cynomolgus monkeys exposed to chronic social stress developed endothelial cell injury and endothelial dysfunction, with a reduction of nitric oxide availability in atherosclerotic arteries [104]. Furthermore, healthy subjects recruited from a population-based cohort of civil servants with no risk factors and no clinical history of cardiovascular disease exhibited blunted endothelium-dependent and flow-mediated dilation at the level of the brachial artery after only a brief episode of mental stress similar to what might easily be encountered in everyday life; and the impairment involving this conduit artery persisted for up to four hours after the resolution of the acute hemodynamic response [105]. As in the subgroup of subjects with diabetes mellitus, no significant impairment in endothelial function, beyond the damage already due to diabetes itself, was seen in response to transient stress exposure. Finally, a similar observation was collected in a cohort of young depressed patients, who were otherwise healthy [106]. There is thus strong evidence that both brief and repeated forms of behavioral and psychological load can initiate or accelerate the atherogenic process by altering the endothelium properties.

Inflammation

Inflammation is another biological mechanism underlying the association between psychological disorders such as depression and cardiovascular morbidity and mortality. It has been demonstrated, both in subjects free of cardiovascular disease [107, 108] and in subjects with established disease [109, 110], that depressive symptoms linearly relate to markers of systemic inflammation, such as C-reactive protein, interleukin-6, and tumor necrosis factor-α. Indeed, there is evidence that depression may be associated with an increase in cardiac mortality [7, 57].

Endocrinological and Metabolic Factors

Psychological disturbances, as well as acute and chronic stress, are believed to act at the level of the central nervous system, not only by activating the sympathetic nervous system, but also by impacting the hypothalamic-pituitary axis. Hypercortisolemia and attenuated feedback control both result from chronic stimulation of the hypothalamic-pituitary axis. In this context, dexamethasone administration does not elicit the expected suppression of cortisol secretion. Additionally, hypercortisolemia has been shown to suppress growth and sex hormone production [57].

The metabolic effects of stress have been well studied in subjects with depression. There is evidence of an increased prevalence of central obesity, insulin resistance and diabetes [111].

Finally, it has been suggested that a combination of endothelial dysfunction and vascular remodeling may explain how acute blood pressure elevations in response to all forms of stress can lead to sustained blood pressure elevation [2]. In this context, the elevation of vascular resistance observed in hypertension results from changes both in vasoconstrictive and vasodilating substances and in the vascular architecture (i.e., decreased lumen vascular diameter and vascular rarefaction). These changes may be responsible for the transition from a state of high cardiac output to a state of high total vascular resistance in sustained hypertension.

◼ Clinical Relevance

As traditional risk factors for cardiovascular disease, such as smoking, family history of coronary artery disease, obesity, diabetes mellitus and hypercholesterolemia, predict no more than 50% of new cardiovascular disease, identification of new potential risk factors, including psychosocial factors, has gained increasing attention in recent years in the hope of broadening the opportunities of intervention. There is a growing body of evidence now linking measures of cardiovascular reactivity to markers of preclinical and clinical cardiovascular disease.

a) Prediction of future increase in blood pressure levels
According to the cardiovascular reactivity hypothesis, normal subjects exhibiting larger increases in blood pressure under psychological stress are more prone to hypertension. Whether cardiovascular reactivity represents simply a marker of hypertension or is causally related, cardiovascular reactivity may help in identifying subjects at risk of cardiovascular disease. A number of prospective studies have investigated the stress-cardiovascular disease link using the cold pressure test in the laboratory in an effort to reproduce daily life stress. Unfortunately, the cold pressure test has proved to be less than ideal for this purpose because it involves nociceptors and does not prompt a β-adrenoceptor-mediated response considered essential in determining early neurogenic hypertension [86, 112]. This may be the reason why, among the main prospective studies using the cold pressure test, the results of four supported the hypothesis [113-116], whereas the results of three did not [117-119].

Studies using other stressors (e.g., mental arithmetic test, video games, anticipation of exercise) have yielded more consistent results regarding the ability of blood pressure reactivity to predict future blood pressure status in young and middle-aged adults with normal blood pressure or with borderline hypertension.

Numerous studies using psychological and psychomotor tasks (video games, mirror-tracing, mental arithmetic test, reaction time) of normotensive children and adolescents have reported an association between blood pressure reactivity and future blood pressure status [114, 120, 121]. In these studies, reactivity to video games where the best predictors of subsequent blood pressure levels.

Over three thousand male and female subjects, aged 19-31 years, enrolled in the CARDIA (Coronary Artery Risk Development in Young Adults) study [122] underwent multi-task reactivity assessment, including the cold pressure test, video games and the mirror star-tracing test. Systolic blood pressure reactivity to cold pressure and the mirror tracing tests was not found to predict systolic blood pressure levels 5 years later, but systolic blood pressure reactivity to video games was found to be predictive, although, on further analysis, only for men. A subsequent report from the CARDIA study [112] that included over

4100 normotensive black and white men and women demonstrated with survival analysis that larger blood pressure responses to each of the cold pressure, star tracing and video game tests were associated with earlier hypertension occurrence at 13-year follow-up, suggesting that blood pressure reactivity to psychological stress reliably identifies young adults at risk for hypertension.

Additionally, in a cohort of Finnish middle-aged men, blood pressure reactivity in anticipation of exercise stress test independently predicted the presence of hypertension (i.e., 165/95 mmHg) 4 years later, after controlling for traditional risk factors [32].

Borderline hypertensives exhibiting an exaggerated diastolic blood pressure response to the mental arithmetic test and a prolonged blood pressure recovery time had a five-year increased risk of developing hypertension [123]. Responses evoked by the mental arithmetic test appeared to be the best ones in predicting future hypertension in borderline hypertensives in a number of studies [124, 125]. In summary, a large body of evidence suggests that cardiovascular responses to very diverse, short-term laboratory stressors predict new cases of hypertension in both young and adult normotensives and in borderline hypertensives. Whether cardiovascular reactivity is causally implicated in the etiology of hypertension, or whether it simply represents a marker of future risk of hypertension, is still a subject of debate. Nevertheless, cardiovascular reactivity is clinically useful and may help in our understanding of the disease processes.

b) Prediction of left ventricular mass
Although left ventricular mass is known to predict cardiovascular morbidity and mortality, only a few studies have addressed the association between measures of reactivity and measures of cardiac volume and structure. The preliminary evidence available suggests that cardiovascular reactivity may, indeed, be a determinant of left ventricular mass in humans. In one investigation [126], mean blood pressure response to a battery of laboratory stressors (video games, parent-child arguments, stressful interviews, postural changes), predicted left ventricular mass/height (2.7) and left ventricular hypertrophy independently of known determinants in a group of adolescents. Another study in the same age group demonstrated that systolic blood pressure reactivity to car driving simulation (but not to the cold pressure test or video games) independently predicted left ventricular mass/body surface area in a follow-up of 2.3 years [127]. A similar observation was made in a small sample of 66 middle-aged men with borderline hypertension: pressure reactivity to mental arithmetic and to isometric exercise explained 15% of variance in left ventricular mass change [128]. In summary, while there is some association between measures of cardiovascular reactivity and left ventricular mass, especially in children and adolescents (although this association has been observed also in adults with elevated blood pressure [30]), it is unclear how strong this association might be. Given the paucity and inconsistency of the available data, the association between cardiovascular responses to stressors and left ventricular mass progression remains a research issue.

c) Prediction of carotid atherosclerosis
Evidence in favor of an association between measures of cardiovascular reactivity and carotid atherosclerosis is accumulating, although there are some discrepancies among studies. In a prospective study, 136 adult unmedicated subjects, either healthy volunteers or patients who had been referred to an outpatient clinic for atherosclerosis prevention, underwent Stroop Color Word Interference task and B-mode carotid ultrasound [129]. In a 2-year follow up, it was found that systolic blood pressure reactivity, independently of traditional risk factors, accounted for an extra 7% of carotid plaque progression, unlike diastolic blood pressure and heart rate reactivity, which showed no predictive power.

Responsiveness to two behavioral stressors, such as public speaking and mirror-image drawing, was evaluated in a sample of 238 middle-aged women [130]. Neither systolic nor diastolic blood pressure responses were found to be related to carotid intima media thickness or number of carotid plaques at 2-year follow-up. However, pulse pressure increase elicited during tasks was associated with carotid disease, independently of resting pulse pressure and known cardiovascular risk factors.

In the Kopi Ischemic Heart Disease Risk Factor study, systolic blood pressure increase in anticipation of bicycle exercise interacting with either high job demands [31] or with low socioeconomic status [63] predicted the development of carotid atherosclerosis in two large samples of Finnish men.

In conclusion, in longitudinal studies, blood pressure reactivity seems to be predictive of carotid disease development and progression, although the association is weak, given (a) that the high-risk patients studied may have already had subclinical disease, and (b) the concomitant effect of psychosocial factors [121].

d) Prediction of new coronary heart disease and of its progression
Overall, the evidence supporting a relationship between reactivity to stress and the prediction of new coronary heart disease is scarce and conflicting, whereas a number of studies have clearly demonstrated an association between stress reactivity and clinical endpoints in patients with pre-existing hypertension or coronary artery disease. In over 1700 hypertensives, blood pressure reactivity was assessed by the difference between doctor-obtained diastolic blood pressure minus nurse-obtained diastolic blood pressure, under the assumption (supported by previous observations on the direct measure of white-coat effect through intra-arterial blood pressure monitoring) that seeing a doctor was more stressful than seeing a nurse [53]. In a 14-year follow up, subjects in the upper tertile for this difference were twice as likely to suffer from a myocardial infarction compared to the others [131]. On smaller samples, these findings were replicated in some [132, 133] but not all investigations [134]. In fact, in a group of 340 post-myocardial infarction patients heart rate reactivity to video game tasks was inversely associated with mortality from cardiac origin.

Conclusion

There is a growing body of evidence linking cardiovascular reactivity to the incidence of cardiovascular disease, despite the wide variation in methodologies used to assess cardiovascular reactivity. Some work [31, 62, 63] suggests that genetic as well as sociodemographic factors may contribute to the impact that cardiovascular reactivity exerts on cardiovascular disease. In other words, subjects with greater cardiovascular reactivity are more prone to developing hypertension and/or coronary artery disease if they are also genetically predisposed and/or are under the influence of chronic psychosocial stress [121]. Given the interest of this issue, and the new possibilities offered by progress in technology in the field of ambulatory blood pressure monitoring over 24 hours, further studies will hopefully clarify the relationship between responses to stress in the laboratory and stress in daily life, and the actual value of cardiovascular reactivity in predicting the development of new disease and/or the risk of their clinical complications.

References

1. Ramachandruni S, Handberg E, Sheps DS et al (2004) Acute and chronic psychological stress in coronary disease. Curr Opin Cardiol 19:494-499
2. Schwartz AR, Gerin W, Davidson KW et al (2003) Toward a causal model of cardiovascular responses to stress and the development of cardiovascular disease. Psychosom Med 65:22-35
3. Parati G, Pomidossi G, Casadei R (1986) Limitations of laboratory stress testing in the assessment of subjects' cardiovascular reactivity to stress. J Hypertens (suppl 6): S51-S53
4. Kamarck TW, Lovallo WR, Kamarck TW et al (2003) Cardiovascular reactivity to psychological challenge: conceptual and measurement considerations. Psychosom Med 65:9-21
5. Hines EA, Brown GF (2006) The cold pressure test for measuring the reactability of the blood pressure: data concerning 571 normal and hypertensive subjects. Am Heart J 11:1-9
6. Hines EA, Brown GF (1932) A standard stimulus for measuring vasomotor reactions: its applications in the study of hypertension. Proc Staff Meet Mayo Clin 7:332-335
7. Rozanski A, Blumenthal JA, Kaplan J et al (1999) Impact of psychological factors on the pathogenesis of cardiovascular disease and implications for therapy. Circulation 99:2192-2217
8. Ayman D, Goldshine AD (1938) Cold as standard stimulus of blood pressure: a study of normal and hypertensive subjects. N Engl J Med 219:650-658

9. Lind AR, Taylor SH, Humphrey PW et al (1964) The circulatory effects of sustained voluntary muscle contraction. Clin Sci 27:229-244

10. Thacker EA (1940) A comparative study of normal and abnormal blood pressures among university students, including the cold pressure test. Am Heart J 20:89-95

11. Shapiro AP, Moutsos SE, Krifcher E (1963) Patterns of pressor response to noxious stimuli in normal, hypertensive and diabetic subjects. J Clin Invest 42:1890-1898

12. Pickering GW, Kissing M (1935) The effects of adrenaline and cold on the blood pressure in human hypertension. Clin Sci 2:201-208

13. Boyer JT, Fraser JRE, Doyle AE (1960) The haemodynamic effects of cold immersion. Clin Sci 19:539-545

14. Remington RD, Lambarth B, Moser M et al (1960) Circulatory reactions of normotensive and hypertensive subjects and of the children of normal and hypertensive parents. Am Heart J 59:58-70

15. Greene MA, Boltax AJ, Lustig GA et al (1965) Circulatory dynamics during the cold pressor test. Am J Cardiol 16:54-60

16. Cuddy RP, Smulyan H, Keighley JF et al (1966) Hemodynamic and catecholamine changes during a standard cold pressor test. Am Heart J 71:446-454

17. Murakami E, Hiwada K, Kokubu T et al (1980) Pathophysiological characteristics of labile hypertensive patients determined by the cold pressor test. Jpn Circ J 44:438-442

18. Mancia G, Parati G (1987) Reactivity to physical and behavioural stress and blood pressure variability in hypertension. In: S. Julius and D.R. Basset (eds.) Handbook of hypertension (Vol 9), Amsterdam: Elsevier

19. Wolff S, Wolf HG (1951) A summary of experimental evidence relating life stress to the pathogenesis of essential hypertension in men. In: Bell ET (ed) Hypertension: a symposium, Minneapolis, Minnesota: University of Minnesota Press

20. Schachter H (1957) Pain, fear, and anger in hypertensives and normotensives: a psychophysiological study. Psychosom Med 19:17-29

21. Engel BT, Bickford AF (1961) Response specificity. Stimulus-response and individual-response specificity in essential hypertensives. Archives of General Psychiatry 5:478-489

22. Hollenberg NK, Williams GH, Adams DF et al (1981) Essential hypertension: abnormal renal vascular and endocrine responses to a mild psychological stimulus. Hypertension 3:11-17

23. Schulte W, Neus H (1983) Hemodynamics during emotional stress in borderline and mild hypertension. Eur Heart J 4:803-809

24. Richter-Heinrich E, Knust U, Muller W et al (1975) Psychophysiological investigations in essential hypertensives. J Psychosom Res 19:251-258

25. Fredrikson M, Dimberg U, Frisk-Holmberg M et al (1985) Arterial blood pressure and general sympathetic activation in essential hypertension during stimulation. Acta Medica Scandinavica 217:309-317

26. Brod J, Fencl V, Hejl Z et al (1959) Circulatory changes underlying blood pressure elevation during acute emotional stress (mental arithmetic) in normotensive and hypertensive subjects. Clin Sci 18:269-279

27. Esler MD, Nestel PJ, Esler MD et al (1973) Renin and sympathetic nervous system responsiveness to adrenergic stimuli in essential hypertension. Am J Cardiol 32:643-649

28. Drummond PD (1983) Cardiovascular reactivity in mild hypertension. J Psychosom Res 27:291-297

29. Fredrikson M, Dimberg U, Frisk-Holmberg M et al (1982) Haemodynamic and electrodermal correlates of psychogenic stimuli in hypertensive and normotensive subjects. Biological Psychology 15:63-73

30. Kamarck TW, Eranen J, Jennings JR et al (2000) Anticipatory blood pressure responses to exercise are associated with left ventricular mass in Finnish men: Kopi Ischemic Heart Disease Risk Factor Study. Circulation 102:1394-1399

31. Everson SA, Lynch JW, Chesney MA et al (1997) Interaction of workplace demands and cardiovascular reactivity in progression of carotid atherosclerosis: population based study. BMJ 314:553-558

32. Everson SA, Kaplan GA, Goldberg DE et al (1996) Anticipatory blood pressure response to exercise predicts future high blood pressure in middle-aged men. Hypertension 27:1059-1064

33. Palatini P, Palomba D, Bertolo O et al (2003) The white-coat effect is unrelated to the difference between clinic and daytime blood pressure and is associated with greater reactivity to public speaking. J Hyperten 21:545-553

34. Light KC, Light KC (2001) Hypertension and the reactivity hypothesis: the next generation. Psychosom Med 63:744-746

35. Parati G, Trazzi S, Ravogli A et al (1991) Methodological problems in evaluation of cardiovascular effects of stress in humans. Hypertension 17:III50-III55

36. Parati G, Pomidossi G, Ramirez A et al (1985) Variability of the haemodynamic responses to laboratory tests employed in assessment of neural cardiovascular regulation in man. Clin Sci 69:533-540

37. Manuck SB, Kamarck TW, Kasprowicz AS et al (1993) Stability and patterning of behaviorally-evoked cardiovascular reactivity. In: J. Blascovich and E.S. Katkin (eds.) Cardiovascular reactivity to psychological stress and disease, Washington, DC: American Psychological Association

38. Kamarck TW, Jennings JR, Debski TT et al (1992) Reliable measures of behaviorally-evoked cardiovascular reactivity from a PC-based test battery: results from student and community samples. Psychophysiology 29:17-28

39. Gerin W, Pickering TG, Glynn L et al (2000) An historical context for behavioral models of hypertension. J Psychosom Res 48:369-377

40. Parati G, Pomidossi G, Casadei R et al (1988) Comparison of the cardiovascular effects of different laboratory stressors and their relationship with blood pressure variability. J Hypertens 6:481-488

41. McKinney ME, Miner MH, Ruddel H et al (1985) The standardized mental stress test protocol: test-retest reliability and comparison with ambulatory blood pressure monitoring. Psychophysiology 22:453-463

42. Turner JR, Sherwood A, Light KC et al (1991) Generalization of cardiovascular response: supportive evidence for the reactivity hypothesis. Int J Psychophysiol 11:207-212

43. Turner JR, Sherwood A, Light KC et al (1994) Inter-task consistency of hemodynamic responses to laboratory stressors in a biracial sample of men and women. Int J Psychophysiol 17:159-164

44. Allen MT, Crowell MD, Allen MT et al (1989) Patterns of autonomic response during laboratory stressors. Psychophysiology 26:603-614

45. Schuler JL, O'Brien WH, Schuler JL et al (1997) Cardiovascular recovery from stress and hypertension risk factors: a meta-analytic review. Psychophysiology 34:649-659

46. Parati G, Bilo G, Mancia G (2004) Blood pressure measurement in research and clinical practice: recent evidence. Curr Opin Nephr Hypertens 13:343-357

47. Parati G, Casadei R, Groppelli A et al (1989) Comparison of finger and intra-arterial blood pressure monitoring at rest and during laboratory testing. Hypertension 13:647-655

48. Pickering TG (1991) Ambulatory monitoring and blood pressure variability. Science Press, London

49. Imholz BPM, Langewouters GJ, van Montfrans GA (1993) Feasibility of ambulatory continuous 24-hour finger arterial pressure recording. Hypertension 21:65-73

49a. Pickering TG (1991) Ambulatory monitoring and blood pressure variability. Science Press, London

50. Parati G, Antonicelli R, Guazzarotti F et al (2001) Cardiovascular effects of an earthquake: direct evidence by ambulatory blood pressure monitoring. Hypertension 39:e22-e24

51. Mancia G, Parati G, Di Rienzo M et al (1997) Blood pressure variability. In: Zanchetti A, Mancia G (eds) Blood pressure variability. Amsterdam, Elsevier Science B.V.

52. Mancia G, Bertinieri G, Grassi G et al (1983) Effects of blood pressure measurement by the doctor on patient's blood pressure and heart rate. Lancet 2:695-698

53. Mancia G, Parati G, Pomidossi G et al (1987) Alerting reaction and rise in blood pressure during measurement by physician and nurse. Hypertension 209-215

54. Mancia G, Di Rienzo M, Parati G (1993) Ambulatory blood pressure monitoring use in hypertension research and clinical practice. Hypertension 21:510-524

55. Lantelme P, Milon H, Vernet M et al (2000) Difference between office and ambulatory blood pressure or real white coat effect: does it mater in terms of prognosis? J Hypertens 18:379-382

55a. Parati G, Ulian L, Santucciu C et al (1998) Difference between clinic and daytime blood pressure is not a measure of the white coat effect. Hypertension 31:1185-1189

56. Kaplan GA, Keil JE (1993) Socioeconomic factors and cardiovascular disease: a review of the literature. Circulation 88:1973-1998

57. Rozanski A, Blumenthal JA, Davidson KW et al (2005) The epidemiology, pathophysiology, and management of psychosocial risk factors in cardiac practice: the emerging field of behavioral cardiology. J Am Coll Cardiol 45:637-651

58. Rosenbaum DS, Jackson LE, Smith JM et al (1994) Electrical alternans and vulnerability to ventricular arrhythmias. N Engl J Med 330:235-241

59. Poulter NR, Khaw KT, Hopwood BE et al (1990) The Kenyan Luo migration study: observations on the initiation of a rise in blood pressure. BMJ 300:967-972

60. Pauletto P, Caroli M, Pessina AC et al (1994) Hypertension prevalence and age-related changes of blood-pressure in semi-nomadic and urban Oromos of Ethiopia. Eur J Epidemiol 10:159-164

61. Nadim A, Amini H, Malek-Afzali H et al (1978) Blood pressure and rural-urban migration in Iran. Int J Epidemiol 7:131-138

62. Light KC, Girdler SS, Sherwood A et al (1999) High stress responsivity predicts later blood pressure only in combination with positive family history and high life stress. Hypertension 33:1458-1464

63. Lynch JW, Everson SA, Kaplan GA et al (1998) Does low socioeconomic status potentiate the effects of heightened cardiovascular responses to stress on the progression of carotid atherosclerosis? Am J Public Health 88:389-394

64. Steptoe A, Cropley M, Johansson M (1999) Job strain, blood pressure and response to uncontrollable stress. J Hypertens 17:193-200

65. Suadicani P, Hein HO, Gyntelberg F (1993) Are social inequalities as associated with the risk of ischaemic heart disease a result of psychosocial working conditions? Atherosclerosis 101:165-175

66. Steptoe A, Roy MP, Evans O et al (1995) Cardiovascular stress reactivity and job strain as determinants of ambulatory blood pressure at work. J Hypertens 13:201-210

67. Kario K, Schwartz JE, Davidson KW et al (2001) Gender differences in associations of diurnal blood pressure variation, awake physical activity, and sleep quality with negative affect. Hypertension 38:997-1002

68. Goldstein IB, Shapiro D, Chicz-DeMet A et al (1999) Ambulatory blood pressure, heart rate, and neuroendocrine responses in women nurses during work and off work days. Psychosom Med 61:387-396

69. TochiKubo O, Ikeda A, Miyajima E et al (1996) Effects of insufficient sleep on blood pressure monitored by a new multibiomedical recorder. Hypertension 27:1318-1324

70. Schwartz AR, Gerin W, Davidson KW (1991) Effects of anger-recall task on post-stress rumination and blood pressure recovery in men and women. Psychophysiology 2000:S12-S13

71. Esler M, Rumantir M, Kaye D et al (2001) The sympathetic neurobiology of essential hypertension: disparate influences of obesity, stress, and noradrenaline transporter dysfunction? Am J Hypertens14:139S-146S

72. Esler M, Jennings G, Lambert G et al (1990) Overflow of catecholamine neurotransmitters to the circulation: source, fate, and functions. Physiol Rev 70:963-985

73. Esler M, Parati G (2004) Is essential hypertension sometimes a psychosomatic disorder? J Hypertens 22:873-876

74. Eide I, Kolloch R, De Q, V et al (1979) Raised cerebrospinal fluid norepinephrine in some patients with primary hypertension. Hypertension 1:255-260

75. Ferrier C, Jennings GL, Eisenhofer G et al (1993) Evidence for increased noradrenaline release from subcortical brain regions in essential hypertension. J Hypertens 11:1217-1227

76. Floras JS (1992) Epinephrine and the genesis of hypertension. Hypertension 19:1-18
77. Rumantir MS, Jennings GL, Lambert GW et al (2000) The 'adrenaline hypothesis' of hypertension revisited: evidence for adrenaline release from the heart of patients with essential hypertension. J Hypertens 18:717-723
78. Johansson M, Rundqvist B, Eisenhofer G et al (1997) Cardiorenal epinephrine kinetics: evidence for neuronal release in the human heart. Am J Physiol 273:H2178-H2185
79. Lampert R, Joska T, Burg MM et al (2002) Emotional and physical precipitants of ventricular arrhythmia. Circulation 106:1800-1805
80. Lown B, Verrier R, Corbalan R et al (1973) Psychologic stress and threshold for repetitive ventricular response. Science 182:834-836
81. Verrier RL, Lown B (1984) Behavioural stress and cardiac arrhythmias. Annu Rev Physiol 46:155-176
82. Lampert R, Jain D, Burg MM (2000) Destabilizing effects of mental stress on ventricular arrhythmias in patients with implantable cardioverter-defibrillators. Circulation 101:158-164
83. Kop WJ, Krantz DS, Nearing BD et al (2004) Effects of acute mental stress and exercise on T-wave alternans in patients with implantable cardioverter defibrillators and controls. Circulation 109:1864-1869
84. Lane RD, Laukes C, Marcus FI et al (2005) Psychological stress preceding idiopathic ventricular fibrillation. Psychosom Med 67:359-365
85. Rozanski A, Bairey CN, Krantz DS et al (1988) Mental stress and the induction of silent myocardial ischemia in patients with coronary artery disease. N Engl J Med 318:1005-1012
86. Jiang W, Babyak M, Krantz DS et al (1996) Mental stress-induced myocardial ischemia and cardiac events. JAMA 275:1651-1656
87. Gottdiener JS, Krantz DS, Howell RH et al Induction of silent myocardial ischemia with mental stress testing: relation to the triggers of ischemia during daily life activities and to ischemic functional severity. J Am Coll Cardiol 24:1645-1651
88. Deanfield JE, Shea M, Kensett M et al (1984) Silent myocardial ischaemia due to mental stress. Lancet 2:1001-1005
89. Giubbini R, Galli M, Campini R et al (1991) Effects of mental stress on myocardial perfusion in patients with ischemic heart disease. Circulation 83:II100-II107
90. Yeung AC, Vekshtein VI, Krantz DS (1991) The effects of atherosclerosis on the vasomotor response of the coronary arteries to mental stress. N Engl J Med 325:1551-1556
91. Gullette EC, Blumenthal JA, Babyak M et al (1997) Effects of mental stress on myocardial ischemia during daily life. JAMA 277:1521-1526
92. Jain D, Burg M, Soufer R et al (1995) Prognostic implications of mental stress-induced silent left ventricular dysfunction in patients with stable angina pectoris. Am J Cardiol 76:31-35
93. Grignani G, Soffiantino F, Zucchella M et al (1991) Platelet activation by emotional stress in patients with coronary artery disease. Circulation 83:II128-II136
94. Levine SP, Towell BL, Suarez AM et al (1985) Platelet activation and secretion associated with emotional stress. Circulation 71:1129-1134

95. Frimerman A, Miller HI, Laniado S et al (1997) Changes in hemostatic function at times of cyclic variation in occupational stress. Am J Cardiol 79:72-75

96. Tsuji H, Larson MG, Venditti FJJ (1999) Impact of reduced heart rate variability on risk for cardiac events; The Framingham Heart Study. Circulation 94:2850-2855

97. Dekker JM, Crow RS, Folsom AR et al (2000) Low heart rate variability in a 2-minute rhythm strip predicts risk of coronary heart disease and mortality from several causes: the ARIC Study. Atherosclerosis risk in communities. Circulation 102:1239-1244

98. Bigger JTJ, Fleiss JL, Steinman RC et al (1992) Frequency domain measures of heart rate period variability and mortality after myocardial infarction. Am J Cardiol 69:891-898

99. Mortara A, La Rovere MT, Pinna GD et al (1997) Arterial modulation of the heart in chronic heart failure: clinical and hemodynamic correlates and prognostic implications. Circulation 96:3450-3458

100. Al-Kubati MA, Fiser B, Siegelova J (1997) Baroreflex sensitivity during psychological stress. Physiol Rev 46:27-33

101. Conway J, Boon N, Jones JV et al (1983) Involvement of the baroreceptor reflexes in the changes in the blood pressure with sleep and mental arousal. Hypertension 5:746-748

102. Fauvel JP, Cerutti C, Quelin P et al (2000) Mental stress-induced increase in blood pressure is not related to baroreflex sensitivity in middle-aged healthy men. Hypertension 35:887-891

103. Fuchs LC, Landas SK, Johnson AK (1997) Behavioural stress alters coronary vascular reactivity in borderline hypertensive rats. J Hypertens 15:301-307

104. Strawn WB, Bondjers G, Kaplan JR et al (1991) Endothelial dysfunction in response to psychosocial stress in monkeys. Circ Res 68:1270-1279

105. Ghiadoni L, Donald AE, Cropley M et al (2000) Mental stress induces transient endothelial dysfunction in humans. Circulation 102:2473-2478

106. Rajagopalan S, Brook R, Rubenfire M et al (2001) Abnormal brachial artery flow-mediated vasodilation in young adults with major depression. Am J Cardiol 88:196-198

107. Miller GE, Stetler CA, Carney RM et al (2002) Clinical depression and inflammatory risk markers for coronary heart disease. Am J Cardiol 90:1279-1283

108. Kop WJ, Gottdiener JS, Tangen CM et al Inflammation and coagulation factors in persons older than 65 years of age with symptoms of depression but without evidence of myocardial ischemia. Am J Cardiol 89:419-424

109. Lesperance F, Frasure-Smith N, Theroux P et al (2004) The association between major depression and levels of soluble intercellular adhesion molecule 1, interleukin-6, and C-reactive protein in patients with recent acute coronary syndromes. Am J Psychiatry 161:271-277

110. Miller GE, Freedland KE, Duntley S et al (2005) Relation of depressive symptoms to C-reactive protein and pathogen burden (cytomegalovirus, herpes simplex virus, Epstein-Barr virus) in patients with earlier acute coronary syndromes. Am J Cardiol 95:317-321

111. Weber-Hamann B, Hentschel F, Kniest A (2003) Hypercortisolemic depression is associated with increased intra-abdominal fat. Psychosom Med 63:619-630

112. Matthews KA, Katholi CR, McCreath H et al (2004) Blood pressure reactivity to psychological stress predicts hypertension in the CARDIA study. Circulation 110:74-78
113. Menkes MS, Matthews KA, Krantz DS et al (1989) Cardiovascular reactivity to the cold pressor test as a predictor of hypertension. Hypertension 14:524-530
114. Wood DL, Sheps SG, Elveback LR et al (1984) Cold pressure test as a predictor of hypertension. Hypertension 6:301-306
115. Kasagi F, Akahoshi M, Shimaoka K (1995) Relation between cold pressure test and development of hypertension based on 28-year follow-up. Hypertension 25:71-76
116. Carrol D, Davey Smith G, Sheffield D et al (1996) Blood pressure reactions to the cold pressure test and the prediction of future blood pressure status: data from the Caerphilly study. Journal of Human Hypertension 10:777-780
117. Harlan WRJr, Osborne RK (1964) Prognostic value of the cold pressure test and the basal blood pressure based on an eighteen-year follow-up. Am J Cardiol 13:832-837
118. Armstrong HR (1950) Rafferty J.A. Cold pressure-test follow-up study and for seven years on 166 officers. Am Heart J 39:484-490
119. Eich RH, Jacobsen EC (2006) Vascular reactivity in medical students followed for 10 yr. Journal of Chronic Diseases 20:583-592
120. Matthews KA, Woodall KL, Allen MT (1993) Cardiovascular reactivity to stress predicts future blood pressure status. Hypertension 22:479-485
121. Treiber FA, Kamarck TW, Schneiderman N (2003) Cardiovascular reactivity and development of preclinical and clinical disease states. Psychosom Med 65:46-62
122. Markovitz JH, Raczynski JM, Wallace D et al (1998) Cardiovascular reactivity to video game predicts subsequent blood pressure increases in young men: The CARDIA study. Psychosom Med 60:186-191
123. Borghi C, Costa FV, Boschi S et al (1986) Predictors of stable hypertension in young borderline subjects: a five-year follow-up study. J Cardiovasc Pharmacol 8 (Suppl 5): S138-S141
124. Borghi C, Costa FV, Boschi S et al (1996) Factors associated with the development of stable hypertension in young borderlines. J Hypertens 14:509-517
125. Falkner B, Kushner H, Onesti G et al (1981) Cardiovascular characteristics in adolescents who develop essential hypertension. Hypertension 3:521-527
126. Murdison KA, Treiber FA, Mensah G et al (1998) Prediction of left ventricular mass in youth with family histories of essential hypertension. Am J Med Sci 315:118-123
127. Kapuku GK, Treiber FA, Davis HC et al (1999) Hemodynamic function at rest, during acute stress, and in the field: predictors of cardiac structure and function 2 years later in youth. Hypertension 34:1026-1031
128. Georgiades A, Lemne C, de Faire U et al (1997) Stress-induced blood pressure measurement predict left ventricular mass over three years among borderline hypertensive men. Eur J Clin Invest 27:733-739
129. Barnett PA, Spence JD, Manuck SB et al (1997) Psychological stress and the progression of carotid artery disease. J Hypertens 15:49-55
130. Matthews KA, Owens JF, Kuller LH et al (1998) Stress-induced pulse pressure change predicts women's carotid atherosclerosis. Stroke 29:1525-1530

131. Alderman MH, Ooi WL, Madhavan S et al (1990) Journal of Clinical Epidemiology. 43:859-866
132. Manuck SB, Olsson G, Hjemdahl P, Rehnqvist N (1992) Does cardiovascular reactivity to mental stress have prognostic value in postinfarction patients? A pilot study. Psychosom Med 54:102-108
133. Krantz DS, Santiago HT, Kop WJ et al (1999) Prognostic value of mental stress testing in coronary artery disease. Am J Cardiol 84:1292-1297
134. Ahern DK, Gorkin L, Anderson JL et al (1990) Biobehavioural variables and mortality or cardiac arrest in the Cardiac Arrhythmia Pilot Study (CAPS). Am J Cardiol 66:59-62

Chapter 4

Mental Stress Ischemia: Characteristics, Pathophysiology, Prognosis and Treatment

M.M. Burg

Mental stress ischemia (MSI) is a recently recognized phenomenon defined by the occurrence of myocardial ischemia during the experience of mentally and/or emotionally stressful circumstances. A substantial research effort has been directed at improving our understanding of this phenomenon, and determining whether it has prognostic significance beyond that associated with the underlying, chronic coronary artery disease (CAD). This effort has also been directed toward determining whether it is possible to specifically treat this phenomenon, and whether treatment improves prognosis. In this chapter, I will first review the literature that describes this phenomenon, relying on both naturalistic and laboratory-based studies. I will then describe the research conducted on the pathophysiology that might underlie MSI, and follow this by a review of the literature concerning prognostic significance and treatment. I will end with a discussion of future directions for research. Rather than provide a comprehensive review of the literature, this chapter will be selective in the literature discussed, the general aim being to inform the reader about MSI.

◼ Mental Stress Ischemia: Recognition of a Phenomenon

The technology for ambulatory electrocardiogram (ECG) monitoring was developed during the early 1960s by Holter [1]. This technology was an important technological breakthrough, as it permitted the examination of ischemic phenomena over prolonged periods of time while patients went about their normal daily activities. Indeed, Holter stated in his original article that the ambulatory monitoring technology should be used for the detection of subclinical angina pectoris or other transient ischemic conditions [1].

One of the earliest studies to utilize Holter monitoring of the ECG in patients with stable CAD was by Bellet et al. [2]. In this study, the ECG of 66 patients was monitored as they drove an automobile. Of these 66 patients, six evidenced episodes of transient ST-segment depression while driving, and of these, two did not report any symptoms. This was the first report of "silent ischemia" during a routine daily activity. Stern and Tsivoni [3] subsequently examined the 24-hour ambulatory ECG record of 140 CAD patients, and found asymptomatic ST-segment and T-wave changes during undisturbed sleep and daily activities. In two studies, Shang and Pepine [4, 5] comprehensively investigated ischemia during ambulatory monitoring in 27 patients with CAD. They found that over 75% of the total ischemic episodes in these patients were during routine activities and without symptom, and that the onset of these silent events occurred at a significantly lower heart rate (HR) than observed with ischemia during exercise stress testing. These findings were subsequently corroborated by others [6].

While these initial naturalistic investigations were being pursued, others were approaching the issue in laboratory settings. In two of the first studies, patients were subjected to emotional stress by having them perform a brief "quiz" that resembled an IQ test, during which HR, blood pressure (BP) and ECG were recorded. During the quiz, ten of 14 patients demonstrated asymptomatic ischemic changes on their ECG [7]. The observed ischemia was at a lower rate-pressure product (HR x systolic BP) than that observed during exercise-induced ischemia for the same patients, which was interpreted by the investigators as evidence of emotionally-induced coronary artery spasm [8]. A more sensitive approach was used by Deanfield et al. [9] in a study of myocardial perfusion (assessed by positron emission tomography-PET) during mental arithmetic and exercise. This approach provided for a direct examination of changes in blood flow through the coronary arteries during laboratory conditions. In the study, 12 of 16 patients evidenced a perfusion defect during the arithmetic task (8 without symptom). The defect observed during mental arithmetic was comparable in size and location to that observed during exercise.

In summary, these early studies took advantage of emerging technologies to study ischemic syndromes during routine activities and during controlled emotional provocation in the laboratory. The picture of ischemic heart disease that emerged from these studies was very different from that obtained previously. This new picture highlighted a much greater frequency and duration of ischemia than had been formerly accepted, and the ischemic episodes were predominantly "silent." Further, this picture revealed the potency of emotional stimuli as provocateurs of ischemia. These studies became the springboard for a comprehensive line of research conducted in several laboratories around the world. As this endeavor progressed, a number of key issues came to be defined, and the descriptor for this phenomenon gradually shifted from "transient" or "silent" myocardial ischemia, to "mental stress ischemia." The key issues were associated with the pathophysiology of the phenomenon, with a particular focus on person-related vulnerabilities, triggering stimuli and physiological mechanisms. Of equal importance were issues related to reproducibility, the prognostic significance of the phenomenon and how best to treat the phenomenon.

Mental Stress Ischemia: Methods of Study

A variety of methods have been developed for the study of MSI. For naturalistic studies of patients during their routine activities, Holter monitoring of the ECG has been combined with comprehensive diaries that provide for recording the type of activity, level of physical and mental arousal experienced, and the type and intensity of accompanying emotions. For laboratory studies, a variety of mental and emotional provocations are used, most notably mental arithmetic, anger recall and personally relevant public speaking. As patients perform these tasks, HR, BP, ECG, ventricular performance, and/or myocardial perfusion are monitored and assessed. Often psychological traits are also assessed, as reported in Figure 1.

- Patients with documented CAD

- Holter monitoring of ECG with detailed diary

- Performance of mentally demanding/emotionally provocative tasks

    - mental arithmetic   - Stroop sensory conflict
    - anger recall / public speaking   - mirror tracing

- Concurrent measurement of CV/myocardial indices:

    - HR / BP   - ECG
    - left ventricular performance   - myocardial blood flow / perfusion

- Assessment of psychological "traits" and state

Fig. 1. Mental Stress Ischemia - Methods

Mental Stress Ischemia: Characteristics

Psychosocial Vulnerability

The ability of emotional and mentally demanding circumstances to provoke ischemia led some researchers to examine the psychological factors that might put patients with CAD at risk for MSI. Taking a laboratory-based approach to this question my colleagues and I [10] studied 30 patients with CAD by having them perform a mental arithmetic task (serial 7 subtraction) and brief exercise while left ventricular (LV) ejection fraction, HR and BP were measured. For this study, a drop in LV ejection fraction of greater than 5% absolute was indicative of LV dysfunction, or ischemia. Patients also completed an assessment battery comprised of multiple measures of trait anger and hostility, including the Videotaped Structured Interview for Type A Behavior Pattern (VSI). Of the 30 patients, 15 demonstrated LV dysfunction (without symptoms) during the arithmetic task. These patients showed a comparable rise in HR and BP to those without ischemia, and they were also comparable on a range of clinical indices, including CAD severity and medications. When we compared the two groups on the psychological measures, we found that those with LV dysfunction during mental arithmetic scored significantly higher on measures of anger and hostility, and lower on a measure of anger control. Others have found this psychological profile to predominate in patients who evidence ischemia (as demonstrated by ambulatory ECG monitoring) during daily activities [11, 12]. Taken together, these studies describe the patient at risk for MSI as one who is routinely emotionally challenged by daily events and readily experiences anger in reaction to these events. Further, this person is likely to express anger aggressively and endorse aggressive behavior as appropriate for regular social interactions [10]. Of note, in our laboratory study, 18 of the 30 patients demonstrated LV dysfunction during the VSI. Furthermore, we found a very high correlation between score on the VSI and the percent of the VSI interview period that the patient was demonstrating LV dysfunction. This becomes important when you realize that the VSI is in many ways a form of anger provocation, and the score on the VSI is largely a function of the degree of anger arousal. Therefore, the greater the degree of anger arousal in these patients, and the longer the anger lasted, the greater the time with LV compromise.

Triggering Stimuli

Exploration of the circumstances and situations that can "trigger" the onset of MSI has been undertaken both in the laboratory and in naturalistic settings. In general, a range of mentally stressful tasks have been used in the laboratory, and these tasks share the common feature of providing a significant cognitive and/or emotional challenge to the patient, including the use of harassment while the patient performs a challenging task. Of greater interest perhaps is the use of more direct emotional provocation. For example, as described above, my colleagues and I found that the discussion of anger-related incidents – an element of the Type A VSI – served to provoke ischemia in over half of our patients with chronic stable CAD [10]. Others have also found anger to be potent in the provocation of ischemia in the laboratory. In one study of 27 CAD patients, the recall of an anger-provoking circumstance was found to be more potent than mental arithmetic or personally relevant public speaking in provoking LV dysfunction [13]. In a second study performed during cardiac catheterization, the degree of anger experienced during recall was significantly correlated with mean decrease in artery diameter in artery segments with significant CAD [14]. Hence, the re-experience of anger related to a prior real-life experience was found to cause a vasoconstriction or spasm in diseased segments of patient's coronary arteries. These studies demonstrate the potency of anger in provoking MSI in the laboratory.

Three studies are exemplars of the approach taken to study triggering in the natural setting. These studies combine Holter monitoring of the ECG over 24-48 hour periods with a comprehensive diary, as described earlier. Patients are instructed to complete a diary entry whenever their activity changes (e.g., answering a phone call, moving from home to the car, driving to work, arriving at work) and/or whenever they experience angina. They record the type of activity, start and stop time, and their location, mood and psychological state during the activity, as well as episodes of angina and taking of nitroglycerin.

In the first study [15], Gabbay and colleagues had 63 CAD patients (60 off medications) undergo 24-48 hours of Holter ECG monitoring with diary. When the ECG record was examined, a relationship was found between total ischemic time and level of mental activity, with the greatest amount of ischemic seen during medium levels of mental activity. Adjusting for the amount of time at each level of mental activity, however, revealed a graded relationship between the level of mental activity and ischemic time: as the level of mental activity increased, the proportion of ischemic time increased, a finding corroborated by others [16]. The researchers then examined the relationship of anger intensity to the occurrence of ischemia. They found that almost twice as much ischemia occurred when anger intensity was rated high as when it was rated low [15].

Gullette et al. [17] also used 48-hour Holter monitoring in combination with diary to study 132 CAD patients off medications. This study specifically examined the importance of key negative emotions in the hour prior to ischemia onset. In unadjusted analyses, it was found that high levels of sadness, frustration and tension were associated with the percent of time during the monitoring period that ischemia occurred. When the researchers adjusted for time of day and activity level, only tension and frustration remained significant. Similar findings have been reported by others [18]. In a subsequent analysis [19], this cohort was divided on the basis of how much variation there was in the emotional responses they recorded in their diary entries. Those patients with a great number of high emotional ratings for tension during the monitoring period were designated as high emotional responders, while the remaining patients were designated as low emotional responders. The 37 high emotional responders were more likely to evidence ischemia during Holter monitoring than the 99 low emotional responders (OR=2.50, p<0.05). Also of note, the high responders were more likely to evidence ischemia during the performance of mentally demanding tasks in the laboratory (OR=3.21, p<0.02). Hence, these studies demonstrate the importance of mental arousal, the range of emotional responsiveness, and the specific emotions of anger and frustration as triggers of ischemia, both during routine activity and during the performance of mentally provocative tasks. These studies also raise important questions as to the pathophysiological mechanisms by which the experience of strong emotion in general, and anger/frustration in particular, is transduced into ischemic syndromes.

Reproducibility

For the study of MSI to progress to the point of effecting clinical practice, it is essential that researchers demonstrate that the effect can be reliably reproduced. Three studies have demonstrated this criterion. In one study [20], CAD patients underwent mental stress testing on two occasions, two weeks apart. Using three different mental stress tasks – mental arithmetic, Stroop Color-Word Conflict and anger recall – researchers demonstrated a high degree of reproducibility across the two testing days, with the anger recall task having the highest degree of reproducibility (90%). These findings have also been replicated in the PIMI study [21], although in PIMI, the Stroop was found to be the more consistent task, and overall reproducibility was not as great (60-68%). Each of these studies utilized left ventricular performance as their index of ischemia. A more recent study [22], utilizing myocardial blood flow to index ischemia, demonstrated 75% reproducibility using a public speaking task wherein the subject is asked to talk about an event that contains real life frustrations and hassles.

Mental Stress Ischemia: Pathophysiology

Questions regarding the pathophysiology of MSI initially focused on the ischemia supply–demand balance – i.e., whether the underlying mechanism was related to significant increases in myocardial oxygen demand during the stressful circumstance (in the laboratory or in the natural environment), or whether it was related to significant reductions in myocardial blood flow during the stressful circumstance. Mental stress *was* associated with significant increases in HR and BP, which is indicative of increased work being done by the heart and, hence, increased myocardial oxygen demand; however, the level of increase in these cardiovascular indices was less than that associated with ischemia during physical stress. Therefore, early in the study of MSI, researchers directed their attention primarily toward supply side mechanisms [23].

In an early study, Chierchia and colleagues [24] examined the effect of beta-blockers on ambulatory ischemia. They found that these agents reduced the frequency of ischemic events overall, and that most events were without symptom and at a lower HR/BP than is normally seen with effort-related ischemia. They concluded that the ischemic events were likely related to transient impairment in regional myocardial perfusion.

In a seminal study of 26 patients with CAD, Yeung et al. [25] examined the vasomotor response of discrete coronary artery segments during mental stress and during infusion of acetylcholine (Ach), an endothelium-dependent vasodilatory agent. They found that arterial segments characterized by the presence of irregularity or frank stenosis responded with paradoxical vasoconstriction during both the mental stress and Ach infusion, thereby demonstrating endothelial dysfunction in the large coronary vessels during mental stress (since the normal response of arterial segments to Ach infusion is vasodilation). The technical approach taken by these investigators also provided for an indirect concurrent assessment of blood flow through these vessels. While blood flow also decreased in the arterial distribution of the irregular and stenosed segments, the investigators were unable to ascertain whether this decrease in flow was due solely to the observed vasoconstriction in the coronary arteries, or whether it was due in part to impairment in the vasodilation response of the capillary bed associated with the diseased coronary artery segment. Interestingly, a subsequent study by a different group also found paradoxical vasoconstriction during mental stress in non-diseased coronary artery segments [26]. At the same time, others were finding that in CAD patients, mental stress was associated with increased arterial pressure (indicative of a more general vasoconstriction) in the periphery [27, 28], thereby hinting at a systemic (rather than focal) dysfunction in endothelial vasomotion. This finding had important methodological implications for the study of MSI, because increased peripheral arterial pressure can produce a state of increased afterload, creating pressure against the left ventricle of the heart, which, as a result, has to work harder to pump blood through the body. Increased afterload can subsequently cause a reduction in left ventricular ejection fraction (EF) that is *not* indicative of ischemia. Hence, in the mid-1990s it became apparent that EF was not a sufficient index of MSI, and coronary blood flow studies using changes in perfusion of the myocardium (indicative of myocardial blood flow) became the method of choice for the study of MSI in the lab.

The study by Yeung et al. [25] indicated a role for vasoconstriction in the large coronary vessels, while hinting at a role for the coronary microvasculature (i.e., the capillary beds). In a study of coronary flow reserve (CFR), which denotes the ability of the microvascular bed to dilate in response to stimulation and thereby augment coronary blood flow, Arrighi and colleagues [29] subjected CAD patients to mental stress in order to observe absolute regional changes in coronary blood flow by PET. They compared the CFR response during mental stress to the response during infusion of Persantine, a pharmacologic agent used to assess the functional severity of CAD. As expected, during the Persantine infusion, the myocardial blood flow response was less in regions with significant coronary artery blockages than in regions without significant blockages. Further, during Persantine infusion, the decreased flow response in areas with significant CAD was associated with a decrease in coronary microvascular resistance (again, as expected); the capillary bed was dilating to compensate for the reduced flow through the blocked coronary artery. Results during the mental arithmetic condition revealed important opposite findings. First, regions with blunted myocardial blood flow/ischemia during mental arithmetic testing did not correspond to regions with blunted myocardial blood flow/ischemia during exercise testing. Rather, during mental stress, myocardial blood flow was lower in regions *without* significant blockages. Second, the regions with lower myocardial blood flow response during mental stress showed increased coronary microvascular resistance. Hence, an expected augmentation of myocardial blood flow in regions without significant blockages during mental stress was blunted instead, and a paradoxical increase in microvascular resistance in the associated coronary bed was seen. These data suggest a prominent role for microvascular dysfunction in MSI.

In a study specifically of endothelial function during mental stress, Sherwood et al. [30] assessed several parameters of cardiovascular performance while healthy subjects performed mental stress tasks. They also assessed the subjects' endothelial function using ultrasound imaging of the brachial artery during reactive hyperemia. Comparing those with high vs. low hyperemic flow response with respect to their systemic vascular resistance (indexed as a function of cardiac output and mean arterial pressure) during mental stress revealed that those with low hyperemic flow response also showed significantly greater systemic vascular resistance (SVR) during mental stress. This finding suggests that the reductions in blood flow during mental stress previously observed by investigators may reflect an underlying and systemic endothelial dysfunction.

In summary, a number of studies from different labs have served to highlight the important role that supply side mechanisms likely play in MSI. Further, these studies demonstrate that the effects occur not only in the large coronary arteries, but in the coronary microvascular beds as well. The importance of endothelial function as a component in the pathophysiology of MSI is also highlighted by this work. Important questions remain as to the reasons for the observed paradoxical response of the studied vasculature, whether at the epicardial level, the microvascular level or, more generally, in the peripheral endothelium.

Mental Stress Ischemia: Prognosis and Treatment

The prognostic significance of MSI has been explored by a number of investigators. The first published report [31] represented a 2-year follow-up of 30 patients who had previously undergone laboratory mental stress testing [10]. For this study, medical endpoints included myocardial infarction and hospital admission for unstable angina and/or revascularization. Within the group of 15 patients who had evidenced MSI, there were a significantly greater (p<0.025) number of events (9 events – 4 MI, 5 unstable angina) than there were within the group of 15 patients who had not evidenced MSI (3 events, all unstable angina).

In a later study, Jiang et al. [32] also reported on the prognostic significance of MSI among the cohort described by Gullette and colleagues [17]. Comparing patients with LV dysfunction during MS to those without revealed a significant effect (Risk ratio=2.40), even after adjusting for age, history of MI and baseline EF. While these reports encountered interest among cardiologists, findings of worse prognosis were based on both hard (e.g., new MI) and soft (e.g., unstable angina) endpoints, and included no deaths. In a larger cohort of 96 patients, Krantz and colleagues [33] also examined the prognostic significance of MSI. Over a 4.4-year follow-up period (median=3.5 years), there were 28 total events. Almost 45% of patients with MSI in the lab experienced an event during follow-up, while fewer than 25% of patients without MSI experienced an event. As with the earlier studies, events included MI and unstable angina; however, in this study there were also five deaths (three among patients with MSI).

Most recently, the PIMI investigators have reported on the prognostic significance of MSI in their multi-center study [34]. In this study of 196 patients who had undergone mental stress testing in the lab, patients were followed for an average of 5.2 years. During the follow-up period there were 17 deaths. Ventricular wall motion abnormalities indicative of MSI had been demonstrated among 40% of those who died, but only 17% of those who survived (rate ratio=3.0; p<0.04). Other indicators of ischemia during MS testing, including LV EF and/or ECG changes, did not predict death, a finding with important implications for future research. This is the only controlled study to show an effect of mental stress on death.

While a great deal of effort has been put forth to promote a greater understanding of the pathophysiology of MSI, and each of the major labs engaged in this work has followed study cohorts to examine prognostic significance, relatively little work has focused on issues of treatment. An exception to this is the work reported by Blumenthal and colleagues [35]. They studied 136 CAD patients, comparing the effects on MSI of an aerobic exercise program (16 weeks, 3 times per week) to a cognitive behavioral stress management program (16 weekly group sessions, 1.5 hours each) and usual care. While patients were randomized to the two treatment conditions, usual care was a convenience assignment of individuals who resided too far from the study site to participate in either treatment condition. Ischemia was measured by ambulatory monitoring of the ECG and by changes in LV wall motion during mental stress. The stress management group, compared with the exercise training and usual care groups, showed significantly greater improvement, both in LV wall motion abnormalities during laboratory mental stress (p<0.001) and in the number of episodes of ischemia during ambulatory monitoring (p<0.003). Blumenthal and colleagues followed their patients for a total of 5 years to assess the prognostic impact of treatment [36]. An effect was found within 1 year (p<0.02), and throughout the follow-up period, patients in the stress management condition showed better outcomes than either of the other 2 groups (p<0.04 at 5-years, compared to usual care). Interestingly, an accompanying assessment of economic impact demonstrated, overall, significantly lower healthcare utilization (and costs) for stress management at 1 year (p<0.001 vs. usual care), at 2-years (p<0.003 vs. usual care, p<0.08 vs. exercise) and at 5 years (p<0.009 vs. usual care). These findings demonstrate the potential effectiveness of a cognitive behavioral stress management program for the treatment of MSI, as well as the pronounced impact such an approach can have on prognosis and healthcare utilization. The findings also raise important questions that relate to pathophysiological mechanisms, particularly as regards the triggering of ischemia by mental stress, and the mode of action of stress reduction approaches.

■ Mental Stress Ischemia: Future Directions

The purpose of this chapter was to provide a focused review of the literature on MSI. Much research in this area has been conducted over the past 30 years. The cumulative work has revealed a great deal regarding MSI – for example, the predominant significance of anger and the associated emotional constructs and circumstances relevant to the provocation of ischemia, as well as the underlying processes by which ischemia is provoked by these emotions and circumstances. The work has also revealed the prognostic importance of MSI and the potential for treating it, both with regard to medical outcomes and to economic considerations. A number of important questions remain, however. For example, studies of MSI in the laboratory have relied on a number of indices of ischemia, including decreases in LV EF, new LV wall motion abnormalities, and reductions in myocardial blood flow. In addition, the specific tasks used to provoke ischemia have included performance of mental arithmetic (e.g., serial subtraction), recall of an anger-inducing event, public speaking on a topic of personal relevance to the patient (e.g., a personal quality that the patient finds objectionable), and the Stroop Color-Word Conflict task. While each of these approaches has been at least partially successful, the acceptance of MSI by the larger cardiologic community and, indeed, the inclusion of clinical mental stress testing for prognostic purposes will require a standardized testing protocol with a "gold standard" means of measurement. Given the importance of anger and frustration in the provocation of ischemia during mental stress, and the apparent importance of personal relevance for the task to provoke ischemia, it may be that some form of matching task to person to insure a level of "ego involvement" will be the most effective. This hypothesis should certainly be tested in future studies of MSI.

Compared with the protocol for exercise stress testing for ischemia, which utilizes an increasingly strenuous gradient and thereby provides for the determination of threshold effects, mental stress testing has been accomplished without such a gradient. Rather, the stressful task is started at its highest level of demand, and ischemia is provoked either within 60 seconds of stress initiation or not at all. This approach does not provide for the "fine grain" analyses of stress thresholds that might be required for future studies of novel treatments. Hence, exploration of differing protocols for stress administration and their effects on the provocation of ischemia is worthy of further conduct.

While the extant literature regarding the prognostic significance of MSI and the impact of treatment shows promise, a great deal of further work is needed in this area. This is particularly the case, given that recent advances in the treatment of ischemic heart disease (e.g., statin therapy for hyperlipidemia) might impact the vascular processes that appear to underlie MSI. Hence, there is an evident need to replicate the prognostic studies conducted to date, and to explore a broader range of treatments for MSI. These studies could be conducted in a more focused manner that also provides for an examination of other possible pathophysiological mechanisms that have shown some degree of promise [37].

■ References

1. Holter NJ (1961) A new method for heart studies. Science 134:1214-1220
2. Bellet S, Roman L, Kostis J, Slater A (1968) Continuous electrocardiographic monitoring during automobile driving: studies in normal subjects and patients with coronary disease. Am J Cardiol 22:856-862
3. Stern S, Tsivoni D (1973) Dynamic changes in the ST-T segment during sleep in ischemic heart disease. Am J Cardiol 32:17-20
4. Pepine CJ, Schang SJ (1975) Antianginal response of coronary heart disease patients on long-term perhexiline maleate. Am J Cardiol 35:168
5. Schang SJ, Pepine CJ (1977) Transient asymptomatic S-T segment depression during daily activity. Am J Cardiol 39:396-402
6. Imperi GA, Pepine CJ (1986) Silent myocardial ischemia during daily activities: studies in asymptomatic patients and those with various forms of angina. Cardiol Clin 4:635-642
7. Schiffer F, Hartley LH, Schulman CL, Abelmann WH (1976) The quiz electrocardiogram: a new diagnostic and research technique for evaluating the relation between emotional stress and ischemic heart disease. Am J Cardiol 37:41-47
8. Schiffer F, Hartley LH, Schulman CL, Abelmann WH (1980) Evidence for emotionally induced coronary arterial spasm in patients with angina pectoris. Br Heart J 40:62-66
9. Deanfield JE, Shea M, Kensett M et al (1984) Silent myocardial ischemia due to mental stress. Lancet 2:1001-1004
10. Burg MM, Jain D, Soufer R et al (1993) Role of behavioral and psychological factors in mental stress induced silent left ventricular dysfunction in coronary artery disease. J Am Coll Cardiol 22:440-448
11. Helmers KF, Krantz DS, Howell RH et al (1993) Hostility and myocardial ischemia in coronary artery disease patients: evaluation by gender and ischemic index. Psychosom Med 55:29-36
12. Helmers KF, Krantz DS, Merz CN et al (1995) Defensive hostility: relationship to multiple markers of cardiac ischemia in patients with coronary disease. Health Psychol 14:202-209
13. Ironson G, Taylor CB, Boltwood M et al (1992) Effects of anger on left ventricular ejection fraction in coronary artery disease. Am J Cardiol 70:281-285
14. Boltwood MD, Taylor CB, Burke MB et al (1993) Anger report predicts coronary artery vasomotor response to mental stress in atherosclerotic segments. Am J Cardiol 72:1361-1365
15. Gabbay FH, Krantz DS, Kop WJ et al (1996) Triggers of myocardial ischemia during daily life in patients with coronary artery disease: physical and mental activities, anger and smoking. J Am Coll Cardiol 27:585-592
16. Barry J, Selwyn AP, Nabel EG et al (1988) Frequency of ST-segment depression produced by mental stress in stable angina pectoris from coronary artery disease. Am J Cardiol 61:989-993
17. Gullette ECD, Blumenthal JA, Babyak M et al (1997) Effects of mental stress on myocardial ischemia during daily life. JAMA 277:1521-1526
18. Freeman LJ, Nixon PGF, Sllabank P, Reaveley D (1987) Psychological stress and silent myocardial ischemia. Am Heart J 114:477-482

19. Carels RA, Sherwood A, Babyak M et al (1999) Emotional responsivity and transient myocardial ischemia. J Consult Clin Psychol 67:605-610

20. Jain D, Joska T, Lee FA et al (2001) Day-to-day reproducibility of mental stress-induced abnormal left ventricular function response in patients with coronary artery disease and its relationship to autonomic activation. J Nucl Cardiol 8:347-355

21. Carney RM, McMahon RP, Freedland KE et al (1998) Reproducibility of mental stress-induced myocardial ischemia in the pathophysiological investigations of myocardial ischemia (PIMI). Psychosom Med 60:64-70

22. Kim CK, Bartholomew BA, Mastin ST et al (2003) Detection and reproducibility of mental stress induced ischemia with Tc-99m sestamibi SPECT in normal and coronary artery disease populations. J Nucl Cardiol 10:56-62

23. Maseri A (1987) Role of coronary artery spasm in symptomatic and silent myocardial ischemia. J Am Coll Cardiol 9:249-262

24. Chierchia S, Muiesan L, Davies A et al (1980) Role of the sympathetic nervous system in the pathogenesis of chronic stable angina: implications for the mechanism of action of β-blockers. Circulation 82(suppl II): 71-81

25. Yeung AC, Vekshtein VI, Krantz DS et al (1991) The effect of atherosclerosis on the vasomotor response of coronary arteries to mental stress. N Engl J Med 325:1551-1556

26. Lacy CR, Contrada RJ, Robbins ML et al (1995) Coronary vasoconstriction induced by mental stress (simulated public speaking). Am J Cardiol 75:503-505

27. Goldberg AD, Becker LC, Bonsall R et al (1996) Ischemic, hemodynamic, and neurohormonal response to mental and exercise stress. Circulation 94:2402-2409

28. Jain D, Shakir S, Burg M et al (1998) Effect of mental stress on left ventricular and peripheral vascular performance in patients with coronary artery disease. J Am Coll Cardiol 31:1314-1322

29. Arrighi JA, Burg M, Cohen IS et al (2000) Myocardial blood flow response during mental stress in patients with coronary artery disease. Lancet 356:310-311

30. Sherwood A, Johnson K, Blumenthal JA, Hinderliter AL (1999) Enothelial function and hemodynamic responses during mental stress. Psychosom Med 61:365-370

31. Jain D, Burg MM, Soufer R, Zaret BL (1995) Prognostic implications of mental stress-induced silent left ventricular dysfunction in patients with stable angina pectoris. Am J Cardiol 76:31-35

32. Jiang W, Babyak M, Krantz DS et al (1996) Mental stress-induced myocardial ischemia and cardiac events. JAMA 275:1651-1656

33. Krantz DS, Santiago HT, Kop WJ et al (1999) Prognostic value of mental stress testing in coronary artery disease. Am J Cardiol 84:1292-1297

34. Sheps DS, McMahon RP, Becker L, Carney RM (2002) Mental stress-induced ischemia and all-cause mortality in patients with coronary artery disease. Circulation 105:1780-1784

35. Blumenthal JA, Jiang W, Babyak MA et al (1997) Stress management and exercise training in cardiac patients with myocardial ischemia. Arch Int Med 157:2213-2223

36. Blumenthal JA, Babyak M, Jiang W, O'Connor C (2002) Usefulness of psychosocial treatment of mental stress-induced ischemia in men. Am J Cardiol 89:164-168

37. Kop WJ, Verdino RJ, Gottdeiner JS, O'Leary ST (2001) Changes in heart rate and heart rate variability before ischemic events. J Am Coll Cardiol 38:742-749

Depression
and Anxiety

Chapter 5

Depression and CHD: Prevalence, Prognosis, Pathophysiology and Treatment

K. Maier ▪ D. Chatkoff ▪ M.M. Burg

▪ Introduction

The comorbidity of depression and coronary heart disease (CHD) has been demonstrated in a broad literature published over the past two decades. In this chapter, we review the current state of this literature, with a particular focus on the prevalence of CHD and depression, the relationship of depression to CHD development and prognosis, and the pathophysiological mechanisms by which these two clinical phenomena may be linked. Key issues relevant to clinical practice and research in this area are also discussed, including assessment and treatment.

Classification and Prevalence of Coronary Heart Disease and Depression

Coronary Heart Disease

CHD is caused by atherosclerosis, or coronary artery disease (CAD), a narrowing of the coronary arteries due to the build-up of fatty plaques that can produce angina pectoris (chest pain) or myocardial infarction (MI) [1, 2], collectively referred to as acute coronary syndrome (ACS). In the US, over 13 million people have a history of ACS. In 2001, there were 502,189 CHD-related deaths, making CHD the single leading cause of death overall. In the year 2000, the annual incidence of MI in Europe was estimated by the World Health Organization (WHO) to be near two million cases [3], with a point prevalence of nearly 10 million for angina [4]. Although death rates from MI have generally declined in recent decades, CHD is still a leading cause of death in the United States and many European countries [5, 6].

CAD is an inflammatory disease, in which each of three stages of plaque development is a response to injury, and in which the associated inflammatory processes can lead to the complicated lesions associated with catastrophic cardiac outcomes [7]. The initial stage of plaque development - the "Type I" lesion - is characterized by endothelial dysfunction, which occurs in response to a range of "irritants" (e.g., tobacco, hypertension, LDL-cholesterol, emotional stress). Increased endothelial permeability, formation of vasoactive molecules, and an overall change of endothelial properties from anticoagulant to procoagulant ensue. The endothelium attracts and absorbs monocytes and activated T-cells in an attempt to respond to damage locally. LDL-cholesterol permeates the endothelial lining, and a fatty streak is formed, provoking further T-cell activation, phagocytosis by macrophages (formation of foam cells), adherence/entry to the endothelium by leukocytes, and proliferation of smooth muscle cells - an inflammatory attempt by the endothelium to rid itself of this offending agent. A cycle of inflammation, lipid modification, and further inflammation follows, maintained by the presence of the lipid "irritants." The lesion gradually grows in size to involve both the endothelium and the intima, and a fibrous cap is eventually formed at the site of the damaged arterial segment. This cap sequesters the lesion from the lumen of the artery, covering the mixture of leukocytes, lipid, and debris that comprise a necrotic core. As CAD progresses to this more advanced stage, physical demands and/or emotional distress can combine with ongoing inflammatory processes to precipitate catastrophic coronary events. The plaque ruptures, leading to hemorrhage, and results in an ACS [8].

Depression

Depression is an episodic clinical syndrome defined by the presence of five out of nine symptoms during the same 2-week period. These symptoms include: 1) depressed mood, 2) diminished interest or pleasure in daily activities, 3) significant unintentional weight change, 4) sleep disturbance, 5) psychomotor retardation or agitation, 6) fatigue or loss of energy, 7) feelings of worthlessness or excessive/inappropriate guilt, 8) decreased ability to concentrate, and 9) thoughts of death or suicide. These symptoms must be present nearly everyday for most of the day, along with either depressed mood or reduced interest, in order to make a diagnosis of major depression. Symptoms of depression usually develop over days to weeks, and an untreated episode of major depression can last up to six months [9, 10]. Less severe clinical presentation is also seen, particularly in patients with comorbid CHD, and, while these less severe clinical presentations do not meet diagnostic criteria for depression, they have been linked to poorer prognosis after ACS.

The point prevalence of depression has been estimated to be over 148 million globally, and over 23 million in Europe [4]. In a recent U.S. sample of over 9000 adults (> 17 yrs of age), the National Comorbidity Survey Replication (NCS-R) found the prevalence for major depression to be 16.2% over a lifetime and 6.6% over a period of 12 months [11]. According to the *DSM-IV* [9], rates of Major Depressive Disorder are twice as common among women as men. For both men and women, rates of depression are highest between ages 25 and 44, whereas individuals over age 65 exhibit the lowest rates [9]. The socioeconomic impact of depression is significant, as indicated by findings from the NCS-R, which show that individuals who suffered from major depression during a 12-month period reported being unable to function in their primary roles (e.g., at work) for an average of 35 days [11].

Depression and CHD

Comorbidity
Considerable epidemiological evidence now shows a fairly reliable association between depression and CHD. Studies have generally found the prevalence of major depression among CHD patients to range between 16-23% [12], with several investigations demonstrating higher rates of clinically meaningful depressive symptoms. For example, Lane et al. [13] found that 31% of participants consecutively admitted for MI in two English hospitals scored 10 or greater on the Beck Depression Inventory (BDI), reflecting a level of symptoms that is clinically relevant. Others have reported that up to 65% of patients have some symptoms of depression following MI. Schleifer and colleagues [14] reported that, among 171 hospitalized MI patients, 45% met criteria for major or minor depression (using Research Diagnostic Criteria) 8-10 days after their MI, and 33% met these criteria 3-4 months later. High rates of depression, ranging from 27-47%, have also been observed among CABG patients prior to surgery [15, 16].

Case studies of MI patients suggest that some degree of depressive symptoms may be expected, given that patients often report feeling guilty over potential lifestyle contributions to their disease, and given that they experience difficulty adjusting to acute physical limitations [17]. Negative mood may be a transient phenomenon for some patients after ACS, with studies reporting improvements in self-report measures of positive and negative mood after 3 months of cardiac rehabilitation [18]. It is notable, however, that almost 1/3 of patients have been found to develop clinically meaningful levels of depressive symptoms within a year following MI [19]. In addition to developing depression in the months following MI, patients who are initially distressed may show limited improvement. For example, Mayou et al. [20] found that, although patients who demonstrated significant levels of anxiety and depression at the time of hospitalization showed improvement over a 3-month period following MI, they did not show continued improvement at 12 months. Taken as a whole, these findings suggest that depression among MI patients is a reactive, transient phenomenon for some, whereas for others, depression is more persistent.

Prognosis
A growing body of research indicates that depression may be prospectively related to the development of CHD, rather than merely a consequence of an ACS event. A recent meta-analysis of 11 prospective studies of initially healthy samples reported a dose-response relationship between depression severity and risk for CHD, with a lifetime clinical diagnosis of depression associated

with greater risk (RR = 2.69) than depressive mood measured by self-report (RR = 1.49) [21].

Such a dose-response relationship is also supported by recent findings that depressive symptoms among Vietnam veterans are associated with greater risk for experiencing an ACS and/or requiring coronary revascularization. It is notable that between 60-80% of the participants in this study reported that the onset of depression predated the development of ACS [22]. Other studies have reported similar associations between lifetime depression and subsequent ACS [23] for both men and women [24].

In addition to increasing risk for the development of ACS, depression has also been found to increase the risk for cardiovascular morbidity and mortality, both in patients with existing CHD and in patients after ACS. This increased risk is different from that associated with standard prognostic indicators such as post-ACS cardiac function or CAD severity. For example, Frasure-Smith et al. [25] found that a diagnosis of clinical depression within days after MI was associated with increased 6-month mortality, while the mere presence of clinically meaningful depressive symptoms (not sufficient to meet diagnostic criteria for major depression) predicted both 18-month and 5-year morbidity and mortality [26, 27]. Similar findings have been reported by Ferketich et al. [24] for men, while Bush et al. [28] found a dose-response relationship between depression and all-cause mortality among MI patients, with even sub-clinical levels of depressive symptoms associated with increased risk of death.

Depressive symptoms among CABG patients have been associated with poorer medical prognosis. For example, Burg and colleagues found that a clinically meaningful level of depressive symptoms in the week prior to CABG was related to 6-month cardiovascular morbidity [29] and 2-year cardiovascular mortality [30]. Similarly, Connerney et al. [31] found that major depression assessed soon after CABG was associated with 1-year medical morbidity, while Blumenthal et al. [32] found that moderate-to-severe depression and depressive symptoms that persisted 6-months beyond surgery predicted up to 5-year mortality.

Mechanisms
A close examination of the pathophysiology of atherosclerosis and depression suggests several common features that could help account for the strong prospective association of depression and CHD. For example, both depression and CHD are associated with alterations in immunological functioning relevant to pro-inflammatory processes. Specifically, depression has been associated with an elevation of interleukin-6 (IL-6), a primary pro-inflammatory cytokine [33, 34]. In addition, experimental injection of IL-6 in laboratory animals results in behaviors resembling depression in humans, such as decreased feeding, psychomotor slowing, and alterations in memory, learning and sleep [35]. In turn, IL-6, and inflammation in general, has been clearly implicated in the pathogenesis of atherosclerosis. In addition to IL-6, other immunological processes have been identified as potential modulators of both diseases. These include increased

levels of acute phase proteins, such as haptoglobin and alpha-1 antitrypsin, increased levels of other pro-inflammatory cytokines, such as IL-1, and activation of some aspects of cell-mediated immunity, along with suppression of other aspects of cell-mediated immunity [34].

Although high-fat diets are problematic in atherosclerosis, there has been some focus on dietary Omega-3 fatty acids for their potential role in mitigating various inflammatory processes that may be associated with CHD and depression. Some authors have suggested that deficiencies in Omega-3 fatty acids could be one causal mechanism linking depression and CHD [36]. Others have presented evidence suggesting that depression may influence the accumulation of adipose tissue, which, in turn, is associated with increased levels of inflammatory markers (such as IL-6) that are implicated in CHD [37, 38]. Although the etiology of obesity is thought to involve biological and genetic factors, in addition to diet and physical activity, it is notable that depression has shown a significant prospective association with obesity among adolescents [39].

In addition to immunological mechanisms, both cardiovascular disease and depression have been associated with increased activation of the HPA axis and with concomitant increases in circulating levels of catecholamines and cortisol. Catecholamines are known to impact the progression of cardiovascular disease through alterations in blood pressure and platelet activation [12] and through direct injury to the vascular endothelial lining of the coronary artery [40]. Notably, enhanced platelet activation and aggregation has been seen in depressed patients, potentially due to 5-HT_{2A} receptor dysregulation [41]. HPA dysregulation is also associated with elevated levels of cortisol, which is known to provoke hyperlipidemia, hypertension and direct endothelial damage [12].

Importantly, these HPA processes are not independent of the immunological pathway described above. For example, it has been suggested that elevation of proinflammatory cytokines, and IL-6 in particular, provoke activation of the HPA axis and a concomitant rise in circulating levels of cortisol and catecholamines [33]. Indeed, one action of cortisol is to down regulate inflammatory processes in a negative feedback loop [37, 38]. The hypercortisolemia seen in depression, however, may have a dysregulating effect on this negative feedback loop. For example, Wirtz et al. [42] report that healthy men with vital exhaustion demonstrate less of a suppressive action from glucocorticoids on the release of IL-6. Like depression, vital exhaustion predicts incident MI, and is characterized by fatigue, loss of energy, and other depressive symptoms [43].

Another pathway that could link depression and CHD is dysregulation of the autonomic nervous system as indexed by heart rate variability (HRV). HRV is a measure of the variability in timing between successive heartbeats [12]. Decreased HRV is thought to reflect decreased parasympathetic contribution to the overall autonomic control of the heart rhythm. Decreased HRV has been associated with increased cardiovascular morbidity and mortality, as well as depression [12, 44]. The possibility that depressive affect might influence HRV is suggested by a novel study showing decreases in HRV in association with feelings of hopelessness and anxiety among championship chess players [45]. Similar findings by Hughes and Stoney [46] also showed that participants with depressed mood demonstrated poorer HRV function during two laboratory stress tasks.

In addition to affecting biological pathways, depression may contribute to CHD and post-ACS prognosis as a function of its relationship with other risk factors. For example, in a large cohort of initially healthy older Americans from the Cardiovascular Health Study, depression among women was significantly related to smoking status at study entry [47]. Current smokers exhibited the greatest levels of depressive symptoms, followed by former smokers and persons who never smoked. Similarly, depressed psychiatric patients have been found to smoke more and have more difficulty quitting than non-depressed patients [48].

In addition to smoking, the Cardiovascular Health Study found that depression was inversely associated with the number of blocks walked in the week prior to study enrollment [47]. Among younger individuals (ages 15-54) in the National Comorbidity Survey, those who engaged in regular physical activity had a lower prevalence of major depression [49], while Rosal et al. [50] found depression to be associated with a greater number of behavioral risk factors, including smoking, sedentary lifestyle and high-fat diet.

Finally, poor adherence to medical advice is a behavioral factor that may contribute to the impact of depression on CHD prognosis. For example, in a 4-month followup study of ACS patients, those reporting mild-to-moderate depression on the BDI were less likely to make prescribed changes to dietary and exercise habits [51]. Patients in this sample with a diagnosis of major depression and/or dysthymia were the least adherent to recommended changes in diet and exercise, and to taking medications as prescribed. Other investigations have documented similar findings of poor adherence in association with depression among ACS patient populations [52]. Studies that have found significant associations between depression and these risk factors have also found that depression predicts CHD morbidity and mortality independently [53], and that depression can potentiate the effects of these risk factors on CHD morbidity and mortality [54].

■ Depression and CHD: Clinical Implications

Assessment of Depression

Assessment of diagnostic depression in CHD populations presents special challenges, in part because most ACS patients are too ill to tolerate lengthy interviews, and they have little unencumbered time during brief hospital stays. Many are also unaccustomed to discussing their emotional problems and have symptoms that are hard to assess in the hospital setting. Lastly, it is often difficult to ascertain whether a physical symptom associated with depression is due instead to some aspect of the patient's CHD. Clinical interviews must therefore be flexible and conducted in a sensitive manner that fosters trust, rapport and disclosure, rather than in the neutral, tightly structured manner of an epidemiologically based interview. Toward this end, the Diagnostic Interview and Structured Hamilton (DISH) was developed for the Enhancing Recovery in Coronary Heart Disease (ENRICHD) Study, a recently completed randomized controlled clinical trial of treatment for depression in post-ACS patients (see below). The DISH incorporates elements of other diagnostic and severity measures of depression, and is well suited for use with this population. It provides for the initial establishment of rapport by allowing the patient to first discuss his or her experiences related to the ACS. It then provides the interviewer with a flexible structure (i.e., using the patient's own way of describing his or her experiences) from which to probe for the presence of symptoms consistent with depression. The scoring takes into account symptom severity and duration in order to facilitate clinical determinations. Lastly, the DISH provides for a brief assessment of lifetime history of depression. The DISH is relatively easy to administer, and it provides a useful diagnostic tool for both clinical and research purposes [55].

Clinicians and researchers also frequently assess the presence of depressive symptoms through the use of self-report questionnaires. Perhaps the most widely used questionnaire for this purpose has been the Beck Depression Inventory [56]. This self-report measure has 21 items grouped by diagnostic symptom (e.g., feelings of guilt, sadness, self-confidence and discouragement, loss of interest, crying, changes in appetite, sleep difficulties, suicidal ideation), and the patient is asked to choose a response that indicates the level of severity for each item. Questionnaire scores, while not directly tied to diagnostic depression, have accepted anchors for depression severity.

Investigations of depression and CHD commonly interpret results using a BDI score of 10 or greater to identify the presence of depression. Research has also found that scores at or above 10 are associated with poorer prognosis, whether for CAD progression [57] or "hard" medical endpoints such as death or myocardial infarction [25, 26]. The predictive nature of BDI scores is independent of important medical prognostic indicators, such as left ventricular function or CAD severity, and the predictive power of BDI scores extends over 5 years [52]. Another symptom-based measure of depression commonly used is the Center for Epidemiologic Studies Depression scale (CES-D) [58]. In clinical research, cutoff scores used in dichotomization for the CES-D to indicate the presence of depression have ranged from 16 or greater, to 21 or greater [21].

Post-ACS Depression Treatment

Psychotherapy
Psychotherapy has long been recommended for patients after ACS, both for those with depression and for those experiencing adjustment difficulties. Until recently, however, there have not been any controlled clinical trials assessing the efficacy of psychotherapy in this population; nor have there been trials examining the impact of psychotherapy on medical prognosis (e.g., reinfarc-

tion, mortality). Previous research has examined the addition of group therapy, relaxation training, and other psychosocial components to ongoing "cardiac rehabilitation," with targets of these treatments including stress reduction, distress management, and health risk behavior change (including reduction of type A behavior). Results of these efforts have been promising for quality of life outcomes, behavior change and overall risk reduction [59].

Two recent randomized clinical trials directly examined the treatment of distress and/or depression in post-MI patients, and the resulting impact of the treatment on the incidence of death or reinfarction. In M-HART [60], acute-MI patients were regularly assessed for levels of distress. Supportive and problem-focused nurse home visits were provided to those randomized to the treatment condition when distress reached at least moderate levels. Although no overall survival benefit was demonstrated for the treatment, increased mortality was seen in older women. Another finding was that some patients evidenced increased distress scores after a nurse visit. Subsequent analyses [61] revealed an enhanced survival effect for those individuals for whom the nurse visits reduced distress. These results highlight the importance of offering depression/distress treatments of known efficacy when working with cardiac patients.

The ENRICHD trial [62, 63] was a multicenter, randomized controlled clinical trial funded by the National Heart, Lung and Blood Institute (NHLBI). ENRICHD was designed to determine the effect on medical prognosis (death, reinfarction) of treating acute MI patients with depression and/or low social support. Patients were randomized to either a usual cardiologic care or intervention condition, and the intervention consisted of up to six months of individual psychotherapy (with up to three months of group psychotherapy where feasible), and up to 12 months of adjunctive pharmacotherapy for patients with severe or unremitting depression. Cognitive therapy [64] was the treatment selected for ENRICHD, in combination with more general behavioral and social learning approaches [62]. This treatment is defined by an active collaboration between patient and therapist and utilizes a relatively structured, agenda-based therapy session. Other defining elements of this approach are the case conceptualization, which is grounded in a cognitive formulation, the use of structured homework assignments, and a treatment focus on behavioral activation, active problem solving and alteration of depressogenic automatic thoughts [64].

ENRICHD demonstrated a modest treatment effect with regard to depression. Those randomized to the intervention condition demonstrated statistically significant reductions both in depression symptoms (49 vs. 33% reduction in BDI score) and in incidence of diagnostic depression. These improvements did not translate into a lower incidence of reinfarction or death overall; however, there was some indication that those with the most severe depression, who additionally showed the greatest benefit from the intervention in terms of fewer depression symptoms, also showed a benefit with regard to reinfarction and/or death [63]. It is important to note as well that those randomized to the usual care condition also demonstrated improvement in depression symptoms, and, at 30-

month followup, no group differences in these symptoms remained. In discussing these findings, the ENRICHD investigators suggest that additional research is needed for determining the threshold effects on depression before improvement can be seen in post-ACS related prognosis. This research must also address the treatment dose necessary to affect the mechanism(s) that link depression to post-ACS prognosis. In addition, the investigators suggest that the effort to identify depression and initiate treatment in the days immediately following MI may have resulted in recruitment of a sizable patient cohort that was merely demonstrating acute adjustment symptoms rather than frank depression. Thus, many of these individuals (in both the intervention and usual care conditions) may have experienced a "spontaneous remission." Hence, research of this kind may necessitate an observation period prior to intervention in order to identify a true depression risk population [63].

Anti-Depressant Medication
Pharmacological treatment of depression in patients with CHD is complex and entails certain limitations and contraindications. For example, tricyclic and monoamine oxidase inhibitor medications are problematic for this population [65, 66], given the effects of these drugs on cardiac conduction, contractility and rhythm, and given their association with orthostatic hypotension. These untoward side effects may be more prevalent in the elderly and in those with unstable coronary disease, poor heart function or persistent arrhythmia. The more benign side-effect profile of the newer selective serotonin reuptake inhibitor (SSRI) medications makes them the class of choice for cardiac patients. SSRIs have been found effective for treating depression in this population, and the recently completed SADHART trial demonstrates their safety [67]. Of note, results from SADHART also indicated that SSRIs might impart some prognostic benefit for cardiac patients, independent of their effect on depression symptoms. This is likely due to the effect of these medications (working through the serotonin receptors on platelets) to affect platelet function.

■ Conclusion

The prevalence of depression among patients with CHD and after ACS is higher than in the general population. Although depression may at times be viewed as a response to the trauma of MI, there is substantial prospective evidence that depression predates and may play a causal role in CHD onset. Despite many unanswered questions about the mechanisms linking depression to CHD, investigations suggest direct biological processes involved in both depression and CAD, and indirect pathways related to health behaviors. Biological mechanisms may include inflammatory and immunological processes, alterations in HPA activation with concomitant increases in cortisol and catecholamine levels, alterations in autonomic nervous system activity, and oxidative processes. Behaviorally, non-adherence to medical regimens and poor health behaviors (such as smoking, atherogenic diets and sedentary lifestyle) are important factors that may also contribute to the observed relationship between depression and CHD.

Despite these plausible mechanisms, effective interventions to improve CHD outcomes by targeting depression remain elusive [68]. The standard treatment of depression with newer antidepressant medications such as SSRIs holds promise with regard to both depression management as well as the potentially direct benefit of reduced platelet activation. Cognitive therapy as used by ENRICHD investigators [63] demonstrates modest improvements in depression among post-MI patients; however, these effects may not be universally beneficial in reducing re-infarction or mortality. Treatment of depression among CHD patients therefore continues to be an area of active investigation. Findings from the ENRICHD study suggest the need for future research to better identify the degree of change in depression needed to impact CHD outcomes. In addition, differentiating patients with adjustment difficulties from those with depressive disorders may further clarify the benefit of cognitive therapy on depression and CHD outcomes.

Ultimately, understanding the many hypothesized behavioral and biological pathways linking depression to CHD outcome will likely facilitate the development of effective interventions. More basic research is therefore needed to elucidate the mechanisms by which depression and CHD are related. Intriguing directions for research in this area include further investigation of inflammatory and oxidative processes, as well as HPAC function and autonomic regulation associated with depression.

References

1. Katzel LI, Waldstein SR (2001) Classification of cardiovascular disease. In: Waldstein SR, Elias MF (eds) Neuropsychology of cardiovascular disease. Mahwah, NJ: Erlbaum, pp 3-14
2. Smith TW, Leon AS (1992) Coronary heart disease: A behavioral perspective. Champaign, Ill: Research Press
3. World Health Organization (2000) Annual incidence for selected causes: by sex, age and WHO subregion: 2000 version 2. Retrieved December 5, 2003, from the World Health Organization Statistical Information System
4. World Health Organization (2000) Point prevalence for selected causes: by sex, age and WHO subregion: 2000 version 2. Retrieved December 5, 2003, from the World Health Organization Statistical Information System
5. American Heart Association (2003) Heart disease and stroke statistics – 2004 update. Am Heart Assoc, Dallas, Texas
6. American Heart Association (2004) Heart attack and angina statistics. Available from the American Heart Association Web site, http://www.americanheart.org
7. Ross R (1991) Atherosclerosis - an inflammatory disease. N Engl J Med 340:115-126
8. Entman ML, Ballantyne CM (1993) Inflammation in acute coronary syndromes. Circulation 88:800-803

9. American Psychiatric Association (1994) Diagnostic and statistical manual of mental disorders (4th ed.). Washington, DC: Author

10. American Psychiatric Association (2000) Diagnostic and statistical manual of mental disorders (4th ed., text revision). Washington, DC: Author

11. Kessler RC, Berglund P, Demler O et al (2003) The epidemiology of major depressive disorder. JAMA 289:3095-3105

12. Musselman DL, Evans DL, Nemeroff CB (1998) The relationship of depression to cardiovascular disease. Arch General Psychiatry 55:580-592

13. Lane D, Carroll D, Ring C et al (2002) The prevalence and persistence of depression and anxiety following myocardial infarction. British J Health Psychol 7:11-21

14. Schleifer SJ, Macari-Hinson MM, Coyle DA et al (1989) The nature and course of depression following myocardial infarction. Arch Intern Med 149:1785-1789

15. Langeluddecke P, Fulcher G, Baird D et al (1989) A prospective evaluation of the psychosocial effects of coronary artery bypass surgery. J Psychosom Res 33:37-45

16. McKhann GM, Borowicz LM, Goldsborough MA et al (1997) Depression and cognitive decline after coronary artery bypass grafting. Lancet 349:1282-1284

17. Ziegelstein RC (2001) Depression in patients recovering from a myocardial infarction. JAMA 286:1621-1627

18. Denollet J (1993) Emotional distress and fatigue in coronary heart disease: The Global Mood Scale (GMS). Psychol Med 23:111-121

19. Lesperance F, Frasure-Smith N, Talajic M (1996) Major depression before and after myocardial infarction: Its nature and consequences. Psychosom Med 58:99-110

20. Mayou RA, Gill D, Thompson DR et al (2000) Depression and anxiety as predictors of outcome after myocardial infarction. Psychosom Med 62:212-219

21. Rugulies R (2002) Depression as a predictor for a coronary heart disease: A review and meta-analysis. Am J Preventive Med 23:51-61

22. Scherrer JF, Xian H, Bucholz KK et al (2003) A twin study of depression symptoms, hypertension, and heart disease in middle-aged men. Psychosom Med 65:548-557

23. Cohen HW, Madhavan S, Alderman MH (2001) History of treatment for depression: Risk factor for myocardial infarction in hypertensive patients. Psychosom Med 63:203-209

24. Ferketich AK, Schwartzbaum JA, Frid DJ, Moeschberger ML (2000) Depression as an antecedent to heart disease among women and men in the NHANES I study. National Health and Nutrition Examination Survey. Arch Internal Med 160:1261-1268

25. Frasure-Smith N, Lesperance F, Talajic M (1993) Depression following myocardial infarction: Impact on 6-month survival. JAMA 270:1819-1825

26. Frasure-Smith N, Lesperance F (1995) Depression and 18-month prognosis after myocardial infarction. Circulation 91:999-1005

27. Frasure-Smith N, Lesperance F (2003) Depression and other psychological risks following myocardial infarction. Arch General Psychiatry 60:627-636

28. Bush DE, Ziegelstein RC, Tayback M et al (2001) Even minimal symptoms of depression increase mortality risk after acute myocardial infarction. Am Cardiol 88:337-341

29. Burg MM, Benedetto MC, Rosenberg R, Soufer R (2003) Presurgical depression predicts medical morbidity 6 months after coronary artery bypass graft surgery. Psychosom Med 65:111-118

30. Burg MM, Benedetto MC, Soufer R (2003) Depressive symptoms and mortality two years after coronary artery bypass graft surgery (CABG) in men. Psychosom Med 65:508-510
31. Connerney I, Shapiro PA, McLaughlin JS et al (2000) In-hospital depression after CABG surgery predicts 12-month outcome. Lancet 358:1766-1771
32. Blumenthal JA, Lett HS, Babyak et al for the NORG Investigators (2003) Depression as a risk factor for mortality after coronary artery bypass surgery. Lancet 362:604-609
33. Kiecolt-Glaser JK, Glaser R (2002) Depression and immune function: central pathways to morbidity and mortality. J Psychosom Res 53:873-876
34. Maes M, Bosmans E, De Jongh R et al (1997) Increased serum IL-6 and IL-1 receptor antagonist concentrations in major depression and treatment resistant depression. Cytokine 9:853-858
35. Dantzer R, Wollman EE, Vitkovic L, Yirmiya R (1999) Cytokines, stress, and depression. Conclusions and perspectives. Advances Experimental Med Biology 461:317-329
36. Severus WE, Littman AB, Stoll AL (2001) Omega-3 fatty acids, homocysteine, and the increased risk of cardiovascular mortality in major depressive disorder. Harvard Review Psychiatry 9:280-293
37. Miller GE, Freedland KE, Carney RM et al (2003) Pathways linking depression, adiposity, and inflammatory markers in healthy young adults. Brain, Behavior, and Immunity 17:276-285
38. Miller GE, Stetler CA, Carney RM et al (2002) Clinical depression and inflammatory risk markers for coronary heart disease. Am J Cardiol 90:1279-1283
39. Goodman E, Whitaker RC (2002) A prospective study of the role of depression in the development and persistence of adolescent obesity. Pediatrics 109:497-504
40. Krantz DS, Manuck SB (1984) Acute psychophysiologic reactivity and risk of cardiovascular disease: A review and methodological critique. Psychological Bulletin 96:435-464
41. Schins A, Honig A, Crijns H et al (2003) Increased coronary events in depressed cardiovascular patients: 5-HT$_{2A}$ receptor as missing link? Psychosom Med 65:729-737
42. Wirtz PH, von Kanel R, Schnorpfeil P et al (2003) Reduced glucocorticoid sensitivity of monocyte interleukin-6 production in male industrial employees who are vitally exhausted. Psychosom Med 65:672-678
43. Appels A, Kop WJ, Schouten E (2000) The nature of the depressive symptomatology preceding myocardial infarction. Behavioral Med 26:86-89
44. Stein PK, Carney RM, Freedland KE et al (2000) Severe depression is associated with markedly reduced heart rate variability in patients with stable coronary heart disease. J Psychosom Res 48:493-500
45. Schwarz AM, Schachinger H, Adler RH, Goetz SM (2003) Hopelessness is associated with decreased heart rate variability during championship chess games. Psychosom Med 65:658-661
46. Hughes JW, Stoney CM (2000) Depressed mood is related to high-frequency heart rate variability during stressors. Psychosom Med 62:796-803
47. Ariyo AA, Haan M, Tangen CM et al (2000) Depressive symptoms and risks of coronary heart disease and mortality in elderly Americans. Circulation 102:1773-1779

48. Glassman AH, Helzer JE, Covey LS et al (1990) Smoking, smoking cessation, and major depression. JAMA 264:1546-1549

49. Goodwin RD (2003) Association between physical activity and mental disorders among adults in the United States. Preventive Med 36:698-703

50. Rosal MC, Ockene JK, Ma Y et al (2001) Behavioral risk factors among members of a health maintenance organization. Preventive Med 33:586-594

51. Ziegelstein RC, Fauerbach JA, Stevens SS et al (2000) Patients with depression are less likely to follow recommendations to reduce cardiac risk during recovery from a myocardial infarction. Arch Intern Med 160:1818-1823

52. Carney RM, Freedland KE, Miller GE, Jaffe AS (2002) Depression as a risk factor for cardiac mortality and morbidity: A review of potential mechanisms. J Psychosom Res 53:897-902

53. Hippisley-Cox J, Fielding K, Pringle M (1998) Depression as a risk factor for ischemic heart disease in men: population based case-control study. British Med J 316:1714-1719

54. Anda R, Williamson D, Jones D et al (1993) Depressed affect, hopelessness, and risk of ischemic heart disease in a cohort of U.S. adults. Epidemiology 4:285-294

55. Freedland KE, Skala JA, Carney R et al, for the ENRICHD Investigators (2002) The Depression Interview and Structured Hamilton (DISH): rationale, development, characteristics, and clinical validity. Psychosom Med 64:897-905

56. Beck AT, Rush AJ, Shaw BF, Emery G (1979) Cognitive therapy of depression. Guilford Press, New York

57. Carney RM, Rich MW, Freedland KE et al (1988) Major depressive disorder predicts cardiac events in patients with coronary artery disease. Psychosom Med 50:627-33

58. Radloff LS (1977) The CES-D Scale: A self-report depression scale for research in the general population. Applied Psychological Measurement 1:385-401

59. Linden W, Stossel C, Maurice J (1996) Psychosocial interventions for patients with coronary artery disease: a meta-analysis. Arch Internal Med 156:745-752

60. Frasure-Smith N, Lesperance F, Prince RH et al (1997) Randomised trial of hme-based psychosocial nursing intervention for patients recovering from myocardial infarction. Lancet 350:473-479

61. Cossette S, Fraser-Smith N, Lesperance F (1999) Impact of improving psychological distress in post-MI patients. Psychosom Med 61:93

62. ENRICHD Investigators (2001)Enhancing Recovery in Coronary Heart Disease (ENRICHD) study intervention: rationale and design. Psychosom Med 63:747-755

63. ENRICHD Investigators (2003) Effects of treating depression and low perceived social support on clinical events after myocardial infarction: the Enhancing Recovery in Coronary Heart Disease Patients (ENRICHD) Randomized Trial. JAMA 289:3106-3116

64. Beck JS (1995) Cognitive therapy: Basics and beyond. Guilford, New York

65. Glassman AH, Roose SP, Bigger JT Jr (1993) The safety of tricyclic antidepressants in cardiac patients. Risk-benefit reconsidered. JAMA 269:2673-2675

66. Cohen HW, Gibson G, Alderman MH (2000) Excess risk of myocardial infarction in patients treated with antidepressant medications: association with use of tricyclic agents. Am J Med 108:2-8

67. Glassman AH, O'Connor CM, Califf R et al Sertraline Antidepressant Heart Attack Randomized Trial (SADHEART) Group (2002) Sertraline treatment of major depression in patients with acute MI or unstable angina. JAMA 288:701-709
68. Frasure-Smith N, Lesperance F (2003) Depression: A cardiac risk factor in search of a treatment. JAMA 289:3171-3173

Chapter 6

Prevalence of Depression in Chronic Heart Failure

E.P. HAVRANEK

Background

Heart failure is a clinical syndrome characterized by the inability of the heart to pump enough blood to meet the demands of the skeletal muscle system during exertion. Heart failure may be the "final common pathway" for many cardiovascular diseases, including coronary artery disease, hypertension and myocarditis, or it may occur as a separate idiopathic entity. It causes functional limitation from dyspnea and fatigue that may be severe; heart failure patients on average report functional limitation nearly two standard deviations from the mean for the normal population [1]. There is a wide variability in disease severity. Some patients may experience symptoms only with unusual exertion outside the boundaries of their usual activity. In its more advanced stages adequate blood flow is impaired at rest, and may result in impaired perfusion of the kidneys, liver and even the cerebrum. Treatment consists of a regimen of multiple drugs that diminish the severity of symptoms and improve survival; curative therapy is not available. There are other options available for a limited subset of the patients with more advanced disease, including cardiac transplantation and mechanical assist devices.

Chronic heart failure is a common condition in Western countries. In the US, approximately 4.9 million individuals have the condition, and 550,000 new cases are diagnosed annually. In 2002 there were approximately 52,000 US deaths and 999,000 hospitalizations resulting from heart failure. It was the leading cause of hospitalization for patients older than 65. In the UK, the prevalence is estimated at 880,000 and the annual incidence is estimated at 63,500 [2]. Prevalence increases markedly with age. Although mortality has declined over the last several decades, it remains high [3].

Comorbidity is common in heart failure patients [4]. Two lines of evidence suggest that depression is likely to be another of these comorbidities.

First, depression has been demonstrated to complicate other chronic illnesses. Diabetes is a prominent example of a chronic illness in which an association with depression has been demonstrated. Anderson et al. [5] performed a quantitative review of 20 studies in which the prevalence of depression in patients with either Type 1 or Type 2 diabetes was compared to a control group of patients without diabetes. There were a total of 2858 diabetic patients examined in these studies. The prevalence of depressive symptoms was 26.1% for diabetic patients versus 14.4% for control patients when self-report scales were used, and 9.0% versus 5.0% when a diagnostic interview was used. Overall, there was a significant odds ratio of 2.0 (95% CI 1.8-2.2) for depression in patients with diabetes. This same group of authors has also performed meta-analyses of the association between depressive symptoms and poor glucose control in diabetic patients [6], and depressive symptoms and diabetic complications [7]. There was a small but significant decrement in glycemic control associated with depression, and diabetic patients with comorbid depression were significantly more likely to have both microvascular and macrovascular complications.

The second line of evidence suggesting an association between depression and heart failure is the link between depression and ischemic heart disease, the most common cause of heart failure in Western countries. The association between depression and acute myocardial infarction has been well described [8]. Patients who are depressed following myocardial infarction have an increased subsequent risk of death. Frasure-Smith and colleagues [9] found that 16% of patients hospitalized with acute myocardial infarction met criteria for major depression. After adjusting for factors known to predict mortality after myocardial infarction, a diagnosis of depression was a significant (OR 5.74, 95% CI 4.61-6.87) independent predictor of mortality. These findings have been confirmed in other studies [10, 11]. In addition, depression appears to be a risk factor for subsequent development of myocardial infarction independent of well-accepted risk factors such as family history, diabetes, smoking, hypertension and hypercholesterolemia [12-14].

▪ Prevalence and Association with Outcomes

Given that depression is common in at least two illnesses predisposing individuals to the development of heart failure, it is not surprising that investigators have found a direct link between depression and heart failure. In one of the first studies to suggest an association, Koenig [15] interviewed 107 patients admitted to an academic medical center with either a primary or secondary diagnosis of heart failure. Of these, 39 (36.5%) were judged to have major depression by Diagnostic and Statistical Manual IV (DSM-IV) criteria. Among a comparison group of 106 patients hospitalized with other cardiac diseases, the prevalence of major depression was 17.0%. Although no data on heart failure severity were given, the author believed the heart failure patients to be more severely ill compared with the comparison cardiac patients. One year following discharge, approximately 40% of those with major depression during hospitalization still had symptoms consistent with major depression.

Havranek, Ware and Lowes [16] studied a group of stable outpatients with heart failure using the Center for Epidemiological Studies Depression case finding instrument (CES-D). Control subjects were selected from patients treated for hypertension in the general medical clinic of the same facility. Outpatients with heart failure were found to have higher CES-D scores than control subjects, indicating a greater burden of depressive symptoms, and they were also more likely (24.4% vs. 9.7%) to have a CES-D score above the usual cutoff (≥16) deemed consistent with a diagnosis of depression. There were no differences between the two groups in functional capacity as measured using a six-minute walk test.

Similarly, Skotzko and colleagues [17] administered the CES-D to a cohort of 33 outpatients with heart failure. They found CES-D scores ≥16 in 42% of patients. Functional capacity was assessed by means of questionnaires (the SF-36 and the Walking Impairment Questionnaire), the six-minute walk test, maximal oxygen consumption (as determined by the cardiopulmonary exercise test) and energy expenditure assessed by both a radioactive tracer technique and a hip accelerometer. There were no differences in functional capacity by CES-D score, implying no relationship between depressive symptoms and heart failure severity. Interestingly, patients with a significant burden of depressive symptoms were less likely to perform a maximal effort during exercise testing, as judged by a mean respiratory quotient less than 1.0. The mean respiratory quotient was consistent with maximal effort (approximately 1.05) for patients without significant depressive symptoms.

Jiang and colleagues [18] used a study design similar to that used by Koenig (both are in the same institution) to assess the prevalence of depression in a patient population hospitalized with heart failure. Jiang and colleagues screened 374 patients using the Beck Depression Index (BDI). Patients with a score greater than the usual cutoff for a clinically significant burden of depressive symptoms (≥ 10) underwent a structured interview to assess for the presence of major depression by DSM-IV criteria. Of the 374 patients assessed, 35.3% had a Beck index score ≥ 10 and 13.9% were given a diagnosis of major depression. Over the ensuing year, patients with major depression were not found have an increased risk of death (OR 2.12, 95% CI 0.94-4.81, p=0.07), but they did have an increased risk of rehospitalization (OR 2.57, 95% CI 1.16-5.68, p=0.02), after controlling for heart failure disease severity with age, left ventricular ejection fraction, New York Heart Association Class, and presence or absence of ischemic etiology for heart failure. Patients with depressive symptoms (Beck score ≥ 10) but without a diagnosis of major depression did not have an increased risk for adverse outcomes.

Vaccarino and colleagues [19] administered the Geriatric Depression Scale (GDS) Short Form to 426 patients admitted to a single hospital with heart failure. Of these patients, 35% were judged to have a mild burden of depressive symptoms, 33.5% were moderate and 9.0% were severe. After adjustment for a broader array of covariates than in Jiang's study, the relationship between GDS score and 6-month mortality was not statistically significant. There was, however, a significant relationship between depressive symptoms and the likelihood of the patient experiencing functional decline as defined by an activities-of-daily-living questionnaire (OR 1.15 for mild symptoms, 1.65 for moderate symptoms, and 2.16 for severe symptoms, p=0.01 for trend).

Rumsfeld and colleagues [20] investigated both the cross-sectional and longitudinal association of depressive symptoms in heart failure patients with health status. Not only did they find depressive symptoms to be the strongest independent predictors of disease-specific quality of life measured with the Kansas City Cardiomyopathy Questionnaire (KCCQ), they found that depressive symptoms predicted short-term decrements in health status.

Using a questionnaire employed in the Studies of Left Ventricular Dysfunction (SOLVD), Konstam and colleagues [21] reported results of health-related quality of life measurements made in conjunction with a major randomized clinical trial of ACE inhibitors for the treatment of heart failure. Designed specifically for the study, the questionnaire was derived from multiple other questionnaires, and was not independently validated. Nevertheless, scores on the subset of the questionnaire that dealt with depression significantly predicted all cause mortality at 3 years (RR 1.065, 95% CI 1.009-1.125, p=0.023).

In summary, studies performed both on patients admitted with heart failure and on stable outpatients demonstrate an increased prevalence of depression. The estimate of prevalence varies widely depending on the method used to identify depressive symptoms and, probably, on unmeasured patient factors. It has not been conclusively demonstrated that depression in heart failure patients is independently associated with mortality. However, the study involving the largest number of patients and the longest follow-up, namely, Konstam and colleagues' analysis of data from SOLVD, does show an association, and smaller studies with shorter follow-ups show a trend in the direction of an association. In addition, there is a clear association between depressive symptoms and subsequent decline in health status in longitudinal studies, and the evidence supports a greater risk of recurrent hospitalization, a greater loss of ability to perform activities of daily living and a greater decline in disease-specific quality of life.

Mechanism of the Association

Although the reasons for the increased prevalence of depression in heart failure are not altogether clear, a few conclusions about mechanisms of action can be drawn based on the available data. Moreover, an understanding of the theoretical models being advanced by investigators is important for moving the field forward.

First, it is necessary to consider whether the relationship between depression and heart failure is mediated through the confounding variables, diabetes and coronary heart disease. My colleagues and I have investigated this question in a cohort of 527 stable outpatients with heart failure and found that neither diabetes nor ischemic heart disease was associated with the presence or absence of a significant burden of depressive symptoms [22]. Because beta-blockers have been implicated as a precipitant of depression and heart failure, and because heart failure patients are now frequently treated with agents from this class, we looked for an association between medication use and depressive symptoms, but found no relationship. Thus, the association between depression and heart failure appears to be direct, and not mediated by confounders.

Although it is tempting to attribute the genesis of depression to the presence of heart failure, an investigation by Abramson and colleagues [23] suggests that depression may contribute to the genesis of heart failure. Abramson and colleagues examined data from a randomized trial, the Systolic Hypertension in the Elderly Program (SHEP), in which patients older than 60 years who had a systolic blood pressure 160-220 mmHg and a diastolic pressure less than 90 mmHg were randomized to stepped, anti-hypertensive treatment or placebo. Patients with a history of heart failure at baseline were excluded from the analysis. The study demonstrated that treatment diminished the incidence of stroke. Patients responded to the CES-D at baseline, and 221 patients (out of a total of 4538 patients randomized) with CES-D score ≥16 were classified as "depressed." During follow-up, heart failure developed in 8.1% of the depressed patients and 3.2% of the non-depressed patients. After adjusting for baseline differences in age, gender, systolic blood pressure, cholesterol, and smoking, depression was a significant predictor of the development of heart failure, with a hazard ratio (2.59, 95% CI 1.57-4.27) greater than for any other variable tested. Depression remained a significant predictor of the development of heart failure after controlling for the occurrence of myocardial infarction during follow-up.

Whether the reverse is true – that the development of heart failure triggers depression – is less clear. If this were the case, one would expect that greater heart failure disease severity is associated with a greater likelihood of depression. In general, data in support of this do not exist.

In the study of outpatients with heart failure by Havranek et al. cited above [16], there was no difference in the 6-minute walk distance between heart failure patients burdened by depressive symptoms and those who were not. This is consistent with the notion that heart failure severity did not differ between the groups. Likewise, the study by Skotzko et al. [17], which employed more rigorous assessments of functional capacity, showed no differences between heart failure patients with positive screening tests for depression and those with negative screening tests with respect to maximal oxygen consumption (14.1 ± 3.4 ml/kg/min vs. 14.4 ± 2.3 ml/kg/min), 6-minute walk distance (1304 ± 370 ft vs. 1307 ± 145 ft), or in estimated daily caloric expenditure.

Another intriguing possibility suggests that it is the onset of heart failure that triggers depression, and that, as the disease progresses, the presence of depressive symptoms become less likely as the patient's intrinsic coping mechanisms that come into play. This view of events is analogous to the data for myocardial infarction, and has not been investigated to date. The link between heart failure and depression thus appears to be complex, with depression interacting with other risk factors to make the development of heart failure more likely. Although, as stated above, it seems reasonable to assume that the occurrence of heart failure could trigger the development of depression, evidence for this is lacking.

Speculations regarding the mechanism of the association can be broadly grouped into two categories that are not mutually exclusive. The first group might be termed psychodynamic. According to this line of thought, the development of depression might be related to a sense of loss surrounding the decrease in functional capacity, fear of death and loss of hope related to having a disease associated with a high mortality. These psychodynamic mechanisms would likely trigger depression in individuals rendered susceptible by genetic or personality factors. These psychodynamic arguments also encompass the notion that depression makes disease severity worse through non-compliance with medications and medical follow-up, and through other poor health habits such as smoking and poor diet. Depressed patients are also less likely to be physically active. Since exercise retards the decline of health-related quality of life in heart failure, and possibly mortality [24], physical inactivity likely contributes to a declining course in heart failure. Depressed individuals are significantly more likely to be divorced and to live in social isolation - conditions also associated with poor health status and poor outcome in heart failure [25].

The second group of speculative mechanisms for the link between heart failure and depression are biological. Depression is accompanied by neurohormonal changes, prominently hypercortisolemia and possibly increased sympathetic activities, both of which contribute to the genesis of heart failure. There appear to be few data, however, to support the notion that the increased levels of circulating catecholamines seen in severe heart failure may cause depression.

Diagnostic Considerations

As alluded to above, the optimal diagnostic strategy for recognizing depression in the setting of heart failure probably consists of screening all patients with a short, self-administered questionnaire with high sensitivity, followed by a specific interview aimed at establishing the diagnosis of major depression by DSM-IV criteria in those with positive screening responses.

The overlap in symptoms between depression and heart failure represents a diagnostic challenge. Both depression and heart failure may cause symptoms of lassitude and easy fatigability. Both screening questionnaires and subsequent interviews should therefore focus on the psychological symptoms of the disease such as hopelessness and sleep disturbance and avoid supporting a diagnosis of depression with symptoms such as fatigue. As noted above, a wide variety of screening instruments are available. These instruments vary significantly in sensitivity and specificity [26] and in their reliance on physical symptoms to support a diagnosis. A thorough review of this topic is beyond the scope of this chapter, but a few remarks are important. The most frequently used instruments in assessing for depression in patients with heart failure have been the BDI, the CES-D, and the closely related MOS-D. In general, the BDI has been demonstrated to be quite sensitive in primary care settings, and may be even more sensitive with heart failure patients given the inclusion of questions assessing for depressive symptoms that overlap with the symptoms of heart failure. This view is supported by the observation that the prevalence of depressive symptoms in heart failure is much greater with this instrument than with others. The CES-D, although less sensitive, has been validated in patients with concurrent medical illness [27-29]. Choice of instrument should be tailored to the setting in which it will be used.

Other more efficient strategies for identifying depression in the setting of heart failure may be proved useful in the future. For example, Brody et al. [30] suggest that patients with major depression can be identified by establishing the presence of at least 3 of 4 of the symptoms of sleep disturbance, anhedonia, low self-esteem and appetite change. Such an approach might mitigate the need for both a screening questionnaire and a diagnostic interview and should be considered in future research. This type of approach may facilitate treatment of depressed heart failure patients by cardiologists and primary care physicians.

■ Treatment Considerations

Although it seems obvious that major depression in patients with heart failure should be treated, as is the case with any other important separate comorbidity, the issue is deserving of future research for the following reasons.

First, the safety of antidepressant drugs in patients with heart failure needs to be explicitly established. Limited data in patients with ischemic heart disease suggest that selective serotonin re-uptake inhibitors (SSRIs) have acceptable levels of adverse events in patients with cardiac disease [31-33]. In at least one study, the side effect profile was better for a drug from this class of agents than for nortriptyline, in part because of the lack of autonomic effects of the SSRI. Of ongoing concern is the establishment of a lack of significant drug interactions with the multiple agents that constitute contemporary heart failure treatment.

Second, the efficacy of antidepressants in patients with heart failure needs to be established. It seems unlikely that treatment of depression will have a major and measurable effect on survival in heart failure. Neither the ENRICHD nor the SADHART studies in post-myocardial infarction depression were able to show significant impact on mortality. Survival, however, should not be the only outcome of interest in patients with a chronic debilitating disease like heart failure [34].

Depression is associated with a significant decrement in health status. Wells and colleagues [35] reported that among patients enrolled in the Medical Outcomes Study those with major depression rated their general health significantly poorer than the general population, and nearly as low as those with congestive heart failure, after each group was adjusted for the presence of comorbidities. Physical function and general health were also lower for depressed patients compared with patients with other chronic diseases such as diabetes and coronary artery disease. Given the significant decrement in health status associated with heart failure, it may be that the improvements associated with treatment of depression will be undetectable by patients. Based on current knowledge, however, this seems unlikely. As noted above, the burden of depressive symptoms seem to be the most significant predictor of health-related quality of life in patients with heart failure.

Conclusions

Congestive heart failure is a highly prevalent disease in Western countries and is associated with a significant burden of morbidity and mortality. Depression is more prevalent in patients with heart failure than in other groups of patients with asymptomatic medical illness. Prevalence estimates vary widely depending on the technique used to identify cases, with best estimates based on diagnostic interviews in the range of 10-15%. The processes linking depression and heart failure are poorly understood. Some evidence suggests that depressed patients with risk factors for heart failure are more likely to go on to develop heart failure. Although conceptually appealing, evidence is lacking that the presence of heart failure triggers depression. Depression appears to act synergistically with heart failure to cause a decline in physical function. Care in the diagnosis of depression is warranted in heart failure patients because of the overlapping symptoms of lassitude and easy fatigability. The effect of treatment of major or mild depression in heart failure patients might therefore be expected to improve health status in these patients, but clinical trials have not been carried out. It would also be useful for clinicians to have the safety of anti-depressant medications established in heart failure patients.

References

1. Ware JE, Kosinski M, Keller SD (1994) SF-36 physical and mental health summary scales: a user's manual. Boston, MA: The Health Institute, New England Medical Center
2. American Heart Association (2003) 2003 Heart and Stroke Statistical Update. Dallas, TX: American Heart Association
3. Levy D, Kenchaiah S, Larson MG et al (2002) Long-term trends in the incidence of and survival with heart failure. N Eng J Med 347(18):1397-1402
4. Havranek EP, Masoudi F, Westfall K et al (2002) The spectrum of heart failure in older patients: results from the National Heart Failure project. American Heart Journal 143:412-417
5. Anderson R, Freedland K, Clouse R, Lustman P (2001) The prevalence of comorbid depression in adults with diabetes: a meta-analysis. Diabetes Care 24:1069-1078
6. Lustman P, Anderson R, Freedland K et al (2000) Depression and poor glycemic control: a meta-analytic review of the literature. Diabetes Care 23:924-942
7. de Groot M, Anderson R, Freedland K et al (2001) Association of depression and diabetes complications: a meta-analysis. Psychosomatic Medicine 63:619-630
8. Fielding R (1991) Depression and acute myocardial infarction: a review and reinterpretation. Social Science & Medicine 32:1017-1027

9. Frasure-Smith N, Lesperance F, Talajic M (1993) Depression following myocardial infarction: Impact on 6-month survival. JAMA 270:1819-1825

10. Barefoot J, Helms M, Mark D, Blumenthal J et al (1996) Depression and long-term mortality risk in patients with coronary artery disease. Am J Cardiol 78:613-617

11. Bush D, Ziegelstein R, Tayback M et al (2001) Even minimal symptoms of depression increase mortality risk after acute myocardial infarction. Am J Cardiol 88:337-341

12. Barefoot J, Schroll M (1996) Symptoms of depression, acute myocardial infarction, and total mortality in a community sample. Circulation 93:1976-1980

13. Ferketich A, Schwartzbaum J, Frid D, Moeschberger M (2000) Depression as an antecedent to heart disease among women and men in the NHANES I Study. Arch Intern Med 160:1261-1268

14. Ford D, Mead L, Chang P et al (1998) Depression is a risk factor for coronary artery disease in men: the Precursors Study. Arch Intern Med 158:1422-1426

15. Koenig H (1998) Depression in hospitalized older patients with congestive heart failure. Gen Hosp Psych 20:29-43

16. Havranek EP, Ware M, Lowes BD (1999) Prevalence of depression in patients with congestive heart failure. Am J Cardiol 84:348-350

17. Skotzko C, Krichten C, Zietowski G et al (2000) Depression is common and precludes accurate assessment of functional status in elderly patients with congestive heart failure. J Card Fail 6:300-305

18. Jiang W, Alexander J, Christopher E et al (2001) Relationship of depression to increased risk of mortality and rehospitalization in patients with congestive heart failure. Arch Intern Med 161:1849-1856

19. Vaccarino V, Kasl S, Abramson J, Krumholz HM (2001) Depressive symptoms and risk of functional decline and death in patients with heart failure. Am Coll Cardiol 38:199-205

20. Rumsfeld JS, Havranek EP, Masoudi M ei al for the Cardiovascular Outcomes Research Consortium (2003) Depressive symptoms are the strongest correlate of quality of life in patients with heart failure. Am Coll Cardiol 42:1811-1817

21. Konstam V, Salem D, Pouleur H et al (1996) Baseline quality of life as a predictor of mortality and hospitalization in 5025 patients with congestive heart failure. Am J Cardiol 78:890-895

22. Havranek EP, Masoudi F, Rumsfeld JS et al (2002) Depression in heart failure patients is not the result of comorbidities or medications. J Card Fail 8:S70

23. Abramson J, Berger A, Krumholz HM, Vaccarino V (2001) Depression and risk of heart failure among older persons with isolated systolic hypertension. Arch Intern Med 161:1725-1730

24. Belardinelli R, Georgiou D, Cianci G, Purcaro A (1999) Randomized, controlled trial of long-term moderate exercise training in chronic heart failure. Effects on functional capacity, quality of life, and clinical outcome. Circulation 99:1173-1182

25. Coyne J, Rohrbaugh M, Shoham V et al (2001) Prognostic importance of marital quality for survival of congestive heart failure. Am J Cardiol 88:526-529

26. Mulrow C, Williams J, Gerety M et al (1995) Case-finding instruments for depression in primary care settings. Ann Intern Med 122:913-921

27. Berkman L, Berkman C, Kasl S et al (1986) Depressive symptoms in relation to physical health and functioning in the elderly. Am J Epidemiol 124:372-388

28. Davidson H, Feldman P, Crawford S (1994) Measuring depressive symptoms in the frail elderly. J Gerontol 49:P159-P164

29. Koenig H, Meador K, Cohen H, Blazer D (1988) Depression in elderly hospitalized patients with medical illness. Arch Intern Med 148:1929-1936

30. Brody D, Hahn S, Spitzer R et al (1998) Identifying patients with depression in the primary care setting: a more efficient method. Arch Intern Med 158:2469-2475

31. Nelson J, Kennedy J, Pollock B et al (1999) Treatment of major depression with nortriptyline and paroxetine in patients with ischemic heart disease. Am J Psychiatry 156:1024-1028

32. Roose S, Glassman A, Attia E et al (1998a) Cardiovascular effects of fluoxetine in depressed patients with heart disease. Am J Psychiatry 155:660-665

33. Roose S, Laghrissi-Thode F, Kennedy J et al (1998b) Comparison of parosetine and nortriptyline in depressed patients with ischemic heart disease. JAMA 279:287-291

34. Havranek E, Masoudi F, Rumsfeld J, Steiner J (2003) A broader paradigm for understanding and treating heart failure. J Card Fail 9:147-152

35. Wells K, Stewart A, Hays R et al (1998) The functioning and well-being of depressed patients: results from the Medical Outcomes Study. JAMA 262:914-919

Chapter 7

Depression in Coronary Artery Disease: Assessment and Treatment

W.J. Kop ▪ D.N. Ader

▪ Introduction

Depression in patients with documented coronary artery disease (CAD) occurs frequently and is associated with elevated risks of cardiac morbidity and mortality. Diagnostic criteria for depression are listed in Table 1 [1].

Table 1. Symptoms for diagnosis of depressive episode

1. Depressed mood
2. Markedly diminished interest or pleasure in activities
3. Weight loss or gain (>5%)
4. Insomnia or hypersomnia
5. Psychomotor retardation or agitation
6. Fatigue or loss of energy
7. Feelings of worthlessness or guilt
8. Diminished ability to concentrate or think
9. Recurrent thoughts of death

Prevalence estimates of depressive disorders in CAD patients range from 15-40% [2-4]. Despite the high prevalence, depression is under diagnosed and hence frequently untreated in CAD [5-7]. Untreated depression is of particular concern because depression is associated with a two to seven fold elevated risk of subsequent cardiac events, which is comparable to traditional cardiovascular risk factors such as hypercholesterolemia and hypertension [2-4, 8]. Biobehavioral mechanisms accounting for these negative outcomes include both biological pathways (e.g., altered sympathetic/parasympathetic balance) and adverse health behaviors (e.g., smoking). This chapter reviews the nature and prevalence of depression in CAD, assessment techniques, the adverse cardiovascular consequences of depression, and treatment options. Adequate assessment and treatment of depression will not only improve patients' quality of life, but may also promote cardiovascular health outcomes in high-risk populations.

The Nature and Prevalence of Depression in Patients with Coronary Artery Disease

Depression is substantially more prevalent among CAD patients (15-40%) than in the general population (estimates ranging from 2.3-9.3%) [9]. Among patients with CAD, higher rates of depression and sub-threshold depressive symptoms are observed in patients with unstable anginal complaints and severe heart failure [10], as well as in those awaiting coronary artery bypass graft (CABG) surgery [11].

The most common types of depressive disorders in cardiac patients are: typical Major and Minor Depressive Mood Disorders, atypical depression, and (vital) exhaustion. Major depression is diagnosed if one of the following primary symptoms is observed: 1) depressed mood and/or 2) markedly diminished interest or pleasure in activities, and a total of five or more symptoms of depression (see Table 1).

The symptomatology of depression in cardiac patients often differs from what is observed in psychiatric patients. Most notably, complaints of tiredness or lack of energy are more frequently observed than melancholy or depressed mood states [3, 4, 12]. Less common symptoms such as irritability and anxiety, are frequent complaints in cardiac patients and tend to occur more often than the typical feelings of guilt and low self-esteem. This different clinical presentation of depression is an important factor in the underdiagnosis of depression among cardiac patients.

Extreme tiredness predicts adverse cardiovascular health outcomes, independent of depressed mood [13, 14]. Based on clinical interviews, this state has been labeled "vital exhaustion" [15] and consists of extreme tiredness, increased irritability, and feelings of demoralization. In the original conceptualization of this construct, the term "vital" was included to reflect the far-reaching consequences of this condition on daily life function (similar to vital depression). The prefix "vital" will not be used in the remainder of this text. Episodes of exhaustion generally last several months, and complaints lasting longer than two years are not regarded as typical for exhaustion. Prevalence estimates of exhaustion in patients with CAD vary between 20-45% [3]. In a recent Italian study, 29% of 130 patients with myocardial infarction (MI) or unstable angina were classified as exhausted [16]. Elevated risks related to exhaustion are reported for MI (OR=2.3) [17], clinical events after coronary angioplasty (OR = 2.7; 95% CI = 1.1-6.3) [18], and sudden cardiac death (OR = 2.2) [13]. As described in detail elsewhere [3], the defining features of depression and exhaustion overlap, but the etiology and biological correlates of these two constructs appear to differ.

The clinical presentation of depression (i.e., melancholic versus atypical) is related to the neurohormonal and hemostatic correlates of the disorder. Typical melancholic depression is associated with increased neuroendocrine activity, whereas atypical depression and exhaustion co-occur with hypocortisolemia [19, 20]. These neurohormonal differences may in part explain why impaired fibrinolysis is observed in exhaustion but not in depression [21, 22], and why cardiovascular risk factors may be differentially associated with depression versus exhaustion [23].

Etiology of Depression in Patients with Coronary Artery Disease

The causes of depression are multifactorial, and include genetic predisposition, history of distressing environmental challenges, and current psychological and biological precipitants. In CAD patients, both psychological and biological factors specifically related to the disease process, such as inflammation, may further contribute to the onset and maintenance of depression.

The psychological antecedents of depression are not fully understood, but often include dysfunctional cognitions and/or a maladaptive response to loss of an important object or person [2, 4]. Exhaustion results frequently from prolonged physical or psychological distress, over which the individual has no control [3, 12].

The biological antecedents of depressive symptoms in CAD patients may differ from depressed individuals in general. It has been argued that depressive symptoms are secondary to coronary disease or its pharmacological treatment, but there is little support for this idea, due to the fact that severity of coronary disease, poor left ventricular pump function or inducibility of ischemia are poor predictors of depressive symptoms [2, 3]. Futhermore, most reports do not support that theory that cardiac medications are the main cause of depressive symptoms in CAD patients [24]. It is possible that depression – in particular, its vegetative components - reflect low-grade inflammation and immune activation [25, 26] or hypothyroidism. The *functional* severity of CAD (e.g., exercise tolerance and severity of dyspnea) appears to be related to depressive symptoms in CAD [24]. Thus, although it cannot be ruled out that underlying coronary disease results in depressive symptoms, most evidence suggests non-cardiac origins of depression in patients with CAD.

Depression often coincides with adverse health behaviors, such as smoking, poor diet, non-adherence to medication regimen, and sedentary life style. For example, a reduced level of regular exercise is common in depressed patients, a fact that is significant given that physical exercise has well-established positive effects on mood [27]. Further studies are needed to disentangle the cause-effect relationships between depression and adverse health behaviors in patients with CAD.

Assessment of Depression and Related Disorders in Patients with Coronary Artery Disease

Depressive disorders can be assessed with questionnaires and structured clinical interviews. The *Diagnostic and Statistical Manual* (DSM-IV) criteria for depression require the presence of depressed mood and/or diminished interest, and a total of 5 out of 9 of the symptoms listed in Table 1 for major depression, and 2 out of 9 for minor depression [1]. Symptoms are required to be present most of the day, almost every day, for at least two weeks. In CAD patients, the 2-week criterion may be omitted for diagnosis of depression if the cardiac event occurred within a shorter time frame [2, 4, 28].

Questionnaires

The advantage of questionnaires is their sensitivity for detecting depression and efficiency of administration. The most commonly used self-report questionnaires for depression in cardiac patients are the Beck Depression Inventory (BDI) [29], the Centers for Epidemiological Studies-Depression (CES-D) scale [30, 31], and the Hospital Anxiety and Depression Scale [32]. Other questionnaires have been used successfully as well, including the Zung depression scale. Most questionnaires assess mood and cognitive components (e.g., sadness, low self esteem, guilt feelings), as well as the "vegetative" components (e.g., sleep problems, appetite changes and lack of energy) of depression. To specifically assess exhaustion, the Maastricht Questionnaire can be used [12?]. Questionnaires are sensitive screening tools for depression, but tend to reveal "false positives." Thus, questionnaire scores indicating depression require further evaluation using structured interviews.

Structured Interviews

Based on the DSM criteria, structured interviews have been developed to assess depression and other psychological disorders. Among the commonly used interviews are the Structured Clinical Interview for DSM-IV Axis I Disorders (SCID), the Composite International Diagnostic Interview (CIDI), the Schedules for Clinical Assessment in Neuropsychiatry (SCAN), and the Diagnostic Interview Schedule (DIS) [28, 33]. A combined self-report and clinical interview technique has been designed to assess depression in patients with medical conditions [34]; the PRIME-MD has an accuracy of 88% for the assessment of depression. Structured interviews are superior to questionnaires in differentiating dysthymia from minor depression. One of the limitations of structured interviews is that they are time-consuming and tend to be resistant to change over time. The Hamilton depression scale is useful for evaluating severity as well as change [28]. For practical purposes, it is generally important that structured interviews allow sufficient flexibility to be amended to the patient's clinical condition, the hospital setting, and the potential of interview administration by individuals without extensive psychological training.

Patients with elevated questionnaire scores, but who do not fully qualify for all DSM major or minor depression criteria based on the structured interview, may still suffer from atypical or subclinical depression, and these patients also may be at risk for adverse cardiovascular events [3, 15].

A strong focus on the mood components of depression in the early phases of the diagnostic assessment may result in under detection of depression because of the atypical nature of depression in patients with cardiac disease. Patients with medical disorders may be reluctant to disclose depressive mood symptoms, due to the fact that the somatic depressive symptoms features often appear salient to them. Some somatic symptoms of depression, such as fatigue, may also reflect angina equivalents and should be treated accordingly. Nonetheless, these complaints should also be counted in the assessment of depression in CAD patients, because it is generally not possible to differentiate the underlying causes of these symptoms. Thus, to adequately assess depression in cardiac patients, it is important to question the patient about *all* items related to depression, starting with the vegetative symptoms [28, 35].

Risk of Future Cardiac Events as Related to Depression

Major depressive disorder, as well as atypical and subclinical depression, increase the risk of first and recurrent MI [3]. Reported risk ratios vary from 2-7, and are thus comparable to well-established CAD risk factors such as hypercholesterolemia, hypertension and obesity [2-4]. The strongest effects of depression are observed for recurrent cardiac events, with risks ranging between 3-7, but first MI is also predicted by depression, with an estimated risk of 1.6 [36]. Psychological risk factors for CAD can be classified into three broad categories, based on their duration and temporal proximity to cardiac events [3]: 1) acute triggers, including mental stress and outburst of anger; 2) episodic factors having a duration of several weeks up to two years, among which are depression and exhaustion; and 3) chronic factors, such as negative personality traits (e.g., hostility) and low socioeconomic status. Because depression is an episodic and often not a chronic condition, the severity of depression and the extent of underlying CAD are not significantly associated [24]. Therefore, depression is primarily a risk factor for adverse cardiac outcome because it affects pathophysiological factors such as blood clot formation, inflammation, plaque rupture, or because it can contribute to life-threatening arrhythmias, all of which promote transformation from stable coronary disease to clinically important and life-threatening conditions.

Indirect cardiovascular consequences of depression are related to the adverse health behaviors and psychosocial correlates of depression. Depression is associated with increased smoking, poor compliance with medication regimens, reduced exercise levels and poor dietary habits [2, 4]. Part of these adverse health behaviors result from the psychosocial consequences of depression, such as social isolation.

Treatment of Depressive Disorders
in Patients with Coronary Artery Disease

Major Depression can be effectively treated with psychological and pharmacological interventions. Atypical depression, subclinical depression, and exhaustion often require intervention as well, particularly if the patient has had prior depressive episodes or a family history of depression. In the United States, fewer than 25% of patients are treated for their clinical depression [9]. Reasons for the underdiagnosis of depression by physicians are summarized in Table 2 [4, 9] and include both the incorrect assumption that depression has no long-lasting effects on clinical outcome and the atypical presentation of depression in many cardiac patients [3].

Table 2. Reasons for underdiagnosis of depression

• Underestimation of adverse effects on clinical cardiovascular outcome
• Atypical nature of depression in cardiac patients
• Belief that depressed mood is "normal," given the patient's medical condition
• Time constraints for appropriate assessment
• Avoidance of social stigma associated with a diagnosis of depression
• Unawareness of treatment options

The management of depression typically has three phases: 1) the acute phase, which focuses on reducing symptoms (6-12 weeks); 2) the continuation phase, focussed on preventing relapse (4-9 months); and 3) the maintenance phase for individuals with known recurrent depression (long-term treatment) [4]. Many depressive episodes associated with acute coronary syndrome (e.g., myocardial infarction) resemble adjustment disorders with high spontaneous recovery rates [37]. Treatment of depression generally requires careful coordination between internal medicine and cardiology with mental health professionals in the cardiac rehabilitation program.

Pharmacological interventions

Selective serotonin reuptake inhibitors (SSRI) tend to be tolerated better than the traditional tricyclic antidepressants (TCA) among CAD patients [38]. In addition, TCAs can have arrhythmogenic side effects and, thus, are less attractive in patients with CAD. Most SSRIs should not be used in combination with class IC anti-arrhythmics or with beta-adrenergic blocking agents, as they may potentiate the effects of these drugs. SSRIs appear to reduce depressive symptoms in cardiac patients as effectively as in depressed individuals referred to psychiatry, but, once treatment is withdrawn, the resumption of depression in patients with CAD is a frequent occurrence. Little is known about the determinants of residual depression or the degree of SSRI efficacy in reducing recurrent cardiac events. Glassman et al. recently conducted a randomized trial examining the benefits an SSRI over placebo in patients with myocardial infarction [37]. The SSRI under investigation was safe and resulted in a significant reduction in depression, primarily in patients with severe or recurrent depression. Some support was found for the notion that SSRIs also prevent recurrent cardiac events during active treatment (14% versus 22%), but the investigation was primarily intended as an efficacy study and not adequately powered to detect this difference at a statistically satisfactory level. Part of the beneficial effects of SSRI may be mediated via their effects on platelet aggregation.

Psychological interventions

Psychological interventions can be provided on an individual basis or in groups, and may range from social support to more intensive cognitive-behavioral therapy. The typical duration of psychological intervention in CAD patients ranges from 8-12 weeks, and efficacy of psychological interventions has been summarized by several authors [39-42].

Cognitive behavioral therapy is often successfully used in the treatment of depressive disorders. The main goal of this approach is to modify dysfunctional thoughts and emotions by structured and empathic questioning of the patient's perceptions and thought processes. The "Enhancing Recovery in Coronary Heart Disease" (ENRICHD) trial recently examined the effects of cognitive behavioral therapy in a large sample (N = 2481) of post myocardial infarction patients with major depression and/or social isolation [43]. The intervention was successful in reducing depression, but there were no beneficial effects in 2-year cardiac events for patients receiving the intervention (24.2%), versus the control group (24.1%). Because dysfunctional cognitions play a relatively minor role in atypical depression, treatments other than cognitive behavioral interventions may be more beneficial to CAD patients with atypical depression or exhaustion.

Evidence suggests that relaxation and breathing therapy are effective in reducing exhaustion in CAD patients. Importantly, these interventions may also successfully prevent recurrent MI and clinical restenosis following coronary angioplasty [44, 45]. At present, the efficacy of relaxation in CAD patients with depression has not been established.

Patient support groups can provide social support, reduce anxiety, and help teach patients how to effectively report symptoms and communicate with their physicians. Social isolation is a risk factor for CAD and is often a concomitant of depression [43]. Social support from family and friends may promote treatment efficacy and recovery from depression. Although social networks generally respond in a supportive manner during early stages of a CAD patient's depression, these resources can be drained as a result of the sustained demands of depressed individuals.

▇ Concluding Remarks and Future Directions

Depression is far more common in CAD patients than in the general population, but often remains undiagnosed and untreated. In CAD patients, depression frequently presents as complaints of fatigue and other vegetative symptoms, rather than as the more typical melancholy that affects the general population. Initial screening of depression can be efficiently conducted in most medical settings using questionnaires; and effective treatment requires the involvement of a multidisciplinary team. The aforementioned ENRICHD trial supports the importance of: 1) careful assessment and treatment of depression in CAD patients, differentiating between major and minor depressive disorder and dysthymia, as well as between related conditions such as exhaustion; 2) assessment of the severity of depression with the aim of detecting cut-off values and/or dose-response relationships; and 3) evaluation of the role of prior depressive episodes and the environmental and social context in which depression occurs [28].

More research is needed on the differentiation between depression and (vital) exhaustion. This distinction may be of particular importance because depression and exhaustion have different neurohormonal correlates [19, 20], and because exhaustion is also one of the defining characteristics of the frailty of aging in the elderly [46]. Research on the differential biobehavioral mechanisms and treatment modules may further our understanding of the relationship between depressive disorders and future cardiac events. Some evidence supports a dose-response relationship between the severity of depression and the risk of adverse cardiovascular outcomes [36], but the evidence is limited and the relationship may be more complex than a linear trend.

Psychosocial risk factors for CAD tend to cluster. Little is known about their additive and synergistic effects. Patients with prior depressive episodes are at increased risk for developing depression when they suffer an acute coronary event. In addition, social isolation may interact with depression to determine an adverse outcome. Classification of psychological characteristics into chronic, episodic and acute risk factors [3] may help elucidate the interrelation of various psychosocial factors and their pathophysiological mechanisms at increasing stages of underlying CAD.

Underdiagnosis has interfered with adequate treatment of depression in CAD patients. Factors involved in the lack of detection of depressive disorders are listed in Table 2, and some solutions to this problem have been discussed in this review. The currently available questionnaires are well suited as initial screening tools, but the subsequent clinical interviews for depression remain time-consuming (approximately 45 min [28]) and require improvements to be generally applicable in general medical practice.

Depression can be treated effectively with a combination of psychological and pharmacological interventions. However, whether this treatment results in improved cardiovascular health remains to be determined. Clearly, the type of treatment needs to be matched with the nature of the depression, and the failure to take this into account may explain why some interventions reveal unsuccessful results [47]. Depression can adversely affect cardiovascular health through both biological processes and adverse health behaviors. Thus, treatment of depressive disorders in CAD will be most effective when symptom management is combined with strategies targeting both the causes, as well as the biological and behavioral concomitants, of depression.

References

1. American Psychiatric Association (1994) Diagnostic and statistical manual of mental disorders. (IV ed.) Washington DC: Am Psychiatric Association
2. Carney RM, Freedland KE, Rich MW, Jaffe AS (1995) Depression as a risk factor for cardiac events in established coronary heart disease: a review of possible mechanisms. Ann Behav Med 17:142-149
3. Kop WJ (1999) Chronic and acute psychological risk factors for clinical manifestations of coronary artery disease. Psychosom Med 61:476-487
4. Lesperance F, Frasure-Smith N (2000) Depression in patients with cardiac disease: a practical review. J Psychosom Res 48:379-391
5. Freedland KE, Lustman PJ, Carney RM, Hong BA (1992) Underdiagnosis of depression in patients with coronary artery disease: the role of nonspecific symptoms. Int J Psychiatry Med 22:221-229
6. Hirschfeld RM, Keller MB, Panico S et al (1997) The National Depressive and Manic-Depressive Association consensus statement on the undertreatment of depression. JAMA 277:333-340
7. Perez-Stable EJ, Miranda J, Munoz RF, Ying YW (1990) Depression in medical outpatients. Underrecognition and misdiagnosis. Arch Intern Med 150:1083-1088
8. Frasure-Smith N, Lesperance F, Talajic M (1995) Depression and 18-month prognosis after myocardial infarction. Circulation 91:999-1005
9. Office of disease prevention and Health promotion, U. D. o. H. a. H. S. (1998) Healthy people 2010 Objectives: draft for public comment Washington, D.C.
10. Freedland KE, Rich MW, Skala JA et al (2003) Prevalence of depression in hospitalized patients with congestive heart failure. Psychosom Med 65:119-128
11. Blumenthal JA, Lett HS, Babyak Ma et al (2003) Depression as a risk factor for mortality after coronary artery bypass surgery. Lancet 362:604-609
12. Appels A (1989) Loss of control, vital exhaustion and coronary heart disease. In: Steptoe A, Appels A (eds) Stress, personal control, and health. John Wiley and Sons, Brussels, Luxemburg, pp 215-235
13. Appels A, Golombeck B, Gorgels A et al (2000) Behavioral risk factors of sudden cardiac arrest. J Psychosom Res 48:463-469
14. Appels A, Kop WJ, Schouten E (2000) The nature of the depressive symptomatology preceding myocardial infarction. Behav Med 26:86-89
15. Appels A (1990) Mental precursors of myocardial infarction. Br J Psychiatry 156:465-471
16. Pignalberi C, Patti G, Chimenti C et al (1998) Role of different determinants of psychological distress in acute coronary syndromes. J Am Coll Cardiol 32:613-619
17. Appels A, Mulder P (1988) Excess fatigue as a precursor of myocardial infarction. Eur Heart J 9:758-764
18. Kop WJ, Appels AP, Mendes de Leon Cf et al (1994) Vital exhaustion predicts new cardiac events after successful coronary angioplasty. Psychosom Med 56:281-287
19. Gold PW, Goodwin FK, Chrousos GP (1988) Clinical and biochemical manifestations of depression. Relation to the neurobiology of stress (1). N Engl J Med 319:348-353

20. Nicolson NA, van Diest R (2000) Salivary cortisol patterns in vital exhaustion. J Psychosom Res 49:335-342
21. Kop WJ, Hamulyak K, Pernot K, Appels A (1998) Relationship between blood coagulation and fibrinolysis to vital exhaustion. Psychosom Med 60:352-358
22. Raikkonen K, Lassila R, Keltikangas-Jarvinen L, Hautanen A (1996) Association of chronic stress with plasminogen activator inhibitor-1 in healthy middle-aged men. Arteriosclerosis Thrombosis and Vascular Biology 16:363-367
23. Kopp MS, Falger PR, Appels A, Szedmak S (1998) Depressive symptomatology and vital exhaustion are differentially related to behavioral risk factors for coronary artery disease. Psychosom Med 60:752-758
24. Kop WJ, Appels A, Mendes de Leon CF, Bar FW (1996) The relationship between severity of coronary artery disease and vital exhaustion. J Psychosom Res 40:397-405
25. Kop WJ (2003) The integration of cardiovascular behavioral medicine and psychoneuroimmunology: new developments based on converging research fields. Brain Behav Immun 17:233-237
26. Kop WJ, Cohen N (2001) Psychological risk factors and immune system involvement in cardiovascular disease. In: Ader R, Felten DL, Cohen N (eds.) Psychoneuroimmunology 3 edn Academic Press, San Diego
27. Blumenthal JA, Babyak MA, Moore KA et al (1999) Effects of exercise training on older patients with major depression. Arch Intern Med 159:2349-2356
28. Freedland KE, Skala JA, Carney RM et al (2002) The Depression Interview and Structured Hamilton (DISH): rationale, development, characteristics, and clinical validity. Psychosom Med 64:897-905
29. Beck AT, Beamesderfer A (1974) Assessment of depression: The depression inventory. In: Pachot P (ed) Modern problems in psychopharmacology Karger, Basel pp 151-169
30. Radloff LS (1977) The CES-D scale: a self-report depression scale for research in the general population. Applied Psychological MeasurementVol. 1(3) Sum
31. Schulz R, Beach SR, Ives DG et al (2000) Association between depression and mortality in older adults: the cardiovascular health study. Arch Intern Med 160:1761-1768
32. Herrmann C (1997) International experiences with the Hospital Anxiety and Depression Scale-a review of validation data and clinical results. J Psychosom Res 42:17-41
33. Robins LN, Helzer JE, Croughan J, Ratcliff KS (1981) National Institute of Mental Health Diagnostic Interview Schedule. Its history, characteristics, and validity. Arch Gen Psychiatry 38:381-389
34. Spitzer RL, Williams JB, Kroenke K et al (1994) Utility of a new procedure for diagnosing mental disorders in primary care. The PRIME-MD 1000 study. JAMA 272:1749-1756
35. Kop WJ, Ader DN (2001) Assessment and treatment of depression in coronary artery disease patients. Italian Heart J 2:890-894
36. Wulsin LH, Singal BM (2003) Do depressive symptoms increase the risk for the onset of coronary disease? A systematic quantitative review. Psychosom Med 65:201-210
37. Glassman AH, O'Connor CM, Califf RM et al (2002) Sertraline treatment of major depression in patients with acute MI or unstable angina. JAMA 288:701-709

38. Roose SP, Laghrissi-Thode F, Kennedy JS et al (1998) Comparison of paroxetine and nortriptyline in depressed patients with ischemic heart disease. JAMA 279:287-291
39. Dusseldorp E, van Elderen T, Maes S et al (1999) A meta-analysis of psychoeducational programs for coronary heart disease patients. Health Psychol 18:506-519
40. Linden W (2000) Psychological treatments in cardiac rehabilitation: review of rationales and outcomes. J Psychosom Res 48:443-454
41. Linden W, Stossel C, Maurice J (1996) Psychosocial interventions for patients with coronary artery disease: a meta-analysis [see comments] [published erratum appears in arch intern med 1996 Nov 11; 156(20):2302]. Arch Intern Med 156:745-752
42. Sebregts EH, Falger PR, Bar FW (2000) Risk factor modification through nonpharmacological interventions in patients with coronary heart disease. J Psychosom Res 48:425-441
43. Berkman LF, Blumenthal J, Burg M et al (2003) Effects of treating depression and low perceived social support on clinical events after myocardial infarction: the Enhancing Recovery in Coronary Heart Disease Patients (ENRICHD) Randomized Trial. JAMA 289:3106-3116
44. Appels A, Bar F, Lasker J et al (1997) The effect of a psychological intervention program on the risk of a new coronary event after angioplasty: a feasibility study. J Psychosom Res 43:209-217
45. van Dixhoorn J, Duivenvoorden HJ, Staal JA et al (1987) Cardiac events after myocardial infarction: possible effect of relaxation therapy. Eur Heart J 8:1210-1214
46. Fried LP, Tangen CM, Walston J et al (2001) Frailty in older adults: evidence for a phenotype. J Gerontol A Biol Sci Med Sci 56:M146-M156
47. Frasure-Smith N, Lesperance F, Prince RH et al (1997) Randomised trial of home-based psychosocial nursing intervention for patients recovering from myocardial infarction. Lancet 350:473-479

Chapter 8

Anxiety and Heart Disease

D.K. Moser ▪ M.J. De Jong

Despite impressive gains made in the treatment of coronary heart disease (CHD), it remains the number one cause of death and a major cause of disability among women and men in the United States (US). By the year 2020, CHD is projected to be the number one cause of death worldwide [1-3]. Coronary heart disease claims more lives each year than the next five causes of death combined [1]. The effect of various demographic (e.g., age, gender) and clinical (e.g., the presence of comorbidities) characteristics on development of cardiac events and on recovery has been well studied [4]. These demographic and clinical characteristics are used commonly in clinical practice to determine patient risk for future events.

Far less attention has been paid to the impact of psychological risk factors despite compelling evidence that they confer equal or, in some cases, greater risk than demographic or clinical risk factors [5-7]. Failure to understand and address psychological risk factors for CHD events may be one reason that CHD morbidity and mortality remain so high. Anxiety disorders are among the most prevalent psychiatric disorders [6]. Given the prevalence of anxiety in the general population and in patients with CHD, the potential public health impact of preventing the development and progression of CHD by appreciating the nature of the relationship between anxiety and CHD is enormous.

▪ Anxiety

Anxiety is a negative affective state resulting from an individual's perception of threat and characterized by a perceived inability to predict, control, or gain the preferred results in given situations [8]. Anxiety is a distinct emotional experience that has cognitive, neurobiological, and behavioral components, and that arises out of the interaction of an individual with the environment [6]. It allows, like other emotions, flexibility in behavioral responses to a changing environment. Anxiety is considered an adaptive process until its magnitude or persistence renders it a dysfunctional response that can have negative consequences.

Anxiety exists on a continuum from normal to pathological, and there are a number of anxiety disorders (i.e., panic disorder, phobic anxiety, generalized anxiety, anxiety reactions, chronic anxiety) [6, 8]. Nonetheless, research to date strongly suggests that anxiety along the continuum from normal anxiety reactions to pathological have comparable cognitive, neurobiological, and behavioral components, and that clinical anxiety and sub-clinical anxiety are not fundamentally different phenomena [6, 8-10]. Thus, the potential link between anxiety and the risk for CHD events has ramifications even for individuals who would not normally be diagnosed with clinical anxiety [6, 10, 11].

■ Anxiety in Individuals with CHD

Anxiety is common among individuals with chronic CHD and among those recovering from acute cardiac events [6, 12-17]. In fact, anxiety is more common than depression [13]. The prevalence of anxiety is approximately 70-80% among patients suffering an acute cardiac event and chronically persists in about 20-25% of individuals with CHD [12, 15, 16]. Even among individuals with CHD who have never had an event, the prevalence of anxiety is 20-25% [13]. Although anxiety is an expected and even normal reaction to an acute cardiac event or the threat of living with a chronic illness, anxiety is not benign if it persists or is extreme [5, 6, 11, 13, 14, 18-21].

Anxiety can hinder psychosocial adaptation to CHD and physical recovery after an acute event. Anxiety predicts poorer quality of life for CHD patients in the short and long term [18, 22-24]. Anxiety hinders psychosocial adaptation by interfering with patients' self-care abilities [14, 25]. Patients who are too anxious frequently are unable to learn or act upon new information about necessary life-style changes [26]. Anxious patients experience problems coping with challenges, and anxiety adversely affects adherence and rehabilitation efforts [22, 25, 26]. Persistent anxiety predicts worse disability, more physical symptoms, and poorer functional status in CHD patients [28, 29]. Anxious CHD patients return to work more slowly or less often than non-anxious patients [30], and have more problems resuming sexual activity after an acute event [31]. Patients with sustained anxiety may suffer from "cardiac invalidism," an older term that still describes a subset of CHD patients whose level of debilitation or disability after a CHD diagnosis or acute event is unexplained by the severity of their physical condition [28, 29, 32].

Despite the importance of anxiety to recovery in patients with CHD, and in particular with acute myocardial infarction (AMI), few investigators have examined the phenomenon. Our research team has focused on studying anxiety in AMI patients and results of our previously published studies are discussed below.

▪ Anxiety after Acute Myocardial Infarction

Prevalence of anxiety in an international sample. Investigators from North America reported that 10-26% of patients with AMI had higher levels of anxiety than patients with a psychiatric disorder [12, 15]. However, the prevalence of anxiety after AMI has not been studied extensively among international populations. Additionally, no investigators have evaluated whether the psychosocial or physiologic factors that are related to anxiety interact with the unique cultures within each country to produce a differential impact on anxiety.

Understanding anxiety from an international perspective is important because anxiety poses a significant risk to patients after AMI. This risk may result from activation of the sympathetic nervous system and hypothalamic-pituitary-adrenal (HPA) axis [17]. Investigators have shown that anxiety after AMI is associated with increased in-hospital complications such as lethal dysrhythmias, continued ischemia, and reinfarction [15]. Furthermore, anxiety has been shown to predict future coronary events and long-term survival after AMI [33-35]. However, individuals from different ethnic and cultural backgrounds may vary in their biological response to anxiety [36].

People from all cultures and countries experience anxiety [37]. Furthermore, culture influences the perception of a stress-producing situation, symptoms of stress, and the expression of emotions [38]. We conducted a study to evaluate whether anxiety after AMI differs across five countries and to determine whether an interaction between country and sociodemographic and clinical variables contributes to variations in the expression of anxiety [39].

This study was a prospective, comparative, cross-cultural investigation of anxiety soon after AMI in five countries. Each participant's anxiety level was assessed within the first 72 hours of hospital admission. Participants were recruited from community hospitals and academic medical centers from the following five countries: Australia, England, Japan, South Korea, and the US. Eligibility criteria for participation in this study included: 1) documented AMI by elevated cardiac isoenzymes and typical ECG changes; 2) onset of AMI outside of the hospital or other institutional setting, such as an extended care facility; 3) hemodynamic stability and absence of pain at the time of interview; and 4) intact cognitive function that allowed the participant to answer questions concerning his or her emotional status. Participants with life-threatening or debilitating co-morbidities were excluded from the study.

Data were collected by experienced cardiovascular nurses who interviewed each participant within 72 hours (mean 53 ± 38 hours) of admission to the hospital. The research assistants collected sociodemographic and clinical data. Anxiety was measured using the Anxiety Subscale of the Brief Symptom Inventory (BSI) to determine patients' perception of their current level of anxiety. Although concise, the 6-item subscale is a reliable and valid measure of state anxiety in acutely ill persons [40]. The Anxiety Subscale of the BSI was selected because it minimizes participant burden, is reliable and valid, was conceptually relatively easy to translate from English into Korean and Japanese, and does not include physical indicators of anxiety. Using a scale of 0 to 4 (0 = "not at all" and 4 = "extremely"), participants rate their level of emotional stress related to six items. The averaged score represents the participant's overall level of state anxiety; thus, mean scores can range from 0 to 4. High standard deviations are common and reflect variability in the samples studied [40]. Native speaking researchers translated the Anxiety Subscale of the BSI from English into Korean and Japanese to ensure linguistic and cultural equivalence. A second native speaking researcher translated the instruments back into English to ensure that the translation process did not distort the meaning of the instruments.

To compare baseline differences in sociodemographic and clinical characteristics among countries, a one-way analysis of variance (ANOVA) or chi-square was used, as was appropriate to the level of measurement. Multifactorial analysis of covariance (ANCOVA) was used to evaluate whether there were differences in mean anxiety scores among the five countries, while correcting for sociodemographic characteristics upon which the countries differed. Additionally, multifactorial ANCOVA was used to evaluate whether sociodemographic and clinical characteristics interacted with country to produce a differential impact on anxiety.

A total of 912 AMI patients participated in this study; 127 from Australia, 144 from England, 136 from Japan, 128 from South Korea, and 377 from the US. Sociodemographic and clinical characteristics of the sample, by country, are presented in Tables 1 and 2.

Table 1. Sociodemographic characteristics in an international sample of 912 AMI Patients

Characteristic	Entire sample N = 912	Australia n = 127	England n = 144	Japan n = 136	South Korea n = 128	United States n = 377
Age, mean ± standard deviation, years*	61 ± 13	62 ± 13	61 ± 13	61 ± 11	57 ± 11	62 ± 14
Education, mean ± standard deviation, years#	12 ± 4	13 ± 4	10 ± 4	13 ± 3	11 ± 5	13 ± 3
Male, n (%)§	658 (72.1)	101 (79.5)	111 (77.1)	109 (80.1)	99 (77.3)	238 (63.1)
Marital status, n (%)						
Married†	684 (75)	87 (68.5)	108 (75)	117 (86)	117 (91.4)	255 (67.6)
Divorced/ widowed/ single	220 (24.1)	40 (31.5)	33 (22.9)	19 (14)	10 (7.8)	118 (31.3)

AMI = acute myocardial infarction; * p = 0.02, South Korea < every other country; # p = 0.004, England and South Korea < every other country; § p = 0.001 U.S, < every other country; † p = 0.001, Japan and South Korea > every other country

Table 2. Clinical characteristics in an international sample of 912 AMI Patients

Characteristic	Entire sample N = 912 N (%)	Australia n = 127 n (%)	England n = 144 n (%)	Japan n = 136 n (%)	South Korea n = 128 n (%)	United States n = 377 n (%)
Current smoker*	419 (45.9)	39 (30.7)	64 (44.4)	93 (68.4)	87 (68)	136 (36.1)
Hypertension#	482 (52.9)	48 (37.8)	59 (41)	74 (54.4)	62 (48.4)	239 (63.4)
Diabetes mellitus§	225 (24.7)	12 (9.4)	37 (25.7)	47 (34.6)	31 (24.2)	98 (26)
Previous AMI#	192 (21.1)	17 (13.4)	29 (20.1)	21 (15.4)	10 (7.8)	115 (30.5)
Killip class						
I†	604 (66.2)	99 (78)	104 (72.2)	116 (85.3)	78 (60.9)	207 (54.9)
II	229 (25.1)	21 (16.5)	29 (20.1)	13 (9.6)	37 (28.9)	129 (34.2)
III-IV	72 (7.9)	7 (5.5)	10 (7)	6 (4.4)	13 (10.2)	36 (9.6)
Treatment in ED						
Fibrinolytic‡	310 (34.4)	34 (26.8)	99 (68.8)	20 (14.7)	36 (28.8)	121 (32.7)
Beta blocker**	320 (35.1)	28 (22.0)	72 (50.0)	11 (8.1)	10 (7.8)	199 (52.8)
Aspirin##	715 (78.4)	103 (81.1)	138 (95.8)	71 (52.2)	103 (80.5)	300 (79.6)
Anxiolytic#	270 (29.6)	30 (23.6)	43 (29.9)	28 (20.6)	33 (25.8)	136 (36.1)

AMI = acute myocardial infarction; ED = emergency department
* p = 0.001, Japan and South Korea > every other country; # p = 0.001, U.S. > every other country; § p = 0.001, Australia < every other country; † p = 0.001, Japan > every other country; ‡ p = 0.001, England > every other country; ** p = 0.001, US and England > Australia > Japan and South Korea; ## p = 0.001, England > US, Australia, South Korea > Japan

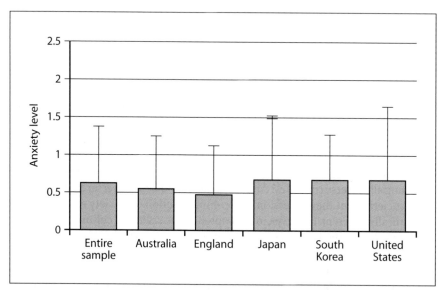

Fig. 1. Mean anxiety levels (with standard deviations) in 912 AMI patients in five countries

The mean level of anxiety in the entire sample was 0.62 ± 0.76 (range 0-3.83), which is 77% higher than the normal mean level of 0.35 reported in a sample of healthy adults levels in each country are illustrated in Figure 1. The mean levels of anxiety in each country were as follows: 0.54 in Australia (this anxiety level is 54% higher than normal); 0.47 in England (34% higher than normal); 0.66 in Japan (89% higher than normal); 0.64 in South Korea (83% higher than normal); and 0.69 in the US (97% higher than normal).

In all countries, patients reported high anxiety levels. A total of 46%, 35%, 43%, 52%, and 50% of patients in Australia, England, Japan, South Korea, and the US, respectively, reported anxiety levels higher than the normal reference mean. A total of 7%, 7%, 15%, 5%, and 10% of patients in Australia, England, Japan, South Korea, and the US, respectively, reported anxiety levels higher than the mean of 1.7 reported for psychiatric in-patients [40].

Although there was a significant difference in anxiety level among the countries ($p = 0.03$) on the overall ANOVA, post hoc testing to discover where the countries differed using the Bonferroni test revealed that only England and the US ($p = 0.03$) differed. Patients in England reported lower levels of anxiety than patients in the US. This difference in anxiety level disappeared after controlling for the sociodemographic variables on which the countries differed.

The following sociodemographic and clinical characteristics were examined to determine whether they interacted with country to influence anxiety: age, gender, marital status, education level, medical history, Killip classification on admission, use of various therapies in the emergency department, and pain level. None of these variables interacted with country to affect anxiety.

The principal findings from this study were that anxiety level early after AMI was high among patients from five diverse countries on four continents and did not differ substantially by country. Although patients from England reported anxiety levels lower than those from the US, there were no differences among any of the other countries, and the difference between English and American patients disappeared after correction for sociodemographic variables on which the countries differed.

To our knowledge, this is the first cross-cultural comparison of anxiety levels in AMI patients soon after the acute event. These findings demonstrate that, despite the potential influence of culture on emotion [38, 41, 42], patients suffering AMI display a similar emotional response to this potentially life-threatening event. If culture influences the experience, expression, and communication of emotion [43], why did we fail to find a difference in the expression of anxiety among patients from these five culturally diverse countries? Anxiety is thought to be a universal emotion found in all societies, but the expression and communication of anxiety are believed to be culturally different. However, in a comprehensive review of cultural variation in emotions, Mesquita & Frijda [44] argue that there are few data from which one can conclusively state that there are cultural variations in emotion. Depending on the theoretical framework from which one's view arises, there are data to support the notion that emotions are universal and data to support the notion that emotions are social constructs [44]. Mesquita and Frijda further note that most of the research on cross-cultural comparisons of emotion considers only abstract representations of emotion, and not concrete representations, such as the specific threat of physical illness. Thus, the expectation that there are cultural differences in the expression of anxiety may be unfounded.

Little cross-cultural research has been conducted to examine the emotions of patients after AMI. Scherer reported that among European, Japanese, and American university students, Japanese students were less fearful and more reserved about expressing their fear, and that they exhibited a diminished physiological response to fear [45]. In contrast, others found that Chinese men who underwent cardiac catheterization and Taiwanese patients with AMI reported similar levels of anxiety as American patients [42, 46]. In an epidemiologic review, Lepine pointed out that anxiety disorders are found in all countries that were studied [47]. Additionally, somatization of anxiety appears to be a common reaction across a variety of cultures [38]. Anticipation of physical danger has been reported as a precursor to anxiety in both non-Western and Western cultures [44]. Therefore, our finding that patients with AMI from five diverse countries expressed similar levels of anxiety suggests that the threatening nature of AMI produces anxiety, regardless of the patient's culture.

The high anxiety level seen among patients in all countries is of concern for a number of reasons. The level of anxiety seen, even in patients from the country with the lowest mean anxiety level, is substantially higher than that seen in healthy individuals [48]. For both humanistic and clinical reasons, it is essential to address this level of anxiety. Anxiety in cardiac patients is associated independently with higher short- and long-term morbidity and mortality [34]. Patients with higher anxiety soon after AMI have a longer stay in the cardiac care unit and hospital [24, 49], report sustained anxiety and long-term distress, suffer more symptoms irrespective of the severity of their physical condition [25], consume more health care resources [25], and report a lower quality of life [18, 24, 50] than patients with lower anxiety.

We investigated the possibility that a number of clinical or sociodemographic factors that might affect anxiety level would interact with country to affect anxiety level. None of the multiple factors examined produced a differential effect on anxiety. This finding suggests that, among AMI patients, anxiety is common regardless of clinical presentation, presence of co-morbidities, or severity of AMI, and that it cannot be predicted by typical sociodemographic or clinical characteristics. Further research is warranted to determine factors that may moderate anxiety in order to better understand the phenomenon among AMI patients and develop effective interventions.

In summary, patients from each country studied experienced high anxiety after AMI. Even though various cultures were represented in this study, culture itself did not account for variations in anxiety after AMI. It appears that anxiety after AMI is a universal phenomenon. Given the potentially negative impact of anxiety on mortality and quality of life after AMI, clinicians and researchers should continue to explore interventions to treat anxiety and minimize its untoward effects.

Gender Differences in Anxiety

Because high anxiety is associated with poorer AMI recovery, it is important that gender differences in anxiety after AMI be explored and interventions to decrease anxiety levels be targeted appropriately to those with the highest levels. It is equally important to explore gender differences internationally to improve planning of international public health initiatives and planning of health priorities and initiatives in the US, which has an increasingly diverse population. Accordingly, we conducted a study to determine whether there are gender differences in anxiety, when measured early after AMI, in an international sample [51].

The sample, measurement and data collection procedures are described above and in the full publication [51]. In this prospective, comparative study, 912 AMI patients were enrolled from Australia, South Korea, Japan, England and the US. Briefly, we used the anxiety subscale of the BSI to assess anxiety level within 72 hours of an admission for confirmed AMI.

Sociodemographic and clinical characteristics of patients at the different sites are compared by gender in Table 3.

Table 3. Demographic and clinical characteristics compared between genders in an international sample of 912 AMI patients

	Australia n = 127		England n = 144		Japan n = 136		South Korea n = 128		United States n = 377	
	M	F	M	F	M	F	M	F	M	F
Age (years)*	60.2± 12.6	71.1± 1185	59.3± 13.3	66.6± 13.9	59.4± 11.4	66.0± 9.1	54.7± 10.8	64.7± 10.3	59.1± 13.3	65.6± 13.2
Education (years)&	14.7± 13.5	10.9± 2.5	10.5± 4.1	8.4± 4.4	13.4± 3.0	10.8± 2.6	12.3± 4.3	8.3± 4.1	13.3± 2.9	12.9± 2.9
% married¶	76%	39%	82%	59%	87%	82%	96%	79%	77%	54%
Admission systolic BP (mmHg)@	138.6± 27.5	140.3± 24.5	142.3± 28.5	143.1± 32.2	131.1± 27.3	128.2± 23.6	129.5± 30.4	124.1± 28.3	141.6± 27.8	142.3± 28.8
Admission diastolic BP (mmHg)@	79.8± 15.9	79.8± 18.4	88.2± 21.3	88.2± 23.3	76.8± 15.6	74.5± 12.6	79.7± 17.6	77.5± 21.2	83.2± 17.5	81.2± 16.3
Admission	73.3± 22.5	80.4± 15.2	78.4± 19.2	80.8± 25.8	78.8± 20.4	76.0± 25.7	75.4± 16.1	73.8± 19.6	77.7± 18.2	83.3± 22.2
Worst AMI pain (0 – 10)#	6.8± 2.4	6.7± 2.9	7.7± 2.3	7.8± 2.8	7.5± 3.0	7.5± 3.0	7.9± 2.7	7.2± 2.6	6.9± 2.6	7.1± 2.6

AMI = acute myocardial infarction; BP = blood pressure; ED = emergency department; * = gender differences in age for all countries ($p < 0.01$); & = gender differences in education level for all countries ($p < 0.01$); # = gender difference in admission pulse ($p = 0.009$) and highest pain level ($p = 0.01$) in US only; ¶ = gender differences for all countries ($p < 0.05$) except Japan; @ = no gender differences

The mean level of anxiety reported for the entire sample was 77% higher than the normative anxiety score for adults. Sixteen percent of women in this sample versus 8 percent of men reported levels of anxiety higher than that seen in psychiatric patients. The range reported was 0-3.83. For reference purposes, the published norm for non-patient subjects is 0.35 ± 0.45; for psychiatric inpatients it is 1.5 ± 1.1; and for psychiatric outpatients it is 1.7 ± 1.0 [40, 48]. Gender-specific values for male and female psychiatric outpatients have been reported at 1.5 ± 0.95 and 1.8 ± 1.0, respectively; and gender-specific values for male and female non-patients have been reported at 0.26 ± 0.31 and 0.44 ± 0.54, respectively. Overall, women reported higher anxiety than men (0.76 ± 0.90 versus 0.57 ± 0.70, p = 0.005). This pattern of higher anxiety in women was seen in each country studied (Fig. 2).

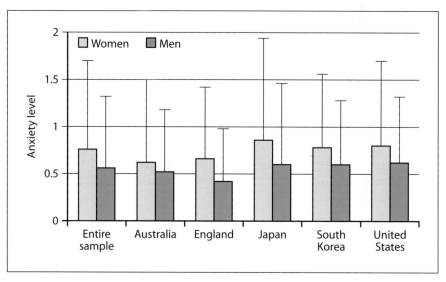

Fig. 2. Gender differences in anxiety overall and in each country

Analyses were performed to determine whether there was an interaction between sociodemographic or clinical variables and gender that would affect the relationship between gender and anxiety. These variables were age, marital status, education level, co-morbidities, pain level, clinical status on admission (i.e., admission vital signs and Killip classification), and medications used in the emergency department and during the hospitalization (e.g., thrombolytics, beta-adrenergic blocking agents, and anxiolytics). None of these variables interacted with gender to affect anxiety.

To summarize, women are more anxious after early AMI than men, and this finding is consistent across a variety of Western and Asian cultural groups. Women reported mean anxiety levels 25% higher than those reported by men, and twice as many women as men in the sample reported anxiety in the extreme ranges. The data also demonstrate that this higher level of anxiety is not the result of the influence of other sociodemographic or clinical characteristics on which men and women suffering AMI frequently differ. All patients should receive adequate assessment and management of their anxiety, but it is important for clinicians to recognize those groups of patients who are at greater risk for higher anxiety. A fruitful area for future research includes an investigation of reasons why women of different cultures all appear to be at higher risk for anxiety after AMI. Other important areas for investigation include determining whether higher anxiety after AMI contributes to the poorer prognosis seen in women, and the best methods for managing anxiety in busy hospitals. Despite the need for such research, the results of the present study are noteworthy for clinicians seeking to improve patient comfort and reduce the potentially harmful consequences of anxiety.

■ Relationship between Anxiety and Cardiac Outcomes in CHD

Despite anxiety being a common psychological response to a diagnosis of CHD or to an AMI, fewer investigators have examined the role of anxiety in cardiac outcomes than have examined the role of depression. Studies of the relationship of anxiety with CHD can be broadly grouped into the two following categories: 1) studies among initially healthy individuals who were followed to detect the occurrence of CHD; and 2) studies among patients with CHD who were followed to detect the occurrence or recurrence of CHD events (Table 4).

Table 4. Studies of the relationship between anxiety and CHD outcomes

Authors	Sample size	Outcome tested	Results
Studies in initially healthy individuals			
Martin et al [52]	60 psychiatric outpatient men and women, 7 years follow-up	CHD mortality	Anxiety not associated with outcome
Haines et al [53]	1457 community-dwelling men, 10 years follow-up	CHD mortality	RR of event for anxious = 3.77; dose response evident
Weissman [54]	3778 healthy men and women, follow-up period not reported	AMI	RR of event for anxious = 4.5
Eaker et al [55]	749 community dwelling women, 20 years follow-up	CHD events	RR of event for anxious = 7.8
Kawachi et al [56]	33,999 health professional men, 2 years follow-up	CHD mortality	RR of event for anxious = 2.45; dose response evident
Kawachi et al [57]	2280 community dwelling men, 32 years follow-up	Sudden death	RR of event for anxious =4.46; dose response evident

Authors	Sample size	Outcome tested	Results
Studies in patients with CHD			
Frasure-Smith et al [34]	220 AMI patients, 1 year follow-up	CHD events	RR of event for anxious = 2.5
Moser et al [15]	86 AMI patients, in-hospital study	Recurrent ischemia, reinfarction, ventricular arrhythmias, death	RR of event for anxious = 4.9
Denollet et al [33]	87 AMI patients, 7.9 years follow-up	MI, cardiac death, unstable angina, sudden death event	RR of event for anxious = 3.9
Herrmann et al [57]	454 patients with medical conditions; 273 CP, 1.9 years follow-up	All-cause mortality	RR of event for anxious = 2.9
Herrmann et al [58]	5057 men and women referred for exercise testing (49% CHD), 5.7 years follow-up	All-cause mortality	RR of event for anxious = 0.75 (increased anxiety associated with increased survival)
Welin et al [59]	255 men and women with MI, 10 years follow-up	CHD and all-cause mortality recurrent infarction	Anxiety not associated with outcome
Mayou et al [18]	347 men and women with MI, 18 month follow-up	CHD mortality	Anxiety not associated with CHD mortality
Lane et al [22, 23]	288 men and women with MI, 4 & 12 month follow-up	CHD and all-cause mortality	Anxiety not associated with mortality outcomes

AMI = acute myocardial infarction; CHD = coronary heart disease; CP = cardiopulmonary; RR = relative risk; MI = myocardial infarction

Among the studies in initially healthy individuals, most [53, 55-57], but not all [52], demonstrated that a variety of anxiety disorders (i.e., panic disorder, self-report phobic anxiety, and self-report anxiety symptoms) predicted future CHD mortality or AMI during a long follow-up period. This relationship was independent of the impact of other major cardiovascular risk factors and there was evidence of a dose-response effect [53, 55-57]. Although these studies provide intriguing evidence of a link between anxiety in individuals without pre-existing disease and the development of CHD events, this body of work has been criticized for failure to control for factors other than cardiovascular risk factors that co-exist with anxiety and that in themselves might explain CHD independently of anxiety [61].

Among studies of the association between anxiety in people who already have CHD and the risk of subsequent CHD events, four have demonstrated that increased anxiety predicted subsequent CHD events (i.e., reinfarction, unstable angina, CHD mortality) [15, 33, 34, 58], three reported no association between anxiety and CHD outcomes [18, 22, 23, 60], and one study reported that anxiety was associated with a survival *advantage* [59]. In all but one of these studies, subjects were patients hospitalized with AMI or other medical problems, or undergoing CHD testing, and followed for months or years to examine CHD outcomes. In rare cases, hospitalized AMI patients were followed only during their hospitalization to examine risk of in-hospital complications [15]. In all of these studies, anxiety was assessed as self-reported symptoms. Although a variety of instruments were used in the studies, all instruments were standardized and psychometrically sound. In all of these studies, a number of factors were controlled, so that the independent contribution of anxiety to CHD outcomes could be determined. Despite these similarities in effort to insure rigor, this group of studies had different findings that left the research and clinical communities unsure of how to interpret the evidence with regard to a possible link between anxiety and CHD outcomes in individuals with pre-existing CHD [61]. Thus, further research is needed in this area.

Relationship between Anxiety and In-Hospital Complications in AMI Patients

Few investigators have examined the relationship between anxiety and in-hospital complications in AMI patients. In order to clarify this issue, we conducted two studies designed to determine 1) the association between early anxiety in the AMI patient and the incidence of subsequent in-hospital AMI complications [15]; and 2) whether perceived control moderates any association between anxiety and in-hospital complications [16].

In the first study, we assessed anxiety level using the anxiety subscale of the BSI within 48 hours of patient arrival at the hospital in 86 confirmed AMI patients. Information about in-hospital complications, including reinfarction, new onset ischemia, ventricular fibrillation, sustained ventricular tachycardia, or in-hospital death were also collected.

Anxiety level as assessed by the BSI in this sample of 86 AMI patients was 1.1 ± 0.93 (range 0-3.3). This is above the norm-referenced score of 0.35 and approaches the norm of 1.7 for psychiatric in-patients. Twenty-six patients (30%) scored at or below the norm of 0.35, while 22 (26%) scored at or above 1.7.

Complications were seen in 22 patients (25.6%). Acute ischemia occurred in 12 patients (14%), reinfarction in 4 (4.7%), sustained ventricular tachycardia in 9 (10.5%), ventricular fibrillation in 8 (9.3%) and in-hospital death in 3 (3.5%). The percentage of patients with complications by anxiety group is presented in Figure 3. Complications were seen in 19.6% of patients with higher anxiety versus 6% of patients with lower levels of anxiety (p = 0.001). Of those patients with complications, one (4.5%) had an anxiety level below 0.35, 7 (31.8%) had an anxiety level between 0.35 and 1.7, and 9 (40.9%) had an anxiety level above 1.7.

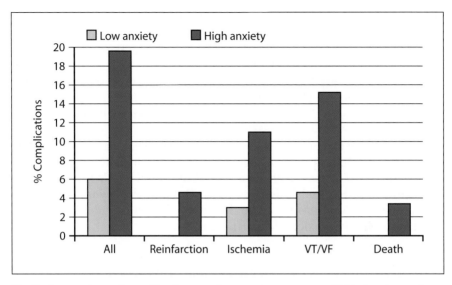

Fig. 3. Comparison of complication rates between acute myocardial infarction patients with low versus high levels of anxiety. VT/VF = sustained ventricular tachycardia/ventricular fibrillation

Multiple logistic regression was used to control for those clinical and sociodemographic factors that can influence the incidence of complications, and it demonstrated that a higher anxiety level was independently predictive of complications. Age, gender, Killip classification, thrombolytic therapy regimen, and worst chest pain score were forced first into the logistic regression model, followed by anxiety. The introduction of anxiety significantly improved the model (p = 0.001). Only Killip classification (odds ratio (OR) 2.7, 95% confidence interval (CI) 1.9-4.7, p = 0.001) and anxiety (OR 4.9, 95% CI 2.1-12.2, p = 0.003) contributed significantly to the model. Patients with Killip class II, compared with Killip class I, had 2.7 times the risk of complications. Controlling for the other factors, patients with higher anxiety (greater than 1.1 on the BSI) had 4.9 times greater risk of complications than patients with lower anxiety.

We conclude that anxiety early after myocardial infarction onset is associated with increased risk of ischemic and arrhythmic complications. This finding suggests that anxiety should be considered among the conventional risk factors for in-hospital AMI complications.

In the second study, we recruited a substantially larger sample and considered the interaction between perceived control and anxiety. We interviewed 536 patients with AMI (age 62 ±14, 34% female) within 72 hrs of admission. Anxiety was measured using the BSI, and perceived control using the Cardiac Attitudes Scale [15]. Complications were defined as reinfarction, ischemia, ventricular tachycardia, ventricular fibrillation, or cardiac death. There were more complications in patients with high versus low anxiety (p <0.001). In multivariate logistic regression analysis, higher anxiety was associated with increased risk for complications (OR = 1.8, 95% CI 1.4-2.2; p = 0.001), independent of age, diabetes, previous AMI, type of AMI, and Killip class. The association between anxiety and complications was moderated by perceived control. For patients with low perceived control, 20% experiencing low anxiety versus 80% experiencing high anxiety had complications (OR = 2.0, 95% CI 1.1-3.9, p = 0.01). For patients with "high perceived control," there was no difference in risk (p > 0.05) based on anxiety level.

We concluded that anxiety predicts risk for complications in AMI patients, but that this relationship is attenuated in patients with "high perceived control." Interventions that increase patient perception of control may help diminish the link between anxiety and poorer outcomes. However, the key to determining the optimal interventions for anxious cardiac patients is understanding the mechanisms linking anxiety with CHD outcomes.

Proposed Mechanisms Linking Anxiety and CHD Outcomes

Although the mechanisms whereby anxiety might be associated with CHD outcomes are not entirely clear [62, 63], evidence suggests that there are two pathways linking anxiety and adverse CHD outcomes - 1) behavioral, and 2) physiological (see Fig. 4) [5-7, 10, 13, 17, 34, 64-66].

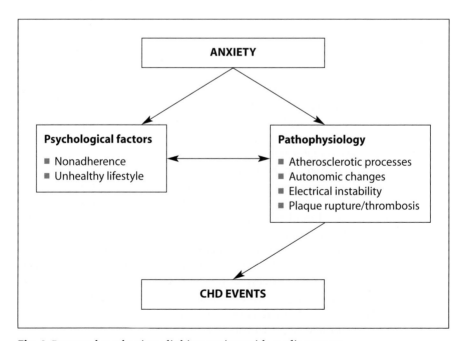

Fig. 4. Proposed mechanisms linking anxiety with cardiac events

■ Physiological Mechanisms

Autonomic nervous system abnormalities. Cardiac function is regulated by the two branches of the autonomic nervous system, the sympathetic nervous system, (SNS) and the parasympathetic nervous system (PNS). The SNS and PNS differ in their anatomy and organization, neurotransmitters, and physiologic effects. In brief, both physiological stressors, such as myocardial ischemia and psychological stressors, such as anxiety, activate the SNS, causing the release of two major catecholamines, epinephrine and norepinephrine. The heart is the first major organ to receive sympathetic input [67, 68]; in fact, the myocardium itself can synthesize norepinephrine [69]. In the short term, this so-called "fight or flight" phenomenon enables individuals to activate internal resources and counteract situations that threaten well-being.

Anxiety and the mental stress associated with it contribute to excessive SNS activation and catecholamine release [70]. There is ample evidence in the literature that anxiety and mental stress activate the SNS for both healthy persons and individuals with poor health. For example, healthy men who were exposed to mental arithmetic and noise stressors had a higher heart rate, and elevated epinephrine and norepinephrine levels upon exposure to a stressor [71]. Similarly, healthy males in another study exhibited an elevated heart rate and blood pressure during a speech stressor [72]. When exposed to mental stress, other healthy persons demonstrated higher sympathetic activity as evidenced by significant changes in heart rate and heart rate variability measures [73]. For patients with CHD who underwent mental stress, there was a positive correlation between plasma epinephrine levels and changes in heart rate, systolic blood pressure, and cardiac output [74].

When considering individuals with cardiac disease, those with elevated anxiety or prolonged stress and a history of AMI had higher plasma norepinephrine levels than healthy volunteers, a finding that is consistent with SNS activation [75]. Likewise, patients undergoing cardiac catheterization manifested higher norepinephrine, but not epinephrine, levels during mental stress testing [76].

In contrast to the SNS, the role of the PNS is to conserve and restore energy. It has been shown that both healthy volunteers with high anxiety and patients with generalized anxiety disorder have lower vagal tone than those with lower anxiety [77, 78]. This weak vagal tone allows sympathetic activity to predominate.

Baroreceptors detect pressure and volume changes and either inhibit or excite the sympathetic and parasympathetic nervous systems. For example, if the baroreceptors sense hypotension, they stimulate the SNS, producing norepinephrine release, tachycardia, vasoconstriction and contractility.

Only recently has anxiety been associated with impaired baroreflex sensitivity for cardiac patients. Watkins and colleagues reported that baroreflex control for patients with AMI and high anxiety was about 20% lower than for patients with AMI and lower anxiety [79].

Cardiovascular reactivity (CVR) refers to a "generalized propensity to respond to behavioral stimuli with cardiovascular reactions of a certain magnitude" [80].

For example, patients with exaggerated CVR experience frequent, pronounced, and sustained changes in blood pressure, heart rate, stroke volume, and total peripheral resistance. Increased CVR may contribute to the development of cardiac disease [10] and be useful in identifying postinfarction patients who are at risk for reinfarction or stroke [81].

Proposed models of the relationship between psychological influences and heart disease generally emphasize the role of the autonomic nervous system [82-84]. One pathophysiologic model accounts for the relationships between acute, episodic, and chronic psychological factors and coronary artery disease (CAD) [83]. According to the model, acute psychological factors, such as anger and mental activity, stimulate autonomic nervous system activity, which in turn triggers production of catecholamines, increases heart rate and blood pressure, decreases plasma volume, constricts coronary arteries, and increases cardiac demand, platelet activity, coagulation, and inflammation. As a result, patients are more prone to thrombogenesis, arrhythmogenesis, altered heart rate variability, increased myocardial oxygen demand, myocardial ischemia, and impaired ventricular function.

Thrombogenesis. High anxiety may contribute to platelet aggregation and recurrent thrombus formation [85, 86]. Evidence suggests that both epinephrine and norepinephrine function as platelet agonists [85, 87] and that epinephrine accelerates hemostasis and fibrinolysis [88]. During mental stress, healthy volunteers had higher norepinephrine and epinephrine levels, increased platelet activation, increased hematocrit levels, and a lower plasma volume [89]. In another study of healthy volunteers, mental stress also increased coagulation and stimulated the fibrinolytic system [90].

Similar results have been reported for patients with cardiac disease. When exposed to mental stress, patients with AMI experienced increased platelet aggregation, formed more circulating platelet aggregates, and developed higher plasma and serum thromboxane B_2 levels than healthy controls [91]. Patients with angina who underwent mental stress testing tended towards platelet activation more than healthy controls [92]. In a review paper, von Kanel concluded that patients with atherosclerosis who experience mental stress may tend towards hypercoagulation due to endothelial dysfunction and reduced fibrinolysis [88]. Ghiadoni and associates [93] reported that healthy persons developed endothelial dysfunction for up to four hours after exposure to mental stress.

Arrhythmogenesis. Enhanced sympathetic stimulation is one cause of cardiac dysrhythmias for patients with cardiac disease [94-96]. In addition, acute psychological insults are capable of causing lethal ventricular dysrhythmias [95, 97, 98]. In research conducted prior to routine beta-blocker use for AMI, patients with AMI and either ventricular dysrhythmias or sinus tachycardia had increased circulating catecholamine levels [99]. Patients with frequent ventricular ectopy but no history of AMI were more anxious than age- and sex-matched medical-surgical patients [100]. An association between high anxiety and prolonged QTc intervals has been reported and may involve high risk for lethal cardiac dysrhythmias [101].

Several researchers have induced mental stress in patients with heart disease. In one study, patients with ventricular dysrhythmias had more ectopy during a mildly stressful interview than during control time periods [102]. In another study, patients had significantly more ventricular dysrhythmias during psychological stress testing than during a control period [98]. For patients with AMI, mental stress contributed to a shorter mean ventricular refractory period, as well as to the onset of nonsustained ventricular tachycardia [103].

Increased myocardial oxygen demand. Mental stress increases heart rate and upsets the balance between myocardial oxygen supply and demand [104, 105]. Many investigators have documented the observation that mental stress increases heart rate [71, 76, 106-110]; however, whether these increases are clinically distinguishable or significant remains questionable. Others have reported that vascular resistance increases when patients with heart disease are exposed to mental stress but decreases in normal controls [111]. Remarkably, patients with heart disease have exhibited larger increases in systemic vascular resistance (SVR) during mental stress than during exercise [74]. In review papers, Rozanski and colleagues compared mental stress-induced ischemia with exercise-induced ischemia, pointing out that mental stress-induced ischemia is often associated with a sudden onset, smaller heart rate elevation, higher blood pressure, and lower double product (heart rate x systolic blood pressure) [105, 112].

Myocardial ischemia. Mental stress is a potent trigger for myocardial ischemia [84, 113]. In fact, mental stress can induce ischemia at lower levels of cardiac demand than exercise [83, 114]. Furthermore, there have been reports of mental stress causing complete coronary artery occlusion [115] or AMI [116]. It is notable that, in fact, patients often report that stress caused their AMI [117, 118].

For patients with atherosclerosis, a catecholamine surge can cause myocardial ischemia due to increased myocardial oxygen demand [84]. Patients with AMI were more anxious 0-2 hours before their AMI than 24-26 hours after the AMI [113]. In a review paper, Kubzansky and associates pointed out that anxiety may cause rapid blood pressure changes and subsequent atherosclerotic plaque rupture [119].

Mental stress should trigger coronary vasodilation due to increased myocardial oxygen demand; however, this compensatory mechanism was absent in patients with Coronary Artery Disease (CAD) [120]. Indeed, mental stress has also been shown to result in the vasoconstriction of coronary arteries, resulting in a decrease in coronary flow velocity in patients with CAD [106]. Yeung and colleagues [76] reported that stenosed or irregular coronary artery segments significantly constrict in response to mental stress, whereas smooth segments remain unchanged or dilated. Legault and colleagues reported that 49% of the patients they examined experienced stress-induced ischemia. They concluded that patients with more severe coronary artery stenoses were the most likely to experience stress-induced ischemia [121]. Furthermore, mental stress has been shown to cause coronary artery vasoconstriction in even normal coronary artery segments for patients with and without CAD [107]. In contrast, other researchers have found that neither normal nor stenotic coronary artery segments changed diameter in response to mental stress [114].

Although the mechanism is not entirely clear, experts have proposed that endothelial dysfunction makes the coronary arteries more sensitive to the constrictor effects of catecholamines [122]. Mental stress increases catecholamine levels and, thus, in the setting of endothelial dysfunction, can cause coronary constriction [115]. Interestingly, others have documented the observation that, during mental stress, coronary flow reserve was lower in myocardial regions without significant epicardial stenosis than in regions with significant stenosis, a finding that also may reflect microvascular dysfunction [123].

Stress-induced ischemic events may occur at relatively low and commonly experienced heart rates, and they may even go unnoticed by patients [109]. The results of another study showed that patients who underwent coronary angiography experienced two time periods of stress: the first while they awaited the results of their procedure, and the second, which was relatively less stressful, while they adjusted to their diagnosis and treatment plan [124]. There were more episodes of silent ischemia during the more stressful time period. Furthermore, patients with a higher norepinephrine level had more of these episodes and experienced longer total ischemic times. Compared to patients without silent ischemia, patients with ischemia reported more social dysfunction, anxiety, dysphoria, and severe depression during the stressful time period.

Finally, patients may hyperventilate in response to acute anxiety. Rasmussen and colleagues reported that hyperventilation can induce coronary artery spasm, a condition that impairs coronary blood flow [125].

In their review paper, Strike and Steptoe emphasized five points: 1) patients with heart disease are more likely to experience mental stress-induced myocardial ischemia (MSIMI), 2) patients with MSIMI are usually asymptomatic, 3) most patients with MSIMI also experience exercise-induced ischemia, 4) the rates of reported MSIMI are highly variable, and 5) most of this research has been conducted with male patients [126]. MSIMI is an important predictor of poor prognosis [126].

Impaired ventricular function. When patients with CHD and exercise-induced, wall-motion abnormalities were exposed to a mental stressor, 72% demonstrated stress-induced wall-motion abnormalities that were similar to exercise-induced wall-motion abnormalities [127]. In addition, 36% of the patients had a 5% or greater drop in their ejection fraction. Yet, 83% of these ischemic patients were asymptomatic, and, as a result, they were unaware that their condition had worsened. In another study, 53% of patients with CHD developed a new wall-motion abnormality when exposed to stress [128]; and, in still another study, patients with cardiac disease whose ejection fraction did not increase by 5% or more during exercise experienced a lower ejection fraction during mental stress [108]. With exposure to mental stress, patients with AMI developed impaired ventricular function as evidenced by a significant increase in pulmonary capillary wedge pressure and decrease in stroke volume [129]. Other authors have also reported wall motion abnormalities or decreased ejection fraction with mental stress [74, 108, 109, 111, 121, 130-132].

Mental stress affects not only systolic function, but also diastolic function. Patients with CAD experienced diastolic dysfunction and increases in blood pressure, heart rate and rate pressure product during a mental stressor [110]. Interestingly, this diastolic dysfunction was not accompanied by either systolic dysfunction or ST-segment ECG changes. In another study, patients with heart failure (HF) showed evidence of increased ventricular stiffness and high left ventricular filling pressures during mental stress [133].

The effects of mental stress extend beyond research settings. Patients with cardiac disease routinely experience stressful situations during the course of everyday life. Blumenthal and colleagues found that patients who developed ischemia and wall motion abnormalities in response to mental stress in a laboratory setting were more likely to experience ambulatory ischemia [134].

Patients with CAD were exposed to a series of mental stresses followed by a physical stressor. During the mental stressor, 21 of 29 patients (72%) with exercise-induced wall-motion abnormalities also demonstrated stress-induced wall-motion abnormalities. Additionally, 36% of the participants had a 5% or greater drop in their ejection fraction [127]. The majority of patients (65%) with exercise-induced wall-motion changes also developed mental stress-induced wall-motion changes.

Behavioral Mechanisms

Experts have hypothesized that behavioral mechanisms are another link between anxiety and cardiac disease. Compared with non-anxious individuals, those with high anxiety may eat an unhealthy diet [135-137], smoke [119, 135-137], consume drugs or alcohol, [135, 137], fail to adhere to therapy [85], sleep poorly [135, 137], and be physically inactive [135-137]. These harmful behaviors are associated with the incidence and progression of cardiac disease [135]. Far less is known about the potential behavioral mechanisms linking anxiety with adverse cardiac outcomes.

Summary

Anxiety is common among cardiac patients and should be treated to enhance recovery and decrease patients' risk of subsequent cardiac events. One of the most important areas for future research is elucidating the mechanisms whereby anxiety causes poorer outcomes in AMI patients. The mechanisms (either physiological or behavioral) whereby anxiety is related to poorer short and long term outcomes in AMI patients have yet to be elucidated. Research in this area is important to help clinicians determine the best ways to manage AMI patients to decrease the negative impact of anxiety. Without understanding the basic underlying mechanisms, it is difficult to know whether treatment should concentrate on pharmacological strategies such as beta-blocker therapy to decrease SNS responses to anxiety or more directly on anti-anxiety drug therapy. The role of nonpharmacologic strategies that decrease psychophysiologic arousal also should be investigated.

Disclaimer Statement

The opinions or assertions contained herein are the private views of the authors and are not to be construed as official or as reflecting the views of the Department of the Air Force or the Department of Defense.

Portions of this chapter have been previously published and are reprinted here with permission.

Acknowledgements

Some of the studies from which the data in this chapter were obtained were funded by the following grants: AACN Sigma Theta Tau Research Grant; Bennett-Puritan AACN Mentorship; Sigma Theta Tau; University of California Pacific Rim Center Grant

References

1. American Heart Association (2002) Heart disease and stroke statistics-2003 update. Dallas: American Heart Association
2. Chockalingam A, Balaguer-Vintro I, Achutti A et al (2000) The World Heart Federation's white book: impending global pandemic of cardiovascular diseases: challenges and opportunities for the prevention and control of cardiovascular diseases in developing countries and economies in transition. Canad J Cardiol 16:227-229
3. Reddy KS, Yusuf S (1998) Emerging epidemic of cardiovascular disease in developing countries. Circulation 97:596-601
4. Breithardt G, Borggrefe M, Fetsch T et al (1995) Prognosis and risk stratification after myocardial infarction. Eur Heart J 16 (Suppl G):10-19
5. Kubzansky LD, Kawachi I (2000) Going to the heart of the matter: do negative emotions cause coronary heart disease? J Psychosom Res 48:323-337
6. Kubzansky LD, Kawachi I, Weiss ST, Sparrow D (1998) Anxiety and coronary heart disease: a synthesis of epidemiological, psychological, and experimental evidence. Ann Behav Med 20:47-58
7. Rozanski A, Blumenthal JA, Kaplan J (1999) Impact of psychological factors on the pathogenesis of cardiovascular disease and implications for therapy. Circulation 99:2192-2217
8. Barlow DH (1988) Anxiety and its disorders. New York: Guilford
9. Lewis MA, Haviland JM (Eds) (1993) Fear and anxiety as emotional phenomena:

Clinical phenomenology, evolutionary perspectives, and information-processing mechanisms. New York: Guilford Press

10. Smith T W, Ruiz JM (2002) Psychosocial influences on the development and course of coronary heart disease: current status and implications for research and practice. J Consult Clin Psychol 70:548-568

11. Kubzansky LD, Kawachi I, Spiro A et al (1997) Is worrying bad for your heart? A prospective study of worry and coronary heart disease in the Normative Aging Study. Circulation 95:818-824

12. Crowe JM, Runions J, Ebbesen LSet al (1996) Anxiety and depression after acute myocardial infarction. Heart and Lung 25:98-107

13. Januzzi JL, Jr. Stern TA, Pasternak RC, DeSanctis RW (2000) The influence of anxiety and depression on outcomes of patients with coronary artery disease. Arch Intern Med 160:1913-1921

14. Malan SS (1992) Psychosocial adjustment following MI: current views and nursing implications. J Cardiovascul Nurs 6:57-70

15. Moser DK, Dracup K (1996) Is anxiety early after myocardial infarction associated with subsequent ischemic and arrhythmic events? Psychosom Med 58:395-401

16. Moser DK, McKinley S, Riegel B et al (2002) Perceived control reduces in-hospital complications associated with anxiety in acute myocardial infarction (abstract) Circulation 106:II-369

17. Sirois BC, Burg MM (2003) Negative emotion and coronary heart disease. A review. Behav Mod 27:83-102

18. Mayou RA, Gill D, Thompson DR et al (2000) Depression and anxiety as predictors of outcome after myocardial infarction. Psychosom Med 62:212-219

19. Moser DK, Dracup K (1995) Psychosocial recovery from a cardiac event: the influence of perceived control. Heart and Lung 24:273-280

20. Rozanski A, Bairey CN, Krantz DS et al (1988) Mental stress and the induction of silent myocardial ischemia in patients with coronary artery disease. N Eng J Med 318:1005-1012

21. Rozanski A, Krantz DS, Bairey CN (1991) Ventricular responses to mental stress testing in patients with coronary artery disease. Pathophysiological implications. Circulation 83(4 Suppl):II-137-144

22. Lane D, Carroll D, Ring C et al (2000) Do depression and anxiety predict recurrent coronary events 12 months after myocardial infarction? QJM 93:739-744

23. Lane D, Carroll D, Ring C et al (2000) Effects of depression and anxiety on mortality and quality-of-life 4 months after myocardial infarction. J Psychosom Res 49:229-238

24. Lane D, Carroll D, Ring C et al (2001) Mortality and quality of life 12 months after myocardial infarction: effects of depression and anxiety. Psychosom Med 63:221-230

25. Mayou R (2000) Research as a basis for clinical care. J Psychosom Res 48:321-322

26. Maeland JG, Havik OE (1989) After the myocardial infarction. A medical and psychological study with special emphasis on perceived illness. Scand J Rehabil Med Suppl 22:1-87

27. Rose SK, Conn VS, Rodeman BJ (1994) Anxiety and self-care following myocardial infarction. Issues in Mental Health Nursing 15:433-444

28. Sullivan MD, LaCroix AZ, Baum C et al (1997) Functional status in coronary artery

disease: a one-year prospective study of the role of anxiety and depression. Am J Med 103:348-356

29. Sullivan MD, LaCroix AZ, Spertus J A, Hecht J (2000) Five-year prospective study of the effects of anxiety and depression in patients with coronary artery disease. Ame J Cardiol 86:1135-1138

30. Havik OE, Maeland JG (1990) Patterns of emotional reactions after a myocardial infarction. J Psychosom Res 34:271-285

31. Rosal MC, Downing J, Littman AB, Ahern DK (1994) Sexual functioning post-myocardial infarction: effects of beta-blockers, psychological status and safety information. J Psychosom Res 38:655-667

32. Sykes DH, Evans AE, Boyle DM et al (1989) Discharge from a coronary care unit: psychological factors. J Psychosom Res 33:477-488

33. Denollet J, Brutsaert DL (1998) Personality, disease severity, and the risk of long-term cardiac events in patients with a decreased ejection fraction after myocardial infarction. Circulation 97:167-173

34. Frasure-Smith N, Lesperance F, Talajic M (1995) The impact of negative emotions on prognosis following myocardial infarction: is it more than depression? Health Psychol 14:388-398

35. Thomas SA, Friedmann E, Wimbush F, Schron E (1997) Psychological factors and survival in the cardiac arrhythmia suppression trial (CAST): a re-examination. Am J Crit Care 6:116-126

36. Lin KM (2001) Biological differences in depression and anxiety across races and ethnic groups. J Clinic Psychiat 62 (Suppl 13):13-19

37. Lepine JP (2001) Epidemiology, burden, and disability in depression and anxiety. J Clinic Psychiat 62 (Suppl 13):4-10

38. Kirmayer LJ (2001) Cultural variations in the clinical presentation of depression and anxiety: implications for diagnosis and treatment. J Clinic Psychiat 62 (Suppl 13):22-28

39. DeJong MI, Chung ML, Roser LP et al (2004) A five-country comparison of anxiety early after acute myocardial infarction. Europ J Cardiovas Nursing 3:129-134

40. Derogatis LR, Melisaratos N (1983) The Brief Symptom Inventory: an introductory report. Psychologic Med 13:595-605

41. Draguns JG, Tanaka-Matsumi J (2003) Assessment of psychopathology across and within cultures: issues and findings. Behav Res Ther 41:755-776

42. Taylor-Piliae RE, Molassiotis A (2001) An exploration of the relationships between uncertainty, psychological distress and type of coping strategy among Chinese men after cardiac catheterization. J Advan Nursing 33:79-88

43. Leff JP (1973) Culture and the differentiation of emotional states. Bri J Psychiat 123:299-306

44. Mesquita B, Frijda NH (1992) Cultural variations in emotions: a review. Psychologic Bull 112:179-204

45. Scherer KR, Wallbott HG, Matsumoto D, Kudoh T (1988) Emotional experience in cultural context: a comparison between Europe, Japan, and the United States. In K. R. Scherer (Ed) Facets of Emotion: Recent Research (pp 5-30) Hillsdale, New Jersey: Lawrence Erlbaum Associates

46. Chiou A, Potempa K, Buschmann MB (1997) Anxiety, depression and coping meth-

ods of hospitalized patients with myocardial infarction in Taiwan. Int J Nursing Stud 34:305-311

47. Lepine JP (2001) Epidemiology, burden, and disability in depression and anxiety. J Clin Psychiat 62(Suppl 13):4-10

48. Derogatis LP (1993) BSI. Brief Symptom Inventory. Administration, scoring, and procedure manual. Minneapolis: National Compute Systems, Inc.

49. Legault SE, Joffe RT, Armstrong PW (1992) Psychiatric morbidity during the early phase of coronary care for myocardial infarction: association with cardiac diagnosis and outcome. Can J Psychiat 37:316-325

50. Brown N, Melville M, Gray D et al (1999) Quality of life four years after acute myocardial infarction: short form 36 scores compared with a normal population. Heart 81:352-358

51. Moser DK, Dracup K, McKinley S et al (2003) An international perspective on gender differences in anxiety early after acute myocardial infarction. Psychosom Me 65:511-516

52. Martin RL, Cloninger CR, Guze SB, Clayton PJ (1985) Mortality in a follow-up of 500 psychiatric outpatients. I. Total mortality. Arch Gen Psychiat 42:47-54

53. Haines AP, Imeson JD, Meade TW (1987) Phobic anxiety and ischaemic heart disease. Bri Med J (Clinical Research Ed) 295:297-299

54. Weissman MM, Markowitz JS, Ouellette R et al (1990) Panic disorder and cardiovascular/cerebrovascular problems: results from a community survey. Am J Psychiat 147:1504-1508

55. Eaker ED, Pinsky J, Castelli WP (1992) Myocardial infarction and coronary death among women: psychosocial predictors from a 20-year follow-up of women in the Framingham Study. Am J Epidemiol 135:854-864

56. Kawachi I, Colditz GA, Ascherio A et al (1994) Prospective study of phobic anxiety and risk of coronary heart disease in men. Circulation 89:1992-1997

57. Kawachi I, Sparrow D, Vokonas PS, Weiss ST (1994) Symptoms of anxiety and risk of coronary heart disease. The Normative Aging Study. Circulation 90:2225-2229

58. Herrmann C, Brand-Driehorst S, Kaminsky B et al (1998) Diagnostic groups and depressed mood as predictors of 22-month mortality in medical inpatients. Psychosom Med 60:570-577

59. Herrmann C, Brand-Driehorst S, Buss U, Ruger U (2000) Effects of anxiety and depression on 5-year mortality in 5,057 patients referred for exercise testing. J Psychosom Res 48:455-462

60. Welin C, Lappas G, Wilhelmsen L (2000) Independent importance of psychosocial factors for prognosis after myocardial infarction. J Intern Med 247:629-639

61. Bunker SJ, Colquhoun DM, Esler MD et al (2003) "Stress" and coronary heart disease: psychosocial risk factors. Med J Aust 178:272-276

62. Hachamovitch R, Chang JD, Kuntz RE et al (1995) Recurrent reversible cardiogenic shock triggered by emotional distress with no obstructive coronary disease. Am Heart J 129:1026-1028

63. Januzzi JL, Jr Stern TA, Pasternak RC, DeSanctis RW (2000) The influence of anxiety and depression on outcomes of patients with coronary artery disease. Arch Intern Med 160:1913-1921

64. Carney RM, Freedland KE, Stein PK (2000) Anxiety, depression, and heart rate variability. Psychosom Med 62:84-87
65. Lesperance F, Frasure-Smith N (1996) Negative emotions and coronary heart disease: getting to the heart of the matter. Lancet 347:414-415
66. Sheps DS, Sheffield D (2001) Depression, anxiety, and the cardiovascular system: the cardiologist's perspective. J Clin Psychiat 62(Suppl 8):12-16
67. Middlekauff HR (1997) Mechanisms and implications of autonomic nervous system dysfunction in heart failure. Curr Opin Cardiol 12:265-275
68. Rundqvist B, Elam M, Bergmann-Sverrisdottir Y et al (1997) Increased cardiac adrenergic drive precedes generalized sympathetic activation in human heart failure. Circulation 95:169-175
69. Mann DL (1999) Mechanisms and models in heart failure: a combinatorial approach. Circulation 100:999-1008
70. Fehder WP (1999) Alterations in immune response associated with anxiety in surgical patients. CRNA 10:124-129
71. Sgoutas-Emch SA, Cacioppo JT, Uchino BN et al (1994) The effects of an acute psychological stressor on cardiovascular, endocrine, and cellular immune response: a prospective study of individuals high and low in heart rate reactivity. Psychophysiol 31:264-271
72. Baggett HL, Saab PG, Carver CS (1996) Appraisal, coping, task performance, and cardiovascular responses during the evaluated speaking task. Personal Soc Psychol Bull 22:483-494
73. Madden K, Savard GK (1995) Effects of mental state on heart rate and blood pressure variability in men and women. Clin Physiol 15:557-569
74. Goldberg AD, Becker LC, Bonsall R et al (1996) Ischemic, hemodynamic, and neurohormonal responses to mental and exercise stress: experience from the Psychophysiological Investigations of Myocardial Ischemia Study (PIMI). Circulation 94:2402-2409
75. Kohn LM, Sleet DA, Carson JC, Gray RT (1983) Life changes and urinary norepinephrine in myocardial infarction. J Hum Stress 9:38-45
76. Yeung AC, Vekshtein VI, Krantz DS et al (1991) The effect of atherosclerosis on the vasomotor response of coronary arteries to mental stress. N Eng J Med 325:1551-1556
77. Thayer JF, Friedman BH, Borkovec TD (1996) Autonomic characteristics of generalized anxiety disorder and worry. Biol Psychiat 39:255-266
78. Watkins LL, Grossman P, Krishnan R, Sherwood A (1998) Anxiety and vagal control of heart rate. Psychosom Med 60:498-502
79. Watkins LL, Blumenthal JA, Carney RM (2002) Association of anxiety with reduced baroreflex cardiac control in patients after acute myocardial infarction. Am Heart J 143:460-466
80. Manuck SB (1994) Cardiovascular reactivity in cardiovascular disease: "Once more unto the breach". Int J Behav Med 1:4-31
81. Manuck SB, Olsson G, Hjemdahl P, Rehnqvist N (1992) Does cardiovascular reactivity to mental stress have prognostic value in postinfarction patients? A pilot study. Psychosom Med 54:102-108
82. Kamarck T, Jennings JR (1991) Biobehavioral factors in sudden cardiac death. Psychol Bull 109:42-75

83. Kop WJ (1999) Chronic and acute psychological risk factors for clinical manifestations of coronary artery disease. Psychosom Med 61:476-487

84. Krantz DS, Kop WJ, Santiago HT, Gottdiener JS (1996) Mental stress as a trigger of myocardial ischemia and infarction. Cardiol Clin 14:271-287

85. Frasure-Smith N, Lesperance F, Talajic M (1995) The impact of negative emotions on prognosis following myocardial infarction: is it more than depression? Health Psychol 14:388-398

86. Hjemdahl P, Larsson PT, Wallen NH (1991) Effects of stress and beta-blockade on platelet function. Circulation 84(6 Suppl):VI-44-VI-61

87. Markovitz JH, Matthews KA (1991) Platelets and coronary heart disease: potential psychophysiologic mechanisms. Psychosom Med 53:643-668

88. von Kanel R, Mills PJ, Fainman C, Dimsdale JE (2001) Effects of psychological stress and psychiatric disorders on blood coagulation and fibrinolysis: a biobehavioral pathway to coronary artery disease? Psychosom Med 63:531-544

89. Patterson SM, Krantz DS, Gottdiener JS et al (1995) Prothrombotic effects of environmental stress: changes in platelet function, hematocrit, and total plasma protein. Psychosom Med 57:592-599

90. Jern C, Eriksson E, Tengborn L et al (1989) Changes of plasma coagulation and fibrinolysis in response to mental stress. Thromb Haemo 62:767-771

91. Grignani G, Soffiantino F, Zucchella M et al (1991) Platelet activation by emotional stress in patients with coronary artery disease. Circulation 83(4 Suppl):II-128-II-136

92. Wallen NH, Held C, Rehnqvist N, Hjemdahl P (1997) Effects of mental and physical stress on platelet function in patients with stable angina pectoris and healthy controls. Eur Heart J 18:807-815

93. Ghiadoni L, Donald AE, Cropley M et al (2000) Mental stress induces transient endothelial dysfunction in humans. Circulation 102:2473-2478

94. Lown B, Verrier RL (1976) Neural activity and ventricular fibrillation. N Eng J Med 294:1165-1170

95. Lown B, Verrier RL, Rabinowitz SH (1977) Neural and psychologic mechanisms and the problem of sudden cardiac death. Am J Cardiol 39:890-902

96. Middlekauff HR, Mark AL (1998) The treatment of heart failure: the role of neurohumoral activation. Int Med 37:112-122

97. Brodsky MA, Sato DA, Iseri LT et al (1987) Ventricular tachyarrhythmia associated with psychological stress: the role of the sympathetic nervous system. JAMA 257:2064-2067

98. Lown B (1987) Sudden cardiac death: biobehavioral perspective. Circulation 76:I-186-I-196

99. Nadeau RA, de Champlain J (1979) Plasma catecholamines in acute myocardial infarction. Am Heart J 98:548-554

100. Katz C, Martin RD, Landa B, Chadda KD (1985) Relationship of psychologic factors to frequent symptomatic ventricular arrhythmia. Am J Med 78:589-594

101. Fava M, Abraham M, Pava J et al (1996) Cardiovascular risk factors in depression: the role of anxiety and anger. Psychosom 37:31-37

102. Lown B, DeSilva RA, Reich P, Murawski BJ (1980) Psychophysiologic factors in sudden cardiac death. Am J Psychiat 137:1325-1335

103. Tavazzi L, Zotti AM, Rondanelli R (1986) The role of psychologic stress in the gen-

esis of lethal arrhythmias in patients with coronary artery disease. Eur Heart J 7(Suppl A):99-106

104. Cordero DL, Cagin NA, Natelson BH (1995) Neurocardiology update: role of the nervous system in coronary vasomotion. Cardiovasc Res 29:319-328

105. Rozanski A, Krantz DS, Bairey CN (1991) Ventricular responses to mental stress testing in patients with coronary artery disease: pathophysiological implications. Circulation 83(Suppl 4):II-137-144

106. Kop WJ, Krantz DS, Howell RH et al (2001) Effects of mental stress on coronary epicardial vasomotion and flow velocity in coronary artery disease: relationship with hemodynamic stress responses. J Am Coll Cardiol 37:1359-1366

107. Lacy CR, Contrada RJ, Robbins ML et al (1995) Coronary vasoconstriction induced by mental stress (simulated public speaking) Am J Cardiol 75:503-505

108. LaVeau PJ, Rozanski A, Krantz DS et al (1989) Transient left ventricular dysfunction during provocative mental stress in patients with coronary artery disease. Am Heart J 118:1-8

109. Mazzuero G, Guagliumi G, Bosimini E et al (1989) Effects of psychophysiological activation on coronary flow, cardiac electrophysiology and central hemodynamics in patients with ischemic heart disease. Biblio Cardiol 47-58

110. Okano Y, Utsunomiya T, Yano K (1998) Effect of mental stress on hemodynamics and left ventricular diastolic function in patients with ischemic heart disease. Jap Circ J 62:173-177

111. Jain D, Shaker SM, Burg M et al (1998) Effects of mental stress on left ventricular and peripheral vascular performance in patients with coronary artery disease. J Am Coll Cardiol 31:1314-1322

112. Rozanski A, Blumenthal JA, Kaplan J (1999) Impact of psychological factors on the pathogenesis of cardiovascular disease and implications for therapy. Circulation 99:2192-2217

113. Mittleman MA, Maclure M, Sherwood JB et al (1995) Triggering of acute myocardial infarction onset by episodes of anger. Circulation 92:1720-1725

114. L'Abbate A, Simonetti I, Carpeggiani C, Michelassi C (1991) Coronary dynamics and mental arithmetic stress in humans. Circulation 83(4 Suppl):II-94-II-99

115. Papademetriou V, Gottdiener JS, Kop WJ et al (1996) Transient coronary occlusion with mental stress. Am Heart J 132:1299-1301

116. Gelernt MD, Hochman JS (1992) Acute myocardial infarction triggered by emotional stress. Am J Cardiol 69:1512-1513

117. Marmot MG (1986) Does stress cause heart attacks? Postgrad Med J 62:683-686

118. Wielgosz AT, Nolan RP (2000) Biobehavioral factors in the context of ischemic cardiovascular diseases. J Psychosom Res 48:339-345

119. Kubzansky LD, Kawachi I, Weiss ST, Sparrow D (1998) Anxiety and coronary heart disease: a synthesis of epidemiological, psychological, and experimental evidence. Ann Behav Med 20:47-58

120. Dakak N, Quyyumi AA, Eisenhofer G et al (1995) Sympathetically mediated effects of mental stress on the cardiac microcirculation of patients with coronary artery disease. American Journal of Cardiology 76:125-130

121. Legault SE, Freeman MR, Langer A, Armstrong PW (1995) Pathophysiology and

time course of silent myocardial ischaemia during mental stress: clinical, anatomical, and physiological correlates. British Heart Journal 73:242-249

122. Vita JA, Treasure CB, Yeung AC et al (1992) Patients with evidence of coronary endothelial dysfunction as assessed by acetylcholine infusion demonstrate marked increase in sensitivity to constrictor effects of catecholamines. Circulation 85:1390-1397

123. Arrighi JA, Burg M, Cohen IS et al (2000) Myocardial blood-flow response during mental stress in patients with coronary artery disease. Lancet 356:310-311

124. Freeman LJ, Nixon PG, Sallabank P, Reaveley D (1987) Psychological stress and silent myocardial ischemia. American Heart Journal 114:477-482

125. Rasmussen K, Ravnsbaek J, Funch-Jensen P, Bagger JP (1986) Oesophageal spasm in patients with coronary artery spasm. Lancet 1:174-176

126. Strike PC, Steptoe A (2003) Systematic review of mental stress-induced myocardial ischaemia. European Heart Journal, 24:690-703

127. Rozanski A, Bairey CN, Krantz DS et al (1988a) Mental stress and the induction of silent myocardial ischemia in patients with coronary artery disease. New England Journal of Medicine 318:1005-1012

128. Gottdiener JS, Krantz DS, Howell RH et al (1994) Induction of silent myocardial ischemia with mental stress testing: relation to the triggers of ischemia during daily life activities and to ischemic functional severity. Journal of the American College of Cardiology 24:1645-1651

129. Mazzuero G, Temporelli PL, Tavazzi L (1991) Influence of mental stress on ventricular pump function in postinfarction patients: an invasive hemodynamic investigation. Circulation 83(4 Suppl):II-145-II-154

130. Bairey CN, Krantz DS, Rozanski A (1990) Mental stress as an acute trigger of ischemic left ventricular dysfunction and blood pressure elevation in coronary artery disease. American Journal of Cardiology 66:28G-31G

131. Burg MM, Jain D, Soufer R et al (1993) Role of behavioral and psychological factors in mental stress-induced silent left ventricular dysfunction in coronary artery disease. Journal of the American College of Cardiology 22:440-448

132. Kuroda T, Kuwabara Y, Watanabe S et al (2000) Effect of mental stress on left ventricular ejection fraction and its relationship to the severity of coronary artery disease. European Journal of Nuclear Medicine 27:1760-1767

133. Giannuzzi P, Shabetai R, Imparato A et al (1991) Effects of mental exercise in patients with dilated cardiomyopathy and congestive heart failure: An echocardiographic doppler study. Circulation 83(4 Suppl):II-155-II-165

134. Blumenthal JA, Jiang W, Waugh RA et al (1995) Mental stress-induced ischemia in the laboratory and ambulatory ischemia during daily life: association and hemodynamic features. Circulation 92:2102-2108

135. Buselli EF, Stuart EM (1999) Influence of psychosocial factors and biopsychosocial interventions on outcomes after myocardial infarction. J Cardiovasc Nursing 13:60-72

136. Hayward C (1995) Psychiatric illness and cardiovascular disease risk. Epidemiol Rev 17:129-138

137. Sirois BC, Burg MM (2003) Negative emotion and coronary heart disease. A review. Behav Modif 27:83-102

Chapter 9

Anxiety, Depressive Symptoms and Heart Transplantation

S. Zipfel ▪ A. Schneider ▪ J. Jünger ▪ W. Herzog

▨ Introduction

For patients suffering from terminal heart failure, orthotopic heart transplantation has become an established means of treatment. So far, over 50000 heart transplantations (HTx) have been performed in 271 transplantation centres around the world. It has been demonstrated that 1-year survival rates are over 80 percent; the mean survival time for HTx-patients has reached nearly 10 years, with a consecutive yearly mortality rate of 4 percent [1]. As a consequence, an increasing number of patients are reaching a long-time survival of more than 10 years [2, 3].

Given that the acute surgical and immunological problems of the transplantation procedure have been largely resolved, interest in the psychosocial implications for the patient and his or her immediate environment has intensified. A number of studies have shown a considerable improvement in quality of life after successful heart transplantation [4, 5]. Nowadays psychological evaluation and psychotherapeutic counselling are integrated in most successful transplant programs.

Over the past 30 years or so, since the early days of transplantation medicine, a dramatic change in the perspective of psychosocial research in heart transplantation has been observed. In the early days, psychosocial research focused on acceptance of the transplanted organ [6]. The major research focus in this field now concentrates on the identification of particular stressors and coping strategies in different phases of transplantation.

The following chapters will focus primarily on anxiety and depressive symptoms in different phases of heart transplantation [7].

Waiting Period

Studies investigating psychosocial aspects of the pre-operative phase have demonstrated enormous distress on patients prior to the operation. During the waiting period, a majority of patients experience a marked worsening in their physical condition, and 30% of the patients die. The already-stressful situation for patients on waiting lists has grown worse in recent years due to the rising demand for organs and a coincidental stagnation or even decline in public willingness to provide them. As a consequence, the waiting period has lengthened and patient survival rate has decreased.

Kuhn et al. [7] described this particular phase as a "dance with the dead." In cases where patients improve and stabilize, they often become ambivalent about whether their decision for HTx is too early; in cases where there is a rapid decline in their somatic condition, they worry about whether an adequate donor organ can be found in time. This ambivalence with respect to their own decision, as well as to the advice of their physicians, creates tremendous psychological stress for both patient and family members. In a cross-sectional study on HTx-patients on the waiting list, Magni and Bogherini [8] found that 35% of the patients studied suffered from anxiety disorders and over 20% suffered from marked depressive symptoms. Kuhn et al. [7] diagnosed at least one psychiatric disorder in 63.8% of their patients on the waiting list for HTx, and Lang et al. [9], in 48% of patients (Review: Zipfel and Bergmann [10]). According to DSM-IV [11], Trumper and Appleby [12] found clinically significant psychiatric symptoms in 39% of their patients waiting for a transplant. Major depressive episodes were the most frequent psychiatric disorder, followed by generalized anxiety disorders. In addition, Triffaux et al. [13] found that 18% of the patients in the sample of waiting patients they investigated had an axis-II-disorder (personality disorder). Bunzel [14] described the situation faced by these patients - i.e., hoping for someone's death in order to get the donor organ - as very burdensome. From her intimate knowledge of HTx patients, she got the impression that a substantial number of the depressive, as well as anxiety, symptoms were motivated by such highly ambivalent feelings. Studies focusing on the distress of the family members of HTx-patients show a high percentage of psychological distress [15]. At least a third of family members have reported that the waiting period resulted in a sustainable negative impact on their lives [16].

Because there has been a lack of reliable data on the course of depressive symptoms during the waiting period before HTx, we carried out a prospective study (Fig. 1) demonstrates that although patients shortly after being scheduled for surgery showed pronounced depressive symptoms (measured with the DS-scale by Zerssen [17]) compared with age matched controls, the level of depressive symptoms was further elevated to a clinically significant level after only four months on the waiting list.

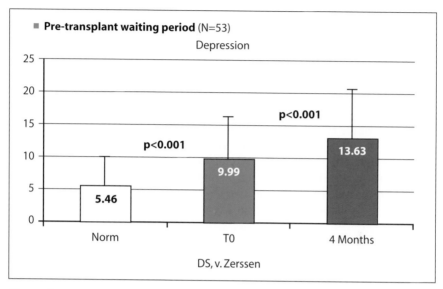

Fig. 1. The course of depressive symptoms during the first 4 months on the waiting list
DS = depression scale, v. Zerssen, T0 = time of pre-transplant evaluation

Peri- and Postoperative Phase

During the period following successful transplantation, HTx-patients often characterize themselves as "flying high," or feeling as though they were on "a second honey moon" [7, 18]. Surviving a life-threatening situation is associated with sub-euphoric feelings. In addition to a sense of understandable relief, part of the euphoria could be due to high doses of corticosteroids for rejection prevention. This well-being, however, is threatened by acute rejection of the donor organ or life-threatening infections from high-dose immuno-suppressant drugs.

The transition from a highly-supervised treatment in a specialised transplant centre to the patient's home environment or a lower-supervised rehabilitation centre marks a critical period. On one hand, there is a strong desire to come home after long-term hospitalisation, but, on the other hand, there are some worries in regard to patient care and a major new responsibility. Patients and families are increasingly confronted with daily tasks they did not have to perform previously, as they assume a more active role.

Kuhn et al. [7] emphasises that in this adaptation period, the HTx-patient has to learn to see himself or herself first as an individual and only second as a transplanted patient. In addition, the adaptation process to gain a stable and reliable body image takes some time and is challenged by postoperative weight gain, mostly due to high doses of immuno suppressant drugs. In terms of their relationships, patients and their partners are required to form a new perspective and reach a new state of equilibrium. This process should not be prolonged, resulting in an unbalanced situation that, according to Bunzel et al. [19], can be characterised as "patient benefit-partner suffer" situation. Overall studies investigating aspects of quality of life [20] show a significant improvement, particularly in terms of functional status and overall quality of life.

Dew et al. [21] used standardised clinical interviews (SCID) [22] to investigate the prevalence of psychiatric disorders in the post-operative period. They found at least one psychiatric disorder in 20.2% of HTx-patients. Major depressive episodes accounted for 17.3% of these, followed by transplant-related, posttraumatic stress disorder (13.7%) and adjustment disorders (10.0%). Interestingly, not a single HTx-patient met the criteria of anxiety disorders.

Family members of HTx-patients also showed transplant-related, posttraumatic stress disorder, with 7.7% of family members meeting all the diagnostic criteria and an additional 11.0% having marked symptoms of PTSD [23]. Risk populations included a) female relatives, b) relatives with a history of psychiatric disorders, and c) relatives with insufficient social support.

Long-Term Course

Thus far, there have been only a few studies investigating the psychosocial impact of long-term survival after HTx. However, a German nationwide survey conducted by cardiologists and heart surgeons [3] agreed unanimously on the relevance of psychosocial aspects to the long-term success of heart transplantation. Studies investigating the overall quality of life showed no significant difference between HTx patients and healthy controls [2]. However, long-term HTx patients showed a significantly reduced somatic functional level, in addition to a reduced sense of role accomplishment, pain and overall general health. It should be noted, that 79% of HTx-patients rated their general health as good to excellent. Compared with the general population, HTx-patients showed no difference regarding their level of anxiety symptoms (Fig. 2). However, long-term survivors

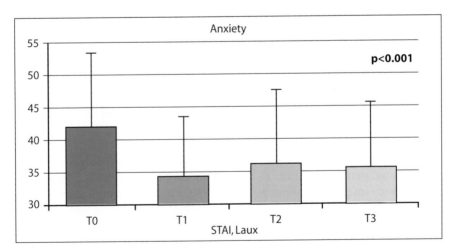

Fig. 2. Long-term course of anxiety in HTx patients (T0: before HTx; T1: 4 months after successful HTx; T2: 1 year after HTx; T3: about 5 years after HTx) STAI = state-trait-anxiety-inventory

considered themselves to be significantly more prone to depression, compared to normal controls. In a small sample, long-term HTx-patients scored relatively high on positive personal bodily feelings a mean of 5-years post-transplant [24]. However, compared with the one-year followup study, a significant decline in emotional well-being was demonstrated.

In our own long-term study of a representative sample of long-term survivors (mean 5.9 years; range 2-10 years; participation rate: 89%), more than one-third reported marked psychological problems. Mainly depressive symptoms, insomnia and psychomotoric disorders were found. With regard to quality of life, HTx patients scored high on nearly every dimension. This particular pattern of scoring seems to be a common finding in HTx-patients [2] and has to be understood as an expression of an idealized picture rather than a representation of the actual status. Some authors argue that this idealized perception may represent in part a marked thankfulness of the long-term HTx-survivors. Nevertheless, the depression scores increased steadily (at 8 weeks, 1 year, and 5.9 years - see Fig. 3) after successful HTx.

Over the long-term course, the level of depressive symptoms reached high preoperative depressive scores. The postoperative depressive symptoms were associated with subjective exhaustion. However, only a small association with the objective exercise tests could be found (ECG-treadmill). In a regression model, the psychological as well as the somatic status, in combination with social life factors, accounted of 77% of the variance of long-term depression scores. This finding underscores the interdependence between the physiological, psychological and social components of this type of depression. The pre-operative depression levels accounted for a third of the variance. Thus we found "state" as well as "trait" markers of long-term depression. In addition, the level of psychosocial support was an important factor in the degree of depressive sympto-

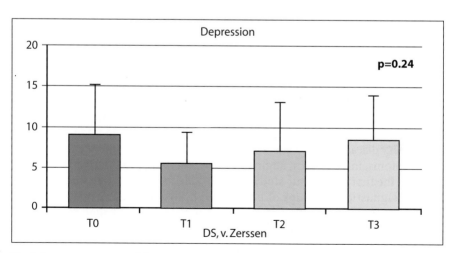

Fig. 3. Long-term course of depression in HTx patients (T0: prior to HTx; T1: 4 months after successful HTx; T2: 1 year after HTx; T3: about 5-years after HTx; DS = depression scale)

matology. Patients who rated their social network as supportive and strong showed the lowest depressive levels and, vice versa. There is an ongoing debate concerning the function of psychosocial support as a protective factor in cardiovascular disease. Psychosocial support can be seen as a link between depressive symptomatology and cardiovascular risk behavior. In this sense, the lack of psychosocial support has also been discussed as a "toxic" component of depressive symptoms [25].

Our findings are in line with studies investigating the course of depressive symptoms after HTx from the US [26] and Austria [8]. Dew et al. [23] investigated HTx-patients prospectively over a three-year-period using standardized clinical interviews (SCID-I) [22]. Their study demonstrated a significant increase in psychiatric disturbances, with an overall prevalence rate of 38.3% after three years. This rate was mainly due to an increase in depression (major depression accounted for 25.5%), as well as to adjustment disorders (which accounted for 20.8% of the psychiatric disturbances). In their study, depression was associated with patients who had a history of psychiatric disorders prior to HTx, and it was more prevalent in female patients who had waited more than six months for HTx. It was also found to be more prevalent in patients who had used an artifical heart prior to HTx. In addition, the level of physical fitness two months after HTx played an important role in the long-term course of depressive symptoms following HTx. The occurrence of a psychiatric disorder was also dependent on the quality of social support. In parallel with our findings, anxiety disorders played a marginal role in long-term HTx patients.

Clinical Subgroups

In our separate studies [27] of the extent and impact of psychological distress for patients with end-stage ischemic (ICMP) and dilated (DCMP) cardiomyopathy, we found that these two types of cardiomyopathy comprise the major distinct entities of patients with terminal heart failure awaiting heart transplantation [1].

Although both cardiomyopathy subgroups showed significantly increased levels of psychological distress compared to healthy controls, the direct comparison between both diagnostic subgroups showed significantly increased levels of depression and anxiety among patients with ischemic cardiomyopathy (ICMP). In addition, the reported levels of physical complaints were significantly increased in both patient groups. ICMP patients with an underlying coronary artery disease showed a tendency towards more pronounced cardiac-related symptoms, in particular, angina pectoris, compared to the DCMP patients. Thus, in the first part of our study, we were able to demonstrate that these two major diagnostic subgroups of patients with severe cardiomyopathy showed differences in psychological distress and, in some cases, in cardiac-related complaints in pre-transplant evaluation. Similar to our study, Trunzo et al. [28] found increased levels of depression among ICMP patients awaiting heart transplantation, compared with a non-ischemic group. The authors concluded that this finding might reflect patients' perception of how they themselves contributed to their illness, as this type of cardiomyopathy may have a more pronounced behavioral component in its pathology compared with the DCMP group. This conclusion is highly speculative, and to our knowledge it is only supported through one recent finding by Alla et al. [29], showing a significantly higher percentage of smokers in their subgroup of ICMP patients, compared with DCMP patients. Majani et al. [30] investigated the relationship between psychological profile and cardiological variables in a sample of patients covering the whole range of severity of chronic heart failure. Compared with DCMP patients, the subgroup of ICMP patients in their study reported lower satisfaction scores with physical functioning and physical appearance. In addition, the authors found a significantly reduced resistance to stress in their ICMP patients.

Psychosocial Predictors for Survival in HTx Patients

To date, there are only a few studies investigating the impact of psychosocial factors on survival in HTx-patients, in contrast to the numerous studies demonstrating the impact of depression on the course of coronary heart disease and in patients with chronic heart failure.

Thus far, only a single study using the "Millon Behavioral Health Inventory," (MBHI) and in particular, the "Life Threat Reactivity Scale", developed by Millon and associates [31], has demonstrated an association between a high score on this scale and an elevated mortality rate prior to transplantation [32]. Using a particular cutoff, the high-risk group showed a mortality rate of 42%, whereas in the low risk group, the mortality rate was only 18%. This scale covers areas like pessimism, sensitivity, trust and alienation. However, it should be noted that the authors did not use survival analyses, and that there was a lack of controlling the results for well known somatic risk factors.

Chacko et al. [33] and Harper et al. [34], from Texas Heart Institute in Houston, were among the first researchers who were able to demonstrate an association between preoperative psychological factors and postoperative survival after HTx. Using a standardised psychiatric interview and additional psychometric testing (e.g., an MBHI), they were able to identify predictors of survival. In particular, a dysfunctional preoperative coping style, as well as a lack of social support, were significant predictors of long-term survival after HTx. An additional axis-I-disorder was associated with prolonged postoperative hospitalization, whereas axis-II-disorder increased the risk of dysfunctional health behavior.

In our own study [27] of the influence of preoperatively assessed clinical and psychological data on pre- and post-transplant outcome, 21% of the entire sample died while waiting for a donor organ. With the exception of the NYHA-functional class for the subgroup of dilated cardiomyopathy, we could find no additional somatic or psychological predictors of survival before heart transplantation. The percentage of survival at one year and 4.4 years for the entire sample was 76.7% and 70.0%, respectively, and was, therefore, slightly higher than the survival rates of a representative German survey with a one-year survival rate of 71% [35]. It was also higher than a recently published one-year survival rate of 62% from a French transplant center [36]. However, our survival rates are lower, compared with the 81% survival rate recently published by the International Society of Heart and Lung Transplantation [1]. With standardized mortality rates in our patient sample of 15.2% for women and 7.7% for men, it is obvious that, even after heart transplantation, patients have a significantly shorter life expectancy than their age and sex-matched counterparts. Higher age of the recipient, as well as higher donor age, was associated with increased risk of post transplant mortality in the subgroup of ischemic cardiomyopathy patients. This finding is in accordance with recently published risk factors for post transplant survival [1].

In addition, the level of preoperative depression (Fig. 4), but not anxiety, was a significant predictor of survival in the subgroup of patients with ischemic cardiomyopathy, but not in the subgroup with dilated cardiomyopathy. This result remained constant even after adjustments for basic socio-demographic and somatic factors were made for both recipient and donor. To our knowledge, this is the first report linking pre-operative depression scores with post transplant survival. This might be due to the fact that the few other studies [33, 34] using hazard proportional models to predict post-transplant survival in heart transplantation did not subdivide their initial sample into the underlying diagnostic groups.

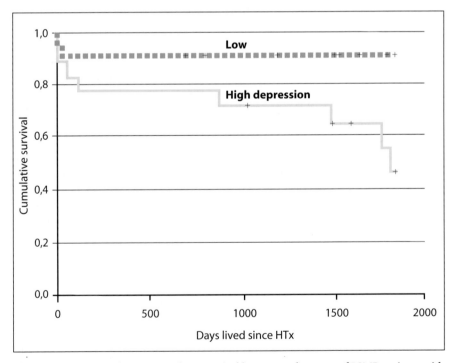

Fig. 4. Comparison of post-transplant survival between subgroups of ICMP patients with high (N = 19) and low (N = 21) preoperative depression scores (log rank: χ^2 = 5.18, p = 0.023)

Although to date our study provides the largest sample of patients for assessing and linking preoperative psychosocial factors and postoperative long-term outcome, we were not able to detect a specific pattern of deaths associated with an increased level of depression. This was most likely due both to the relatively small sample size in the various subgroups and to a variety of different causes of death after transplantation. Therefore, it remains speculative as to whether an increased level of depression is associated with a specific pathogenetic pathway.

However, Dew et al. [21] recently showed that postoperative depression was an independent predictor for cardiac allograft disease. Although transplant vasculopathy and native atherosclerosis are clinically and pathologically different entities, the pathogenesis of both diseases exhibits some common mechanisms. Deng et al. [37] state that both may be regarded as responses to injury within a broadened concept of the immune system. Alloantigens (e.g., on donor endothelial cells) or autoantigens (e.g., oxidized LDL-cholesterol) can be obtained from antigen- presenting cells by the T cells of the body's immune system. This may be one of the reasons why Aziz et al. [38] found a significantly higher incidence of coronary artery disease in patients with a former ICMP compared with DCMP patients, even 10 years after heart transplantation (35% vs. 9%, p = 0.02).

Over the past few years, an increasing number of studies have identified specific mechanisms known to increase the risk of death in patients with coronary heart disease (CHD), such as decreased vagal and increased sympathetic tone [39, 40], as well as affection of the platelets [41] or a possible association with inflammation processes [42]. However, heart transplant patients with a history of ischemic cardiomyopathy differ in many ways from patients with CHD. Shapiro et al. [43] showed that in HTx patients with a denervated heart, no functional reinnervation or other compensatory adaptation occurred up to one year after heart transplantation. Salmon et al. [44] found that the disrupted responses to a psychological stressor after HTx were due to the functional deficit in the innervation of the heart and a greater reliance on a hormonal response. However, recent findings [45] have shown significant sympathetic as well as parasympathetic reinnervation in long-term transplant patients. Further studies are needed to investigate the effect of depression in long-term transplanted patients on the autonomic nervous system.

A general point that applies to all patients with organ transplantation is the need for life-long immunosuppression as a prerequisite for good graft function. However, rates of noncompliance range between 20-50% in these patients, often leading to graft loss and death [46]. In a recent meta-analysis it was shown that depressed patients had a 3 times greater risk of noncompliance with medical treatment recommendation, compared with non-depressed patients [47]. In particular, Ziegelstein et al. [48] showed that patients with depression are less likely to follow recommendations to reduce cardiac risk factors during recovery from myocardial infarction. These findings may in part explain why ICMP patients with high depressive symptoms may experience a higher risk of post-HTx mortality. However, they do not explain the difference in susceptibility for depression and mortality between the two groups of cardiomyopathy patients.

Central Nervous Complication after HTx

After HTx, 30-60% of patients show neurological complications, due to the primary disease, intraoperative complications, metabolic encephalopathy, or to the neurotoxic side effects of the different immuno suppressants, as well as opportunistic infections. Particularly during a heart transplant operation, there is a certain risk for embolic complications as well as hypoxic problems [49]. Older studies have shown that up to 9% of HTx-patients develop a central embolic complication or cerebral bleeding with consecutive epileptic seizures [50]. In another study, Inoue et al. [51] compared central complications in patients with HTx, bypass surgery and cardiac valvular replacement. HTx-patients showed the highest complication rates (19.8%), followed by ACB-surgery (9.5%) and elective valvular replacement surgery (3.5%). A particular risk factor was preoperative circulation assistance.

Due to the need for high doses of glucocorticoids for rejection prevention after HTx , some HTx patients react with agitation, anxiety, sleep disturbances or major problems with cognitive function. In rare cases, a steroid-induced psychosis is observed [52]. In addition, some immuno suppressants, e.g., Cyclosporin-A, impact concentration and cognitive function [53].

■ Psychiatric and Psychosocial Interventions in HTx-Patients

There is a marked discrepancy between the number of studies demonstrating the prevalence of psychiatric comorbidity in HTx patients prior to and after HTx and few reports of structured psychosocial intervention programs.

Occasionally, there are reports varying in scope from the instruction of basic relaxation techniques necessary for attenuating agitation, anxiety and sleep disturbances [54], to more encompassing family interventions programs for fostering self-efficacy and family cohesion [55], and, finally, even more comprehensive psychoeducative, preoperative teaching programs [56]. A recent paper by Cupples and Streslow [57] summarised the initial results of the effectiveness of cognitive behavior in increasing patient compliance.

In Heidelberg, we implemented a "stepped" care program for HTx-patients and their family members. Every patient (and most of the time, their family as well) are contacted and seen personally for an intensive evaluation involving psychological testing prior to being scheduled for HTx. Our primary goal in making early, regular contact is the early identification of problematic areas. Our intent is not to exclude the patients from being scheduled for transplantation, but early on, to provide an effective psychosocial support for patients and their family members during the difficult periods of the transplantation process. Another element of our psychosocial intervention program is a regular outpatient meeting every four weeks for patients on the waiting list and their families. Besides practical information concerning the HTx procedure and living with a transplanted organ, psychological and social support is one of the most important issues. These groups are well accepted by the patients and their families.

In some circumstances, patients and whenever needed relatives get additional support by trained psychotherapists. Another important component of our program is a guided self-help group, particularly for patients after successful HTx. Besides organizing social events and providing mutual emotional support, the support group uses the Internet as a communication platform both within the self-help group and beyond the region affiliated to the Heidelberg transplant centre. This information platform has a high attraction for affected and interested people [58, 59].

There is far more research on the pharmacological side effects of antidepressive therapy in HTx patients. An observational trial found severe side effects in 20% of patients treated with a tricyclic antidepressant [60]. However, there are much more positive data on the rate of side effects in HTx-patients treated with SSRI, particularly Fluoxetine [61]. It should be noted, however, that there is a risk of severe interaction between SSRI and the anticoagulant Warfarin, a drug often used in patients with severe heart failure prior to transplantation.

For the antidepressant Nefazodone, which has a potentially sedative effect, an interaction with the immuno suppressant Cyclosporin A has been shown, leading to a 10-fold increased serum level of Cyclosporin-A [62]. Due to dangerous "drug-drug" interactions, patients taking immunosuppressants were strongly advised not to take Hypericinium as an herbal remedy [63, 64]. Triggered by strong interactions with the Cytochrom-450 3A4 enzyme, a dramatic decrease of Cyclosporin serum levels has been observed, creating the related danger of donor organ rejection. Herbal medications are particularly dangerous due to the fact that anyone can buy them over-the-counter, and to the fact that, increasingly, they are used to self-medicate for depressive symptoms.

In a recent German multicenter project, we changed our focus slightly to incorporate more preventative strategies. The aim of the study was, early on, to enhance the quality of life and healthy behavior in patients with milder forms of heart failure. Success in this type of endeavor is possible only by means of a very intensive interdisciplinary approach, including cardiologists, psychotherapists, cardiothoracic surgeons, and last but not least, by focusing in particular on the needs of patients and their families.

References

1. Hosenpud JD, Bennett LE, Keck BM et al (2000) The registry of the international society for heart and lung transplantation: seventeenth official report-2000. J Heart Lung Transplant 19:909-931
2. Hetzer R, Albert W, Hummel M et al (1997) Status of patients presently living 9 to 13 years after orthotopic heart transplantation. Ann Thorac Surg 64:1661-1668
3. Pethig K, Besser K, Heublein B, Wahlers T et al (1999) Koronare Vaskulopathie nach Herztransplantation-Einfluss von zeitlichem Auftreten, Schweregrad und Progredienz auf die Prognose im Langzeitverlauf. Z Kardiol 88:498-506

4. Grady KL, Jalowiec A, White WC et al (1996) Predictors of quality of life in patients with advanced heart failure awaiting transplantation. J Heart Lung Transplant 14:2-10

5. Frierson R, Tabler J, Spears R (1992) Heart transplantation. In: Craven J, Rodin G. Psychiatric aspects of organ transplantation. Oxford University Press 12:164-176

6. Castelnuovo-Tedesco P (1973) Organ transplant, body image, psychosis. Psychoanal Quart 42:349-363

7. Kuhn WF, Myers B, Brennan AF et al (1988) Psychopathology in heart transplant candidates. J Heart Transplant 7:223-226

8. Magni G, Bogherini G (1992) Psychosocial outcome after heart transplantation. In: Walter PJ (Ed) Quality of life after open heart surgery. Dordrecht: Kluwer Academic Press

9. Lang T, Klaghofer R, Buddeberg C (1997) [Psychiatric comorbidity and psychosocial markers in patients before heart, liver or lung transplantation]. Schweiz Med Wochenschr 127:1950-1960

10. Zipfel S, Bergmann G (1999) Psychosomatische Aspekte bei Herzschrittmacher und Herzoperation. In: Studt HH, Petzold ER (Eds) Psychotherapeutische Medizin. Berlin: de Gruyter 135-137

11. American Psychiatric Association (APA) (1994) Diagnostic and statistical manual of mental disorders (DSM-IV). Fourth edition. Washington, DC

12. Trumper A, Appleby L (2001) Psychiatric morbidity in patients undergoing heart, heart and lung, or lung transplantation. J Psychosom Res 50:103-105

13. Triffaux JM, Wauthy J, Bertrand J et al (2001) Psychological evolution and assessment in patients undergoing orthotopic heart transplantation. Eur Psychiatry 16:180-185

14. Bunzel B (1993) Herztransplantation: psychosoziale Grundlagen und Forschungsergebnisse zur Lebensqualität. Stuttgart, New York: Thieme

15. Nolan MT, Cupples SA, Brown MM et al (1992) Perceived stress and coping strategies among families of cardiac transplant candidates during the organ waiting period. Heart Lung 21:540-547

16. Collins EG, White WC, Jalowiec A (1996) Impact of the heart transplant waiting process on spouses. J Heart Lung Transplant 15:623-630

17. Zerssen D (1975) Depressionkala (D-S). Beltz, Weinheim

18. Christopherson LK (1987) Cardiac transplantation: a psychological perspective. Circulation 75:57-62

19. Bunzel B, Laederach HK, Schubert MT (1999) Patients benefit-partners suffer? The impact of heart transplantation on the partner relationship. Transpl Int 12:33-41

20. Dew MA (1998) Quality-of-life studies: organ transplantation research as an exemplar of past progress and future directions. J Psychosom Res 44:189-195

21. Dew MA, Roth LH, Schulberg HC et al (1996) Prevalence and predictors of depression and anxiety-related disorders during the year after heart transplantation. Gen Hosp Psychiatry 18(6 Suppl):48-61

22. Spitzer RL, Williams JB, Gibbon M, First MB (1992) The Structured Clinical Interview for DSM-III-R (SCID). I: History, rationale, and description. Arch Gen Psychiatry 49:624-629

23. Stukas AAJ, Dew MA, Switzer GE et al (1999) PTSD in heart transplant recipients and their primary family caregivers. Psychosomatics 40:212-221

24. Bunzel B, Laederach HK (1999) Long-term effects of heart transplantation: the gap between physical performance and emotional well-being. Scand J Rehabil Med 31:214-222

25. Fraser-Smith N, Lesperance F, Gravel G et al (2000) Social support, depression, and mortality during the first year after myocardial infarction. Circulation 101:1919-1924
26. Dew MA, Kormos RL, DiMartini AF et al (2001) Prevalence and risk of depression and anxiety-related disorders during the first three years after heart transplantation. Psychosomatics 42:300-313
27. Zipfel S, Schneider A, Wild B et al (2002) Effect of depressive symptoms on survival after heart transplantation. Psychosom Med 64:740-747
28. Trunzo JJ, Petrucci RJ, Carter A, Donofrio N (1999) Use of the MMPI and MMPI-2 in patients being evaluated for cardiac transplant. Psychol Rep 85:1105-1110
29. Alla F, Briancon S, Juilliere Y et al (2000) Differential clinical prognostic classifications in dilated and ischemic advanced heart failure: the EPICAL study. Am Heart J 139:895-904
30. Majani G, Pierobon A, Giardini A et al (1999) Relationship between psychological profile and cardiological variables in chronic heart failure. The role of patient subjectivity. Eur Heart J 20:1579-1586
31. Millon T, Green C, Meager R (1982) Millon Behavioral Health Inventory Manual, 3rd ed. Minneapolis, MN: National Computer Systems Inc.
32. Coffman KL, Brandwin M (1999) The Millon Behavioral Health Inventory Life Threat Reactivity Scale as a predictor of mortality in patients awaiting heart transplantation. Psychosomatics 40:44-49
33. Chacko RC, Harper RG, Gotto J, Young J (1996) Psychiatric interview and psychometric predictors of cardiac transplant survival. Am J Psychiatry 153:1607-1612
34. Harper RG, Chacko RC, Kotik HD et al (1998) Self-report evaluation of health behavior, stress vulnerability, and medical outcome of heart transplant recipients. Psychosom Med 60:563-569
35. Deng MC, De Meester JM, Smits JM et al (2000) Effect of receiving a heart transplant: analysis of a national cohort entered on to a waiting list, stratified by heart failure severity. Comparative Outcome and Clinical Profiles in Transplantation (COCPIT) Study Group. BMJ 321:540-545
36. Kirsch M, Baufreton C, Naftel DC et al (1998) Pretransplantation risk factors for death after heart transplantation: the Henri Mondor experience. J Heart Lung Transplant 7:268-277
37. Deng MC, Plenz G, Erren M et al (2000) Transplant vasculopathy: a model for coronary artery disease? Herz 25:95-99
38. Aziz T, Burgess M, Rahmann AN et al (2001) Cardiac transplantation for cardiomyopathy and ischemic heart disease: differences in outcome up to 10 years. J Heart Lung Transplant 20:525-33
39. Carney RM, Freedland KE, Stein PK (2000) Anxiety, depression, and heart rate variability. Psychosom Med 62:84-87
40. Gorman JM, Sloan RP (2000) Heart rate variability in depressive and anxiety disorders. Am Heart J 140:77-83
41. Camacho A, Dimsdale JE (2000) Platelets and psychiatry: lessons learned from old and new studies. Psychosom Med 62:326-336
42. Appels A, Bär FW, Bruggeman C, Baets M (2000) Inflammation, depressive symptomatology, and coronary artery disease. Psychosom Med 62:601-605

43. Shapiro PA, Sloan RP, Bagiella E et al (1996) Heart rate reactivity and heart period variability throughout the first year after heart transplantation. Psychophysiology 33:54-62

44. Salmon P, Stanford C, Mikahil G et al (2001) Hemodynamic and emotional responses to a psychological stressor after cardiac transplantation. Psychosom Med 63:289-99

45. Überfuhr P, Frey AW, Reichart B (2000) Vagal reinnervation in the long term after orthotopic heart transplantation. J Heart Lung Transplant 19:946-50

46. Bunzel B, Laederach HK (2000) Noncompliance in organ transplantation: a review. Wien Klin Wochenschr 12:423-440

47. DiMatteo MR, Lepper HS, Croghan TW (2000) Depression is a risk factor for non-compliance with medical treatment: meta-analysis of the effects of anxiety and depression on patient adherence. Arch Intern Med 160:2101-2107

48. Ziegelstein RC, Fauerbach JA, Stevens SS et al (2000) Patients with depression are less likely to follow recommendations to reduce cardiac risk during recovery from a myocardial infarction. Arch Intern Med 160:1818-1823

49. Padovan CS, Sostak P, Straube A (2000) Neurological complications after organ transplantation. Nervenarzt 71:249-258

50. Adair JC, Call GK, O'Connell JB, Baringer JR (1992) Cerebrovascular syndromes following cardiac transplantation. Neurology 42: 819-823

51. Inoue K, Luth JU, Pottkamper D et al (1998) Incidence and risk factors of perioperative cerebral complications. Heart transplantation compared to coronary artery bypass grafting and valve surgery. J Cardiovasc Surg 39:201-208

52. Wolkowitz OM, Reus VI, Canick J et al (1997) Glucocorticoid medication, memory and steroid psychosis in medical illness. Ann NY Acad Sci 82:381-396

53. Grimm M, Yeganehfar W, Laufer G et al (1996) Cyclosporine may affect improvement of cognitive brain function after successful cardiac transplantation. Circulation 94:1339-1345

54. Riedel-Keil B, Strenge H (1994) Psychologische Betreuung Herztransplantierter: Interventionsmethoden. In: Strenge H, Strauß B, Stauch C (editors) Ein neues Herz. Göttingen: Hogrefe 120-125

55. Johann B, Richter-Görge H (1999) Familientherapeutische Interventionen in der Betreuung von Transplantationspatienten. In: Johann B, Lange R (Eds) Psychotherapeutische Interventionen in der Transplantationsmedizin. Lengerich: Pabst Science Publishers 119-125

56. Berron K (1986) Transplant patients' perceptions about effective preoperative teaching. J Heart Transplant 5:162-165

57. Cupples SA, Streslow B (2001) Use of behavioral contingency contracting with heart transplant candidates. Prog Transplant 11:137-144

58. Schlehofer B, Zipfel S, Siwinska J et al (2001) A prospective follow-up study of the EUROPACT study group on psychosocial aspects in heart transplantation. Acta Chir Austriaca 33(Suppl):126

59. Hoevels R, Schlehofer B, Zipfel S et al (1999) Psychotherapeutische und psychosoziale Betreuung von Herztransplantationspatienten. In: Johann B, Lange R (editors) Psychotherapeutische Interventionen in der Transplantationsmedizin. Lengerich: Pabst Science Publishers 106-118

60. Kay J, Bienenfeld D, Slomowitz M et al (1991) Use of tricyclic antidepressants in recipients of heart transplants. Psychosomatics 32:165-170
61. Strouse TB, Fairbanks LA, Skotzko CE, Fawzy FI (1996) Fluoxetine and cyclosporine in organ transplantation: failure to detect significant drug interactions or adverse clinical events in depressed organ recipients. Psychosomatics 37:23-30
62. Wright DH, Lake KD, Bruhn PS, Emery RW (1999) Nefazodone and cyclosporine drug-drug interaction. J Heart Lung Transplant 18:913-915
63. Armstrong SC, Cozza KL (2001) Consultation-liaison psychiatry drug-drug inter-actions update. Psychosomatics 42:157-159
64. Turton-Weeks SM, Barone GW, Gurley BJ et al (2001) St John's Wort: a hidden risk for transplant patients. Progress in Transplantation 11:116-120

Chapter 10

Psychological Factors in Hypertension Development and Treatment

T. Rutledge

Introduction

This chapter begins with the ambitious aim of reviewing the evidence for psychosocial factors in the development and treatment of hypertension. The literature base is now nearly a century old, and comprises well over a thousand empirical and narrative manuscripts. The methodologies employed, psychological constructs of interest, and theoretical underpinnings in this research are many and varied, reflecting the numerous trends and cultural zeitgeists of the previous decades. At the time of this writing, the relationship between psychological factors and hypertension is a topic of growing interest, spurred by recent reviews and the continuing influx of prospective data from several large US-based cohort studies [1-4]. It is not the purpose of this paper to comprehensively review this extensive database. Rather, the intention is to provide a) an overview of the primary theories, methods of study and evidence for emotional factors in hypertension, with an emphasis on recent findings; b) a review of the multiple behavioral and physiological mechanisms proposed by researchers to bridge the association between psychological characteristics and blood pressure regulation, and c) a discussion of the evidence and implications for the treatment of psychological factors among patients with current or elevated risk for hypertension.

Overview

Hypertension, as readers will readily acknowledge, is a complex, heterogeneous entity with contributions from genetic and environmental sources. Even without considering the implications of the recent decision by the Joint National Committee (JNC) to create a new "prehypertensive" category [5] for individuals with systolic and diastolic blood pressures, falling between, respectively, 120-

139 mm Hg and 80-89 mm Hg, hypertension rates in modernized countries are alarmingly high. Current epidemiological estimates suggest that hypertension accounts for more than 10 million annual hospital visits in the US alone, and affects more than 40% of European adults [6]. The clinical relevance of these statistics will become clearer in the years ahead, but the prevalence of the condition is all the more disturbing in light of the poor awareness and undertreatment of hypertension in both Europe and North America [7].

The most common diagnosis of hypertension is essential or primary hypertension, in both cases inferring the lack of a specific biological cause for the condition. Treatments, pharmacological and otherwise, continue to evolve with medical advances, but remain of moderate efficacy in many cases, and are frequently accompanied by side effects that can significantly impair quality of life [8]. Treatment programs for high blood pressure are also long-term by default. Most medication-based treatments, in fact, are akin to life sentences. Although typically asymptomatic, the health consequences of hypertension are very serious, with virtually unassailable evidence suggesting a direct relationship between hypertension and the incidence of coronary artery disease and stroke. Combined with the release of the recent, empirically driven, JNC guidelines recognizing that cardiovascular risk begins as low as 115 mm Hg for systolic blood pressure, the impact and opportunity for behavioral health researchers may be stronger than at any time in the history of our field.

Theoretical Models

Psychological theories of hypertension development fall largely into one of three categories [2]. One of the oldest perspectives is the view that chronic elevations in negative affect have a direct and causal effect on blood pressure levels. From this model, blood pressure increases over time can be explained in direct proportion to the severity of affective characteristics such as anger or Type A behavior. Although the simplicity of this theory is attractive, the inability to consider moderator relationships (for example, racial differences in hypertension) and the absence of mechanistic pathways make it difficult to reconcile with biomedical theories of hypertension. A modernized version of this perspective, however, is currently the dominant behavioral theory of hypertension development, and will be discussed shortly.

Another theoretical position held by researchers is the view that psychological characteristics are largely epiphenomenal in nature in relation to blood pressure. According to this view, statistical associations are purely correlative and lacking in substance. Needless to say, this is not a position often lauded by behavioral researchers, but it does account for a large segment of published findings concerning relationships between psychological variables and blood pressure. For example, there exist dozens of case-control studies in which psychological distress was shown to be higher among hypertension patients relative to normotensive controls. While these differences are consistent with a causal model of hypertension, the psychological predictors are inherently confounded by the participant's awareness of their health status. Other papers demonstrate that awareness, and not blood pressure status, can better explain differences in self-reported distress [9], findings that are consistent with studies showing that negative affect levels are almost invariably higher among participants with known medical conditions. In short, this second theoretical perspective contends that third variables - including health awareness, physiological signs and symptoms of the disease, side effects of medication, functional impairments from illness, or other factors such as low socioeconomic status that may increase hypertension risk and impact mental health - can explain observed blood pressure associations with psychological variables. In each case, the third variable perspective gains strength by the inability in most studies to disentangle the temporal sequence of psychological variables and blood pressure risk. This is a significant methodological shortcoming, and one that is not easily addressed in a field in which correlational studies are the primary source of knowledge.

Temporal confounds are a primary criticism in behavioral reviews of hypertension [10, 11], but this shortcoming is no longer the barrier to progress that it once seemed to be. Supplementary evidence from three alternative research paradigms have brought renewed credibility to the argument that psychological factors may independently affect blood pressure regulation. Two of these sources, involving animal models of psychosocial stress and laboratory studies of mental stress and cardiovascular reactivity, will be examined in more detail in the discussion of mechanisms.

The final paradigm is represented by the still modest but rapidly growing collection of prospective findings [12-14]. Prospective studies, by design, follow a collection of normotensive participants over a period of years to measure relationships between baseline-measured factors and the development of hypertension over follow-up. In comparison to the cross-sectional and case-control designs that make up the majority of the behavioral medicine research of hypertension, prospective models confer important methodological advantages. One of the most significant advantages is the ability to link the incidence of hypertension to psychological characteristics measured well before the onset of high blood pressure, thereby eliminating temporal confounds to causation. Statistical methods for analyzing cohort data also lend themselves to more complex multivariate modelling to control for other known risk factors, and for quantifying clinical significance.

Prior to the turn of the 21st century, prospective studies were simply too rare to make a sweeping impact on the field, in spite of their advantages. At the time of this writing, at least 17 published cohort studies exist [4, 11], and that number is expected to grow significantly in the next decade. Table 1 provides a list of the major categories of psychological factors measured in these studies. Among the listed factors, anger, hostility, and Type A characteristics are the most common, and this is true not only for the prospective results but also for the psychology-hypertension field as a whole. Various synonyms for these terms exist. Vital exhaustion, for example, has shown associations with cardiovascular disease outcomes in several studies [15], but relationships with blood pressure are less well known at this time. Most critically for current purposes, a quantitative review of the prospective outcomes [11] concluded that the collected results are strongly in favor of an association between negative affect and hypertension development. This is especially true for anger, anxiety and depression, and several prospective studies, with less longitudinal evidence, suggest hypertension relationships after controlling for biomedical covariates and, to a lesser extent, for defensiveness, social isolation and personality variables.

Table 1. Primary psychological factors linked to hypertension

Anger expression	*Anger-in*
	Anger-out
Anxiety	
Defensiveness	*Defensive-hostility*
Depression	*Hopelessness*
Hostility	*Suppressed hostility*
Social support/Social isolation	*Social networks*
Stress	
Type A behavior pattern	

In the initial description of theoretical models of hypertension development, it was suggested that the majority of psychological evidence could be categorized into one of three paradigms. Two of these, the direct effects and third variable models, were summarized above. The final paradigm, one that now influences nearly all areas of health psychology research, is the biopsychosocial model [16]. The strength of the biopsychosocial model, in comparison to the above theories, is that it is best able to incorporate information from other sciences into a behavioral theory of hypertension development. Psychological factors, based on biopsychosocial theory, can act directly or indirectly on blood pressure levels through a number of behavioral and pathophysiological mechanisms, and these relationships can themselves be moderated by factors such as age, gender, family history and race, as well as properties of the psychological factor itself. Figure 1 (Appendix A) provides a graphic illustration of the biopsychosocial model of hypertension. This illustration demonstrates some of the many suggested moderator and mechanism variables, and it is not intended to be exhaustive. Even this simplified model, however, shows that no single study can hope to include all of the relevant contributing variables.

In addition to the potential moderator and mechanistic variables from a biopsychosocial perspective, the clinical properties of the psychological factor, a consideration that is often under-appreciated, is of central importance. Based on our biological understanding of the hypertension process, it is highly unlikely that transient or infrequent periods of negative emotions are significant contributors to long-term blood pressure patterns. Rather, we believe that chronic or recurrent episodes are the most likely contributors to hypertension. This not only has implications for the researcher, suggesting, for instance, that even in prospective studies the measurement of psychological predictors should occur at more than one time period, it also has implications for clinicians who may question the necessity or impact of intervening in their patients' mental health status. At present, even the more rigorous cohort studies available do not provide data on this issue.

Research Design Considerations

Our review of the psychological theories of hypertension thus far has identified a number of criticisms and methodological shortcomings in each theoretical model. Many of these limitations can be tied to the use, or, in some cases, overuse, of particular research designs for testing psychological-hypertension relationships. Although it is impossible for researchers to carry out a true randomized, controlled study of hypertension due to our inability "to assign" mental health conditions to participants, it is important that investigators be aware of the primary strengths and drawbacks that accompany commonly used research designs.

Table 2 offers a breakdown of the four most commonly used designs for testing psychological factor-hypertension associations. As shown, each of these models possesses particular strengths and weaknesses. In some cases, the weaknesses inherent in one model can be compensated for by the advantages of another, whereas, in other cases, the limitations are difficult to compensate for using any of the other paradigms. Fundamentally, each design in Table 2 is correlational in nature, meaning that causal inferences can be supported only with the converging results of multiple studies that address alternative explanations. In the behavioral study of hypertension, cross-sectional studies of college student populations and experimental studies of mental stress reactivity are the most common forms of investigation; as a result, the majority of our evidence is based on normotensive participants without a history of psychiatric illness. The continued reliance on such low-risk samples, without follow-up, is unlikely to strengthen our current knowledge base. What is needed are creative experimental designs that help clarify mechanisms of risk, additional prospective studies - including an improved focus on the clinical properties of proposed psychological risk factors - and treatment efforts that ascertain changes in hypertension risk, based on modifications in mental health. These are our most valuable stratagems for advancing psychological factor-hypertension relationships into mainstream medicine.

Table 2. Characteristics of research designs assessing relationships between psychological factors and hypertension

	Description	Strengths	Weaknesses
Cross-sectional study	Self-reported psychological characteristics are measured in association with blood pressure or blood pressure status	Convenient and inexpensive Clinical samples not required Can measure multiple factors	Chicken and egg dilemma Possible third variables Self-reporting biases
Case-control study	Matched pairs of normotensive and hypertensive patients are compared on one or more psychological measures	Includes clinical cases Controls for matched factors Can measure multiple factors	Health awareness bias Unmeasured third variables Self-reporting biases
Experimental study	Participants of varying blood pressure status complete self-report measures and one or more laboratory challenges	Standardization Includes physiological data Randomization of variables	Health awareness biases Chicken and egg dilemma Unmeasured third variables
Prospective study	Normotensive cohort measured at baseline and tracked for hypertension development over time	Temporal sequence clear Control for many variables Comparison to other factors	No causation implied History effects Unmeasured third variables

Clinical Significance

Concerns over the clinical importance of psychological relationships in published research reside in much of the behavioral medicine literature [17, 18]. Efforts to provide a compelling demonstration of clinical significance have been an elusive goal. This is due in large part to the private nature of psychological information, the complex and poorly understood relations between cognition and physiological functions, the research methods we employ to study psychological phenomena, and the statistical techniques we use to analyze and express relationships. These drawbacks create an imposing obstacle for behavioral researchers seeking to communicate their findings to colleagues in medicine and epidemiology. Despite the many hundreds of papers suggesting relationships between psychological characteristics and blood pressure, traditionally there has been little momentum to recognize mental health variables as a primary risk factor for hypertension. The lack of criteria by which to determine the clinical significance of psychological data, combined with the inconsistent results of behavioral treatments for hypertension, are the most important contributors to this ongoing impasse.

Changing this state of affairs will likely require a concerted effort on the part of behavioral researchers to modify their traditional means of collecting, assessing and communicating their results. A sizable body of literature exists on the clinical significance of testing [19, 20], and, although the recommendations from this collection extend well beyond the limits of this chapter, we can, nevertheless, summarize some of the most important themes as they apply to the behavioral study of hypertension. Perhaps the most universal limitation in our research literature is the near exclusive reliance on statistical methods that translate poorly into real world quantities. A survey of individual studies, narrative reviews, and meta-analyses returns a massive database of correlation and linear regression coefficients, and a smaller set of "effect size" terms, such as Cohen's d, with barely a mention of the practical implications for the millions at risk for developing high blood pressure. In the context of hypertension risk, what does a correlation value of 0.20 with depression confer? Does it become any more intelligible when this 0.20 statistic is confirmed by 10 such studies? How does the assessment change if the result of one or more studies is nonsignificant by statistical criteria? Finally, what is the practicing physician to make of these numbers in his or her discussion with hypertension patients?

In the face of such questions, our challenge becomes clearer. As it turns out, the clinical ramifications of a correlation value are less determined by statistical significance values than by the design of the study and the base rate of the outcome measure. In the case of comparatively rare outcomes, such as mortality and hypertension, the incidence even of a very small correlation can have a considerable real world impact [19, 21]. But such inferences are impossible to determine at face value. In the fields of medicine and epidemiology, the presentation of health statistics in the format of correlation values or regression coefficients is rare. By far, the preferred format for results in these fields is the language of epidemiological statistics, such as odds ratios, risk ratios and other public health measures. These measures, particularly in the context of longitudinal data collection, provide a more direct means of quantifying the risk conferred by a factor (e.g., a risk ratio of 2.0 for hypertension based on depression status at baseline suggests that depressed patients have double the risk of developing hypertension, compared with those without depression). They also provide a direct means of making comparisons between risk factors. Even in studies in which results are expressed as correlations, efforts to associate hypertension relationships with established risk factors (such as smoking, obesity, a positive family history or physical inactivity) can offer a baseline for judging associations with psychological factors.

Efforts to demonstrate clinical significance can also be assisted by formulating our research questions into outcome measures and quantities that have clinical meaning. A typical study of blood pressure change, for example, may report a set of standardized regression coefficients to support the hypotheses that blood pressure changes are greater among patients with higher hostility scores. These results would be virtually impossible to translate into a practical application for patients due to limitations inherent to the statistical presentation [22]. If instead the researcher supplemented the regression results with statistics or graphs displaying outcomes, such as the proportion of participants showing blood pressure increases in lower and higher scoring hostility scores, or the hostility of participants with blood pressure increases above 5 or 10mm Hg, or the severity of the hostility score associated with a clinically significant increase in blood pressure, the results would become much clearer for the practically inclined reader. Importantly, such an improvement does not necessarily require learning new statistical procedures or purchasing expensive software. Many of the most useful descriptions of clinical impact can be derived with basic statistics; the most important elements are more often creativity and interest in demonstrating practical applications. In cases in which researchers do wish to incorporate public health or other statistical measures into their results, useful guides for translating correlation values into risk and odds ratios are available [19]. Most of these conversions can be completed by hand or using a hand calculator. In our later discussion of psychological treatments for hypertension, we will touch on methods for improving the presentation of clinical significance in treatment outcome reporting.

Mechanisms

Proposed psychological mechanisms for hypertension risk can be characterized in several ways. In Figure 1, for example, mechanisms are categorized primarily either as behavioral or pathophysiological. In the former category, factors such as obesity, physical activity level and smoking represent established risk factors for both hypertension and cardiovascular disease. The majority of pathophysiological mechanisms thought to mediate psychological relationships with hypertension are also commonly cited as pathways to cardiovascular disease; these include heightened sympathetic activity, vascular remodeling, vasoconstriction and alterations in neuroendocrine regulation. The inclusion of theoretical mechanisms in behavioral studies of hypertension is far from common, and even in cases in which such factors are measured they are typically treated as control variables or moderators rather than mediating links. The distinction between moderating and mediating roles for variables, as well as the appropriate testing procedures for these very different approaches, has been well described [23, 24]. Mediators represent necessary variables in a causal relationship. The release of testosterone and human growth hormone, for example, are known to partly mediate changes in muscle strength and compositions in response to resistance exercise. In many relationships there can exist multiple mediator variables. In any description of hypertension mechanisms in relation to psychological variables, mediator analyses are the implied method of testing.

Another means of discussing mechanisms for hypertension risk in the behavioral sciences is to base our categorization on the quality and quantity of evidence we have for each proposed explanatory process. In this system of evaluation, theory becomes somewhat less important than empirical support, although the two are always linked. Mechanisms with the greatest degree of supporting evidence include behavioral risk factors and cardiovascular reactivity.

Behavioral Risk Factors

Relationships between measures of negative affect and behavioral risk factors for hypertension and cardiovascular disease have been well established, and they appear to be sufficient in magnitude to warrant continued attention from public health researchers and interventionists. Independent studies of varying gender, age and ethnic composition suggest that the risk of smoking, obesity, substance abuse, poor dietary habits and physical inactivity is substantially higher among individuals reporting high levels of psychological stress [25-27]. In many cases, relationships between mental health and behavioral risk are bidirectional, with the presence of each increasing the risk of developing other behavioral and affective conditions. Because these behaviors are among the most accepted risk factors for hypertension, demonstrations that health behaviors are causally linked to psychological factors and that the treatment of psychological factors can effectively improve health behaviors are each indirect but powerful methods for strengthening the psychological relationships with hypertension.

Although studies indicating associations between psychological measures and health behaviors are numerous, the majority are cross-sectional. The limitation of this design is the inability to establish the temporal relationship between the affective characteristic and the behavior pattern, which makes associations with blood pressure status difficult to determine. In an ideal study, investigators would follow a cohort of normotensive participants with few behavioral risk factors, periodically measuring psychological, behavioral and blood pressure variables over a period of years. Evidence that psychological stress predicted the onset of behavioral risk habits, and that these participants were likely to develop hypertension, would represent some of the strongest evidence available for a behavioral theory of hypertension. Unfortunately, no such study exists at present.

Adherence behaviors, particularly in light of the new JNC guidelines that support interventions at blood pressure levels below traditional diagnostic levels, represent another behavioral pathway by which psychological factors may increase hypertension risk and disrupt treatment efforts. Poor adherence to medication and rehabilitation regimens is believed to be a primary mediator of cardiovascular disease outcomes [28]. Although anti-hypertensive medications are well-known to have a negative effect on quality of life - resulting in appreciable implications for adherence - there is substantial evidence that high levels of negative affect undermine attempts to modify behavioral risk factors and thereby maintain anti-hypertensive treatment [29, 30]. The evidence also shows that this can be directly linked to health outcomes [31]. From the perspective of hypertension development, the relationship between psychological factors and adherence behaviors can manifest in a couple of ways: 1) by decreasing the motivation to modify hypertension risk factors such as smoking; and 2) by predisposing poor treatment results and increasing drop-out rates, resulting in either blood pressure increases or poor control of existing hypertension. As implied, lack of adherence is likely of greatest significance as a behavioral risk factor for patients with a family history of hypertension, or for ethnic groups (such as African-American) that have higher rates of hypertension. Lack of adherence is also a significant risk factor for those whose existing blood pressure places them in the "pre-hypertensive" risk category (>120 mm Hg systolic and/or >80 mm Hg diastolic).

Many of the higher quality prospective studies reported in recent years include behavioral and biomedical risk factors as control variables in their measurement protocols [11]. In most cases, findings from these studies suggest that associations between anger, depression, hostility and other psychological factors cannot be explained on the basis of traditional risk variables. Importantly, even this support for independent relationships with hypertension does not undermine the possibility of an important role with respect to health behaviors. Mediators are not always all-or-none pathways. A risk variable can function as a partial mediator of a relationship, for example, in which case a predictor may have evidence for an independent connection to hypertension, as well as a pathway through one or more mediating behavioral factors. Results from existing prospective efforts generally do not present data in this format, however. With regard to known behavioral risk factors for hypertension, we believe that their high prevalence in modernized countries and consistent connections to psychological stress characteristics is suggestive as a primary mechanism, but the overall evidence supports the position that psychological associations with hypertension are at best only partially explained by known behavioral risk factors.

Finally, the importance of relationships between psychological characteristics and known behavioral risk factors for hypertension is significantly strengthened by evidence from the cardiovascular disease literature, in which major coronary risk factors such as smoking and obesity are believed to be critical variables linking negative affect and psychosocial stress to coronary artery disease incidence and outcomes [32-35]. In a larger context, both emotional and behavioral precursors to hypertension and cardiovascular disease are thought to exert their influence by disposing changes in underlying cardiovascular structure and function.

Cardiovascular Reactivity

Without question, the pathophysiological measure of greatest interest to behavioral investigators of blood pressure is cardiovascular reactivity under periods of mental or emotional stress [36]. Reactivity is defined as the magnitude of the physiological response - most commonly measured in terms of blood pressure and heart rate changes relative to resting levels - during the performance of a short-term stressor. Reactivity responses are usually, but not always, collected in the course of a laboratory exercise, and most often in regard to standardized challenges, such as mental arithmetic or public speaking, that are predominantly psychological in nature [37]. A pattern of heightened reactivity to stress suggests a strong sympathetic nervous system response to stress. Over time, theorists contend that exaggerated sympathetic nervous system activity to daily demands places an increased load on the cardiovascular system, leading to functional, and eventually, structural changes that promote and maintain an increase in resting blood pressure.

Initial concerns about reactivity responses were addressed by controlled laboratory studies demonstrating that reactivity patterns varied significantly across individuals, but were stable over time and consistent across different forms of mental stress testing [38]. Research findings also suggested that reactivity patterns could be predicted by self-reported psychological characteristics, such as anger expression, hostility and Type-A behavior patterns, and reactivity responses were associated with hypertension in several prospective studies [39, 40]. There remain numerous controversies and questions regarding the status of reactivity as an independent risk factor for hypertension. This area of research is one of the fastest growing in the behavioral medicine field.

The strongest support for the continued focus on cardiovascular reactivity as a risk factor for hypertension and cardiovascular disease comes from a series of primate studies completed in the 1980s [41]. By standardizing the diets of male cynomolgus monkeys exposed to varying levels of social disruption, researchers showed that monkeys in a high stressed condition showed the greatest evidence of atherosclerosis on autopsy. This provided very compelling support for the effects of psychosocial stress on cardiovascular disease risk. Furthermore, an additional manipulation introducing a beta-blocker (propranolol) to the high stress monkey group counteracted the progression of atherosclerotic lesions, suggesting that the effects of psychosocial stress were mediated by increases in sympathetic nervous system activity [42]. Predictably, this elegant series of studies led to a surge of interest in studying psychosocial connections to cardiovascular disease in human populations.

There is no parallel breakthrough study for hypertension development in the animal or human literature. One recent longitudinal study of college-age adults showed that reactivity responses to mental stress testing in the laboratory statistically mediated 3-year increases in blood pressure based on defensiveness scores [43], but relatively few studies include simultaneously measures of psychological status, reactivity and hypertension outcomes by which to assess this process. A number of additional field and laboratory studies also indicate that factors such as the presence of social support can reduce blood pressure reactivity to stress [44, 45], and that reactivity responses captured in the laboratory generalize to reactivity patterns that occur in reaction to stressors in real life circumstances as measured by ambulatory monitoring [46]. Both findings have implications for reactivity as an important variable for psychological characteristics.

Within the body of prospective evidence supporting the position that psychological factors are predictors of hypertension, cardiovascular reactivity patterns have been measured in only a handful, and reactivity responses as control variables or mediators of psychological predictors are reported in only a single study [43]. Overall, however, the view that reactivity responses function as a mechanism by which psychosocial variables may increase the risk of hypertension is stronger than ever. This despite the fact that negative associations between reactivity patterns and hypertension risk continue to appear, suggesting that important questions remain concerning our understanding in this area [47].

Treatment

Very different approaches have been used in the behavioral or nonpharmacological interventions for the prevention or treatment of hypertension. Interventions that focus strictly on behavioral outcomes, such as lifestyle modification programs that foster exercise habits and dietary changes (described, e.g., by Appel and colleagues [48]), are not typically considered "psychological treatments," a category that traditionally focuses on relaxation therapy, biofeedback and stress management. For behavioral medicine researchers, the distinction between psychological and behavioral treatment alternatives to medication for the management of hypertension is artificial, and possibly counter productive. As the research we have reviewed indicates, the behavioral factors that serve as the primary targets in lifestyle modification studies are highly influenced by psychological factors. A successful behavioral modification program for diet, smoking or exercise will, by necessity, have components of the treatment protocol that address mood, motivation and stress management, as well as other important psychosocial characteristics. Similarly (as shown by Everson and colleagues [25]), changes in health behavior risk factors will likely mediate the psychological effects of cardiovascular outcomes. Based on our theoretical understanding of the psychological effects of hypertension, and on the empirical evidence for mechanistic pathways, it is therefore more accurate to conceptualize psychological and behavioral treatment models for hypertension as intrinsically linked efforts that fundamentally target very similar processes in improving blood pressure.

Even limited to the accepted definition for psychological treatments, however, the literature examining intervention efforts with hypertension is large, with the number of published papers numbering in the hundreds [49, 50]. There is no consensus in this field at present. Reviews by recognized blood pressure panels [5] are generally critical of psychological interventions, citing numerous studies with results suggesting nonsignificant differences between randomly assigned control and treatment groups, or blood pressure differences of insufficient magnitude to warrant widespread practice with hypertension patients. In contrast, several narrative and meta-analytic reviews suggest that psychological treatments appear effective to a degree rivalling that of the common medication-based protocols when protocol differences and patient characteristics are considered [51].

A limitation of many psychological treatment studies is that they frequently sacrifice treatment efficacy for treatment standardization, employing interventions that allow for straightforward statistical comparisons with minimal consideration given to the appropriateness of the treatment for individual patients. Treatment efforts that include a greater focus on matching treatment goals to patients - and intervening with patients with relatively higher blood pressure levels - have shown more impressive results. Findings from a pair of recent, carefully designed, randomized, controlled trials demonstrate this difference in methodological focus. In the first one, a large study of stress management interventions [52], the results suggested mostly small and nonsignificant blood pressure reductions in a group-based, 18-month protocol. This investigation targeted pre-hypertensive patients, with diastolic blood pressure in the range of 80-89 mm Hg. The investigators concluded that the role of stress-management in blood pressure treatment was unsupported by their findings, despite a large and well-standardized treatment trial.

In the second study, Linden and colleagues [53], conducted an individually tailored, 10-session stress management program for hypertensive patients. Eligible patients - those demonstrating 24-hour ambulatory blood pressure readings exceeding 140/90mm Hg - experienced sizeable and sustained improvements in blood pressure as measured by ambulatory monitoring post-treatment and at 6-month follow-up. The control group was crossed-over to the individualized treatment at a designated interval and demonstrated similar gains. Their results further suggested that blood pressure changes were associated with measured treatment gains in the form of anger coping styles and self-reported stress reductions, findings highly consistent with the biopsychosocial model of hypertension development.

The extent to which differences in the protocols of these studies can account for their divergent findings, or explain the numerous other cases of inconsistent findings in the psychological treatment literature, remains to be established. At minimum, however, the protocols offer specific and testable methodological features that should be closely considered in the design of future investigations and treatment efforts. Moreover, it cannot be denied that incorporating features that allow for an assessment of clinical significance and cost-effectiveness would enhance the value of any investigation. Some of the features that could be incorporated are considered in more detail in the subsequent discussion of treatment reporting.

Clinical Significance in Treatment Reporting

Previously, we discussed some of the difficulties inherent in determining the clinical significance of the majority of published studies evaluating the psychological predictors of hypertension development. Several specific statistical and methodological issues were described, and we argued that not only is it possible to present our findings in ways that are more easily interpreted in practical terms, but that the effort of doing so would be of great benefit to our current knowledge base.

Similar concerns and opportunities are present within the literature evaluating behavioral treatments of hypertension. The methodologies employed in nonpharmacological treatment studies of hypertension vary significantly, as do the presentation of findings. In many cases, results are described using common inferential statistics such as T-tests or variance analyses. Typically, these are accompanied by a probability value for determining the credibility of the observed differences. Meta-analytic reviews of this literature (see, e.g., [51]), while suggesting an overall effectiveness of behavioral treatments, tend to summarize effects in terms that are not easily translated into clinical value. Combined with the considerable inconsistency in effects between studies, behavioral interventions for hypertension are not widely recommended by physician panels or frequently practiced in medical settings [5].

Given the fact that quantitative reviews are typically favorable in their appraisal of behavioral interventions, and fact that there are promising results from a randomized controlled trial of stress-management for hypertension [53], the argument can be made that at least a portion of the resistance to behavioral treatments comes from our own methods of communicating research findings. Greater attention by investigators to important clinical outcome measures, and the inclusion of additional statistical results could dramatically improve our ability to extrapolate the practical worth of behavioral treatments relative to standard medical interventions.

Table 3 describes several categories of outcomes that can enhance the presentation of findings from studies describing behavioral treatments for hypertension. Rarely will all categories be applicable to a given investigation, but at least some of the outcomes listed should be standard components of any results section describing treatment. For example, in addition to the usual reporting of statistical significance, which, in almost all cases, relies on mean values, the inclusion of central tendency measures, such as the median and mode, would allow the reader to identify what the most common treatment outcomes were for patients in the study, without concerns that a subgroup of high or low responders is responsible for the statistical results. Creative researchers will also likely identify categories or examples of clinical outcome applications beyond those presented in Table 3.

Other suggestions include explicit presentation of the percentages of patients with blood pressure reductions meeting minimum guidelines for clinically acceptable improvements, expanding the definition of treatment effects to include outcomes such as quality of life measures, exploring factors that help identify which patients are most likely to respond to a particular treatment program, and discussing implications for real-world costs and benefits of an intervention. As is the case with respect to the clinical significance of efforts aimed at improving our understanding of the psychological factors in hypertension development, few of these additional outcome measures require outside consultation (cost-effectiveness assessment probably being the most glaring exception), and some do not even require the collection of additional information from participants.

Table 3. Statistics and outcome measures enhancing the clinical interpretation of treatment studies

Method	Description
1. Blood pressure changes over treatment intervals	Present mean, median and modal change values, 3 and 6-month post-treatment
2. Treatment mortality statistics	Drop-out percentages and proportion of non-responders over treatment intervals
3. Clinical significance criteria	Percentage of patients showing blood pressure reductions of at least 5mm Hg post-treatment and at follow-up
4. Quality of life statistics	Reductions in medications required and side-effects, improvements in mood and anxiety symptoms
5. Predictors of treatment change	Associations between measured baseline medical, demographic and psychosocial variables that predict a positive response to treatment
6. Cost-effectiveness/cost-benefit	Describe time, personnel and treatment costs analyses for behavioral program, relative to medication alternative

Conclusions

This chapter examined the relationship between psychological factors and hypertension, with an emphasis on recent research and methodology issues. Findings from three areas were reviewed: 1) studies addressing possible relationships between psychological characteristics and hypertension development; 2) research exploring potential mechanisms; and 3) studies examining the effects of psychological treatments for blood pressure reduction and hypertension management. This chapter will conclude by summarizing some of the major themes from these areas.

Psychological Factors and Hypertension

The factors most consistently associated with hypertension include anger, anxiety, depression, defensiveness, hostility and other Type-A behavior characteristics. Considerable variability exists, both in the terminology used across studies (making aggregation efforts challenging) and in the type and quality of the psychological measures employed. Findings from the recent (and still accumulating) prospective studies are promising and have created renewed enthusiasm with regard to psychological effects. Longitudinal studies, because they can better control for temporal confounds, offer a stronger design alternative for supporting causal associations between psychological variables and hypertension risk. An equally important result is that, when quantified in the form of risk ratio statistics, the effects of psychological factors appear comparable to established behavioral risk factors such as smoking, obesity, and physical inactivity. Finally, separate findings support psychological-hypertension associations across gender, ethnic and age subgroups.

Taken collectively, the evidence for a primary role of psychological factors in hypertension risk has never been stronger. Recommendations for future research include additional prospective studies that incorporate validated psychological measures, a greater emphasis on temporal and clinical features of psychological characteristics, and experimental models that elucidate mechanistic pathways.

Mechanisms

Empirically supported mechanisms include established cardiovascular risk factor behaviors, low socioeconomic status, and pathophysiological processes such as cardiovascular reactivity. Social support and other measures of relationship quality are additional factors of interest to mechanism researchers. The currently prevailing theory of hypertension development among behavioral medicine researchers emphasizes biopsychosocial contributions to disease. From this perspective, psychological influences on blood pressure can manifest in several pathways, including health behaviors, physiological changes, and through indirect mechanisms such as poor treatment adherence. Our understanding of psychosocial mechanisms has benefited from animal models, experimental studies, longitudinal efforts, and from parallel research efforts in cardiovascular disease.

Treatment Considerations

This chapter was critical of artificial distinctions made between "behavioral" treatments such as lifestyle modification programs and "psychological" treatments such as relaxation and stress-management. In a variety of forms, behavioral treatments for hypertension date back to the middle of the 20th century, and the general consensus by medical experts is that the magnitude of behavioral interventions is modest. Quantitative reviews of behavioral interventions, however, cast a more favorable light on effect sizes, and it is suggested that methodological differences between studies may account for some of the inconsistency in treatment outcomes. Psychological interventions appear to be most effective for patients with relatively higher blood pressure levels, and efforts to improve the match between treatment and individual patient goals may further enhance their effectiveness.

The recent focus on the risk of blood pressure below traditional levels for hypertension is an opportunity for behavioral medicine researchers to play a role in primary prevention efforts. An additional treatment issue remains the almost entirely unexplored possibility that psychosocial treatments among distressed but normotensive groups may reduce their later risk for hypertension. This issue, largely the product of prospective findings that provide longitudinal associations between psychological characteristics and hypertension development, suggest that early modification of at risk characteristics can alter the course of hypertension.

Future Research Issues

Despite continued progress, a number of thorny methodological issues remain that limit the recognition of the importance of psychological factors in hypertension development and treatment. Among the most pressing issues are an over reliance on cross-sectional studies of low-risk college populations, a comparatively small literature addressing mechanisms, inconsistent standards for measuring and validating hypertension status, and data analysis and presentation methods that obscure possible clinical significance. In regard to the latter obstacle, this chapter highlighted a number of specific methods that can improve the translation of psychological findings into practical effects and enable more effective reviews.

References

1. Gerin W, Pickering TG, Glynn L et al (2000) An historical context for behavioral models of hypertension. J Psychosom Res 48:369-377
2. Jorgensen R S, Johnson B T, Kolodziej ME, Scheer GE (1996) Elevated blood pressure and personality: A meta-analytic review. Psychol Bull 120:293-320
3. Steptoe A (2000) Psychosocial factors in the development of hypertension. Ann Behav Med 32:371-375
4. Yan LL, Lio K, Matthews KA, Daviglus ML et al (2003) Psychosocial factors and risk of hypertension. JAMA 290:2138-2148
5. Chobanian AV, Bakris GL, Black HR et al (2003) The Seventh Report of the Joint National Committee on Prevention, Detection, Evaluation, and Treatment of High Blood Pressure. The JNC 7 report. JAMA 289:3560-3572
6. Wolf-Maier K, Cooper RS, Banegas JR et al (2003) Hypertension prevalence and blood pressure levels in 6 European countries, Canada, and the United States. JAMA 289:2363-2369
7. Hajjar I, Kotchen TA (2003) Trends in prevalence, awareness, treatment, and control of hypertension in the United States, 1988-2000. JAMA 290:199-206
8. Cote I, Gregoire JP, Moisan J (2000) Health-related quality-of-life measurement in hypertension. A review of randomised controlled drug trials. Pharmacoeconomics 18:435-450
9. Irvine MJ, Garner DM, Olmstead MP, Logan AG (1989) Personality differences between hypertensive and normotensive individuals: influence on knowledge of hypertension status. Psychosom Med 51:537-549
10. Diamond EL (1982) The role of anger and hostility in essential hypertension. Psychol Bull 92:410-433
11. Rutledge T, Hogan BE (2002) A quantitative review of prospective evidence linking psychological factors with hypertension development. Psychosomatic Medicine 64:758-766
12. Davidson K, Jonas BS, Dixon KE, Markovitz JH (2000) Do depression symptoms pre-

dict early hypertension incidence in young adults in the CARDIA study? Arch Intern Med 160:1495-1500

13. Everson SA, Kaplan GA, Goldberg DE, Salonen JT (2000) Hypertension incidence is predicted by high levels of hopelessness in Finnish men. Hypertension 35:561-567

14. Jonas BS, Franks P, Ingram DD (1997) Are symptoms of anxiety and depression risk factors for hypertension? Longitudinal evidence from the National Health and Nutrition Examination Survey I epidemiologic follow-up study. Arch Fam Med 6:43-49

15. Kopp MS, Falger PR, Appels A, Szedmak S (1998) Depressive symptomatology and vital exhaustion are differentially related to behavioral risk factors for coronary artery disease. Psychosom Med 60:752-758

16. Brownley KA, Hurwitz BE, Schneiderman N (1999) Ethnic variations in the pharmacological and nonpharmacological treatment of hypertension: biopsychosocial perspective. Hum Biol 71:607-639

17. Rosenthal R, Rubin DB (1979) A note on percent variance explained as a measure of the importance of effects. J App Soc Psychol 9:395-396

18. Schmidt FL (1996) Statistical significance testing and cumulative knowledge in psychology: implications for training of researchers. Psychol Method 2:115-129

19. Rosenthal R, Rosnow RL, Rubin DB (2000) Contrasts and effect sizes in behavioral research: A correlational approach. New York, NY: Cambridge University Press

20. Willenheimer R (2001) Statistical significance versus clinical relevance in cardiovascular medicine. Prog Cardiovasc Dis 44:155-167

21. Abelson RP (1985) A variance explanation paradox: When a little is a lot. Psychol Bull 97:129-133

22. Greenland S, Schlesselman JJ, Criqui MH (1986) The fallacy of employing standardized regression coefficient and correlations as measures of effect. Am J Epidemiol 123:203-208

23. Baron R M, Kenny DA (1986) The moderator-mediator variable distinction in social psychological research: Conceptual, strategic, and statistical considerations. J Pers Soc Psychol 51:1173-1182

24. Holmbeck GN (1997) Toward terminological, conceptual, and statistical clarity in the study of mediators and moderators: Examples from the child-clinical and pediatric psychology literatures. J Consult Clin Psychol 65:599-610

25. Everson S, Kauhanen J, Kaplan G et al (1997) Hostility and risk of mortality and acute myocardial infarction: the mediating role of behavioral risk factors. Am J Epidemiol 146:142-152

26. Rutledge T, Reis SE, Olson M et al (2001) Psychosocial variables are associated with atherosclerosis risk factors among women with chest pain: the WISE study. Psychosom Med 63:282-288

27. Sielger IC, Peterson BL, Barefoot JC, Williams RB (1992) Hostility during late adolescence predicts coronary risk factors at mid-life. Am J Epidemiol 136:146-154

28. McDermott MM, Schmitt B, Wallner E (1997) Impact of medication nonadherence on coronary heart disease outcomes. Arch Intern Med 157:1921-1929

29. Glassman AH, Covey LS, Stetner F, Rivelli S (2001) Smoking cessation and the course of major depression: a follow-up study. Lancet 16:1929-1932

30. Wang PS, Bohn RL, Knight E et al (2002) Noncompliance with antihypertensive

medications: the impact of depressive symptoms and psychosocial factors. J Gen Intern Med 17:504-511

31. Zigelstein RC, Bush DE, Fauerbach J (1998) Depression, adherence behavior, and coronary disease outcomes. Arch Intern Med 158:808-809

32. Frasure-Smith N, Lesperance F, Talajic M (1995) The impact of negative emotions on prognosis following myocardial infarction: is it more than depression? Health Psychol 14:388-398

33. Kamarck T, Jennings JR (1991) Biobehavioral factors in sudden cardiac death. Psychol Bull 109:42-75

34. Rozanski A, Blumenthal JA, Kaplan J (1999) Impact of psychological factors on the pathogenesis of cardiovascular disease and implications for therapy. Circulation 99:2192-2217

35. Williams JE, Nieto FJ, Sanford CP et al (2002) The association between trait anger and incident stroke risk: the Atherosclerosis Risk in Communities (ARIC) Study. Stroke 33:13-19

36. Lovallo WR, Gerin W (2003) Psychophysiological reactivity: Mechanisms and pathways to cardiovascular disease. Psychosom Med 65:36-45

37. Schwartz AR, Gerin W, Davidson KW et al (2003) Toward a casual model of cardiovascular responses to stress and the development of cardiovascular disease. Psychosom Med 65:22-35

38. Kamarck T, Lovallo WR (2003) Cardiovascular reactivity to psychological challenge: Conceptual and measurement considerations. Psychosom Med 65:9-21

39. Knox SS, Hausdorff J, Markovitz JH (2002) Coronary Artery Risk Development in Young Adults Study. Reactivity as a predictor of subsequent blood pressure: racial differences in the Coronary Artery Risk Development in Young Adults (CARDIA) Study. Hypertension 40:914-919

40. Matthews KA, Salomon K, Brady SS, Allen MT (2003) Cardiovascular reactivity to stress predicts future blood pressure in adolescence. Psychosom Med 65: 410-415

41. Kaplan JR, Manuck SS, Clarkson TB et al (1983) Social stress and atherosclerosis in normocholesterolemic monkeys. Science 220:733-735

42. Kaplan JR, Manuck SB, Adams MR et al (1987) Inhibition of coronary atherosclerosis by propranolol in behaviorally predisposed monkeys fed an atherogenic diet. Circulation 76:1365-1372

43. Rutledge T, Linden W (2003) Defensiveness and prospective blood pressure increases: the mediating effect of cardiovascular reactivity. Ann Behav Med 25:34-40

44. Allen K, Blascovich J, Mendes WB (2002) Cardiovascular reactivity and the presence of pets, friends, and spouses: the truth about cats and dogs. Psychosom Med 64:727-739

45. Karlin WA, Brondolo E, Schwartz J (2003) Workplace social support and ambulatory cardiovascular activity in New York city traffic agents. Psychosom Med 65:167-176

46. Kamarck TW, Janicki DL, Shiffman S et al (2002) Psychosocial demands and ambulatory blood pressure: a field assessment approach. Physiol Behav 77:699-704

47. Fauvel JP, M'Pio I, Quelin P et al (2003) Neither perceived job stress nor individual cardiovascular reactivity predict high blood pressure. Hypertension (in press)

48. Appel LJ, Champagne CM, Harsha DW et al (2003) Writing Group of the PREMIER Collaborative Research Group. Effects of comprehensive lifestyle modification on blood pressure control: main results of the PREMIER clinical trial. JAMA 289:2083-2093
49. Jacob RG, Chesney MA, Williams DM et al (1991) Relaxation therapy for hypertension: design effects and treatment effects. Ann Behav Med 13:5-17
50. Linden W (1988) Biopsychological barriers to the behavioral treatment of essential hypertension. In: Linden W (Ed) Biological Barriers in Behavioral Medicine. New York, NY: Plenum Press 163-192
51. Linden W, Chambers LA (1994) Clinical effectiveness of non-drug therapies for hypertension: a meta-analysis. Ann Behav Med 16:35-45
52. Batey DM, Kaufmann PG, Raczynski JM et al (2000) Stress management intervention for primary prevention of hypertension: detailed results from Phase I of Trials of Hypertension Prevention (TOHP-I). Ann Epidemiol 10:45-58
53. Linden W, Lenz JW, Con AH (2001) Individualized stress management for primary hypertension. Arch Intern Med 161:1071-1080

Appendix A

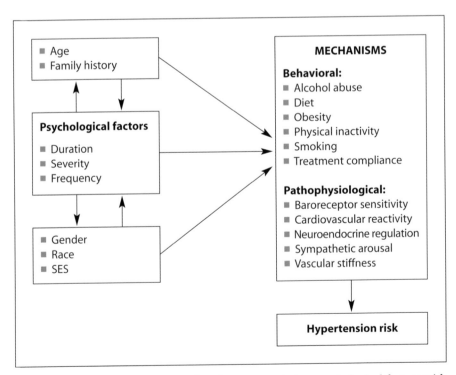

Fig. 1. Model illustrating theoretical pathways associating psychological factors with the development of hypertension SES = socioeconomic status

Personality
and Relational Aspects

Chapter 11

Type A, Type D, Anger-Prone Behavior and Risk of Relapse in CHD Patients

A. COMPARE ▪ G.M. MANZONI ▪ E. MOLINARI

▪ Introduction

The association between personality and physical illness is supported by many different empirical studies and, as Panzer and Viljoen [1] maintain, numerous clinicians and many researchers who belong to different areas and scientific disciplines are in agreement about the existence of complex and stable bio-psychosocial associative patterns.

The basis for this hypothesis is a vision of personality that can be viewed, as Salivini puts it, as a "mecanomorphic" type; in other words, this view considers personality to be an objective entity, a psychological entity identifiable with specific biological and social conditioning [2].

This theoretical assumption can be seen especially in the field of developmental research conducted in the neuroanatomic and neurophysiologic spheres, according to which personality is viewed as an emerging psychological property of an underlying dynamic neural structure, which establishes itself in a flexible way during its development, in relation both to genetic predisposition and the interaction of individuals with their surrounding social environment [1, 3]. In particular, the influence that modeling has in the first experiences of education and attachment with the primary caregiver has often been emphasised [4-6].

These are the premises on which the connection between personality and physical illnesses is based. It is derived from studies in neuroscience, according to which there should be a constitutional vulnerability towards stress, a dysfunctional neuro-cognitive and neuro-emotive functioning, which co-determines the onset of physical illness, and an inadequate handling of difficult and stressful situations, which is the developmental result of a particular genetic development in conjunction with a person's life experiences [1].

For example, the research done on animals (monkeys in particular) demonstrates that maternal behavior towards her offspring programs their neuroendocrine responses to stress, acting as a modulator of their physiological activation, and that this modeling has a strong influence on their behavior and immunologic functioning even as adults [1]. Luecken holds that this happens also in the case of human development. He maintains that the modulating influence that the primary caregiver exhorts on the physiological activation of the child determines the type and the sensibility of his/her responses to stress, both on a short-term and, especially, on a long term basis; these responses are a combination of emotive, cognitive and physiological reactions, and they vary in their capacity to handle stress, acting either as a protection or causing the development of a physical illness during adulthood [6].

Coronary heart disease (CHD) is one of the pathologies that have been studied the most in relation to personality and psycho-emotive stress. The etiological and prognostic independent link between stress (acute or chronic) and various clinical cardiovascular outcomes, including the onset of CHD, infarction (lethal and non-lethal) and coronary artery disease (CAD), which can be divided into different categories of seriousness, is recognised both in the medical and psychological spheres [7-9].

The literature dealing with the relationship between psychological stress and CHD in the areas of epidemiological research, behavioral medicine, psychosomatic science and, recently, health psychology, is vast. Even the scientific literature on the role of personality in the etiology and prognosis of heart disease is extensive, especially with respect to the type A behavior pattern (TABP), although the enormity of this literature is not universally recognised. As Pedersen and Denollet assert, for example, in an article that appeared in 2003, "Little research on the interface between cardiology and psychology includes personality traits" [10].

However, this realisation is valid only inside a "mecanomorphic" paradigm, according to which personality is made up of traits, dispositions and temperaments. It loses its meaning if considered in light of a paradigm which Salvini defines as "anthropomorphic," in which personality is not a reality that is naturally and objectively given, but the totality of psychological processes (mental states, auto-perceptive constructs, interactive schemes) produced by people who interact with the environment, within symbolic, normative and sociocultural contexts. According to Salvini, these processes, varying in their degree of self awareness, are generated by actors who are dynamically engaged in the construction of the reality which concerns them, while being affected by its effects, predefined by themselves or others [2].

The theoretic contribution of Thorensen and Powell regarding the TABP is very clear on this matter. In fact, the authors state that there is a tendency to assign the status of a personality profile to a construct that has received a lot of attention through the years, and on which a vast amount of research has been done, but which does not correspond to stable and global traits of the "mecanomorphic" personality and which, on the contrary, is a pattern of psycho-emotive and behavioral processes produced actively by the person in response to specific environmental events, which, themselves, are created by the person. This definition can be assimilated by either an "anthropomorphic" vision of personality or a transactional one, according to the authors [11].

The expression *Type A Behavior Pattern* was introduced in the late 50s, in a behavioral context, when a group of American cardiologists, including Jenkins, Rosenman and Friedman, hypothesised that one of the independent etiological factors of heart disease was a specific behavioral and emotive modality in response to certain environmental prodding [12]. The realisation that the traditional coronary risk factors (age, hypertension, diabetes, smoking, high level of cholesterol) were not enough to explain the alarming increases in the major cardiac diseases during those years led to this conclusion. The contemporary discovery of specific associations between specific physiological variables, including an increase in the level of cholesterol and blood coagulation in reaction to an acute sense of urgency, encouraged further research, finally resulting in a specific emotive and behavioral pattern that increased the risk of heart disease and which they called Type A Behavior Pattern. This was contrasted with the Type B Behavior Model, which was simply defined as the absence of the extreme characteristics of the A type[13].

Pedersen and Denollet [10] point out that the TABP was purposely defined in order to avoid any association with personality traits, even though in practice it ended up adhering to the dominant "mecanomorphic" paradigm, and was even referred to as "type A personality."

As Friedman [14] maintains, the TABP immediately became what in the 30s was called "coronary-prone behavior," after some famous scholars with a psychoanalytic orientation, including Menninger [15], observed that some behaviors were associated with specific physiological events in patients affected by heart diseases. For example, an association between high blood pressure and a strong motivation to reach a high social status, together with the tendency to inhibit emotions and thoughts of anger in a defensive way, was observed [16].

The TABP was welcomed with great enthusiasm by the scientific community. The enthusiasm was so immense that, according to Chesney, the type A behavior model should be considered a milestone in behavioral medicine, since it was the first construct that was really able to associate behavior with a serious physical illness [17].

In fact, the first American and English prospective studies demonstrated that people characterised by the TABP have a high incidence of CHD, and that this is significantly higher than the incidence of CHD in people characterised by the type B behavior pattern [18].

A large part of the research that followed obtained similar results, and a large amount of evidence was obtained - so much evidence that, in 1981, a work group was appointed by the National Heart, Lung and Blood Institute, an American agency, to revise all the works that had been produced on the etiological factors of CHD to recognise the TABP as an independent risk factor for CHD, on the same level as smoking, high cholesterol and hypertension [18].

Four years later, however, the enthusiasm started to wane after some important studies failed to demonstrate a relationship between the TABP and cardiovascular disease [11]. Nonetheless, a subsequent meta-analysis managed to demonstrate a modest, but still significant, association [19].

The resulting controversy that occurred became so intense that many researchers changed their approach in studying TABP. In the attempt to discover which type A subjects really risked developing CHD, researchers branched off in two different directions. The first, based on the distinction made between toxic and non-toxic components of TABP, focused on the examination of components that demonstrated a significant association with the development of cardiac disease. Of these, the one that received the most attention was the hostility/anger dimension, followed by competitiveness and time urgency. The second direction of research focused on discovering the environmental situations mainly implicated in the elicitation of TABP and the possible physiological risks [20].

According to Fred and Hariharan [18], the peak of the controversy was reached when Lachar affirmed that the coronary-prone behavior and the TABP were not synonyms. In other words, that the coronary-prone behavior should not be seen as being characterised by an extreme motivation to reach objectives and an extreme involvement at work, but, rather, as a physical and emotive reactivity towards challenging situations, in particular, ones capable of eliciting anger, cynicism, distrust and hostility [13] (see page 149).

Finally, in 1995, in the confusion which still surrounds TABP concerning its predictive power with respect to cardiac disease, especially with respect to whether it is a trait or state, a new psycho-social factor of cardiac risk appeared on the scene of psychosomatic research, the type D personality, where "D" stands for "Distressed personality" [21]. Unlike the TABP, the type D personality was explained from the beginning as a global conjunction of traits inside the "mecanomorphic" paradigm. According to those who wrote on the subject, type D personality characterised those with a tendency to experience negative emotions and inhibit their expression, and it was demonstrated that the patients who are affected by heart disease and who also have a type D personality are four times more prone to death, compared with patients who are not considered type D [22].

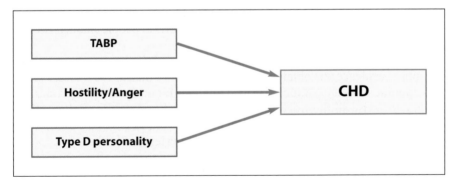

Fig. 1. Personality patterns partially recognised as cardiac risk factors. TABP, type A behavior pattern; CHD, coronary heart disease

◼ The Type A Behavior Pattern

Friedman and Rosenman have defined the type A behavior model as an emotive and behavioral pattern elicited by certain environmental events promoted by the western culture, which rewards people who think, act, communicate and, in general, live more rapidly and aggressively [13]. This behavior model can be seen in people aggressively struggling to do more in less time, even against obstacles put there by other people or by situations beyond their control [23].

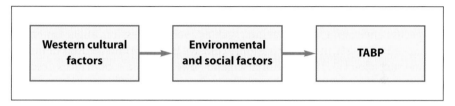

Fig. 2. Cultural conceptualisation of TABP

The characteristics of the TABP are: impatience, aggression, an intense motivation to reach their objectives which become ever greater, a sense of urgency with regard to time and a desire to make progress and be recognised. The counterpart of the TABP is the type B pattern, characterised by patience and tranquillity, a moderated sense of urgency with regard to time and little aggression or competition [13]. As Ray and Bozek state, the labels "Type A" and "Type B," in and of themselves, deliberately have no meaning [23].

Pedersen and Denollet affirm that the TABP was not conceived as a stable personality profile [10]. Friedman and collaborators defined it explicitly as a reaction behavior to situations, perceived as difficult, that are encountered in the course of everyday life, a behavior characterised by anger, hostility, explosive language, urgency and specific motor characteristics. This assumption is evident in the way in which the TABP was and is still evaluated, ie through a structured interview purposely formulated to research situations able to cause specific behavioral responses, measured in terms of frequency, intensity and modality [13].

Nevertheless, according to Thorensen and Powell [11], the TABP was understood as a conjunction of personality traits. As a result, the term "type A personality" appeared simultaneously with "type A behavior pattern." This happened in the positivist and empiricist scientific spirit in which the TABP was born, the object of which was to pinpoint a behavioral and emotive typology capable of explaining the aspects of the etiology of cardiac disease that remained unknown, abstracting it from the single individual.

In fact, from the theoretic point of view, even though the various terminologies utilised then are still utilised today, the construct referred to by all authors is the same, because it was born in the same spirit of research. The only things that differ are the aspects the authors refer to. The nomenclature "TABP" emphasises the reactive behavioral components that emerge in the "here and now" during the structured interview, whereas "Type A personality" highlights the dispositional components and the recurrence of the behaviors over time.

In line with this setup, two conceptualisations of the construct, which, for the sake of simplicity we will call uniquely TABP, currently exist. The first refers to what is measured from the self-administered questionnaires, and is mainly directed to the evaluation of personality traits. The primary characteristics of the type A personality are extreme competition and ambition, an excessive involvement in work, and a strong sense of impatience and urgency in activities. Conversely, the second version, which is associated with the structured interview (SI), refers to specific environmental behaviors, such as social aggression, anger (intensity and speed of onset), motor activation, explosive language and feelings of hostility and suspicion [11, 13]. As Thorensen and Powell [11] state, both faces describe a similar phenomenon, even though they represent two different aspects.

In many studies, it is not clear which of the two senses of the term is related to the clinical outcome[11, 14, 19]. Hence, differences are attributed mainly to two different modalities of measurement. There are significant problems associated with self-administered questionnaires, due to the fact that they assume subjects can accurately observe and remember their behavior [13].

The confusion in the definitions, evaluations and results has pushed many authors to doubt the validity of the construct and question its value in further research [14]. This uncertainty is illustrated by Dimsdale's definition of TABP as a "hodgepodge" [24].

A theoretic synthesis was performed by Thorensen and Powell [11], according to whom the confusion that surrounded the TABP for so long was determined by an insufficient theoretic elaboration of the construct, in part linked to the dominant influence of the epidemiological research. They advanced a transactional conceptualisation of TABP and proposed a view of the construct in terms of how a person's perceptions, thoughts, emotions, behaviors and the physiological processes develop and function interactively in a circular relationship with respect to environmental situations (Fig. 3).

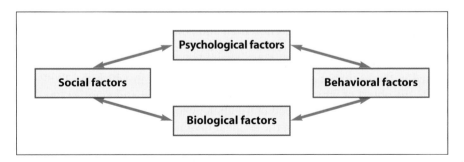

Fig. 3. Multifactorial model of TABP

In the theoretic model the two authors proposed, psychological, social, behavioral and biological factors are interdependent. For example, certain environmental stimuli can elicit the TABP and its physiological correlates in a person after he/she has behaved in a certain way – eg utilising particular language and facial expressions – which, in turn, leads to further type A behaviors. At the basis of this are particular schemes of the self and others, beliefs with which persons with a TABP use to construct their personal and social reality. The uncertainty of their own ability to be successful in situations perceived as important and, in particular, ambiguous and incontrollable, should, according to the model proposed by Thorensen and Powell, stimulate the TABP [25].

There are three basic beliefs that subjects with a type A pattern use to constitute their reality: (1) I have to constantly prove myself to be worthy by reaching important, socially recognised goals; (2) I don't believe in the existence of universal moral principles that guarantee honesty, justice and goodness; and (3) I believe that my resources for being successful are scarce and insufficient. These cognitive schemes set the stage for typical behaviors of the TABP (extremely competitive behavior, impatience, hostility and anger), and they also should be expected to influence the physiological responses [11].

From a psychological point of view, the model postulates that people demonstrating the TABP harbour a deep sense of insecurity and inadequacy. The never-ending race to be successful serves to avoid and reduce the negative judgements from others, as well as from themselves. In fact, these cognitive auto-evaluation processes seem to be at the heart of the TABP [26], even though, for the most part, they do not appear to be conscious [11]. For this reason, according to Thorensen and Powell, the self-administered questionnaires designed to measure TABP are unreliable, whereas methods of evaluation that use non-verbal performance, such as the SI, should be more reliable [11].

Instruments of Evaluation

As mentioned previously, the evaluation of the TABP can be carried out through two principal modalities: the structured interview (SI) and the self-administered questionnaire. The SI was created by Friedman and Rosenman in 1959[12]. It is made up of questions formulated to investigate the behavioral reactions experienced in everyday life in response to difficult situations, including the frequency, intensity and expressive modalities of anger and hostility. The investigators, expressly trained for this purpose, try to provoke the subject and observe his or her behavioral responses, especially language (eg. explosive language), sense of time (urgency and impatience) and the psychomotor signals. The findings of SI are therefore evaluated from the behaviors, rather than the content of the answers.

The final classification consists of a scale made up of four categories:
- complete development of A (A extreme),
- incomplete development of A,
- incomplete development of B,
- complete development of B (B extreme).

Twenty years after the definition of the SI, the videotaped structured interview (VSI) was developed by Friedman and colleagues. The addition of video recording has permitted additional diagnostic research, as well as the ability to follow possible future changes in the intensity of type A behavior.

Currently, in order to diagnose the TABP, the "video recorderd clinical exam" (VCE) is utilised, and the presence of symptoms, traits and psychomotor signs relative to two principle components is investigated:
1) a sense of time urgency;
2) fluctuating hostility.

This new diagnostic instrument was developed by Friedman and colleagues as an attempt to improve the sensibility, specificity and efficiency of previous ways of researching the TABP.

The VCE consists of a series of flexible questions that can be varied as examiners judge necessary. The most important aspect is the effort to investigate the psychomotor signs of the TABP with the same attention given to other behaviors. With respect to the VSI, six previously defined symptoms and four new psychomotor signs observed in type A subjects have been added for the diagnosis. The assessment can detect 3 levels of type A behavior:
- very serious (150-400 points);
- serious (100-149 points);
- not serious to moderately serious (0-99 points).

Video recorded clinical exam:	
Manifestation of a sense of urgency with regard to time	**Manifestation of fluctuating hostility**
Symptoms and traits	*Symptoms and traits*
- Awareness of one's own hurry - Reprimanding others for slowing down - Hurrying while walking, eating and leaving the table - An intense aversion to having to wait in a queue - Extreme punctuality - A rare recollection of memories, observation of natural events or day dreaming	- Frequently getting angry while driving - Disbelief in altruism - Insomnia caused by anger or frustration - Chronic difficulty in the relationship with one's children - Tension or competition with one's partners - Grinding of teeth - Irritability that is easily provoked and discomfort when having to face petty mistakes

Psychomotor signs	Psychomotor signs
- Chronic facial tension - Eyebrow elevation (tic) - Lifting or pulling away shoulders (tic) - Tense posture - Quick speech - Snapping of the tongue - Forced inhaling of air - Excessive facial sweat - Frequent batting of the eyelids	- Facial hostility - Periorbital pigmentation - Retraction of the eyelid (tic) - Hostile quality of the voice - Bilateral retraction of the muscles of the mouth (tic) - Tightening the hand during a conversation - Hostile laughter

The second evaluative modality is represented by a series of self-administered questionnaires: the Jenkins Activity Survey (JAS) [27], the Bortner Type A Scale [28], the Framingham Type A Scale [29], the Multidimensional Type A Behavior Scale (MTABS) [30], the Student Toxic Achievement Questionnaire (STAQ) and the Working Adult Toxic Achievement Questionnaire (WATAQ), these last ones both constructed by Birks and Roger [31].

The JAS, which is used globally, has demonstrated construct validity and includes three factors (speed and impatience, task involvement and highly motivated behavior). In a few prospective studies, the third factor – that is, highly motivated, objective-oriented behavior – emerged as being associated with positive and protective indexes, such as satisfaction and a good performance, and this has resulted in its being considered a "non-toxic" component, in contrast to the other two, which represent "toxic" components and are associated with negative clinical indexes [31]. The JAS does not evaluate aggression and hostility [13].

The MTABS was purposely created to provide a complete evaluation of the multidimensional nature of TABP. This instrument includes five factors: hostility, impatience/irritability, achievement striving, anger and competitiveness. According to the authors, the factors related to achievement striving represent a non-toxic component, whereas all the others measure toxic components. However, the validity analysis has demonstrated that the factor considered as non-toxic does not measure a distinct component because it is positively correlated with the other four, particularly anger and impatience/irritability [31].

In order to distinguish the toxic part of achievement striving from its non-toxic component, the probable source of negative results obtained with MTABS, Birks and Roger constructed two questionnaires, the STAQ and the WATAQ, both of which demonstrate a bi-dimensional structure coherent with the authors' initial intentions. From the correlation analysis, a negative association between the two factors emerged, and these factors subsequently became known as "strong toxic motivation" and "strong non-toxic motivation." The convergent and discriminant validity analysis confirmed this distinction, highlighting indexes of association with other scales, which are perfectly coherent with the different natures of the two constructs [31].

Studies on the TABP

The first empirical evidence of an association between TABP and cardiac illness came in 1975 with the publication of the final results of a prospective study conducted on the American population and called Western Collaborative Group Study (WCGS) [32]. In the sample, 3.154 healthy men between the ages of 39 and 59 were evaluated with respect to the TABP using of the SI. After 8-1/2 years, 257 men had developed a cardiovascular illness. After controlling for the effects of traditional risk factors, it became apparent from the analysis that subjects classified as type A had double the probability of having a diagnosis of angina pectoris or heart attack of the myocardium, compared with those classified as type B.

Another prospective study conducted on the American population, the JAS [33] showed similar results. However, in this study, a self-administered questionnaire, the JAS, was utilised to evaluate the TABP. The data gathered after four years of follow-up showed that the scores obtained from 120 subjects who developed a cardiovascular illness were significantly greater than the scores of the 524 subjects who remained healthy.

In 1980, the results of a prospective study on the English population were published. Referred to as the Framingham Heart Study [29], the research effort focused the psychosocial factors linked to the onset of the CHD. In the sample, both healthy men and healthy women were included (i.e. no subject was affected by cardiovascular disease). Also in this case, the instrument utilised to evaluate the TABP was a self-administered questionnaire, the Framingham Type A Scale. After eight years of follow-up, the Framingham Type A Scale was demonstrated to be an independent predictor of cardiac disease and heart attack of the myocardium in middle-aged men, as well as an independent predictor of angina pectoris in women between the ages of 45 and 64.

The first prospective study on the European population was the French-Belgian Cooperative Group Study, published in 1982 [34]. Using another self-administered questionnaire, the Bortner Rating Scale, this study, after a follow-up of five years, demonstrated once again that the TABP was an independent risk factor for cardiovascular illness. In 1985, results from another prospective study, this one lasting eight years and including about 2.200 Japanese men resident in Hawaii between the ages of 57 and 70, was published. However, the Honolulu Heart Project [35] failed to demonstrate a relationship between the TABP, measured with the JAS, and cardiovascular illness.

Nevertheless, in 1981, the work group appointed by the National Heart, Lung and Blood Institute to revise all the works produced on the etiological factors of CHD concluded that the TABP, as defined by the SI and the JAS, as well as by the Framingham Type A Scale, was associated with a greater risk of cardiac illness in middle-aged American workers [36].

It is significant that, even though the greater part of the prospective studies on the population gave positive results, many studies conducted on subjects who were at a high risk of cardiovascular illness did not arrive at the same conclusions. Only one (the WCGS, which included 67 men who had already experienced a cardiac event) demonstrated a significant association between TABP, as measured with the JAS, and heart attack [37].

The Multiple Risk Factor Intervention Trial recruited about 3,000 men who were at risk for a CHD. The risk was linked to the presence of at least two to three cardiac risk factors: smoking, hypertension and high cholesterol. The TABP was evaluated both through the JAS and the SI, but neither evaluation demonstrated a link between the TABP and the onset of cardiac illness [37, 38].

The same results were obtained from the Aspirin Myocardial Infarction Study, a clinical trial designed to evaluate the effect of aspirin on the risk of heart attack. The TABP, measured with the JAS, could not be related either to the risk of heart attack or even to the risk of mortality [39].

The results of the study by Dimsdale and collaborators for one year on a sample of 189 subjects who underwent a cardiac surgical intervention were particularly surprising. The Type B behavior pattern emerged as predictor of successive cardiac events [40].

Also, the Multicenter Post Infarction Program [41], conducted on 548 patients who had suffered a non-fatal heart attack failed to demonstrate an association between the TABP, as measured by the JAS, and the successive mortality rate.

Additional negative results come from angiographically studies, which show inconsistent associations in most cases between the TABP and CAD, in particular arteriosclerosis [42]. Interestingly, however, the meta-analysis of Miller and collaborators [19] identified important methodological problems in this type of study, mostly resulting from the flawed selection of subjects. The meta-analysis revealed that the comparison groups utilised – in theory, comprised of subjects who had no degree of coronary disease – included in reality a percentage of persons with a subclinical form of CAD much greater than that expected in the general population. In other words, the number of healthy subjects who were included was very low.

The coup de grace, however, occurred in 1988, with the publication of the study by Ragland and Brand [42]. This study examined the incidence of mortality over a period of 22 years in 257 men affected by cardiac disease who had participated to the WCGS. The investigators discovered that subjects, both young and old, who had been classified as type A at the beginning of the study had 10% fewer deaths from CAD, compared with subjects who had been classified as type B. These results suggested that the TABP could have a protective effect on subjects affected by cardiovascular disease, and they led the investigators to hypothesise that the TABP could promote more healthy behaviors in subjects who were aware of their illness [43, 44].

The weight of these failures to establish a clear connection between the TABP and cardiovascular illness created a great deal of doubt concerning the TABP as a risk factor. Successive revisions attempted to conciliate the positive results obtained in the first studies with the negative results that later emerged, and investigators concluded that the evidence supported TABP as a risk factor for the CHD in studies of healthy populations, but not in studies where cardiac risk was already present [13, 19].

There were other clinical trials that contradicted these results. For example, the Recurrent Coronary Prevention Project showed that the patients who had suffered from a heart attack who had attended a counselling treatment for TABP in addition to a cardiac counselling treatment had a recurrence of heart attack which was 44% lower, compared with those who had had attended only the cardiac counselling treatment. The protective effect of counselling for TABP remained even after 4 $^{1}/_{2}$ years [45].

Nevertheless, scepticism spread in the scientific community, and led many many researchers, as well as clinicians, to focus on the components considered to be the most toxic-namely, hostility and anger [24].

A recent meta-analysis of all the prospective studies published through 1998 in which the hypothetical association between TABP, hostility and cardiovascular disease was tested, both in healthy subjects and in subjects affected by a heart disease, showed, once again, the negative results obtained previously, highlighting a significant relationship only when it came to hostility. These results have led authors to doubt the significance of the TABP, as well as both its predictive and preventive implications [46].

Despite this, studies on the TABP continue to appear in the literature, always with controversial results. For example, a prospective study of 25 years conducted on 1.806 healthy men published in 2004 demonstrated a significant association between TABP, measured with JAS, and the onset of cardiac illness in after a follow-up of 16 years [47], whereas another prospective study of 10 years conducted on 3.873 men and women published in the same year failed to demonstrate any association at all between TABP and the onset of CHD [48].

■ Pathophysiological Mechanisms

The physiological processes which have been considered and examined as being responsible for the pathogenesis of the cardiovascular disease in relation to the TABP are four: an elevated production of catecholamine and elevated cardiac reactivity, an excessive level of testosterone, high levels of corticosteroids and a reduced antagonism of the parasympathetic system in comparison to the activation of the sympathetic system [13] (Fig. 4).

Many laboratory studies have tested the hypothesis of an association between the TABP and a major cardiovascular reactivity in response to stressful stimuli, and the majority of them have obtained positive results [20]. In addition, studies conducted on animals (monkeys) have demonstrated a significant association between elevated cardiac reactivity and arteriosclerosis. During autopsy, the monkeys classified as "highly reactive" showed nearly twice as much arteriosclerosis, compared with those characterised by low cardiovascular reactivity [49, 50]. The role of the sympathetic nervous system in raising blood pressure, increasing catecholamines and otherwise stimulating cardiac reactivity has been emphasised a great deal, and it could be that these processes damage the endothelium, in addition to promoting blood platelet aggregation [51].

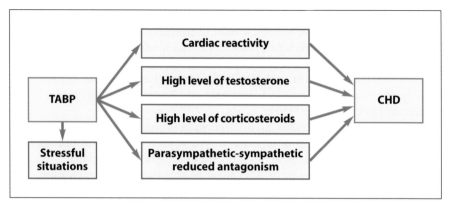

Fig. 4. Pathophysiological links between TABP and CHD

A significant amount of research identifies cardiac reactivity as the connection between TABP and CHD, highlighting the fact that the frequency of reactions to stressful events may be more significant than the intensity [13, 20].

However, the revisions of Contrada and Krantz [52] and Lyness [20] emphasised the fact that the relationship between TABP and the various measures of cardiac reactivity (catecholamine level, heart rate, arterial blood pressure and cortisol level) depend on a series of moderating factors, such as gender, method of evaluation of the TABP and the nature of the stressful condition (Fig. 5). The authors demonstrated that in subjects classified as type A through the structured interview, it is more likely that elevated sympathetic-adrenomedullary levels result from stress, and that the relationship between the TABP and cardiac reactivity is stronger in (a) laboratory studies that supply an incentive to performance, (b) stressful situations that provoke hostility and (c) cognitive tasks of moderate difficulty. Also, there was a negative association, especially in men, in both young subjects and adults. The reasons

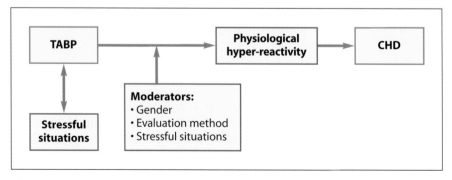

Fig. 5. Moderators influencing the link between TABP and CHD

could be linked both to biological diversity and to the different sociocultural influences that affect the way men tend to perceive difficult situations. The males with a type A pattern responded to environmental challenges with elevated sympathetic-adrenomedullary activity and activation of the pituitary adrenal-cortical system. Stimulation of the sympathetic nervous system, conversely, should cause a rise in blood pressure, increased heart rate and the release of catecholamines [52].

In some laboratory studies, no differences in sympathetic reactivity towards difficult situations were found between type A pattern subjects and subjects with a type B pattern, except at baseline, suggesting that the cognitive processes of evaluation play an important causative role in elevated activation [20]. However, a study by Williams and collaborators [53], conducted on healthy male subjects, demonstrated a chronic rise in sympathetic reactivity in subjects with a type A pattern under all conditions, also in the baseline. This result suggests the existence of chronic sympathetic hyperactivity in subjects with a type A pattern, in which cognitive evaluations of situations do not play a decisive role. A chronic elevated level of corticosteroids should contribute to the formation of arteriosclerosis through increased enzyme activity and catecholamine synthesis, and the reduction of enzymes needed for their degradation.

Subjects with the type A pattern should also have elevated levels of testosterone, compared with type B subjects, after carrying out cognitive tasks [54]. Testosterone is implicated in increased aggression and cardiac reactivity and decreased HDL cholesterol levels in males. Testosterone can also be associated with hostile behavior and the process of arteriosclerosis formation [13].

In another study, type A subjects demonstrated low vagal activity in their parasympathetic response, in contrast to the effects of sympathetic activation [55]. Suarez and collaborators, however, observed an association between TABP and the level of basal cholesterol with heart rate and catecholamine and cholesterol levels, measured during the mental execution of an arithmetic task [56]. In this last study, the middle-aged male subjects classified as type A who had an elevated basal level of cholesterol experienced a significant increase in heart rate and catecholamine and cholesterol levels while performing a mental test, in contrast to type B subjects. This result highlights the fact that behavioral factors could increase the risk of coronary diseases even more in those subjects who have an elevated level of cholesterol [56].

▪ Hostility and Anger

Studies of hostility and anger as autonomous cardiovascular risk factors began to rise from the ashes of the TABP, or rather, from the dismantling process the TABP was subjected to after many studies obtained negative and contradictory results [9, 13]. What motivated the research on the role of hostility in the etiology of cardiac illness was the discovery that some components of the TABP could be more toxic than others. In particular, the negative effects on cardiovascular health of anger could be traced back to the formulation of the psychoanalytic concept of "repressed anger" [16].

Hostility and anger have been mainly studied together as a single cardiac risk factor. In this context, the hostility component represents a personality trait linked to interpersonal behavior, and it is characterised by a pessimistic orientation to interpersonal interactions and life in general, a cynical lack of trust generalised toward other people, negative opinions and attitudes towards others (cynicism, distrust, denigration etc), frequent fits of rage and clear expression of aggressive behavior. The component of anger, in contrast, is generally thought of as falling under the emotional experience profile, indicating a tendency to chronically experience strong feelings of anger [57].

Secondarily, the relationship of the expressive modalities was also examined. For example, Dembrosky and collaborators [58] investigated two specific elements in the anger/hostility construct: the Potential for Hostility and Anger-In. The Potential for Hostility was defined as the relatively stable tendency to react to frustrating events with anger, disgust, irritation and resentment; it was also thought to manifest itself as a critical attitude, antagonism and non-cooperation. The Anger-In element, on the other hand, was referred to as the incapacity to express feelings of irritation and anger towards sources of frustration and a tendency to direct these feelings inward. Siegman and collaborators [59] distinguish between hostility associated with the experience of anger and hostility associated with the expression of anger.

As Smith and collaborators affirm, even though hostility and anger, both meant as personality characteristics, are conceptually related, they are not so intensely related as to represent interchangeable labels for a single construct [57]. In fact, the concept of hostility mostly implies cognitive and transitional factors: the belief that people are primarily motivated by egoistic intentions and are frequently a source of mistreatment, the tendency to attribute to others an aggressive intent, and the relational perspective of being at odds with and different from others. The concept of anger, on the other hand, implies an emotive reaction, one that is primarily unpleasant and varies in intensity from irritation to rage. However, it is often difficult to maintain a clear distinction, due to the fact that anger also implies cognitive and relational factors, and, like hostility, can refer to the tendency to act aggressively towards others.

Studies on Anger/Hostility

On the basis of some of the data from the WCGS, Matthews and collaborators demonstrated a significant association between the incidence of cardiac disease over a period of four years and the dimension Anger/Hostility, as evaluated through the SI [60].

On the basis of a revision of the codification system of the SI, Dembroski and collaborators divided Anger/Hostility into two parts: the "potential for hostility" and "internalised anger" [58]. The authors found an association between the two constructs and the severity of cardiac disease, even after controlling for traditional risk factors. In addition, a reanalysis of the data collected by Dimsdale in 1979 [40], which did not demonstrate any association between the TABP and a series of blocked blood vessels in 103 male patients, found instead that both the potential for hostility and the internalised anger were significantly associated with angiographic results [61].

Another reanalysis, this one conducted on data from in the Multiple Risk Factor Intervention Trial, demonstrated that the two components (i.e., "potential for hostility" and "internalised anger") evaluated with the SI were able to predict cardiovascular disease independently of the traditional risk factors [62]. Positive results were derived also from studies that did not use the SI, but instead a self-report questionnaire specifically designed to measure hostility.

The Cook-Medley Hostility Scale (Ho), a scale of the Minnesota Multiphasic Personality Inventory (MMPI), was utilised extensively and found to be significantly associated both with cardiac morbidity and mortality [63]. Hostility, as measured with the Ho, was also found to predict the severity of coronary disease in cardiac patients of both sexes [64]. In a prospective study of 10 years performed on 1.877 middle-aged male workers, an independent association between the scores obtained on the Ho and the cardiac events which followed, including death, was demonstrated [65]. In another prospective study of 255 doctors, Barefoot and collaborators found a relationship between hostility, measured with the Ho in 1950, and subsequent cardiac events that occurred up until 1980. This association was independent of other risk factors, such as smoking, age, hypertension or obesity. In addition, subjects with scores above the median on the Ho had a mortality index six times greater than subjects whose scores were below the median [66]. In another prospective study covering 29 years, the same authors replicated the preceding results with a sample of 128 university students; in addition, they discovered that a combination of about 50 items – related to cynicism, hostile affect and style, and an aggressive style of answering – was more predictive than the Ho scale [67]. This last result suggests that hostility, like the TABP, is a multidimensional construct composed of subparts that are toxic in varying degrees.

Not all studies on hostility have produced results demonstrating a relationship with cardiac dysfunction. Siegman and collaborators [68] noticed a negative association between the scores on the Ho and the severity of coronary illness. In addition, Ho scores did not predict cardiovascular illness in a prospective study over a period of 25 years conducted on 478 doctors; nor did they do so in studies over periods of 30 and 33 years, conducted on 280 men and 1.400 university students, respectively [13].

In addition to the Ho the Buss-Durkee Hostility Inventory [69], another self-report instrument, has been frequently used in the evaluation of hostility as a cardiac risk factor. A factors analysis of this psychometric instrument isolated two components: "expressive or antagonistic hostility" and "neurotic or experiential hostility." The first one refers to an open verbal and/or physical expression of aggression, and it has demonstrated a positive correlation with the coronary illness. Conversely, the second component, which represents the subjective experience (such as resentment, suspicion, diffidence and irritation), has demonstrated an association with anxiety and an inverse relationship with the severity of the coronary illness [13].

More recently, in an analysis of the Multiple Risk Factor Intervention Trial, Matthews and collaborators found that subjects who had scores, as assessed by the Interpersonal Hostility Assessment Technique (IHAT), higher than the median were characterised by a significant increased (60%) risk of cardiac death at follow-up (which was 16 years), compared with subjects who had lower scores, after controlling for traditional risk factors. At baseline these subjects were not affected by CHD, but characterised instead by an elevated risk relative to traditional risk factors [70] .

A prospective study conducted on a sample of 1,305 elderly men followed for over seven years demonstrated that subjects with an elevated baseline level of anger, measured with a scale derived from the MMPI-2, were three times more likely than subjects with a low score to die from cardiac illness or have a non-fatal heart attack, even after controlling for demographic, medical and behavioral risk factors [71].

In another prospective study, high scores on a scale of three items used to assess anger as a trait were significantly associated with cardiac disease and heart attack in a sample of 1,000 men followed for a period of over 30 years. In this study, anger was shown to increase risk by three to six times [72].

With respect to the nonexpressive component of anger, a study conducted by Gallacher and collaborators on a sample of 3,000 middle aged men demonstrated that the suppression of anger (low anger externalised and high anger internalised), as measured with some of the Framinghan scales, was associated with a significant increased risk of cardiac illness over a period of 9 years, independently from a long series of other demographic, medical and behavioral variables [73].

In the Atherosclerosis Risk in Communities Study (ARIC), elevated scores of anger as a trait measured with the questionnaire developed by Spielberger and colleagues [74] were associated with a significant increase (50-75%) of cardiac risk during a period of 4 $^{1}/_{2}$ years [75]. A subsequent analysis also demonstrated that, in the angry temperament, one of the two components of anger as a trait conceptualised by Spielberger was more intensely related to the incidence of CHD than the other factor, relative to the anger provoked by negative events [76]. In both studies, gender and ethnicity had no affect on the results.

Two other prospective studies on the relationship between anger and cardiac illness yielded negative results. In a sample of more than 20,000 healthy men, the scores obtained on the scale of externalised anger in Spielberger's questionnaires did not predict the development of CHD during the two-year period of the study [77]. Similarly, in a sample of more than 9,000 healthy French and Irish men, Sykes and collaborators could not demonstrate an association between hostility and the incidence of cardiac illness over a period of 5 years [78].

In conclusion, despite some negative results, the majority of studies show that the various measures of anger and hostility are significantly correlated with elevated cardiac disease risk and reduced longevity, and that the risk is greatest when traditional risk factors are also present [57].

Instruments of Evaluation

The two most common modalities for the evaluation of hostility and anger are the SI, of which there are a few different versions, and self-administered questionnaires [57].

The most important SI for the behavioral evaluation of hostility is the IHAT, developed by Barefoot and collaborators, based on the structured interview utilised for the evaluation of the TABP [79,80]. Hostile behavior is evaluated on the basis of the expressive style, not on the content of the answers, and it is divided into four types: (1) a direct or indirect challenging attitude towards the interviewers, (2) hostile with holding of information (3) evasion of the question and (4) irritation. The interview has proved reliable, stable over time and significantly associated with the incidence of CHD and various indices of CAD [79].

The self-report instruments for measuring hostility are essentially two: the Ho [81] and the Buss-Durkee Hostility Inventory [69].

The Ho is a part of the MMPI, and it measures cynical hostility, suspiciousness, resentment and cynicism. However, it has also been shown to be significantly associated with characteristics other than hostility, such as anxiety and depression, and to have an ill-defined organisational structure [57].

The Buss-Durkee Hostility Inventory is made up of two distinct scales: the expressive or antagonistic hostility scale and the neurotic or experiential hostility scale. The first identifies verbal and/or physical aggression, whereas the second evaluates more subjective experiences, such as resentment, suspicion, diffidence and irritation. Both scales have demonstrated good construct validity [57].

The instrument for measuring anger is the State-Trait Anger Inventory (STAXI) [74]. The STAXI evaluates both the experience and the expression of anger. The experience of anger includes anger as a state – defined as an emotive experience characterised by subjective feelings of variable intensity – and anger as a trait or disposition to perceive a large number of situations as annoying and to respond with increased anger as a state. The STAXI distinguishes between two forms of expressed anger: anger expressed outwardly toward others; and anger directed inward (with the aim of keeping it in or suppressing it). The STAXI is composed of 44 items, divided into six different scales. They include: Anger as a state (S-Anger), Anger as a trait (T-Anger) - which is constituted by two subscales: Anger Temperament (T-Anger/T), which evaluates the general predisposition for feelings of anger and unmotivated anger, and Anger Reactivity (T-Anger/R), which refers to the predisposition of experiencing anger when one is criticised or attacked - Anger directed internally (AX/In), Anger directed externally (AX/Out), Control of anger (AX/Con) and, finally, the Expression of anger (AX/EX), intended as a general frequency index [74].

Pathophysiological Mechanisms

Many studies have demonstrated that hostility is related to cardiac illness through an exaggerated cardiovascular and neuroendocrine reaction towards stressful events, and an increasing number of scientific works support the hypothesis that these exaggerated responses can contribute to the onset and the progression of CAD and to the manifestation of CHD [8, 82].

The relationship between hostility and cardiac and neuroendocrine reactivity, however, seems to be mediated by demographic and situational factors [13]. In fact, some studies have demonstrated the existence of a relationship between hostility and physiological reactivity in cases of harassment suffered in interpersonal or social situations, especially in young men [13, 83]. Besides an exaggerated reactivity to negative events, the recollection of passed events lived with anger, discussions or debates on current events and the viewing of anger-provoking films were found to induce anger in subjects classified as hostile [57, 84].

Recently, other mechanisms have been identified as responsible for the association between hostility and cardiac disease. Hostile subjects have a significant rise in lipids in the blood in response to stressful stimuli, as well as a significant activation of blood plaques [57]. Other mechanisms involving inflammatory processes and other components of the immune system have also been discovered [85].

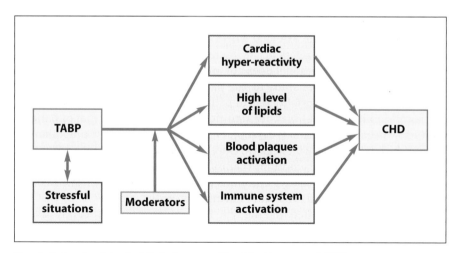

Fig. 6. Pathophysiological links between Hostility/Anger and CHD

Type D Personality

The type D personality (Distressed Personality) was introduced in 1996 by Johan Denollet and his work group as an important and stable psychosocial coronary risk factor [18].

The construct originated from a study of the relationship between personality traits and cardiac risk (morbidity and mortality) in cardiac patients, and it was identified both deductively based on personality theories already in existence, as well as inductively, based on empirical evidence and factors analysis [10, 86].

Type D personality characteristics can be summarised as negative affection and social inhibition. The first denotes the tendency to experience strong negative emotions consistently over time and in different situations, whereas the second refers to the tendency to inhibit the expression of negative emotions in social interactions [86].

From the clinical point of view, people with a type D personality tend to worry, have a pessimistic vision of life and feel anxious and unhappy. They are more readily irritated and, in general, experience fewer positive emotions. At the same time, they tend not to share their negative emotions because they are afraid of being rejected or disapproved of. These people tend to have few friendships and to feel uncomfortable in the presence of strangers [10].

The role of negative emotions and psychological distress in the pathogenesis of CHD had already been extensively studied [3]. For example, it had been demonstrated that negative emotions can interfere with the capacity to face physical illness positively and that depression and social detachment are predictive of death in cardiac patients independently of the severity of the illness [87-89].

However, the construct defined by Denollet and his research group does not refer to transitory emotive experiences that can repeat themselves in time, but to chronic emotive tonalities that "colour the relationship a person has with him/herself and with the external world during his/her life" [3] (page 414). Moreover, the construct refers to the interaction of two factors, negative affection and social inhibition, and it does not imply only the first. In reference to this, Denollet, in a prospective study of 202 patients suffering from heart disease, demonstrated that the mortality rate of patients with high negative affection, but low social inhibition (6%), was not significantly different from that of patients with a low negative affection (7%) [86]. These results highlight the fact that the way in which people deal with negative emotions can be as important a prognostic indicator as the negative emotions themselves, and the fact that the combined effect of experiencing negative emotions and dealing with them in a manner that is not healthy can be even more harmful to cardiac health.

It was also demonstrated that the type D personality is significantly associated to a few emotive and social pathologies such as depression, vital exhaustion, anger, pessimism and social detachment, which are in turn recognised as important prognostic risk factors [86]. As Denollet [10] states, these results support another important aspect of the type D personality, which is the hypothesis that psychological risk factors of a chronic type, such as the type D personality, could

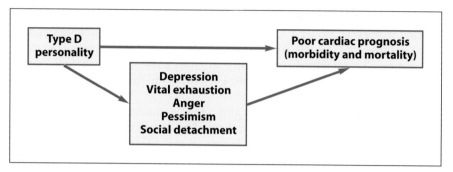

Fig. 7. Direct and indirect links between type D personality and poor cardiac prognosis

promote the development of psychological and behavioral cardiac risk factors of a transitory type, acting both directly and indirectly (Fig. 7).

Instruments

The DS14 is the psychometric instrument used to measure the type D personality [90]. It consists of 14 items, divided into two subscales: Negative Affection (NA) and Social Inhibition (SI). A score of ≥ 10 in both the scales characterises subjects with a type D personality. The DS14 has demonstrated adequate internal validity (Cronbach's $\alpha = 0.88$ for NA and 0.86 for SI) and good reliability (test-retest $r = 0.72$ for NA and 0.82 for SI).

However, in the first studies, the measurement of the construct was carried out with two questionnaires already in existence, the STAI (State-Trait Anxiety Inventory) of Spielberger and the scale of social inhibition, which belongs to the Heart patients psychological questionnaire [86].

Studies of Risk Factors for Cardiac Events

The first prospective study suggesting an association between the type D personality and a negative cardiac prognosis was published in 1995. The results demonstrated that 73% of the deaths that occurred in a sample of 105 cardiac patients involved subjects who had been evaluated as having a type D personality at the beginning of the study. The type D personality emerged as being associated with a risk of death from cardiac causes 6 times greater than non-D type cardiac patients. The study demonstrated that the type D personality could predict mortality independently of the conventional biomedical risk factors, such as physical weakness, progressive or successive myocardial infarction, smoking and age [21].

These results were confirmed a year later in a study that was an extension of preceding studies, both with respect to the sample considered (303 patients with cardiac illnesses) and with respect to the follow-up period (6-10 years). The mortality rate was greater for patients with a type D personality, compared with those without it (27 vs. 7%, p<0.00001), and the impact of the type D personality on mortality remained significant even after removing the variance due to the ventricular ejection fraction, physical weakness and the lack of a medical therapy after infarction [86].

In 1998, a study of a homogenous group of 87 patients who had had an infarction with a negative prognosis, as indicated by a level of ventricular ejection fraction of 50%, was published. In a follow-up at 6-10 years, the type D personality, in combination with a ventricular ejection fraction level of 30%, was demonstrated to be an independent predictive factor of mortality and non-fatal infarction. In this study, anxiety, depression and anger were also measured: none of these variables significantly increased the independent predictive power of the type D personality on the mortality of the patients with a low ventricular ejection fraction [22].

In 2000, the results obtained in the preceding studies of heterogeneous patients with cardiac illnesses were replicated on an independent sample of 319 patients. In a 5 year follow-up, the type D personality emerged as being an independent predictive factor of mortality and non-fatal heart attack, as well as a composite outcome including mortality, non-fatal heart attack, coronary artery bypass and percutaneous transluminal coronary angioplasty [91].

Also in 2000, an independent research group studied the role of the type D personality in a sample of people who had died from sudden cardiac arrest. Measurements were obtained through interviews with relatives close to the victims. The results demonstrated that, after controlling for the effects of conventional biomedical risk factors, the patients characterised by negative affection and social inhibition (post-hoc evaluation) were at seven times greater risk than other patients for sudden cardiac arrest [92].

Recently, a study conducted on 875 patients treated for percutaneous coronary intervention who were included in the registry of the Rapamycin-Eluting Stent Evaluated At Rotterdam Cardiology Hospital (RESEARCH) demonstrated that patients with a type D personality, evaluated six months after the intervention, had an elevated cumulative risk for suffering an adverse cardiac event (heart attack and death), compared with patients who were not classified as having a type D personality (5.6% vs. 1.3%; p<0.002) in a nine month follow-up. The type D personality remained an independent predictive risk factor of an adverse cardiac event even after controlling for the effects of the biomedical variables, including the interventions the patients had undergone [93].

Pathophysiological Mechanisms

Studies examining the psycho-physiological links between the type D personality and the pathogenesis of cardiac disease have identified mechanisms related to the immune system and hyper-reactivity.

In a cross-sectional study conducted on a sample of 42 men suffering from chronic cardiac insufficiency, an independent, significant association between type D personality and a major level of proinflammatory cytokine TNF-α, and its soluble receptors 1 and 2, emerged, after controlling for the effects linked to the ischaemic etiology and severity of the insufficiency. In other studies, the level of TNF-α and its soluble receptors have been associated with the pathogenesis of cardiovascular illness, and the receptor 1 emerged as a stronger and more accurate predictor of mortality, independently of the duration of the follow-up and other clinical variables [94].

In another cross-sectional study conducted on 173 healthy students, Habra and collaborators demonstrated that the social inhibition component was associated with high blood pressure reactivity toward stress induced from the execution of a mathematical task in association with repeated harassment, and that both social inhibition and negative affection were correlated with major cortisol reactivity [95]. Denollet downplays this correlation by asserting that, even if this result contradicts what is found in other studies of patients affected by cardiac illness, it is possible that the synergistic effect of negative affection and social inhibition could have a positive relationship with age [10].

Conclusions

A lot of scientific research conducted in different areas of study, especially epidemiology, attempted and still attempts to find a relationship between cardiovascular disease and personality traits, as well as stable behavioral patterns. From the beginning until nowadays, three constructs consecutively emerged from research as risk factors for CHD and subsequent relapse: Type A Behavioral Pattern (TABP), Anger/Hostility-prone behavior and Type D personality.

The TABP emerged in the late 50s, in a behavioral context, when a group of American cardiologists hypothesised that one of the independent etiological factors of heart disease was a specific behavioral and emotive modality in response to certain environmental prodding [12].

Pedersen and Denollet [10] point out that the TABP was purposely defined in order to avoid any association with personality traits, even though in practice it ended up being referred to as "type A personality."

The characteristics of the type A behavior pattern identified by the authors are: impatience, aggression, an intense motivation to reach their objectives which become ever greater, a sense of urgency with regard to time and a desire to make progress and be recognised.

According to Chesney (1988), the Type A behavior model should be considered a milestone in behavioral medicine, since it was the first construct that was really able to associate behavior with a serious physical illness [17].

However, this enthusiasm started to wane after some important studies failed to demonstrate a relationship between the TABP and cardiovascular disease [11]. The resulting controversy led many researchers to attempt discovering which Type A subjects really risked developing CHD. A distinction was made between toxic and non-toxic components of TABP. Of these, the one that received the most attention was the hostility/anger dimension, followed by competitiveness and time urgency.

Finally, in 1995, in the confusion which still surrounds TABP concerning its predictive power with respect to cardiac disease, especially with respect to whether it is a trait or state, a new psycho-social factor of cardiac risk appeared on the scene of psychosomatic research, the type D personality, where "D" stands for "Distressed personality" [21]. According to those who wrote on the subject, type D personality characterises those with a tendency to experience negative emotions and inhibit their expression, and it was demonstrated that the patients who are affected by heart disease and who also have a type D personality are four times more prone to death, compared with patients who are not considered type D [22].

In conclusion, as Panzer and Viljoen [1] maintain, nowadays numerous clinicians and many researchers who belong to different areas and scientific disciplines are in agreement about the existence of complex and stable bio-psychosocial associative patterns. Along the years, authors labelled them Type A, Type D and Anger/Hostility-prone behavior. Each showed and still shows empirical evidence about the links with the cardiovascular outcome, even if results are sometimes controversial. More well conducted research is needed again in order to completely validate, modify or totally refuse the constructs described above, even towards the identification of new and more predictive ones.

■ References

1. Panzer A, Viljoen M (2003) Associations between psychological profiles and diseases: examining hemispheric dominance and autonomic activation as underlying regulators. Med Hypotheses 61:75-79
2. Salvini A (1995) Gli schemi di tipizzazione della personalità in psicologia clinica e psicoterapia. In: Pagliaro G, Cesa-Bianchi M (Eds) Nuove prospettive in psicoterapia e modelli interattivo-cognitivi. FrancoAngeli, Milan, Italy, pp 63-105
3. Lesperance F, Frasure-Smith N (1996) Negative emotions and coronary heart disease: getting to the heart of the matter. Lancet 347:414-415
4. Fonagy P (2001) The human genome and the representational world: the role of early mother-infant interaction in creating an interpersonal interpretive mechanism. Bull Menninger Clin 65:427-448
5. Joseph R (1999) Environmental influences on neural plasticity, the limbic system, emotional development and attachment: a review. Child Psychiatry Hum Dev 29:189-208
6. Luecken LJ (1998) Childhood attachment and loss experiences affect adult cardiovascular and cortisol function. Psychosom Med 60:765-772
7. Hemingway H, Marmot M (1999) Evidence based cardiology: psychosocial factors in the aetiology and prognosis of coronary heart disease. Systematic review of prospective cohort studies. BMJ 318:1460-1467
8. Rozanski A, Blumenthal JA, Kaplan J (1999) Impact of psychological factors on the

pathogenesis of cardiovascular disease and implications for therapy. Circulation 99:2192-2217

9. Strike PC, Steptoe A (2004) Psychosocial factors in the development of coronary artery disease. Prog Cardiovasc Dis 46:337-347

10. Pedersen SS, Denollet J (2003) Type D personality, cardiac events, and impaired quality of life: a review. Eur J Cardiovasc Prev Rehabil 10:241-248

11. Thorensen CE, Powell LH (1992) Type A behavior pattern: new perspectives on theory, assessment and intervention. J Consult Clin Psychol 60:595-604

12. Friedman M, Rosenman RH (1959) Association of specific overt behavior pattern with blood and cardiovascular findings; blood cholesterol level, blood clotting time, incidence of arcus senilis, and clinical coronary artery disease. JAMA 169:1286-1296

13. Lachar BL (1993) Coronary-prone behavior. Type A behavior revisited. Tex Heart Inst J 20:143-151

14. Friedman HS, Booth-Kewley S (1988) Validity of the type A construct: a reprise. Psychol Bull 104:381-384

15. Menninger KA, Menninger WC (1936) Psychoanalitic observations in cardiac disorders. Am Heart J 11:10

16. Siegman AW (1993) Cardiovascular consequences of expressing, experiencing, and repressing anger. J Behav Med 16:539-569

17. Chesney MA (1988) The evolution of coronary-prone behavior. Ann Behav Med 10:43-45

18. Fred HL, Hariharan R (2002) To be B or not to be B-is that the question? Tex Heart Inst J 29:1-2

19. Miller TQ, Turner CW, Tindale RS et al (1991) Reasons for the trend toward null findings in research on type A behavior. Psychol Bull 110:469-485

20. Lyness SA (1993) Predictors of differences between type A and B individuals in heart rate and blood pressure reactivity. Psychol Bull 114:266-295

21. Denollet J, Sys SU, Brutsaert DL (1995) Personality and mortality after myocardial infarction. Psychosom Med 57:582-591

22. Denollet J, Brutsaert DL (1998) Personality, disease severity, and the risk of long-term cardiac events in patients with a decreased ejection fraction after myocardial infarction. Circulation 97:167-173

23. Ray JJ, Bozek R (1980) Dissecting the A-B personality type. Br J Med Psychol 53:181-186

24. Dimsdale JE (1988) A perspective on Type A behavior and coronary disease. N Engl J Med 318:110-112

25. Strube MJ, Boland SM, Manfredo PA, Al-Falaij A (1987) Type A behavior pattern and self-evaluation of abilities: empirical tests of the self-appraisal model. J Pers Soc Psychol 52:956-974

26. Matthews KA (1982) Psychological perspectives on the type A behavior pattern. Psychol Bull 91:293-323

27. Jenkins CD, Rosenman RH, Friedman M (1967) Development of an objective psychological test for the determination of the coronary-prone behavior pattern in employed men. J Chronic Dis 20:371-379

28. Bortner RW (1969) A short rating scale as a potential measure of pattern a behavior. J Chronic Dis 22:8791

29. Haynes SG, Feinleib M, Kannel WB (1980) The relationship of psychosocial factors to coronary heart disease in the Framingham study. III. Eight-year incidence of coronary heart disease. Am J Epidemiol 111:37-58

30. Burns W, Bluen SD (1992) Assessing a multidimensional type A behavior scale. Personality and Individual Differences 13:977-986

31. Birks Y, Derek R (2000) Identifying components of type A behavior: "toxic" and "nontoxic" achieving. Personality and Individual Differences 28:1093-1105

32. Rosenman RH, Brand RJ, Jenkins D et al (1975) Coronary heart disease in western collaborative group study. Final follow-up experience of 8 1/2 years. JAMA 233:872-877

33. Jenkins CD, Rosenman RH, Zyzanski SJ (1974) Prediction of clinical coronary heart disease by a test for the coronary-prone behavior pattern. N Engl J Med 290:1271-1275

34. French-Belgian-Collaborative-Group (1982) Ischemic heart disease and psychological patterns: Prevalence and incidence studies in Belgium and France. Adv Cardiol 29:25-31

35. Cohen JB, Reed D (1985) The type A behavior pattern and coronary heart disease among Japanese men in Hawaii. J Behav Med 8:343-352

36. Coronary-prone behavior and coronary heart disease: a critical review (1981) The review panel on coronary-prone behavior and coronary heart disease. Circulation 63:1199-1215

37. Jenkins CD, Zyzansky SJ, Rosenman R (1976) Risk of new myocardial infarction in middle-aged men with manifest coronary heart disease. Circulation 53:342-347

38. Shekelle RB, Hulley SB, Neaton JD et al (1985) The MRFIT behavior pattern study. II. Type A behavior and incidence of coronary heart disease. Am J Epidemiol 122:559-570

39. Shekelle RB, Gale M, Norusis M (1985) Type A score (Jenkins activity survey) and risk of recurrent coronary heart disease in the aspirin myocardial infarction study. Am J Cardiol 56:221-225

40. Dimsdale JE, Hackett TP, Hutter AM et al (1979) Type A behavior and angiographic findings. J Psychosom Res 23:273-276

41. Case R.B, Heller SS, Case NB, Moss AJ (1985) The multicenter post-infarction research group. Type A behavior and survival after acute myocardial infarction. N Engl J Med 312:737-741

42. Pickering TG (1985) Should studies of patients undergoing coronary angiography be used to evaluate the role of behavioral risk factors for coronary heart disease? J Behav Med 8:203-213

43. Ragland DR, Brand RJ (1988) Coronary heart disease mortality in the western collaborative group study. Follow-up experience of 22 years. Am J Epidemiol 127:462-475

44. Ragland DR, Brand RJ (1988) Type A behavior and mortality from coronary heart disease. N Engl J Med 318:65-69

45. Friedman M, Thoresen CE, Gill JJ, Ulmer et al (1986) Alteration of type A behavior and its effect on cardiac recurrences in post myocardial infarction patients: Summary results of the recurrent coronary prevention project. Am Heart J 112: 653-665

46. Myrtek M (2001) Meta-analyses of prospective studies on coronary heart disease, type A personality, and hostility. Int J Cardiol 79:245-251

47. Gostautas A, Perminas A (2004) [impact of the relationship between smoking and

stressogenic behavior (type A behavior) and their cumulative effect on development of myocardial infarction and mortality (25-year follow-up data)]. Medicina (Kaunas) 40:265-271

48. Eaker ED, Sullivan LM, Kelly-Hayes M et al (2004) Anger and hostility predict the development of atrial fibrillation in men in the Framingham offspring study. Circulation 109:1267-1271

49. Manuck SB, Kaplan JR, Clarkson TB (1983) Behaviorally induced heart rate reactivity and atherosclerosis in cynomolgus monkeys. Psychosom Med 45:95-108

50. Manuck SB, Kaplan JR, Clarkson TB (1983) Social instability and coronary artery atherosclerosis in cynomolgus monkeys. Neurosci Biobehav Rev 7:485-491

51. Manuck SB, Kaplan JR, Matthews KA (1986) Behavioral antecedents of coronary heart disease and atherosclerosis. Arteriosclerosis 6:2-14

52. Krantz DS, Contrada RJ, Hill DR, Friedler E (1988) Environmental stress and biobehavioral antecedents of coronary heart disease. J Consult Clin Psychol 56:333-341

53. Williams RB, Jr, Suarez EC, Kuhn CM et al (1991) Biobehavioral basis of coronary-prone behavior in middle-aged men. Part I: Evidence for chronic SNS activation in Type As. Psychosom Med 53:517-527

54. Williams RB, Jr, Lane JD, Kuhn CM et al (1982) Type A behavior and elevated physiological and neuroendocrine responses to cognitive tasks. Science 218:483-485

55. Muranaka M, Monou H, Suzuki J et al (1988) Physiological responses to catecholamine infusions in type A and type B men. Health Psychol 7:145-163

56. Suarez EC, Williams RB, Jr, Kuhn CM et al (1991) Biobehavioral basis of coronary-prone behavior in middle-age men. Part II: Serum cholesterol, the type A behavior pattern, and hostility as interactive modulators of physiological reactivity. Psychosom Med 53:528-537

57. Smith TW, Glazer K, Ruiz JM, Gallo LC (2004) Hostility, anger, aggressiveness, and coronary heart disease: An interpersonal perspective on personality, emotion, and health. J Pers 72:1217-1270

58. Dembroski TM, MacDougall JM, Williams RB et al (1985) Components of Type A, hostility, and anger-in: relationship to angiographic findings. Psychosom Med 47:219-233

59. Siegman AW, Anderson R, Herbst J et al (1992) Dimensions of anger-hostility and cardiovascular reactivity in provoked and angered men. J Behav Med 15:257-272

60. Matthews KA, Glass DC, Rosenman RH, Bortner RW (1977) Competitive drive, pattern a, and coronary heart disease: a further analysis of some data from the western collaborative group study. J Chronic Dis 30:489-498

61. MacDougall JM, Dembroski TM, Dimsdale JE, Hackett TP (1985) Components of type A, hostility, and anger-in: further relationships to angiographic findings. Health Psychol 4:137-152

62. Dembroski TM, MacDougall JM, Costa PT Jr, Grandits GA (1989) Components of hostility as predictors of sudden death and myocardial infarction in the multiple risk factor intervention trial. Psychosom Med 51:514-522

63. Hardy JD, Smith TW (1988) Cynical hostility and vulnerability to disease: social support, life stress, and physiological response to conflict. Health Psychol 7:447-459

64. Williams RB Jr, Haney TL, Lee KL et al (1980) Type A behavior, hostility, and coronary atherosclerosis. Psychosom Med 42: 539-549

65. Shekelle RB, Gale M, Ostfeld AM, Paul O (1983) Hostility, risk of coronary heart disease, and mortality. Psychosom Med 45:109-114

66. Barefoot JC, Dahlstrom WG, Williams RB Jr (1983) Hostility, CHD incidence, and total mortality: a 25-year follow-up study of 255 physicians. Psychosom Med 45:59-63

67. Barefoot JC, Dodge K A, Peterson BL et al (1989) The cook-medley hostility scale: item content and ability to predict survival. Psychosom Med 51:46-57

68. Siegman AW, Dembroski TM, Ringel N (1987) Components of hostility and the severity of coronary artery disease. Psychosom Med 49:127-135

69. Buss AH, Durkee A (1957) An inventory for assessing different kinds of hostility. J Consult Psychol 21:343-349

70. Matthews KA, Gump BB, Harris KF et al (2004) Hostile behaviors predict cardiovascular mortality among men enrolled in the multiple risk factor intervention trial. Circulation 109:66-70

71. Kawachi I, Sparrow D, Spiro A, 3rd et al (1996) A prospective study of anger and coronary heart disease. The normative aging study. Circulation 94:2090-2095

72. Chang PP, Ford DE, Meoni LA et al (2002) Anger in young men and subsequent premature cardiovascular disease: the precursors study. Arch Intern Med 162:901-906

73. Gallacher JE, Yarnell JW, Sweetnam PM et al (1999) Anger and incident heart disease in the Caerphilly study. Psychosom Med 61:446-453

74. Spielberger CD, Reheiser EC, Sydeman SJ (1995) Measuring the experience, expression, and control of anger. Issues Compr Pediatr Nurs 18:207-232

75. Williams JE, Paton CC, Siegler IC et al (2000) Anger proneness predicts coronary heart disease risk: prospective analysis from the atherosclerosis risk in communities (aric) study. Circulation 101:2034-2039

76. Williams JE, Nieto FJ, Sanford CP, Tyroler HA (2001) Effects of an angry temperament on coronary heart disease risk: the atherosclerosis risk in communities study. Am J Epidemiol 154:230-235

77. Eng PM, Fitzmaurice G, Kubzansky LD et al (2003) Anger expression and risk of stroke and coronary heart disease among male health professionals. Psychosom Med 65:100-110

78. Sykes DH, Arveiler D, Salters CP et al (2002) Psychosocial risk factors for heart disease in France and Northern Ireland: the prospective epidemiological study of myocardial infarction (prime). Int J Epidemiol 31:1227-1234

79. Brummett BH, Maynard KE, Haney TL et al (2000) Reliability of interview-assessed hostility ratings across mode of assessment and time. J Pers Assess 75:225-236

80. Haney TL, Maynard KE, Houseworth SJ et al (1996) Interpersonal hostility assessment technique: description and validation against the criterion of coronary artery disease. J Pers Assess 66:386-401

81. Cook W, Medley D (1954) Proposed hostility and pharisaic-virtue scales for the MMPI. J Appl Psychol 38:414-418

82. Treiber FA, Kamarck T, Schneiderman N et al (2003) Cardiovascular reactivity and development of preclinical and clinical disease states. Psychosom Med 65:46-62

83. Smith TW (1992) Hostility and health: current status of a psychosomatic hypothesis. Health Psychol 11:139-150

84. Christensen AJ, Smith TW (1993) Cynical hostility and cardiovascular reactivity during self-disclosure. Psychosom Med 55:193-202

85. Kop WJ (2003) The integration of cardiovascular behavioral medicine and psychoneuroimmunology: New developments based on converging research fields. Brain Behav Immun 17:233-237

86. Denollet J, Sys SU, Stroobant N et al (1996) Personality as independent predictor of long-term mortality in patients with coronary heart disease. Lancet 347:417-421

87. Frasure-Smith N, Lesperance F, Talajic M (1995) Depression and 18-month prognosis after myocardial infarction. Circulation 91:999-1005

88. Frasure-Smith N, Lesperance F, Talajic M (1995) The impact of negative emotions on prognosis following myocardial infarction: is it more than depression? Health Psychol 14:388-398

89. White RE, Frasure-Smith N (1995) Uncertainty and psychologic stress after coronary angioplasty and coronary bypass surgery. Heart Lung 24:19-27

90. Denollet J (2002) Type D personality and vulnerability to chronic disease, impaired quality of life and depressive symptoms. Psychosom Med 64:101

91. Denollet J, Vaes J, Brutsaert DL (2000) Inadequate response to treatment in coronary heart disease: adverse effects of type D personality and younger age on 5-year prognosis and quality of life. Circulation 102:630-635

92. Appels A, Golombeck B, Gorgels A et al (2000) Behavioral risk factors of sudden cardiac arrest. J Psychosom Res 48:463-469

93. Pedersen SS, Lemos PA, van Vooren PR et al (2004) Type D personality predicts death or myocardial infarction after bare metal stent or sirolimus-eluting stent implantation: A rapamycin-eluting stent evaluated at Rotterdam cardiology hospital (research) registry substudy. JAMA 44:997-1001

94. Denollet J, Conraads VM, Brutsaert DL et al (2003) Cytokines and immune activation in systolic heart failure: the role of type D personality. Brain Behav Immun 17:304-309

95. Habra ME, Linden W, Anderson JC, Weinberg J (2003) Type D personality is related to cardiovascular and neuroendocrine reactivity to acute stress. J Psychosom Res 55:235-245

Chapter 12

Defensive Hostility and Cardiovascular Disease: Theoretical and Empirical Bases for an Interpersonal Approach-Avoidance Conflict Perspective

R.S. Jorgensen ▪ R. Thibodeau

For thousands of years and across different cultural contexts, social, psychological, and physical well-being has been associated with the balance versus imbalance of natural forces within the person [1, 2]. As suggested by such ancient physicians as Hippocrates, a linkage between physical health and personality/emotional factors has been evident [3]. During the late nineteenth century, a defense against unconscious, psychological conflict was seen as a cause of the psychosomatic disorder of conversion hysteria (e.g., limb paralysis in the absence of a discernible organic cause; [3]). With respect to the cardiovascular system, William Harvey, in 1628, noted that a "mental disturbance" that induces either pleasant or painful affective states influences activity of the heart, and Sir William Osler, in 1910, characterized cardiac patients as ambitious men who constantly pushed the machinery of the body to its limits [4]. Alexander [5] posited the theory that high blood pressure of unknown origins (essential or primary hypertension) was prevalent among persons oriented to social status and the defensive inhibition of the cognitive and emotive aspects of anger in an effort to avoid interpersonal conflict. With theoretical and methodological advances in physiology, psychology, medicine and sociology, pre-scientific and 19-20th century speculations evolved to a rigorous examination of the scientific basis for the role of the experience, management and expression of emotion in the etiology and pathophysiology of disease. Although inconsistent findings have been reported, a substantial body of evidence shows a link between stressors and cardiovascular disease (CVD). Research further implicates such psychosocial factors as hostility, social defensiveness and the experience and expression of anger as mediators of this link [6-10].

In the current chapter, following a discussion of the evolution of the defensive hostility (DH) construct, the conflict model (which has its origin in the desire for social approval on the one hand, and the experience of defense and anger-related feelings on the other), is discussed in the context of cardiovascular disease - viz., coronary heart disease (CHD) and primary hypertension, a major CHD risk factor - as well as in the context of possible stress-related physiological processes. Methodological issues are examined in relation to predicting cardiovascular disorders with the sole use of summary scores derived from participant responses to questionnaires concerning the experience of agonistic reactions. Additionally, for the purpose of ferreting out somatogenic (i.e., disease processes inducing psychological changes), psychogenic (psychological factors inducing states of health) and biopsychosocial synergistic relations (bi-directional pathways involving both psychogenic and somatogenic factors), a research design with possible results implicating each paradigm is presented. The chapter closes with a discussion of future research directions from the perspective of "biopsychosocial synergy" and a multi-method approach to the assessment of the DH typology.

Hostility and Anger

Due to the major impact of cardiovascular disorders on morbidity and mortality and to the fact that traditional risk factors (e.g., cholesterol, smoking, obesity) cannot account for all incidences of CHD, a large literature, accumulated across decades, points to the role of cognitive, affective and behavioral factors in the development of heart disease and high blood pressure [4, 6, 10-12]. As a result of a distinguished group of scientists reviewing the 1977 proceedings of the "Forum on Coronary-Prone Behavior" (sponsored by the National Heart, Lung and Blood Institute of the USA), the Type-A Behavior Pattern (TABP) – an action-emotion complex characterized by impatience, exaggerated competitiveness, a chronic sense of time urgency, aggressive drive and hostility – was the first psychosocial variable to receive authoritative recognition as a risk factor for CHD [13]. In subsequent years, however, failure to replicate the TABP's prediction of markers for CHD in prospective epidemiological research and cross-sectional angiography studies of coronary artery disease (CAD) encouraged researchers to search for the toxic components of coronary-prone behavior. Due to its covariation with CHD and CAD, hostility emerged as a key toxic component [4, 6, 8, 10, 11]. "Cynical hostility" or the "potential for hostility" are two constructs discussed in the literature on heart disease and hostility.

In terms of mental outlook, hostility has been construed as a cognitive set characterized by a cynical mistrust and suspiciousness of others [6, 9, 14, 15]. In an interpersonal context, this cognitive set appears to increase the likelihood of experiencing angry affect, including resentment, disgust, irritability and contempt, as well as the coextensive behavioral expression of aggression - e.g., verbal attack, physical assault, and indirect actions such as gossip and character assassination [9, 11]. Anger expression has been further divided into a) anger-out (overt behavior that is visible to others), b) anger-in (the suppression of the overt expression of anger) and c) constructive anger expression (an assertive and mature discussion of the interpersonal triggers of the experience of anger) [6, 7].

In their meta-analytic review of the correlation of hostility with heart disease,

Miller and colleagues [8] compared interview-based assessments of hostility with self-assessments. Compared with the MMPI-derived Cook and Medley Hostility scale (Ho) [16], the Potential for Hostility (POHO) measure, derived from the structured interview (SI) for the TABP, demonstrated a significantly stronger association with heart disease. However, the Ho scale showed a significantly greater association with mortality in general than the interview approach. Whereas the Ho scale assumes the ability of respondents to present an accurate characterization of themselves with items varying in content (e.g., resentful feelings versus paranoid perceptions of others), POHO relies on the ability of trained individuals to rate, from the highly interpersonal and challenging context of the SI, a respondent's potential for the frequent experience of anger-laced affect and cognition with coextensive antagonistic, disagreeable and uncooperative behavior. Similarly, for the covariation of elevated blood pressure (BP) with measures of hostility and anger, the meta-analysis by Jorgensen and colleagues [7] showed that measures grounded in an interpersonal context (e.g., role-playing, projective tests administered by another person, use of interpersonal vignettes and interviews) manifested a stronger correlation than self-report measures of hostility, anger expression and anger experience.

As discussed by Jorgensen [6], a number of reasons may account for why a focused incorporation of participants' interpersonal orientation improves prediction. First, measures provided by constructs such as the Ho scale and anger expression and experience scales [17] do not provide a unitary, summed score centering on a specific interpersonal context(s). Given the importance of the interpersonal context in hostility and anger, it is possible that an overall self-report score basically captures, in large part, an affective experience and does not adequately tap salient interpersonal orientations and behaviors. Second, respondents are asked to report on socially undesirable attributes. That is, respondents may either knowingly (impression management) or unknowingly (defensive, self-deception) under-report the experience of covert anger, overt anger expression and a hostile mental outlook. These measures typically correlate negatively with measures of social defensiveness, such as, the Marlowe-Crowne Social Desirability Scale [18]. Moreover, measures of covert agonistic reactions (e.g., anger held in and the Ho scale) also have been shown to correlate with measures of neuroticism (e.g., trait anxiety and depressed mood). It is noteworthy that neuroticism has been found to a) not correlate with heart disease, b) positively correlate with angina symptoms in persons without CHD, and c) be inversely related to blood pressure elevations among persons unaware of their BP status but directly related in persons aware of their BP status. Hence, depending on sample composition (e.g., inadvertent selection of a high proportion of persons with a high neuroticism score), scores of experiential, covert anger and hostility may be elevated because of the neuroticism factor, which may mask relationships by itself or in combination with other dimensions (e.g., BP status awareness or persons with symptoms of angina without underlying disease).

Consequently, to optimize the prediction of cardiovascular diseases from measures of hostility and anger, the work of Jorgensen et al. [7] and Miller et al.

[8] strongly advocates the utilization of indicators designed to show how participants engage in their interpersonal lives. For decades, the construct of a defensive need-for-approval has been proposed as a predictor of cardiovascular health status, and recently this has emerged as a potential way of isolating those persons scoring high on cynical hostility as being at greatest risk for CVD. The following section discusses the interactive framework.

■ Defensive Hostility: A Conflict Model

Model Development
As stated above, the "cynical-hostility" construct emerged as a major description of a hostile cognitive set predisposing an individual to frequent bouts of interpersonal strife and conflict [8, 19]. This cognitive set includes the belief that, in general, people cannot be trusted, due to their selfish motives, and the likelihood of being provoked and harmed by them [19]. To assess cynical hostility, the 50-item Cook and Medley Hostility Scale (Ho) of the MMPI [16] has been used frequently [8, 19]. Although both prospective [20-22] and cross-sectional [23, 24] studies exist showing an association between Ho scores and CAD, other prospective [25, 26] and cross-sectional [27, 28] studies failed to replicate the association. Although Siegman and colleagues [29] found a significant association of Ho scores with CHD, this relation became non-significant following statistical adjustment for socioeconomic status, hypertension and diabetes. Nevertheless, recall that the meta-analysis by Miller et al. [8] demonstrated a weak association between the Ho and coronary heart disease but a more robust correlation between the two in predicting all-cause mortality. Recent epidemiological studies employing an abbreviated form of the Ho [30-32] also provide some support for the conclusions of Miller and colleagues regarding an association between cynical hostility and heart disease. Further, Knox et al. [32] have shown that the association between cynical hostility and heart disease can relate to other factors associated with social functioning as well - namely, gender and social support. It is possible that the inconsistent findings involving cynical hostility, in part, relate to an inconsistent investigation of the combined influence of cynical hostility with other theoretically relevant psychosocial variables.

Recently, social defensiveness has emerged as a potential moderator variable that, in conjunction with cynical hostility, is thought to categorize persons at risk for stress-related cardiovascular disease [33-35]. This defensive orientation toward interpersonal relationships has been conceptualized as safeguarding self-esteem by turning away, either behaviorally or cognitively, from interpersonal conflict and evaluative threat in order to maintain social approval [18, 34, 36, 37]. Specifically, this defensive striving for social approval is thought to mark a defensive avoidance of the recognition, reporting and behavioral display of angry feelings [7, 18, 34, 36, 37].

As indicated above, the defensive need for approval, when combined with cynical hostility, has been implicated as a contributing factor in CHD-prone individuals, in both a psychosocial and physiological sense [15, 34, 35]. Some CHD-prone people have been characterized as harboring a cynical mistrust of others that conflicts with the desire to be validated through the reception of affection and love [15, 34, 35, 38], which is tantamount to an "approach-avoidance" conflict, focusing on a wish for the approval of others while distrusting the same people capable of providing the desired approval, love, acceptance and reassurance. Theoretically, this habitual state of social conflict induces a chronic state of physiologic activation that fosters cardiovascular disease development [15, 33-35].

Before the introduction of the cynical hostility/high social defensiveness category (defensive hostility=DH), Weinberger et al. [39] used the Marlowe-Crowne Social Desirability Scale or MCSDS [18] as a measure of social defensiveness, together with the tendency to manifest anxiety in order to create categories of repressors, including: "high MCSDS and low anxiety;" "low MCSDS and low anxiety" (usually referred to as "low anxious"); "low MCSDS and high anxiety" (usually referred to as "high anxious"); and "high MCSDS and high anxiety" (usually referred to as "defensive high anxious"). In a similar fashion, Jamner and colleagues [34] introduced the DH type in an ambulatory blood pressure monitoring (ABPM) study of 33 male paramedics; specifically four groups were created by using median splits to parse the men into the categories of DH (high MCSDS and high Ho), high social-defensive (SD; high MCSDS but low Ho), high hostile (HH; low MCSDS but high Ho), or non-defensive low hostility (LRisk; low on both dimensions).

Research Findings

Cardiovascular reactivity (CVR) to lab stressors and ecological stressors (e.g., ABPM while at work) has been presented as a marker of risk for cardiovascular disease; thus, CVR has been a major focus of research activity [40]. In their study of male paramedics, Jamner et al. [34] showed that within the high interpersonal stress of the hospital context, the highest heart rate (HR) and diastolic blood pressure (DBP) levels obtained by ABPM were associated with the DH profile. Among healthy men and women categorized according to the above median split procedures, Helmers and Krantz [33] found a "gender by defensiveness by hostility interaction" that approached significance. Perusal of systolic blood pressure (SBP) means across a baseline and two stress periods (mental arithmetic without harassment and a speech concerning negative personal characteristics) were consistent with the highest levels being associated with the DH profile, but only for men; however, the computation of post-hoc comparisons revealed that the DH male group differed significantly from the HH and SD males only with respect to baseline SBP. For a group of male university students, Jorgensen and colleagues [35] reported that the MCSDs correlated with HR and SBP reactivity to a mental arithmetic task with harassment only for the high Ho group (that is, those scoring above the Ho median). Similarly, among male university students undertaking a reaction time task with threat of shock, high levels of stressor-induced additional HR (that is, HR levels in excess of that predicted from the covariation of oxygen consumption and HR during exercise, thereby indicating HR levels in excess of metabolic demand) was associated with the DH group [41]. However, Shapiro and colleagues [42] found that heart rate reactivity to a math stressor was significantly related to high Ho within low MCSDS males; this association was not obtained for females. In other words, compared with other studies of cardiovascular response, the results of Shapiro and colleagues [42] showed that HR reactivity, at least for male participants, correlated with a profile of defensive underreporting of hostility (low Ho, high MCSDS) in lieu of a DH profile. In discussing the differing results between the paramedic and lab reactivity studies, Shapiro et al. [42] speculated that the defensive/low hostility males were more reactive in the lab due to a diminished capacity to deploy the coping style of disengaging from interpersonal stress, which could be deployed in the field; however, the nature of the task could be another reason why CVR was not associated with DH. As reported by Suarez and associates [43], high sympathetic nervous system reactivity associated with cynical hostility is triggered by abrasive harassment (e.g., "Stop mumbling, I can't understanding your answers," p. 79). The study by Shapiro et al., however, used challenges for increased speed; consequently, it is possible that correlation of DH with CVR was not obtained because these investigators utilized behavioral challenge rather than abrasive harassment.

It is noteworthy that the Jorgensen et al. study used a series of harassing statements delivered in an officious, fault-finding manner (e.g., "Please keep up with the metronome and stop making so many mistakes," p. 158). It also is noteworthy that for a correlate of cynical hostility, the self-report of "anger-out" [19], al' Absi et al. [44] obtained only a non-significant trend for the high anger-out/high MCSDS males to manifest high heart rate reactivity to a mental arithmetic task with minimal social interaction (viz., participants were instructed, from a separate control room, to begin again after a mistake through an intercom).

Interestingly, relative to the other males, al'Absi et al. [44] report that the "high anger out/high MCSDS" males showed the highest levels of salivary cortisol thirty minutes following a very interpersonal public speaking task (consisting of three 4-minute speeches involving a defense against the accusation of shop-lifting, a discussion of whether homosexuals should be allowed in the military, and a discussion on a paper concerning the causes of gray hair, as the speeches were videotaped, and as two white-coated experimenters stood in the room). All in all, the results of the psychophysiological studies indicate that, at least for males, interpersonal harassment characterized by evaluative threat and aggravation is key to inducing relationships between DH and physiological reactivity.

In terms of severity of CAD, promising results were reported by two groups that utilized the typing procedures of Jamner et al. [34]. For three different samples of cardiac patients, Helmers and colleagues [45] showed that the DH profile, in comparison to the other three profiles, manifested the longest duration of ischemia during daily activities (assessed by ambulatory monitoring), the most pronounced ischemia during mental stress, and the most perfusion defects during thallium exercise scintigraphy. In terms of the composition of their three samples, one sample consisted only of males, and there were more males than females in the two other samples. (A test for gender by DH was not reported.) Jorgensen and colleagues administered the Ho and MCSDS scales to 59 male patients at a Veterans Administration Medical Center the day prior to their angiographic procedures. An *a priori* contrast showed that the DH group's mean number of arteries with at least a 50% blockage (mean = 2.5) differed significantly from the combined means of the other groups. Moreover, the HH and SD groups did not differ from the Lrisk group. This promising study sampled mostly white participants, and like the Helmers et al. studies, focused on men. Hence, the impact of socio-cultural and biological factors related to gender and race are unknown. Another shortcoming of the above studies pertains to examining persons with suspected or actual CAD. The potential impact of disease or the mere awareness of the presence or potential presence of CAD makes it impossible to rule out a somatogenic basis (whereby the disease might alter the psychosocial factors) for the obtained findings. For example, it is possible that a history of vitiated health status and knowledge of greater risk for mortality could elevate cynical hostility and social defensiveness. Additional research is required to assess whether the same pattern of results would emerge in females, non-white samples, and persons without diagnosed CVD undergoing non-invasive assessments (e.g., echo-cardiography). Given the retrospective nature of both studies, somatogenic causes cannot be differentiated from psychogenic factors (namely, the possibility that psychosocial factors could alter health status). However, as with other diseases (e.g., primary hypertension), the DH and CAD association is likely to reflect a biopsychosocial synergistic model, in which behavior, affect, mental states, physiology, constitution and environmental factors create causal matrices of complex, bi-directional linkages in the development of stress-related diseases [7, 10, 46, 47].

Investigating Psychogenic, Somatogenic and Biopsychosocial Synergy: a Proposed Design

To study the relative impact of somatogenic, psychogenic and biopsychosocial synergistic factors, it is essential to combine cross-sectional and prospective research designs in which both initially disease-free participants and disease-diagnosed participants, matched for salient individual differences (e.g., gender, race, blood pressure, cholesterol and so forth), are studied across time. In such a study, the somatogenic paradigm would be supported if, e.g., a) the association of DH with CHD results from longitudinal studies showed increases in the Ho and MCSDS following diagnosis among initially healthy people, and if b) the Ho and MCSDS scores increased longitudinally in individuals diagnosed initially with CHD and whose disease worsened. A psychogenic paradigm would be supported if a) the DH/CHD association relates to the development of disease, with the Ho and MCSDS remaining stable among the initially healthy group, and if b) an augmentation of the DH/CHD association occurred, with the MCSDS and Ho remaining stable across time among initially diagnosed CHD patients. The bi-directional influences of psychogenic and somatogenic factors would be implicated (supporting a biopsychosocial synergistic paradigm) if a number of cross-sectional and longitudinal results were found. First, for the longitudinal tracking of the initially disease-free, a) the DH type should show the prospective association with CHD, b) a DH subgroup should show stable Ho and MCSDS and stable CHD severity and c) another DH subgroup should show increases in the Ho and MCSDS with a coextensive increase in CHD severity. Second, for the longitudinal study of the initial group of CHD patients, a) an initial association of CHD with the DH type should be obtained and b) increases in the Ho and MCSDS should covary with increases in disease severity [7, 10, 46].

Approach-Avoidance Conflict and Coactivation

Cacioppo and Berntson [48], in their review of evaluative processes, detailed the concept of "coactivation" in the context of approach-avoidance conflicts [49]. In essence, both approach and avoidance tendencies are thought to be activated at the same time in the appropriate eliciting context, and this coactivation induces high levels of the cognitive, behavioral and physiological components of arousal [48, 50]. In the case of DH, it is proposed that in the eliciting context of social conflict, the coactivation of avoidance tendencies (basic mistrust, resentment and negative appraisals of others) and approach tendencies (seeking approval) generate contemporaneous tendencies of fight/effort and fear associated with possible loss of control/subordination. In other words, at risk DH males may oscillate between a) subordination in the service of keeping social approval and b) agonistic behavior intended to "ward off" the anticipated interpersonal onslaught, thereby simultaneously triggering the physiological responses characteristic of both behavioral patterns. Furthermore, the simultaneous activation of the sympathoadrenal-medullary axis associated with agonistic reactions and the pituitary adrenocortical axis associated with the loss of control/subordination may arise not only during the actual encounter, but during subsequent ruminative, revivifications of the event [47, 51]. Over time, frequent evocations of this coactivation could foster CAD development or worsen the disease status. Recurrent and excessive perturbations of the sympathoadrenal-medullar axis may contribute to endothelial damage and atherosclerotic lesions by means of such factors as high levels of cardiovascular reactivity (e.g., high levels of turbulent blood flow where arteries bifurcate) and high circulating catecholamines [10, 47, 52-54]. Concurrent with the effects of recurrent sympathoadrenal-medullar axis reactivity, excessive and frequent pituitary adrenocortical axis reactivity may cultivate atherosclerotic lesions by means of cortisol's ability to liberate free fatty acids and augment sympathetic nervous system (SNS) responsiveness [52, 55].

A Matrix of Possible Physiological Mechanisms: Biopsychosocial Synergy

Recall that, in the paramedic study of males, Jamner and associates [34] found that a DH profile was linked with high HR and DBP. Recall also, that other investigators studying males have observed stressor-evoked HR and SBP reactivity [35], stressor-evoked HR in excess of metabolic demand [41], and elevated baseline SBP [33]. Interestingly, epidemiological studies have shown that in men high resting HR prospectively predicts CVD, CVD-related mortality or both [56-58]. Kannel et al. [58] also reported a prospective relationship between high HR and CVD among their female participants, although the relationship they observed was weaker than that observed among men. Similarly, high HR prospectively predicted mortality among older women with disability [59]. It is also noteworthy that results from cross-sectional studies show associations between high resting HR and atherogenic lipid levels in men [60, 61] and in women [60]. Taken collectively, these epidemiological and lab results are consistent with the notion that high levels of sympathoadrenal-related cardiac activity may place DH males, if not DH females, at greater risk for CVD.

Involvement of the autonomic nervous system in the association of cardiovascular activity with lipid levels is supported by research showing that stressor-induced tachycardia (that might result, for example, from activities such as race car driving and public speaking) and the rise in plasma free fatty acids were blunted by beta-blockade [62, 63]; autonomic nervous system involvement also is supported by research showing HR, serum cholesterol and triglycerides to be higher in people assessed after an earthquake relative to those assessed before the earthquake [64]. Among a group of men with unmedicated, mild-hypertension, Jorgensen and colleagues [65] showed that stressor (video-game and a color-word task) -induced HR acceleration correlated with total serum cholesterol and triglycerides. However, as discussed by van Doormen [66], associations between cardiovascular reactivity and lipid levels are found inconsistently, which may relate to use of small samples and the moderating influences of age, medication status, and patient cardiac status (high BP or CHD). Consistent with the conclusions of their literature review, van Doormen [66] reported that cardiac responsivity (pre-ejection period, cardiac out-put and stroke volume), aggregated across two stressors (mental arithmetic and a reaction time task), was positively correlated with cholesterol for a subgroup of middle-aged males (no such relationship was found for adolescents or females). In a review of epidemiological findings, Palatini [67] concludes that increased cardiovascular morbidity relates to a clustering of high HR, high resting blood pressure, high lipid values, and markers of insulin resistance, all of which are influenced by sympathetic overactivity. Given the decades of epidemiological findings, the preliminary research on DH, and research suggesting a matrix of cardiac and neuroendocrine bi-directional influences in the pathophysiology of cardiovascular disease, it is possible that a frequent "co-activation" of the sympathetic-adrenal axis and pituitary adrenal axis could contribute to frequent bouts of cardiac and vascular responses that damage arteries, through high levels of circulating stress hormones (e.g., epinephrine and cortisol), high levels of atherogenic serum lipids, and elevated resting blood pressure in the at-risk DH male. Moreover, given the conclusions of Palatini [67], this stress reactivity, along with life-style factors (e.g., atherogenic diet, being overweight, sedentary life-style) and genetic risk (e.g., family history of hypertension, heart disease and/or diabetes), could contribute to a clustering of insulin resistance, high-blood pressure and dyslipidaemia. Such a clustering is characteristic of syndrome X and its high risk for cardiovascular disorders. Thus, an examination of the linkages of life-style behaviors, genetic risk, biological processes, gender and social conflict-related physiological reactivity may provide biopsychosocial synergistic pathways for CVD development in a subgroup of DH people (e.g., white, middle-aged males of a Western cultural background).

In recent years, a consensus has emerged that atherosclerosis reflects a chronic infectious disease [68, 69]. For example, in a discussion of the relationship between cardiovascular disease and immune functioning across the human lifespan, Kop [70] theorizes that the chronic condition of dispositional hostility triggers acute stress reactions (e.g., angry reactions) and that episodic stress reactions (e.g., depressed mood and exhaustion) are linked to alterations in immune functioning (such as immune suppression, susceptibility to infection, phagocytosis or pro-inflammatory cytokines) conducive to atherogenesis. It is noteworthy that low density lipoproteins (LDL) and hypertension are capable of stimulating inflammatory responses [68, 69], and that C-reactive protein, a marker of inflammation and risk for cardiovascular disease, has been associated with an adverse lipid profile in children (low high density lipoprotein in both genders, as well as total cholesterol in boys [71]). Interestingly, there is also evidence of an association between cynical hostility and elevated levels of LDL [72, 73]. Regarding markers of inflammatory processes, two studies, albeit showing different relationships, have demonstrated that cynical hostility is moderated by depressive symptoms. Suarez [74] showed high levels of the cytokine of Interlukin-6 (a marker of inflammatory status) to be associated with high cynical hostility and high levels of depressed symptoms; whereas Miller and associates [75] showed high levels to be associated with high cynical hostility but low reports of depressed mood. In discussing the different patterns found by Miller et al. [75] and Suarez [74], Miller and colleagues suggest that the latter study's use of only male, non-smokers and the former study's use of a clinical sample could contribute to the observed discrepancy. However, there is another possible explanation. High cardiovascular reactivity has been associated with a self-report of low depressed mood and high levels of distress (based on the clinical evaluations of judges); this discrepancy has been interpreted as reflecting defensiveness [76]. Therefore, it is possible that, in order to maintain social approval, the sample investigated by Miller and colleagues contained enough persons associated with the subgroup of cynical hostile individuals prone to a defensive underreporting of distress, which is consistent with the DH category.

Conclusions

In some DH individuals prone to stress-related heart disease, research and theory implicate an approach-avoidance conflict. On the one hand, the DH person distrusts others and expects to be the recipient of social harm and, consequently, may frequently experience a mental state of vigilance for the predatory social acts of others, which is likely to increase bouts of anger experience and expression, in addition to the associated sympathoadrenal-medullary reactions. On the other hand, the desire to be approved of by those who are construed as having the potential for attack and domination often seems to induce a mental state of subordination, distress (anxiety and depressed mood), and responses characteristic of the pituitary-adrenal-medullary axis. Over the course of a lifetime, the coactivation of both systems of the autonomic nervous system could induce vascular hypertrophy and atheroma conducive to CVD. From a biopsychosocial synergistic perspective, the psychophysiological and anatomical changes could induce further changes conducive to disease progression. For example, acute stressor-related cortisol activation could a) suppress immune function and increase vulnerability to infection, thus contributing to arterial damage [68, 70], b) augment reactivity of the SNS, and c) foster excess liberation of free fatty acids. Frequent and chronic SNS activation may create vascular injury, contribute to vascular hypertrophy, or both. In combination with a high dietary intake of fat, the actions of both these mechanisms could then result in the development of high levels of LDL and, as a result, foster inflammation related to atherosclerotic lesions. With respect to the central nervous system, research suggests that a) glucocorticoids (e.g., cortisol) can damage the memory function of the brain [77] and b) hypertension and diffuse atherosclerotic disease adversely affects a variety of domains of cognitive function [78]. Because the optimal modulation of emotion and coping with stress is thought to be intimately connected to cognitive function [79], it is possible that impaired cognitive functioning, for example, could slow information processing and the efficacious recall of past effective coping mechanisms, the net result being less efficacious coping. This hypothesized decrement in coping related to anatomical changes then may contribute to an increase in agonistic transactions and thereby reinforce the DH pattern and its associated cascade of physiological, emotive and behavioral adjustments conducive to disease development.

In closing, a relatively small body of research has supported the construct of DH as a contributor to stress-related CVD. Consequently, little is known about the possible moderating influences of gender, ethnicity, cultural background, socioeconomic status, education or risk factors, including both lifestyle and genetic. A combination of prospective and cross-sectional designs is warranted to ferret out the psychogenic, somatogenic and biopsychosocial synergistic influences. There are other research questions as well, particularly related to the use of multimethod approaches in the assessment of defense and hostility. These include the use of interpersonally grounded assessments (e.g., POHO), self-reported measures of hostility (e.g., Ho), and ecological measures of physiology (ABPM) and perceived stress/negative affect (ecological momentary assessment or EMA - see also the research of Brosschot & Thayer [80] and Smyth and associates [81]. Such a multi-method approach would enable investigators to examine converging versus discrepant responses with respect to the "profiling process" (e.g., DH people scoring high on Ho, low on POHO, and reporting low levels of EMA). The evidence supporting the theory that defensive strivings are marked by a discrepancy between self-judgements and the judgements of others having to do with psychosocial functioning - as discussed by Horowitz & Znoj [82] and by Shedler and associates [76] - may provide researchers with a more accurate categorization of the DH profile. Finally, given the accumulating evidence linking CAD to activity of the immune system, such factors as immune suppression and inflammatory processes appear to be an exciting avenue for future research, particularly in view of the fact that the nature of the immune system's involvement is likely to change throughout the human lifespan [70].

References

1. Cohen KS (1999) The way of Qigong: the art and science of chinese energy healing. Ballantine Publishing Group, New York
2. Kagan J (1994) Galen's prophecy: temperament in human nature. Basic Books, New York
3. Alexander F (1954) The scope of psychoanalysis: the selected papers of Franz Alexander. New York: Basic Books, Inc.
4. Williams RB, Barefoot JC (1988) Coronary-prone behavior: the emerging role of the hostility complex. In: Houston BK, Snyder CR (Eds) Type A behavior pattern: research, theory, and intervention. New York: Wiley, pp 189-211
5. Alexander F (1939) Emotional factors in essential hypertension. Psychosom Med 1:175-179
6. Jorgensen RS (2005) Issues in the measurement of anger and hostility: cardiovascular disease as an illustrative case. In: Anderson NB, Salovey P (Eds) Encyclopedia of heath and behavior. Thousand Oaks, CA, Sage
7. Jorgensen RS, Johnson BT, Kolodziej ME, Schreer GE (1996) Elevated blood pressure and personality: a meta-analytic review. Psychological Bull 120:293-320
8. Miller TQ, Smith TW, Turner CW et al (1996) Meta-analytic review on hostility and physical health. Psychological Bull 119:322-348
9. Smith TW (1994) Concepts and methods in the study of anger, hostility and health. In: Siegman AW, Smith TW (Eds) Anger, hostility, and the heart. Hillsdale, NJ, Erlbaum, pp 23-42
10. Williams RB, Barefoot C, Schneiderman N (2003) Psychosocial risk factors for cardiovascular disease: more than one culprit at work. JAMA 290:2190-2192
11. Dembroski TM, Costa PT (1987) Coronary prone behavior: components of the Type A pattern and hostility. J Personality 55:212-235
12. Rosenman RH, Swan GE, Carmelli D (1988) Definition, assessment, and evolution of the Type A behavior pattern. In: Houston BK, Snyder CR (Eds) Type A behavior pattern: research, theory, and intervention. Wiley, New York, pp 8-31

13. Houston BK (1988) Introduction. In: Houston BK, Snyder CR (Eds) Type A behavior pattern: research, theory, and intervention, Wiley, New York, pp 1-7
14. Houston BK, Vavak CR (1991) Cynical hostility: developmental factors, psychosocial correlates, and health behaviors. Health Psychol 10:9-17
15. Jorgensen RS, Frankowski JJ, Lantinga LJ et al (2001) Defensive hostility and coronary heart disease: a preliminary investigation of male veterans. Psychosom Med 63:463-469
16. Cook WW, Medley DM (1954) Proposed hostility and pharisaic virtue scales for the MMPI. J Applied Psychol 38:414-418
17. Buss AH, Durkee A (1957) An inventory for assessing different kinds of hostility. J Consult Psychol 21:343-349
18. Crowne DP, Marlowe D (1964) The approval motive: studies in evaluative dependence. Wiley, New York
19. Smith TW (1992) Hostility and health: current status of a psychosomatic hypothesis. Health Psychol 11:139-150
20. Barefoot JC, Dahlstrom WG, Williams RB (1983) Hostility, CHD incidence and total mortality: a 25-year follow-up study of 255 physicians. Psychosom Med 45:59-64
21. Barefoot JC, Dodge KA, Peterson BL et al (1989) Cook-Medley hostility scale: item content and ability to predict survival. Psychosom Med 51:46-57
22. Shekelle RB, Gale M, Ostfeld AM, Paul O (1983) Hostility, risk of coronary heart disease, and mortality. Psychosom Med 45:109-114
23. Helmers KF, Krantz DS, Howell RH et al (1993) Hostility and myocardial ischemia in coronary artery patients: evaluation by gender and ischemic index. Psychosom Med 55:29-36
24. Williams RB, Haney TL, Lee KL et al (1989) Type A behavior, hostility, and coronary atherosclerosis. Psychosom Med 42:539-549
25. Hearn MD, Murray D, Luepker RV (1989) Hostility, coronary heart disease, and total mortality: a 33-year follow-up study of university students. J Behav Med 12:105-121
26. McCranie EW, Watkins LO, Brandsma JM, Sisson BD (1986) Hostility, coronary heart disease (CHD) incidence, and total mortality: lack of an association in a 25-year follow-up study of 478 physicians. J Behav Med 9:119-125
27. Dembroski TM, MacDougall JM, Williams RB et al (1985) Components of type A, hostility, and anger-in: relationship to angiographic findings. Psychosom Med 47:219-233
28. Helmer DC, Ragland DR, Syme SL (1991) Hostility and coronary artery disease. Am J Epidem 133:112-122
29. Siegman AW, Townsend ST, Civelek AC, Blumenthal RS (2000) Antagonistic behavior, dominance, hostility, and coronary heart disease. Psychosom Med 62:248-257
30. Barefoot JC, Larsen S, von der Lieth L, Schroll M (1995) Hostility, incidence of acute myocardial infarction, and mortality in a sample of older Danish men and women. Am J Epidemiol 142:477-484
31. Everson SA, Kauhanen J, Kaplan GA et al (1997) Hostility and increased risk of mortality and acute myocardial infarction: the mediating role of behavioral risk factors. Am J Epidem 146:142-152
32. Knox SS, Siegmund KD, Weidner G et al (1998) Hostility, social support, and coronary heart disease in the National Heart, Lung, and Blood Institute Family Heart Study. Am J Cardiol 82:1192-1196

33. Helmers KF, Krantz DS (1996) Defensive hostility and cardiovascular levels and responses to stress. Annals Behav Med 18:246-254
34. Jamner LD, Shapiro D, Goldstein IB, Hug R (1991) Ambulatory blood pressure and heart rate in paramedics: effects of cynical hostility and defensiveness. Psychosom Med 53:393-406
35. Jorgensen RS, Abdul-Karim K, Kahan TA, Frankowski JJ (1995) Defensiveness, cynical hostility and cardiovascular reactivity: a moderator analysis. Psychother Psychosom 64:156-161
36. Jorgensen RS, Gelling PD, Kliner L (1992) Patterns of social desirability and anger in young men with a parental history of hypertension: association with cardiovascular reactivity. Health Psychol 11:403-412
37. Weinberger DA (1990) The construct validity of the repressive coping style. In: Singer JL (Ed) Repression and dissociation: implications for personality theory, psychopathology, and health. Chicago, University of Chicago Press, pp 337-386
38. Fontana AF, Kerns RD, Blatt SJ et al (1989) Cynical mistrust and the search for self-worth. J Psychosom Res 33:449-456
39. Weinberger DA, Schwartz GE, Davidson RJ (1979) Low-anxious, high-anxious, and repressive coping styles: psychometric patterns and behavioral and physiological responses to stress. J Abnorm Psychol 88:369-380
40. Linden W, Gerin G, Davidson K (2003) Cardiovascular reactivity: status quo and a research agenda for the new millennium. Psychosom Med 65:5-8
41. Larson MR, Langer AW (1997) Defensive hostility and anger expression: relationship to additional heart rate reactivity during active coping. Psychophysiol 34:177-184
42. Shapiro D, Goldstein IB, Jamner LD (1995) Effects of anger/hostility, defensiveness, gender, and family history of hypertension on cardiovascular reactivity. Psychophysiol 32:425-435
43. Suarez EC, Kuhn CM, Schanberg SM et al (1998) Neuroendocrine, cardiovascular, emotional responses of hostile men: the role of interpersonal challenge. Psychosom Med 60:78-88
44. al'Absi M, Bongard S, Lovallo WR (2000) Adrenocorticotropin responses to interpersonal stress: effects of overt anger expression style and defensiveness. Intern J Psychophysiol 37:257-265
45. Helmers KF et al (1995) Defensive hostility: relationship to multiple markers of cardiac ischemia in patients with coronary disease. Health Psychol 14:202-209
46. Engel GL (1977) The need for a new medical model: a challenge for biomedicine. Science 196:129-136
47. McCabe PM, Sheridan JF, Weiss JM et al (2000) Animal models of disease. Physiol Behav 68:501-507
48. Cacioppo JT, Berntson GG (1994) Relationship between attitudes and evaluative space: a critical review, with emphasis on the separability of positive and negative substrates. Psychologic Bull 115:401-423
49. Miller NE (1951) Comments on theoretical models illustrated by the development of a theory of conflict behavior. J Personality 20:82-100

50. Lang PJ, Bradley MM, Cuthbert BN (1997) Motivated attention: affect, activation, and action. In: Lang PJ, Simons RF, Balaban MT (Eds) Attention and orienting: sensory and motivational processes. Lawrence Erlbaum Associates, Mahwah NJ, pp 97-135

51. Henry JP (1986) Neuroendocrine patterns of emotional response. In: Plutchik R, Kellerman H (Eds) Emotion: theory, research and experience, vol. 3. Academic Press, Orlando FL, pp 37-60

52. Herd JA (1986) Neuroendocrine mechanisms in coronary heart disease. In: Matthews KA, Weiss SM, Detre T et al (Eds) Handbook of stress, reactivity, and cardiovascular disease. Wiley, New York, pp 49-70

53. Kaplan JR, Botchin MB, Manuck SB (1994) Animal models of aggression and cardiovascular disease. In: Siegman AW, Smith TW (Eds) Anger, hostility, and the heart. Lawrence Erlbaum Associates, Hillsdale, NJ pp 127-148

54. Rozanski A, Blumenthal JA, Kaplan J (1999) Impact of psychological factors on the pathogenesis of cardiovascular disease and implications for therapy. Circulation 99:2192-2217

55. Lovallo WR (1997) Stress and Health: biological and psychological interactions. Sage Publications, Thousand Oaks, CA

56. Dyer AR, Persky V, Stamler J et al (1980) Heart rate as a prognostic factor for coronary heart disease and mortality: findings in three Chicago epidemiologic studies. Am J Epidem 112:736-749

57. Friedman GD, Klatsky AL, Siegelaub AB (1975) Predictors of sudden cardiac death. Circulation 51(Suppl III):164-169

58. Kannel WB, Kannel C, Paffenbarger RS, Cupples LA (1987) Heart rate and cardiovascular mortality: the Framingham study. Am Heart J 113:1489-1494

59. Chang M, Havlik RJ, Corti MC et al (2003) Relation of heart rate at rest and mortality in the women's health and aging study. Am J Cardiol 92:1294-1299

60. Boona KH, Arnesen E (1992) Association between heart rate and atherogenic blood lipid fractions in a population: the Tromso Study. Circulation 86:394-405

61. Williams PT, Haskell WL, Vranizan KM et al (1985) Associations of resting heart rate with concentrations of lipoprotein subfractions in sedentary men. Circulation 71:441-449

62. Taggart P, Carruthers M (1972) Suppression by oxyprenolol of adrenergic response to stress. Lancet 2:256-258

63. Taggart P, Carruthers M, Sommerville W (1973) Electrocardiogram, plasma catecholamines and lipids, and their modification by oxyprenolol when speaking before an audience. Lancet 2:341-346

64. Trevisan M, Celentano E, Meucci C et al (1986) Short-term effect of natural disasters on coronary heart disease risk factors. Arteriosclerosis 6:491-494

65. Jorgensen RS, Nash JK, Lasser NL et al (1988) Heart rate acceleration and its relationship to total serum cholesterol, triglycerides, and blood pressure reactivity in men with mild hypertension. Psychophysiol 25:39-44

66. van Doornen LJP, Snieder H, Boomsma DI (1998) Serum lipids and cardiovascular reactivity to stress. Bio Psychol 47:279-297

67. Palatini P (1999) Elevated heart rate as a predictor of increased cardiovascular morbidity. J Hypertension 17(Suppl 3):S3-S10
68. Fahdi IE, Gaddam V, Garza G et al (2003) Inflammation, infection and atherosclerosis. Brain, Behavior, and Immunity 17:238-244
69. Ross R (1999) The pathogenesis of atherosclerosis: an inflammatory disease. N Engl J Med 340:115-126
70. Kop WJ (2003) The integration of cardiovascular behavioral medicine and psychoneuroimmunology: new developments based on converging research fields. Br Behav Imm 17:233-237
71. Wu DM, Chu NF, Shen MH, Chang JB (2003) Plasma C-reactive protein levels and their relationship to anthropometric and lipid characteristics among children. J Clin Epidemiol 56:94-100
72. Brindley DN, McCann BS, Niaura R et al (1993) Stress and lipoprotein metabolism: modulators and mechanisms. Metabolism 42:3-15
73. Suarez EC, Bates MP, Harralson TL (1998) The relation of hostility to lipids and lipoproteins in women: evidence for the role of antagonistic hostility. Ann Behav Med 20:59-63
74. Suarez EC (2003) The joint effect of hostility and severity of depressive symptoms on plasma interleukin-6 concentration. Psychosom Med 65:523-527
75. Miller GE, Freedland KE, Carney RM et al (2003) Cynical hostility, depressive symptoms, and the expression of inflammatory risk markers for coronary heart disease. J Behav Med 26:501-515
76. Shedler J, Mayman M, Manis M (1993) The illusion of mental health. Am Psychologist 48:1117-1131
77. Sauro MD, Jorgensen RS, Pedlow TC (2003) Stress, glucocorticoids, and memory: a meta-analytic review. Stress 6:235-245
78. Waldstein SR, Tankard CF, Maier KJ et al (2003) Peripheral arterial disease and cognitive function. Psychosom Med 65:757-763
79. Lazarus RS (1993) From psychological stress to the emotions: a history of changing outlooks. Ann Rev Psychol 44:1-21
80. Brosschot JF, Thayer JF (2003) Heart rate response is longer after negative emotions than after positive emotions. Intern J Psychophysiol 50:181-187
81. Smyth J, Ockenfels MC, Porter L et al (1998) Stressors and mood measured on a momentary basis are associated with salivary cortisol secretion. Psychoneuroendocrinology 23:353-370
82. Horowitz M, Znoj H (1999) Emotional control theory and the concept of defense: a teaching document. J Psychother Practice Res 8:213-223

Chapter 13

In Sickness and In Health: Interpersonal Risk and Resilience in Cardiovascular Disease

J.M. Ruiz ▪ H.A. Hamann ▪ J.C. Coyne ▪ A. Compare

Charles Jacobs and his wife were going through their normal Saturday morning routine when he experienced sudden and severe chest pressure, radiating pain, nausea, and shortness of breath. Mrs. Jacobs quickly called for paramedics before returning to monitor and comfort her husband while experiencing her own emotional reactions. In the days that followed, Mr. Jacobs was diagnosed with CAD and significant occlusion in several vessels. He underwent coronary artery bypass grafting (CABG) surgery and was given a post-surgical regimen of medications, exercise, and diet before being discharged a week after the initial event. Due to the surgical incision and recovery process, Mr. Jacobs must adhere to a number of behavioral restrictions, which limit his ability to do household chores, drive a car and go to his job (he is an independent auto mechanic). In addition to his health and medical regimen concerns, Mr. Jacobs struggles with worries about his family's financial situation. He is also concerned about the prospect of being a burden to his wife, who must help in his care while managing their household and family. Mrs. Jacobs has always been somewhat of a worrier, and this incident has left her concerned about her husband's health and the possibility of life without him. Now her day revolves around her husband, watching what he eats and how he takes his medications, asking him to "slow down," and vigilantly monitoring for signs of physical problems. In response to his wife's concerns, Mr. Jacobs tries to convince her of his health by pushing himself to resume his normal activities, while denying his own concerns and suppressing any illness behaviors. However, his wife's worry and vigilance has him wondering whether he is more vulnerable than he has been willing to admit.

The Jacobs' case illustrates what we all experience on a daily basis: we influence other people and they influence us. Quite often, our relationships are dynamic, give-and-take experiences that can take on lives of their own. These interactions and, more specifically, the individuals themselves may be important influences on health and well being [1, 2]. Traditionally, researchers have dichotomized the study of psychosocial risk factors into individual/psychological factors and social/environmental factors. This approach has been effective in identifying important sources of non-traditional risk, but it has not fully elucidated the characteristics of these risk factors. For example, the traditional approach to risk factor identification would highlight Mr. Jacobs' personality, coping styles and available social support as determinants of his recovery and future health. However, it would fail to identify his wife's personality and behaviors, as well as Mr. Jacobs' responses to his wife, as potential influences on his health.

The interpersonal approach provides an integrative framework for conceptualizing individuals as active risk/benefit influences on one another [3, 4]. This emphasis on individuals also redefines, in a couple of different ways, how we conceptualize so-called social factors. First, it re-characterizes social risk factors as individuals rather than abstract groupings, allowing the researcher to consider the unique attributes each person brings to the interaction. For example, Mr. Jacobs is not just married, he is in a marriage to Mrs. Jacobs - a loving but anxious and vigilant individual. Second, while the interpersonal approach does not abandon the individual difference approach, it emphasizes its role within the interpersonal context. One aim of this chapter is to review interpersonal theory and models for understanding the interplay between individuals and their social environments. A second aim is to focus on the literature identifying interpersonal influences in cardiovascular health and disease.

A Primer on Interpersonal Theory and Concepts

The interpersonal approach is based on a long tradition, formulated in the works of such theorists and researchers as Sullivan [5], Leary [6], Carson [7], Benjamin [8, 9], Wiggins [10], Kiesler [11], Kelley [12], Dewey and Bentley [13], Thibaut and Kelly, [14], and Wachtel [15, 16]. Founded as a reaction to Freud's intrapsychic view of the individual, Sullivan's approach shifted the emphasis to the importance of interpersonal interactions and conceptualized individual personality as "the relatively enduring pattern of recurrent interpersonal situations which characterize a human life" [5]. Inherent in the interpersonal view is the notion that individuals are defined by their social behaviors and these behaviors represent the units of interpersonal communication. This reduction to observable behaviors makes the interpersonal approach well suited for psychosocial risk factor research [1, 4, 17, 18]. Moreover, the importance of social behaviors is consistent with most models of psychosocial risk, which assume that individual factors reflect social attributes and that social environments are key to the expression of those attributes [3, 19-21].

Conventional personality theorists tend to posit the ideas that personality "is" something and personality "does" something [22, 23]. The "is" notion reflects the idea that personality can be characterized. The "does" notion suggests that the expression of those characteristics influence the person's experience. The interpersonal approach locates the "is" in recurring patterns of interaction [5], rather than within the isolated individual, and it emphasizes what is being done in those interactions. The interpersonal approach also provides specific tools for translating psychosocial factors into their interpersonal units of behavior. It thus provides a process model for examining how those behaviors influence interpersonal interactions. The first of these tools is the *interpersonal circumplex* (IPC) [6, 11], which characterizes psychosocial factors explicitly in terms of their social behaviors and attributes. The second is the *transactional cycle*, which models the process of interpersonal interactions [7, 11, 24]. Together, these tools help researchers capture the dynamics of the interpersonal interactions in specific relationships.

The Interpersonal Circumplex

According to interpersonal theory, social behaviors vary along two broad dimensions - affiliation (ranging from interpersonal warmth and friendliness to coldness and hostility) and control (ranging from interpersonal dominance to submissiveness) [6, 10, 11]). Leary [6] made these dimensions more accessible by organizing them orthogonally into a circle or interpersonal circumplex (IPC; see Fig. 1). In the IPC, all social behaviors reflect a blend of these two broad dimensions. For example, a parent's nurturing behavior toward his or her child would reflect a blend of friendliness (as opposed to hostility) and dominance (as opposed to submissiveness). The IPC can be used to characterize specific social

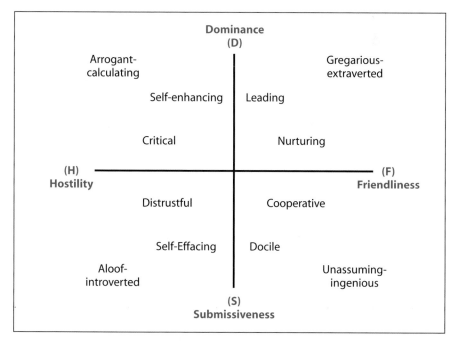

Fig. 1. The interpersonal circumplex (from [11, 17])

behaviors, as well as provide a common conceptual framework for the organization and comparison of related constructs [25-27]. This ability to capture the interpersonal correlates of a particular trait has led some to characterize the IPC as the "dispositional model" [4].

In addition to behaviors, many researchers suggest that the dimensions of the IPC also reflect other important social attributes. For example, several researchers suggest that the dimensions of the IPC reflect exchanges of social resources [7, 28]. In this view, interpersonal interactions involve exchanges of status (i.e., control) and acceptance. Interpersonal interactions are thus reflections of efforts to obtain, as well as grant, status and acceptance [11, 29]. For example, a supervisor may praise one of his or her workers and appoint that individual to manage a group project. The supervisor's actions reflect maintenance of control over all the workers, while at the same time granting status and preference to one worker over the others. Wiggins [28, 30] and others [31, 32] also suggest that the dimensions of affiliation and control in the IPC reflect broad motivational states of communion and agency, respectively. Communion is hypothesized to reflect a desire for intimacy and harmony, whereas agency reflects a striving for autonomy and power. These conceptualizations have led to the suggestion that the dimensions of the IPC may reflect important gender differences (agency reflects masculinity, communion reflects femininity) and that these differences tell us something about the types of challenges men and women are more likely to perceive and react [31, 33].

A number of circumplex-based measures have been developed for the assessment of interpersonal behaviors [10, 34, 35], interpersonal goals [36], perceived interpersonal problems [37], perceived interpersonal messages from others ("impact messages"; [38-40]) and perceived social support [11, 41]. In addition, several tools are available for validating circumplex structure in newly developed measures [27, 34, 42]. Perhaps one of the most useful advances comes from the integration of the IPC with the five-factor model (Revised Interpersonal Adjective Scales-Big Five; IASR-B5; [26, 43]. Using this approach, the two principle circumplex dimensions of dominance and affiliation are substituted for the interpersonally oriented traits in the five-factor model (i.e., extraversion and agreeableness, respectively), and the three remaining factors are used to complete the model [26, 28]. The resulting interpersonal taxonomy has two important uses. First, it provides a common conceptual space for characterizing and comparing traits [44, 45]. Second, this characterization tells the researcher something about the interpersonal preferences resulting from certain traits, while, at the same time, highlighting the "less desirable" behaviors (or situations leading to less preferable behaviors) in relation to those traits. For example, dominant individuals are more likely to be comfortable in leadership positions, compared with more submissive individuals; hostile individuals are more likely to be comfortable reprimanding someone than friendly people. Hence, the dispositional model is an important tool for understanding the interpersonal correlates of particular traits and behaviors and for identifying potential behavioral challenges or stressors.

Interpersonal Interactions

In addition to identifying interpersonal characteristics, it is important to understand what those characteristics "do" in interpersonal interactions. For example, in the above scenario, Mrs. Jacobs is an anxious person and her anxious behavior has consequences in her interactions with Mr. Jacobs. Although we would expect that people generally behave in a dispositionally congruent manner, there may be instances where people take on relationship-specific behaviors. For example, a hostile individual may generally behave in a defensive, antagonistic manner, yet be friendly, trusting, and even vulnerable in a close romantic relationship. Interpersonal theorists posit two conceptualizations of interpersonal interactions. In the *interactional perspective*, individuals come together and influence one another yet remain distinct entities [46]. In contrast, the *transactional perspective* posits that in some interactions, individuality is lost in favor of relationship-specific characteristics [13]. The interactional perspective is useful for conceptualizing most interpersonal interactions, whereas the transactional perspective may be more applicable to understanding the complexities of established relationships - i.e., those in which some of the emergent characteristics of the relationship are no longer reducible to the characteristics the individuals brought to the relationship [47]. Because the vast majority of interpersonal health research is best characterized as falling within the interactional perspective, we will focus on this aspect in our review. However, we will briefly discuss the merits, and potential health applications, of the transactional perspective later in the chapter.

Interpersonal interactions are guided by two principles. The first is the principle of "reciprocal determinism," most notably explicated in contemporary social cognitive research [48-50]. Reciprocal determinism states that individuals influence, and are influenced by, their interactions with others. For example, a hostile person who vigilantly watches a benign stranger may communicate suspicion and defensiveness, which in turn pulls for a less friendly, colder response from the interpersonal target. As a result, the hostile person creates (influences) an interpersonal interaction of mistrust that serves to validate his or her initial hostile cognitions. Put another way, reciprocal determinism functions as a causal loop akin to a self-fulfilling prophesy [7, 51, 52], in which individuals create their own mood-congruent realities by influencing and restricting the responses of others in their social environment [53-57].

The response of the interpersonal target is guided by the principle of complementarity [7, 11, 58-60], which suggests that for each action there is a predictable interpersonal response. Kiesler states, "our interpersonal actions are designed to invite, pull, elicit, draw, entice, or evoke 'restricted classes' of reactions from persons with whom we interact" [58]. Putting the IPC into action, interpersonal complementarity is characterized by similarity or correspondence on the affiliation dimension (e.g., friendliness pulls for friendliness) and reciprocity on the control dimension (e.g., dominance pulls for submissiveness). There is little debate that this principle applies to the affiliation dimension. You can walk outside and be fairly sure that smiling at the next person who walks by will evoke a friendly interpersonal response. However, if you attempt to assert dominance over the next person (e.g., forcefully moving into their personal space), you will probably, but not necessarily, get the reciprocal submissiveness (moving away from you). Although highly probable, complementarity along the control dimension remains controversial [58, 59, 61].

The Transactional Model. Complementing the dispositional IPC model, the *transactional model* (see Fig. 2) is a *process model* for understanding how individual psychosocial factors influence the interpersonal give-and-take process of interactions [4, 11]. Importantly, and despite the unfortunate terminological similarities, the transactional model *is not* related to the transactional perspective [13], to which we alluded earlier in this section. The transactional model is consistent with the interactional perspective in that persons are conceptualized as individuals who reciprocally influence one another. Each person begins with a unique, *covert state*, composed of their personality, goals, tactics, experiences, and current mood [4, 11, 23]. As seen in Figure 2, the interaction begins with Person A's covert state influencing his or her overt behavior towards Person B (Pathway A). For example, a happy individual may smile at Person B, while an angry individual may frown. This overt behavior impacts Person B, constricting that individual's covert experience (Pathway B). In other words, a smile is more likely to be interpreted by Person B as a friendly gesture than a threat or challenge. Person B's constricted covert experience then produces a congruent overt response (Pathway C) which impacts Person A (Pathway D). Although there are few examples of the full transactional cycle in health research, the model has proven useful for understanding the acute effects of one person's personality and social behaviors on a second person [62].

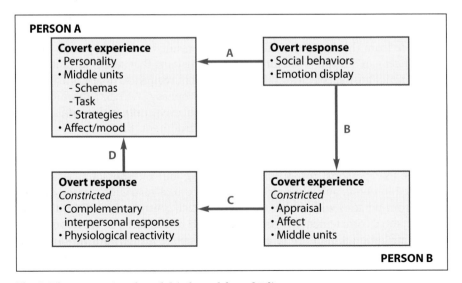

Fig. 2. The transactional model (adapted from [17])

The transactional model predicts that negative personality traits evoke more stressful interpersonal interactions in what can become recursive, self-perpetuating patterns [16, 53, 54]. Substantial research suggests that such interactions are associated with acute psychological and physiological consequences, as well as biobehavioral disease mechanisms [21, 63]. Although a single event may not be a plausible trigger for disease, the cumulative effect of repeated interactions, either for the negative individual or a person in a relationship with such an individual, may have important health consequences. As demonstrated in Figure 3, repeated negative interactions, conceptualized as transactional cycles, contribute to cumulative stress or allostatic load with direct health consequences [64]. Because personality is characterized by patterned behavior [5, 12, 14], negative individuals should be expected to instigate and engage in repeated negative interactions. This stressful interactional pattern may maintain the individual's view of the world as threatening, while eroding social resources such as social support. Moreover, a stressful interactional history may engender a more wary social audience, who reciprocally see the individual as a threat. In contrast, positive traits might be expected to evoke more positive interpersonal experiences, increases in social resources, and a less threatening social world.

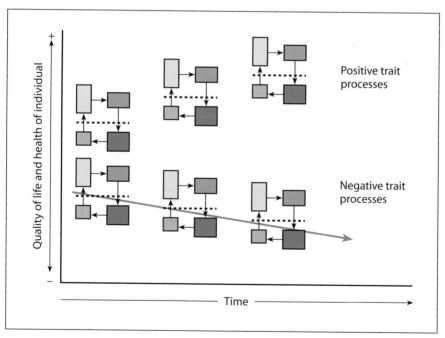

Fig. 3. Personality as transactional cycles over time (from [64]). Positive traits engender positive interpersonal interactions, which reduce interpersonal stress, strengthen social relations and reduce acute physiological reactivity. Negative traits engender more stressful interpersonal interactions, erode social relations and increase physiological reactivity

In a recent experience sampling study, Hawkley and colleagues [65] found that participants reported being among other people during 56% of sampling episodes over a 7-day period. These data and other statistics [66] suggest that we spend a significant proportion of our daily lives in interpersonal environments. Hence, investigating interactions between personality risk factors and the social environment may be critical to understanding how such risk factors influence health and wellness. To accomplish this goal, it is important to examine the social properties of traits, as well as the dynamic of the interaction. The dispositional (IPC) model can help by characterizing the interpersonal attributes of a given psychosocial factor and suggesting interpersonal conditions that could be perceived as more challenging or stressful. The process (transactional) model is useful for putting traits and behaviors in action to understand how interactions unfold. Importantly, this model may help understand not only the effects on the individual during and following such interactions, but also the effects of such traits on social targets. These models are particularly well suited for understanding general interpersonal behaviors and acute interactions.

The Special Case of Enduring Interpersonal Relationships

In addition to novel interactions with strangers, people spend a significant percentage of time with co-workers, friends, family members, and significant others [65]. For example, in the momentary sampling study by Hawkley and colleagues [65], college students reported being with friends and roommates during almost 40% of the sampling episodes over the course of the week. In addition, a recent momentary assessment study of time-use among nearly 12,000 respondents showed that, on average, married, working couples spend 2 hours per day together, whereas retired couples spend closer to 3.5 hours together [67]. Compared with daily chance interactions with strangers, known relationship partners may represent stable, long-term interpersonal influences.

As discussed earlier, there are two approaches for conceptualizing interpersonal interactions. The interactional perspective conceptualizes relationships as repeated interactions between distinct individuals [46]. However, relationships involve prior experiences, dependence and shared goals, not the least of which may be a desire to maintain the viability of the relationship. These relationship-specific factors may moderate the impact of individual factors. For example, Mr. Jacobs' reaction to his wife's vigilance may be moderated by his degree of happiness in the marriage. If he is satisfied with his relationship he may respond to his wife's vigilance by noting to himself, "She's just showing that she cares about me. This helps me to feel safe if I suffer another heart attack." Likewise, if he is less satisfied in the marriage, he may be more likely to have a negative interpretation of her behaviors, which could lead to more tense interpersonal transactions. Consistent with the interactional perspective, Mrs. Jacobs retains her individual personality, yet its impact is moderated by Mr. Jacobs' relationship quality. Hence, relationship quality may be useful for conceptualizing relationships from the interactional perspective.

One approach to modeling longitudinal relationship risk within the inter-actional perspective is shown in Figure 4. The *Transitive Model* [68] illustrates 3 types of effects. First, it shows how an individual's own personality traits influ-ence his or her own health over time ("within person" effects; Pathways A and B). Second, it shows how the current affect of one person influences the current affect of his or her relationship partner (the so called "contagion" effects; Path-way C) [69, 70)]. Third, it illustrates how an individual's personality influences his or her partner's health over time ("transitive" effects, Pathways D and E). Consistent with the preceding discussion, relationship satisfaction moderates the transitive effects of personality (Pathway F). This approach may be particular-ly appropriate for researchers who are interested in prospective research with cou-ples undergoing medical procedures [71]. In general, it may be of interest in studying longitudinal relationship effects outside of the laboratory, when gen-eral interaction patterns, rather than specific acute interactions, are the mech-anisms of interest. Notably, the model is appropriate for the study of co-work-ers, friends, enemies, family members, spouses, healthcare providers or any other dyadic relationship hypothesized to influence health and well-being.

An alternative to the interactional perspective is the possibility that rela-tionships lead to the emergence of new, relationship-specific characteristics, which influence the health of the individual and relationship partner. Interde-pendence theories suggest that repeated interactions between individuals become crystallized as habitual patterns of social behavior between those individuals [12, 14, 72, 73]. Sporadic longitudinal research suggests that couples become more similar over time, adopting similar behaviors and mannerisms [74-76].

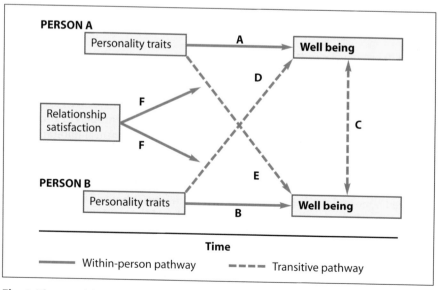

Fig. 4. The transitive model of interpersonal relationships (adapted from [68])

Dewey and Bentley [13] posit the idea that through repeated interactions, individuals "shape" one another, or develop "co-traits" [77], leading to loss of individuality in favor of relationship-specific behaviors (i.e., transactional perspective). For example, two otherwise friendly individuals may conflict over various issues, such as household chores, finances or child-rearing. Over time, these conflicts may lead to a general conflictual pattern where each predictably behaves in a hostile, antagonistic manner, but only in the context of their relationship. Hence, individual behavior in the context of this relationship departs from more typical personality and social behaviors observed in other contexts. For health researchers interested in the influence one person has upon a relationship partner, the transactional perspective suggests that relationship-specific behaviors, as opposed to general social behaviors and personality, may be the better predictor of influence.

Regardless of the specific conceptual framework, the interpersonal approach maintains that people are health risk and resilience factors for one another. The approach includes models for characterizing the social attributes of psychosocial risk factors (IPC) and tools for comparing and contrasting those factors. It also makes predictions about situations that may be more or less interpersonally stressful and evocative. In addition, the approach offers models for conceptualizing acute interpersonal interactions (transactional model), demonstrating individual interpersonal risk over time (transactional trajectory), and understanding interpersonal risk in the context of existing relationships (transitive model). Next, we turn to the evidence regarding interpersonal risk, including an examination of specific psychosocial risk factors, types of relationships, and phenomenon associated with cardiovascular health and disease.

■ Evidence of Interpersonal Risk in Cardiovascular Disease

Social Status and Cardiovascular Risk

Animal Models. Because of their propensity to arrange in social hierarchies and develop atherosclerosis, primates have been useful in the study of social status, interpersonal interactions and atherogenesis. Two lines of research are particularly useful in this regard. The first consists of laboratory models of social risk, and the second of ecological studies of animals in their natural habitat.

In a series of laboratory studies, Kaplan and Manuck developed a paradigm for examining how individual differences in social status behaviors influence the development and progression of atherosclerosis [78-81]. The paradigm involved cynomolgus macaques (*Macaca fascicularis*) housed in small groups and fed an atherogenic (high-fat) diet. Once placed in housing groups, the animals established dominance hierarchies through aggression. Groups were then randomly assigned to one of two conditions. In the stable condition the same animals were housed together for the duration of the study, limiting the need to exhibit dominance due to the established social hierarchy. In the unstable condition, groups were mixed multiple times over the course of the study, resulting in repeated interpersonal conflict, as hierarchies were re-established. Individual animals in each condition were classified as dominant or subordinate, based on outcomes of dyadic confrontations or fights [78]. Results showed that dominant males developed more atherosclerosis than subordinates, but only in the unstable conditions [78, 79, 81]. Follow-up studies revealed that this relationship was mediated by increased sympathetic arousal [81] and that dampening of sympathetic responses with chemical blockade (propranolol) reduced both aggressive behavior and the rate of atherogenesis [82, 83]. This research illustrates two important aspects of interpersonal risk. First, individual differences in social status are associated with atherogenesis. Second, this association is mediated by environmentally evoked dominance behaviors.

An important caveat to these findings is the role of ovarian function in females. Normal ovarian functioning prior to menopause appears to buffer against atherogenesis presumably through the cardio-protective effects of estrogen [84, 85]. Conversely, infrequent ovulation is associated with increased risk prior to menopause. In a series of studies, Kaplan examined the role of social status on ovulation dysfunction and disease development. Using the basic paradigm, female macaques were fed an atherogenic diet, housed in small social groups, and classified as dominant or subordinate [86, 87]. Compared with matched males, female macaques developed less atherosclerosis. As expected, there was an interaction with status. Dominant females ovulated more regularly and developed less atherosclerosis than submissive females. Subsequent studies demonstrated that dominant females who were oophorectomized at the beginning of the study, developed atherosclerosis at a similar rate to subordinates [88], and that the provision of exogenous estrogen to subordinates mitigated status differences [89, 90]. These findings suggest that, unlike dominance in males, submissiveness in female macaques confers increased risk through the mechanism of decreased estrogen production.

Animal societies are complex. Organizations range from egalitarian, where members share in resources regardless of social rank, to top-down hierarchies, where resource allocation is skewed towards dominance and power [91]. Societies also vary in terms of the relative stability of the hierarchy [91, 92], with the least stable hierarchies resulting in greater stress and disease risk [81]. Ecological studies of primates in unstable social situations mirror laboratory findings; physiological stress effects are most evident among dominant males [92]. However, ecological studies of stable groups suggest that subordinate primates are at higher risk for disease [91, 93, 94]. For example, a recent quantitative analysis of multiple species and societies found that subordinates in stable, hierarchical societies had significantly higher basal cortisol levels than their more dominant counterparts [95]. Two social mechanisms were identified as integral to these effects. First, subordinates in these groups are subject to more daily stressors resulting from less access to food, shelter, and mating opportunities, as well as from greater likelihood of attack by more dominant members of the society and vulnerability to environmental hazards such as predators [95]. Second, subordinates in these groups have less access to social support, such as grooming, which may promote health by dampening stress responses [91, 96, 97]. Hence, ecological studies suggest that subordinates in stable social hierarchies and dominants in unstable hierarchies are at greatest health risk.

Sapolsky recently wrote, "Rank means different things in different species and populations" [91]. This comment underscores the importance of social context as a moderator of rank, as it pertains to social functioning and health. Both laboratory and ecological studies of rank in primates support the role of social stability as a key environmental characteristic. Unstable environments challenge social order, evoking individual differences in dominance behaviors and leading to interpersonal conflict, stress and more pronounced atherogenesis. This effect is qualified by gender, as dominant females competing for mating opportunities experience more regular ovulation, leading to lower disease risk. In stable social situations, rank or "pecking order" is associated with resource allocation, which differentiates risk. Sapolsky [91] likens this scenario to the negative health effects of lower socio-economic status (SES) in humans [98]. However, both stable and unstable effects may apply to humans, who typically occupy a variety of different social environments (e.g., family, neighborhood, community, and work), any of which could be more or less stable.

Status and Risk in Humans. Social dominance is an emerging psychosocial risk factor for coronary heart disease (CHD) and all-cause mortality in humans [2, 99]. This association is increasingly supported by prospective research. For example, Houston and colleagues [100] found that higher dominance predicted CHD events and all-cause mortality over a 22-year follow-up. Whiteman et al. [101] and Siegman et al. [102] reported similar findings over 5 and 8-year follow-ups, respectively. Additional evidence links higher social dominance with physiological risk markers (e.g., cholesterol abnormalities; [103]). Interestingly, in contrast to ecological primate studies, human investigations suggest that submissiveness, not dominance, is a greater health risk factor in stable societies. One potential explanation for the discrepancy between literatures may be the lack of social stability measurement in human studies. Alternatively, it is possible that more dominant humans perceive the environment - real or imagined - as more threatening or unstable.

Laboratory investigations of social dominance have focused on cardiovascular reactivity (CVR) as a mechanism for disease [1, 63, 104, 105]. Two types of studies characterize this literature. The first are studies of attempts to exert social influence, usually through giving a persuasive speech [106, 107]. Several studies have demonstrated that such behavioral dominance efforts evoke significant increases in blood pressure and heart rate [108, 109]. Moreover, larger incentives to gain control are associated with more pronounced physiological responses [106, 108, 109]. These findings are consistent in interactions with strangers and in established relationships. For example, husbands attempting to influence their wives during a discussion exhibit larger increases in interpersonal hostility and CVR than husbands not attempting to influence their partners [62, 110].

To our knowledge, only one study has contrasted efforts to appear more vs. less dominant (submissive). Smith and colleagues [107] used a job interview scenario to elicit persuasive behavior. Participants were told that they were interviewing for one of two positions - a supervisory position (requiring dominant, forceful qualities) or a customer service position (requiring submissive, "good listener" qualities). Results showed a condition-by-gender effect, in which men in the dominant condition and women in the submissive condition displayed the largest blood pressure increases. Although both results are consistent with the animal models of risk, it is possible that the female finding reflects a mismatch [111, 112] between preferred behaviors (submissiveness) and task demands (assertiveness). Despite this ambiguity, the evidence supports a relationship between efforts to influence others and heightened physiological reactivity.

A second type of investigation focuses on individual differences in dominance. For example, healthy Type-A men, high in need for control, are more interpersonally cold and display larger increases in CVR than Type Bs, when attempting to persuade their wives [113]. Interestingly, these responses are more pronounced for couples in which the wife has obtained a higher level of education. This finding suggests that high status similarities in couples are an interpersonal risk factor for men, independent of the risk conferred by the trait alone. More generally, these couple effects are consistent with the earlier animal literature emphasizing the relevance of interpersonal context on the expression of individual differences in social status and, hence, on cardiovascular risk.

Finally, individual differences have interpersonal consequences. Consistent with the transactional model, individual differences in one spouse are expected to have consequences for the partner during interactions. For example, Brown and colleagues [114] found that people who perceived their spouse to be high in dominance displayed larger increases in CVR during preparation and expression of their opinions to this spouse, compared with people who perceived their spouse to be more submissive.

To summarize, animal and human studies increasingly support social dominance as a risk factor for CVD and all-cause mortality. Importantly, this risk factor is interpersonal in nature, with a body of animal and human evidence demonstrating the interpersonal context as relevant to the expression social dominance and vulnerable to its effects. The evidence suggests that dominance in men and submissiveness in women are associated with greater disease risk. A number of issues remain to be addressed. For example, more is known about the dominance as opposed to the submissive end of the control spectrum, and the range of measured physiological mechanisms is limited. Despite these limitations, interpersonal status and control are relevant to the work of researchers and clinicians alike. Next, we examine the relevance of interpersonal affiliation to CVD.

Affiliative Behavior and Cardiovascular Risk

Affiliation in Animal Models. Unlike interpersonal status, there is no clear programmatic research model investigating the cardiovascular consequences of affiliation. In addition, the animal literature is skewed towards the study of warm and friendly social behaviors (e.g., grooming). This may be due to conceptual difficulties in distinguishing interpersonal hostility, and to the fact that aggression is confounded by interpersonal control. Nevertheless, primate research does shed light on the use of pro-affiliative behaviors in response to stressful events, and it points to potential biological mediators of cardiovascular stress responses.

A recent review of 81 studies covering 60 primate species found that animals engage in social interactions for approximately 10% of their active, awake time [115]. Agonistic behaviors constituted less than 1% of that awake time, suggesting that benign and warm, affiliative interactions (e.g., grooming) accounted for the bulk of the remainder. Friendly encounters among adult primates involve all combinations of gender and social rank, contradicting the hypothesis that such behaviors predominantly reflect tactical mating strategies [116-118]. Adults appear to engage in affiliative behavior for a number of reasons, including social bonding ([119, 120], enlisting allies [118, 121, 122], post-conflict reconciliation with fellow combatants [123-126] and assistance in rearing young [127].

Although friendly interactions occur throughout primate troops, individuals spend a majority of their time with specific others (i.e., preferential affiliation). Preferential matches occur between animals of the same gender that share similar age, or they reflect affiliative behaviors and hierarchical position [117, 118, 127]. These pro-affiliative relationships may have important health benefits. First, the presence of a preferred counterpart appears to buffer stress responses during aversive events. For example, Gust and colleagues [128] removed a sample of captive female rhesus monkeys from their social groups and placed them either alone or with a preferred companion in a novel environment. Although both conditions exhibited significant initial immune responses, these responses were attenuated over time among animals in the companion as opposed to the alone condition. Second, limited evidence suggests that primates seek out and "console" preferred counterparts who experience stressors such as being the victim of aggression [129]. Hence, like social support in humans, affiliative bonds in primates appear to dampen stress responses, which may have important implications for physical health.

An emerging animal model of affiliation and stress regulation comes from the attachment literature. This model emphasizes the central role of two neuropeptides, oxytocin and vasopressin, in the mediation of affiliative social behaviors [130-132]. Oxytocin's role in maternal behavior is well known, as it stimulates both contractions during labor and lactation [133]. However, new evidence suggests that oxytocin may also facilitate adult-adult pair bonding [119, 134]. In addition, oxytocin is linked to dampened cardiovascular and hypothalamic-pituitary adrenalcortex (HPA) reactivity, which may have important beneficial effects for cardiovascular disease [135-137]. In contrast, vasopressin is less understood, although some evidence suggests its role in more cold and hostile social behaviors, including vigilance and aggression [138]. Vasopressin is also associated with increased sympathetic and HPA activation [139]. Hence, oxytocin and vasopressin may influence health both indirectly, through affiliative interpersonal behaviors, and directly, through their actions on autonomic and endocrine arousal.

Unlike the primate studies of social status and atherosclerosis, there is no analogous animal model of interpersonal affiliation and cardiovascular disease risk. Despite this shortcoming, studies of animal affiliation do suggest important interpersonal pathways and factors that may be relevant in humans. These pathways and factors include supportive and provocative actions of one individual on the acute stress of another, as well as the moderating roles of relationship quality and similarity between support giver and recipient. In addition, emerging evidence suggests a neurobiological basis for affiliative behaviors that may have implications for the interpersonal and physiological regulation of stress responses. These topics are examined more closely in humans in the next section.

Affiliation and Risk in Humans. Human studies of interpersonal affiliative risk are more definitive than in animal literature. For example, research clearly supports low hostile environments, such as SES neighborhoods, with more negative life events, higher levels of stress, more negative emotions, and higher rates of cardiovascular disease and early mortality [98, 140, 141]. In what Powell [142] refers to as a "next step" investigation, Reiff and colleagues [143] examined associations between chronic stress due to hostile interpersonal environments (i.e., crime) and cardiovascular health in a cross-sectional study of an urban community. Participants reported high rates of exposure to drug use and violent crime, with a quarter of the sample reporting being the victim of violent physical assault or rape. These experiences contributed to chronic stress levels, which were independently associated with hypertension status after controlling for traditional risk factors and depression.

Gallo and Matthews [98] argue that hostile environments affect health through two pathways. First, hostile environments influence health directly by evoking increases in vigilance, negative affectivity and stress. Second, stressful environments erode one's "reserve capacity" of social resources (e.g., social support), resulting in increased vulnerability. Conversely, higher social capital communities - characterized by higher levels of interpersonal trust, bonding and mutual aid - are associated with health benefits [144]. For example, Kawachi and colleagues [145] found that individuals living in states with wider participation in pro-affiliative activities, such as church groups, unions, sports leagues, fraternal and civic organizations and parent-teacher associations, lived significantly longer than people living in less affiliative states. Thus, the affiliative quality of the interpersonal environment appears to be an important determinant of physical health.

Laboratory manipulations of interpersonal affiliation suggest that this relationship may be mediated by acute changes in physiological response. At one end, hostile interpersonal environments exacerbate CVR to lab stressors [109, 146, 147]. For example, harassment during a speech task evokes significantly larger blood pressure increases than benign or supportive comments [148]. At the other end of the affiliation dimension, a large body of evidence shows that warm, supportive environments appear to dampen emotional and physical responses to stress, including CVR, endocrine and immune response [149, 150]. More recently, adult-adult bonding has been shown to elicit increases in oxytocin [151, 152], although its role in stress regulation remains unknown.

Social support research has been dichotomized into "passive" and "active" paradigms [149]. The passive paradigm posits that the mere presence of a support person will attenuate reactivity in the support recipient. In the context of a stressful event, passive support from strangers [153, 154], acquaintances [155], friends [156], significant others [157] and even pets [158, 159] reliably dampens acute cardiovascular responses in support recipients. Moreover, simply imagining a close friend, as opposed to a less well-known acquaintance, produces similar benefits [160, 161].

Active support paradigms hypothesize that effortful behavioral support, including emotional, tangible and informational support, will also attenuate stress responses in support recipients [162]. For example, Lepore and colleagues [162] instructed participants to give a short speech under one of three conditions - alone in a room, in the presence of an inattentive confederate or in the presence of an actively supportive confederate. Participants in the active support condition displayed significantly less CVR relative to the other conditions. Although there is little data comparing active and passive support in the same study, independent investigations demonstrate the transitive interpersonal benefits of warm interpersonal communication.

Four key moderators qualify the effectiveness of support behaviors from one person in mitigating the stress responses in another. The first two moderators involve characteristics of the relationship between the support giver and receiver. First, more trusted and satisfying relationships better attenuate stress responses than unfamiliar or less satisfying relationships [163-165]. For example, Fontana and colleagues [164] demonstrated that support offered by friends was superior to that offered by strangers, but only when the quality of the friendship was judged by the support recipient to be high. Similarly, Kiecolt-Glaser has programmatically demonstrated that people in more satisfying marriages report feeling more supported and display less cardiovascular, endocrine and immune reactivity to marital conflict than less satisfied couples [166-171]. Second, the gender match between support giver and receiver may be important, as men and women differ in their support behaviors and needs [31, 172]. Fritz and colleagues [172] found that when discussing a problem with a friend, female supports were more likely to provide communal support such as empathic listening, while men were more likely to engage in agentic support such as advice-giving. Results suggest that the relative match between support style and support needs is an important determinant of support efficacy.

The second two moderators are focused on evaluative threat and support receiver perceptions of the support giver. First, evaluative environments undermine the effectiveness of affiliative support and may potentiate greater reactivity [109, 164, 173]. This may be an important confound; as few studies recognize that intended support givers may also be unintended evaluative threats. For example, one might benefit from the encouragement of a friend during a challenge, but also be self-conscious about underperforming in the presence of that friend. Second, support is often in the eye of the beholder. Individual differences, such as hostility, may bias one's perception of another person's behaviors. This may have implications for how one receives intended support [174, 175]. For example, hostile individuals benefit less from support in laboratory paradigms; they exhibit less CVR attenuation and report more anger than less hostile participants receiving or imaging support [176-177]. These four factors suggest that the efficacy of support is contingent on the relationship between the support giver and receiver. These factors may also impact the receiver's potential for perceiving the supporter's behavior as non-evaluative and well -intentioned.

A fundamental issue in health-affiliation research concerns the dichotomy between cold hostility vs. warm friendliness [178, 179]. Substantial research suggests that interpersonal hostility is associated with greater stress, larger physiological responses, disease progression and poor adaptation. However, it is unclear whether warm, positive environments promote resilience, or whether it is simply the absence of hostility that matters most. Simply put, does being nice matter more than not being nasty? Few studies have attempted to disentangle this dichotomy, and most of them have attempted to do so in the context of coping with a major stressor, yielding mixed findings [179, 180]. However, recent work has begun to focus on the health effects of positive, enjoyable - as opposed to stressful - situations. For example, Light and colleagues [151] recently demonstrated that receiving more frequent hugs is associated with oxytocin release and lower basal blood pressure. This issue remains an important challenge to psychosocial researchers, as it may determine whether interventions should focus simply on reducing interpersonal negativity or also on teaching proactive positive social behaviors.

In summary, interpersonal affiliation characteristics, ranging from warm-friendliness to hostile-provocation, are important moderators of stressful experiences. Primate and human research demonstrates that cold and hostile interpersonal environments heighten emotional and physiological reactivity, whereas warm and supportive environments dampen such responses. Several factors, including the relationship type and quality, evaluative threat and individual differences in negativity (and, theoretically, positivity), moderate the affiliation - reactivity association. As is the case with interpersonal status (refer to previous section), the literature supports the basic dimensions of interpersonal behavior as important determinants of stress, emotional and physiological response, cardiovascular disease and mortality.

Relationships and Longitudinal Risk

Relationships such as friendships and marriage represent chronic sources of interpersonal influence that should, in theory, be important determinants of physical health (see Fig. 3). Prospective investigations of healthy participants support the relationship between social connectedness and the lower incidence of cardiovascular disease and all-cause -mortality [181-186]. However, the health benefits of relationships are moderated by their affiliative quality [187, 188]. Closer, more supportive relationships are associated with lower incidence of MI [189]. For example, marriage is associated with lower risk of cardiovascular morbidity and all-cause mortality [190, 191], but only when the relationship is experienced as supportive and satisfying [179, 192-196]. Distressing and unsatisfying relationships are associated with a worse prognosis and earlier mortality. The toll of relationship strain may be evident prior to clinical manifestations of disease. For example, Kiecolt-Glaser and colleagues [168] compared married women to separated/divorced women and found that disrupted marriages were associated with significantly poorer immune functioning, which may be indicative of increased vulnerability.

In addition to their role in the development and expression of disease, relationships are particularly important in times of illness [177, 188, 197, 198]. As illustrated in the opening vignette, the emotional impact of illness often extends beyond the patient to affect close network members such as spouses [199-204]. Emotional reactions among support persons are common throughout the course of an illness. For example, spouses commonly experience shock reactions during and following their husband or wife's myocardial infarction (MI; [205]). Similar responses are seen in the context of cardiac procedures such as coronary artery bypass surgery (CABG). Support persons report significant distress, irritability, depressive symptoms and problems with sleep during the waiting periods prior to CABG procedures [203, 206], with continued affective disturbance during acute [199, 207] and long-term [208] recovery phases. Although spouses adjust over time, longitudinal evidence suggests that cardiac events continue to affect quality of life and behavior 10 years later [209]. Despite some evidence suggesting that spouse distress is greater than patient distress [210-213], recent work suggests that this finding is more likely a result of gender [214-217]. Resolution of this issue requires greater attention to the effects of gender, versus role (patient vs. spouse), and alertness to the possibility that being a woman confronting illness in a close relationship may have greater implications for well being and level of distress than who has the illness. Regardless of who is more affected in terms of distress, evidence unequivocally demonstrates that intimate relationships strongly influence the course and outcome of illness.

Factors Influencing Support Person's Adjustment to Partner's Illness. A support person's adjustment to a loved one's illness is influenced by contextual factors, resources and stable premorbid factors, including aspects of their personality [218]. In particular, higher neuroticism is associated with greater distress and caregiving burden [219-222]. Conversely, positive traits such as optimism are associated with lower perceived caregiving burden and predict less depressive symptoms over time [220, 223, 224]. Caregiving burden is important because, in interdependent relationships, close supports and spouses are often charged with the care of patients who are restricted by illness or during the recovery process. In addition, prospective studies and quantitative reviews have demonstrated that higher caregiving burden predicts higher caregiver morbidity and early mortality [225-227].

Patient Effects on Supports. The social behaviors of patients - in addition to influencing their own psychosocial risk factors - can also influence their supporters' adaptation and health. For example, studies across illness domains demonstrate that higher patient distress predicts greater caregiving burden among their support persons [228-231]. In addition, patient personality traits also influence partner adaptation. In a prospective study of male CABG patients and their spouses, patient presurgical neuroticism predicted higher spouse depressive symptoms. In addition, patient presurgical optimism predicted fewer spouse depressive symptoms 18 months after CABG, independent of the spouse's own presurgical traits [232]. These findings support the transitive properties of personality (see Fig. 4, Pathways D and E) and suggest that in the context of illness, patients can heighten, as well as reduce, the burden on their caregiving supports.

Support Effects on Patient. Support persons can also influence patients' emotional and physical adaptation to disease. The term "support" in relation to affiliative networks suggests that members of the network can benefit patients during times of illness. Indeed, the social support literature clearly shows the benefit to survival of having engaged affiliative networks. At the interpersonal level, supports can reduce patient stress and burden through emotional (listening, consoling, rallying), tangible (assistance with activities of daily living, also referred to as ADLs) and informational (interpreting physician discussions, seeking out information) means [69, 97, 221, 225, 230, 233, 234].

Unfortunately, supports can also have negative effects on patients. Patients' perceptions of the quality of spouse support predict adjustment to disease [235, 236] and survival following cardiac events [237]. However, not all support is appreciated. For example, in a non-cardiac sample, Newsome and Schulz [238] found that loss of control to caregiver assistance predicted increased depressive symptoms over a one-year period. In addition, supports can also communicate hostility in the context of caregiving [239]. Among families coping with cancer, spouse criticism of patient coping efforts predicted increases in distress, intrusive thoughts and depressive symptoms [240-243]. In addition, spouse withdrawal and avoidance of the topic of illness in conversation is also associated with increased patient distress among couples coping with illness [240, 242-244]. These relationships are important, as pre and post-surgical distress in CABG patients predicts increases in depressive symptoms, greater functional impairment and slower return to work [245-248]. Depressive symptoms, in particular, may be critical to future health among cardiac patients. For example, depressive symptoms in CABG and MI survivors are predictive of future cardiac events and mortality [249-252]. Although the findings regarding negative spouse behaviors and patient distress are modest (most data suggest that supportive behaviors far outnumber unsupportive behaviors), the importance of the relationship is a consistent finding. It is possible that negative spouse behaviors are symptomatic of other, more substantial interpersonal influences.

Distressed and anxious social network members are particularly important sources of interpersonal risk for patients. In couples coping with illness, higher spouse distress following diagnosis predicts poorer patient adaptation and higher patient distress [213, 229, 240, 244, 253-257]. In addition, spouse personality traits such as neuroticism predict patient depressive symptoms over time [232]. Evidence suggests that this transference is related to the frequency in which distressed spouses engage in negative behaviors such as patient-focused vigilance [204, 258, 259] and avoidant coping [240, 242-244]. These behaviors may reflect attempts by the distressed spouse to regulate his or her emotions through approach/withdrawal efforts [260]. However, they may have emotional as well as compensatory behavioral consequences (avoidance, protective buffering) for patients. Protective buffering - hiding worries from others - may benefit the "protected" person [261], but at a cost of increased distress and impaired adaptation in the "protector" 1 [255, 262].

At this point, we should offer some clarification regarding spousal over-involvement and over-protectiveness which, based on clinical observations and anecdotal accounts, are often hypothesized to undermine patient adaptation [211, 213, 263-265]. However, a body of empirical research suggests either no relation or one contrary to the popular notion: moderate levels of "over-protectiveness" actually have benefitsfor the ill partner [180, 266, 267]. For example, in a study of 56 couples, Fiske and colleagues [266] found that over-protectiveness was associated with couples developing closer ties after MI. These findings suggest caution in making assumptions about interpersonal influence, and they emphasize the need for conclusions to be based in empirical data.

Three important qualifications to the findings of negative support behaviors deserve mention. First, open communication between patients and supports is associated with better adjustment [242, 243, 268]. Second, social network members can compensate for spouse shortcomings [269]. Third, relationship quality and satisfaction moderate the interpersonal influence of social network members' behaviors on one another [242, 243, 270, 271]. These points suggest potential opportunities for intervention that go beyond an exclusive focus on the patient.

In summary, available evidence strongly supports the position that relationships are important influences on physical health. Higher social integration is generally more beneficial relative to isolation. However, specific relationships can either be beneficial or damaging, depending on the quality of the relationship and the level of relationship satisfaction. In the context of illness, social network members share the illness experience with the person who is affected. A review of evidence across illness domains suggests that both patients and supports can influence one another's experiences, adaptation and health over time. These findings support the interpersonal conceptualization of interpersonal risk.

Future Directions

The review of specific relationship behaviors as longitudinal interpersonal risk factors demonstrates the evolution of psychosocial research. One of the running themes in this review has been the emphasis of *specificity*, as opposed to *generality*, in conceptualizing social risk. For example, is risk most influenced by the work environment itself or by the individuals within that environment? Is a social network beneficial in and of itself, or are some individuals in the social network more beneficial than others? Furthermore, can the beneficial members also be sources of stress in certain situations? Generality has important advantages, including identification of general types of social risk, but it is less useful in answering questions focused on why some people do well in certain situations and others do not. The advantage of the interpersonal approach is its ability to conceptualize specific relationships and interpersonal encounters. In doing so, the approach helps us understand how each individual influences, and is influenced by, those with whom he or she interacts.

Future interpersonal research should begin to address a number of social relationships that may be instrumental in understanding cardiovascular risk. For example, researchers should address not only close network relationships but also other important interpersonal influences on patients. For example, do certain status and affiliative qualities among physicians engender lower distress, higher confidence and faster recovery in patients and their family members? Are particular interpersonal qualities more effective at engendering behavioral change following myocardial infarction? Does the similarity or match between the interpersonal styles of the healthcare provider and patient produce better results than mismatches between those interpersonal characteristics? Answers to these questions may help practitioners improve the health of patients who can be medically treated, but, for unknown reasons, are not amenable to engaging in those treatments.

As noted earlier, the evidence regarding relationships and health largely fits with the interactional perspective [46], which emphasizes individuality. Consistent with Dewey and Bentley's [13] transactional perspective, future research should also consider the health implications of emergent relationship-specific characteristics that develop over repeated interactions between individuals, and that may not be representative of each individual's general characteristics. Importantly, the interactional and transactional perspectives should be considered complimentary in that, together, they may offer a more comprehensive picture of the person, the relationship and the person in the relationship, as all three factors may be relevant to understanding psychosocial influences in health.

Racial and Ethnicity-Related Health Disparities and Interpersonal Behaviors. Another important direction that may benefit from an interpersonal research approach concerns the issue of race and ethnicity-related health disparities. National statistics repeatedly highlight differences between the life -expectancy and health status of ethnic minorities, compared with the non-Hispanic White majority in the United States [272, 273]. Although these differences are observed across illness domains, longevity differences are largely driven by cardiovascular and cerebrovascular disease disparities, particularly among Blacks, who experience the largest and most pervasive differences in health compared with Whites [272, 274].

Schnittker and McLeod [275] suggest that understanding race-related health disparities requires a consideration of both "upstream" and "downstream" mechanisms. Upstream mechanisms refer to higher-order constructs, such as socio-structural and cultural factors that influence risk. For example, lower socio-economic neighborhoods tend to have higher rates of violent crime, lower quality housing, more dense population distributions, fewer healthy food choices, fewer exercise opportunities and less access to quality healthcare Kaplan and Keil, 1993 [98, 140, 276-278]. These socio-structural characteristics may engender the development of downstream individual factors, such as hostility and negative affectivity, poor coping, increased physiological reactivity, health-damaging behaviors and conflictual social behaviors - all of which contribute to health risk [275, 279-282].

In addition to traditional structural and individual risk factors, investigators hypothesize that racism and discrimination may be important contributors to physical health, particularly among traditionally stigmatized groups such as Blacks [283]. Discrimination can occur at the macro-societal level, as a result of segregation or unfair resource distribution, or it can occur simply through the marginalization of one group by the rest of society. In contrast, health psychologists are becoming more interested in individual experiences of racism, and research increasingly supports an association between higher perceived racism and health [284, 285]. Although evidence is limited, higher perceived racism is associated with important cardiovascular outcomes such as higher resting blood pressure [286-288], and, more recently, with subclinical-carotid artery disease [289].

In addition to overt acts, implicit attitudes may moderate experiences of discrimination. The transactional perspective of Kiesler [11] suggests that these interpersonal experiences can be shaped by either party in an interpersonal encounter. For example, an individual who harbors discriminatory views can transactionally create interpersonal tension in a neutral individual, ranging from mild vigilant behavior to overt expression. Likewise, an individual who perceives himself or herself to be stigmatized (or has "stigma consciousness" [290, 291]) may communicate defensiveness in interpersonal interactions, potentially evoking or exacerbating complementary defensiveness and suspicion in an otherwise neutral or ambivalent target [292, 293]. Finally, awareness of others' stigma may be associated with compensatory behaviors to avoid the appearance that one is discriminatory, which may also contribute to interpersonal tension [294]. In addition to overt acts, these more subtle interpersonal processes may also be important to understanding potential cardiovascular risk associated with stigma and discrimination.

In contrast to negative disparities, lessons may also be learned from further study of groups who are at the positive end of the disparities continuum. For example, one of the most intriguing questions in Hispanic health is the phenomenon referred to as the "Latino" or "Hispanic Paradox." The Hispanic Paradox refers to the relatively good health and longevity among Hispanics relative to Whites [295]. These differences exist despite generally lower socioeconomic status and obvious deprivation among Hispanics. In addition, epidemiological evidence suggests that among Hispanics, foreign-born Latinos have lower early mortality rates than U.S. born Latinos, suggesting a potential acculturation effect [296, 297]. These differences are not explained by problems with data reliability [298], or by the "Salmon Bias" hypothesis (i.e., the hypothesis that Hispanics return to their home country in old age, and, hence, are never recorded as deceased in the death index) [295]. Nor are the differences explained by the possibility that healthier Latinos migrate to the U.S. [295]. An interpersonal hypothesis is that cultural differences in social capital, including large family support, involvement in neighborhood, clubs, and religious organizations, and respect and rallying around elder family members (e.g., respect for elders) may influence not only illness risk, but also support recovery. Hence, the interpersonal approach may be useful for investigating social aspects of both health-damaging, as well as health-resiliency, phenomena contributing to race and culture-related health disparities.

Developmental. Animal and human evidence support early-life social deprivation as a strong determinant of emotional, behavioral and biological dysregulation [299-303]. However, is status (presence/ absence of a parent) alone the determinant of these effects or, like marriage, does the quality of the relationship influence future risk? [304] In a 35-year followup of the Harvard Mastery of Stress Study, Russek and Schwartz [305] found that, compared with only 25% of college students who had rated their parents as warm and caring, 87% of undergraduates who had rated both parents as interpersonally cold were diagnosed with serious health challenges (CAD, hypertension, ulcers) as older adults. If parental affiliative qualities are stable, these findings suggest that the affiliative quality of early social relationships may be an important determinant of future cardiovascular risk.

Interpersonal analysis of the developmental antecedents to disease risk is aided by an excellent rodent model of variances in maternal behaviors and hypothalamic-pituitary-adrenal feedback development central to stress regulation [306, 307]. Meaney and colleagues [306] have demonstrated that female rats vary in the frequency, duration and quality of care they exhibit towards their young. These behaviors are expressed as licking and grooming and arched back nursing (LG/ABN). In a systematic program of research, Meaney has demonstrated that pups of mothers high in LG/ABN develop denser glucocorticoid receptor fields (GCRs), compared with pups of low LG/ABN mothers. GCRs are a critical part of the negative feedback loop necessary for regulating biological stress responses and approach/avoidance behaviors.

An important issue is whether or not these differences are hardwired. Two lines of research address this question. First, Meaney has demonstrated that offspring of low LG/ABN mothers placed with high LG/ABN mothers receive more maternal attention and that denser GCR development results, relative to their unadopted siblings. Second, human handling of pups increases LG/ABN behaviors toward those pups. This handling manipulation resulted in denser GCR fields in pups of naturally low LG/ABN mothers who were handled and returned to the same mother. These findings suggest that stress system development varies as a function of maternal attention rather than genetic determinism. Taken as a whole, the available evidence suggests that variations in the affiliative quality of the early social environment can influence risk trajectories for disease in adulthood.

In Closing

Imagine for a moment that you have two tickets to college basketball's Final Four games (if you don't like basketball, imagine a large event that you would like to see). Who would you take? What is his or her relationship to you, and how might that individual influence your experience at the games? Picture yourself in your seat at the event. Are you experiencing the crowd in general or are you more likely experiencing the individuals seated close by? How would those individuals influence your experience? If they were rooting for the same team as you were, would your enjoyment of the experience be heightened? Imagine that those around you were intoxicated and belligerent. How would they affect your experience and how would the person you brought with you moderate that experience?

Psychosocial researchers are increasingly interested in examining the individual in social environments. The interpersonal concepts and models provide a framework for identifying interpersonal risk factors for health. Finally, the interpersonal approach to risk factor identification highlights individual and relationship factors that can be addressed by practitioners. Patient appointments can be opportune moments for assessing traditional risk factors, as well as interpersonal risk factors, that play an important role in patient adaptation.

References

1. Smith TW, Gerin W (1998) The social psychophysiology of cardiovascular response: an introduction to the special issue. Ann Behav Med 20:243-246
2. Smith TW, Ruiz JM (2002) Psychosocial influences on the development and course of coronary heart disease: current status and implications for research and practice. Consult Clin Psychol 70:548-568
3. Smith TW (1994) Concepts and methods in the study of anger, hostility, and health. In: Siegman AW, Smith TW (Eds) Anger, hostility and the heart. Lawrence Erlbaum, Hillsdale, NJ pp 23-42
4. Smith TW, Gallo LC, Ruiz JM (2003) Toward a social psychophysiology of cardiovascular reactivity: interpersonal concepts and methods in the study of stress and coronary disease. In: Suls J, Wallston K (Eds) Social psychological foundations of health and illness. Blackwell, Malden, MA pp 335-366
5. Sullivan HS (1953) The interpersonal theory of psychiatry. Norton, New York
6. Leary T (1957) Interpersonal diagnosis of personality. Ronald, New York
7. Carson RC (1969) Interaction concepts in personality. Aldine, Chicago
8. Benjamin LS (1974) Structural analysis of social behavior. Psychol Rev 81:392-425
9. Benjamin LS (1994) SASB: A bridge between personality theory and clinical psychology. Psychol Inquiry 5:273-316
10. Wiggins JS (1979) A psychological taxonomy of trait-descriptive terms: the interpersonal domain. J Pers Soc Psychol 37:395-412
11. Kiesler DJ (1996) Contemporary interpersonal theory and research: personality, psychopathology, and psychotherapy. John Wiley & Sons, New York

12. Kelley HH (1983) The situational origins of human tendencies: a further reason for the formal analysis of structures. Pers Soc Psychol Bull 9:8-30
13. Dewey J, Bentley AF (1949) Knowing and the known. Beacon, Boston
14. Thibaut JW, Kelley HH (1959) The social psychology of groups. Wiley, New York
15. Wachtel PL (1977) Psychoanalysis and behavior therapy: toward an integration. Basic Books, New York
16. Wachtel PL (1997) Psychoanalysis, behavior therapy, and the relational world. American Psychological Association, Washington, DC
17. Gallo LC, Smith TW (1999) Patterns of hostility and social support: conceptualizing psychosocial risk as a characteristic of the person and the environment. J Res Pers 33:281-310
18. Smith TW, Gallo LC (2001) Personality traits as risk factors for physical illness. In: Baum A, Revenson T, Singer J (Eds) Handbook of health psychology pp 139-172
19. Blascovich J, Tomaka J (1996) The Biopsychosocial model of arousal regulation. In: Zanna MP (Ed) Advances in experimental psychology, vol. 29. Academic Press, New York pp 1-51
20. Carver CS, Scheier MF (1998) On the self-regulation of behavior. Cambridge University Press, New York
21. Obrist PA (1981) Cardiovascular psychophysiology: a perspective. Plenum Press, New York
22. Allport GW (1937) Personality: a psychological interpretation. Holt, Rinehart & Winston, New York
23. Cantor N (1990) From thought to behavior: having and doing in the study of personality and cognition. Am Psychol 45:735-750
24. Kiesler DJ (1986) Interpersonal methods of diagnosis and treatment. In: Michels R, Cavenar JO Jr (Eds) Psychiatry, vol. 1. Lippincott, Philadelphia pp 1-23
25. Pincus AL, Gurtman MB (1995) The three faces of interpersonal dependency: structural analyses of self-report dependency measures. J Pers Soc Psychol 69:744-758
26. Trapnell PD, Wiggins JS (1990) Extension of the interpersonal adjective scales to include the big five dimensions of personality. J Personali Soc Psychol 59:781-790
27. Wiggins JS, Broughton R (1991) A geometric taxonomy of personality. Eur J Pers 5:343-365
28. Wiggins JS, Trapnell PD (1996) A dyadic-interactional perspective on the five-factor model. In: Wiggins JS (Ed) The five-factor model of personality. Guilford Press, New York pp 88-162
29. Bakan D (1966) The duality of human existence: isolation and communion in western man. Beacon Press, Boston
30. Wiggins JS (1991) Agency and communion as conceptual coordinates for the understanding and measurement of interpersonal behavior. In: Grove W, Cichetti D (Eds) Thinking clearly about psychology: essays in honor of Paul Everett Meehl, vol 2. Personality and psychopathology. University of Minnesota Press, Minneapolis pp 89-113
31. Helgeson VS (1994) Relations of agency and communion to well-being: evidence and potential explanations. Psychol Bull 116:412-428
32. Nealey JB, Smith TW, Uchino BN (2002) Cardiovascular responses to agency and communion stressors in young women. J Res Pers 36:395-418

33. Taylor SE, Klein LC, Lewis BP et al (2000) Biobehavioral responses to stress in females: tend-and-befriend, not fight-or-flight. Psycholog Rev 107:411-429

34. Gurtman MB, Pincus AL (2003) The circumplex model: methods and research applications. In: Schinka JA, Velicer WF (Eds) Handbook of psychology: research methods in psychology, vol. 2. John Wiley & Sons, Inc, New York pp 407-428

35. Wiggins JS, Trapnell P, Phillips N (1988) Psychometric and geometric characteristics of the revised interpersonal adjective scales (IAS-R). Multivariate Behav Res 2:517-530

36. Horowitz LM, Dryer DC, Krasnoperova EN (1997) The circumplex structure of interpersonal problems. In: Plutchik R, Conte HR (Eds) Circumplex models personality emotions. American Psychological Association, Washington, DC pp 347-384

37. Alden LE, Wiggins JS, Pincus AL (1990) Construction of circumplex scales for the inventory of interpersonal problems. J Pers Assess 55:521-536

38. Kiesler DJ, Schmidt JA, Wagner CC (1997) A circumplex inventory of impact messages: an operational bridge between emotion and interpersonal behavior. In: Plutchik R, Conte HR (Eds) Circumplex models of personality and emotions. American Psychological Association, Washington, DC pp 221-244

39. Schmidt JA, Wagner CC, Kiesler DJ (1993) DSM-IV Axis II: dimensionality ratings? "Yes"; Big Five? "Perhaps later." Psychological Inquiry 4:119-121

40. Schmidt JA, Wagner CC, Kiesler DJ (1999) Psychometric and circumplex properties of the octant scale impact message inventory (IMI-C): a structural evaluation. J Counsel Psychol 46:325-334

41. Trobst K (2000) An interpersonal conceptualization and quantification of social support transactions. Pers Soc Psychol Bull 26:971-986

42. Gurtman MB (1994) The circumplex as a tool for studying normal and abnormal personality: a methodological primer. In: Strack S, Lorr M (Eds) Differentiating normal and abnormal personality. Springer, New York pp 243-263

43. Wiggins JS, Broughton R (1985) The interpersonal circle: a structural model for the integration of personality research. In: Hogan R, Jones WH (Eds) Perspectives in personality: JAI. Press, Inc, Greenwich, CT pp 1-47

44. Gallo LC, Smith TW (1998) Construct validation of health-relevant personality traits: interpersonal circumplex and five-factor model analyses of the aggression questionnaire. Int J Behav Med 5:129-147

45. Ruiz JM, Smith TW, Rhodewalt F (2001) Distinguishing narcissism and hostility: similarities and differences in interpersonal circumplex and five-factor correlates. J Pers Assess 76:537-555

46. Watzlawick P, Beavin JB, Jackson DD (1967) Pragmatics of human communication. A study of interactional patterns, pathologies, and paradoxes. W.W. Norton & Company, New York

47. Coyne, JC, Lazarus RS (1980) Cognitive style, stress perception, and coping. In: Kutash IL, Schlesinger LB (Eds) Handbook on stress and anxiety. Jossey-Bass, San Francisco

48. Bandura A (1978) The self-system in reciprocal determinism. Am Psychol 33:1175-1184

49. Caspi A, Bem DJ, Elder GH (1989) Continuities and consequences of interactional styles across the life course. J Pers 57:375-406

50. Mischel W, Shoda Y (1999) Integrating dispositions and processing dynamics within in a unified theory of personality: the cognitive-affective personality system. In: Per-

vin LA, John OP (Eds) Handbook of Personality: Theory and research, 2 ed. Guilford Press, New York pp197-218
51. Merton RK (1948) The self-fulfilling prophecy. Antioch Rev 8:193-210
52. Merton RK (1957) Social theory and social structure. Collier-MacMillan, London
53. Coyne JC (1976a) Toward an interactional description of depression. Psychiat 39:28-40
54. Coyne JC (1976b) Depression and the response of others. J Abnorm Psychol 85:186-193
55. Darley JM, Fazio RH (1980) Expectancy confirmation processes arising in the social interaction sequence. Am Psychol 35:867-881
56. Jussim L (1986) Self-fulfilling prophecies: a theoretical and integrative review. Psychol Rev 9:429-445
57. Miller DT, Turnbull W (1986) Expectancies and interpersonal processes. In: Rosenzweig MR, Porter LW (Eds) Annual Review, Palo Alto. Ann Rev Psychol 37:233-256
58. Kiesler DJ (1983) The 1982 interpersonal circle: a taxonomy for complementarity in human transactions. Psychol Rev 90:185-214
59. Orford J (1986) The rules of interpersonal complementarity: does hostility beget hostility and dominance, submission? Psychol Rev 93:365-377
60. Wiggins JS (1982) Circumplex models of interpersonal behavior in clinical psychology. In: Kendall PC, Butcher JN (Eds) Handbook of research methods in clinical psychology Wiley, New York pp 183-221
61. Gurtman MB (2001) Interpersonal complementarity: integrating interpersonal measurement with interpersonal models. J Couns Psychol 48:97-110
62. Smith TW, Brown PC (1991) Cynical hostility, attempts to exert social control, and cardiovascular reactivity in married couples. J Behav Med 14:581-592
63. Manuck SB (1994) Cardiovascular reactivity and cardiovascular disease: "once more unto the breach." Int J Behav Med 1:4-31
64. Smith TW, Spiro A (2002) Personality, health, and aging: prolegomenon for the next generation. J Res Pers 36:363-394
65. Hawkley LC, Burleson MH, Berntson GG, Cacioppo JT (2003) Loneliness in everyday life: cardiovascular activity, psychosocial context, and health behaviors. J Pers Soc Psychol 85:105-120
66. Bolger N, DeLongis A, Kessler RC, Schilling EA (1989) Effects of daily stress on negative mood. J Pers Soc Psychol 57:808-818
67. Gatenby R (2004) Married only at the weekends? A study of the amount of time spent together by spouses. Analysis from the UK 2000 time use survey. National Statistics Online: *www.statistics.gov.uk*
68. Ruiz JM, Matthews KA, Scheier MF, Schulz R. Does whom you marry matter for your health? Influence of patient's and spouse's personality on their partner's psychological well-being following coronary artery bypass surgery. Unpublished manuscript
69. Nieboer AP, Schulz R, Matthews KA et al (1998) Spousal caregivers' activity restriction and depression: a model for changes over time. Soc Sci Med 47:1361-1371
70. Schulz R, Bookwala J, Knapp JE et al (1996) Pessimism, age, and cancer mortality. Psychol Aging 11:304-309
71. Coyne JC, Smith DA (1991) Couples coping with a myocardial infarction: a contextual perspective on wives' distress. J Pers Soc Psychol 61:404-412

72. Johnson DW (2003) Social interdependence: the interrelationships among theory, research, and practice. Am Psychol 58:931-945
73. Rusbult CE, Van Lange PAM (2003) Interdependence, interaction, and relationships. Ann Rev Psychol 54:351-375
74. Gruber-Baldini AL, Schaie KW, Willis SL (1995) Similarity in married couples: a longitudinal study of mental abilities and rigidity-flexibility. J Pers Soc Psychol 69:191-203
75. Surra CA, Longstreth M (1990) Similarity of outcomes, interdependence, and conflict in dating relationships. J Pers Soc Psychol 59:501-516
76. Zajonc RB, Adelmann PK, Murphy ST, Niedenthal PM (1987) Convergence in the physical appearance of spouses. Motivation Emotion 11:335-346
77. Patterson SP (1988) Relationships within the family: a systems perspective on development. In: Hinde RA, Stevenson-Hinde J (Eds) Relationships within families: mutual influences. Oxford University Press, New York pp 7-26
78. Kaplan JR, Manuck SB, Clarkson TB et al (1982) Social status, environment, and atherosclerosis in cynomolgus monkeys. Arteriosclerosis 2:359-368
79. Kaplan JR, Manuck SB, Clarkson TB et al (1983) Social stress and atherosclerosis in normocholesterolemic monkeys. Science 220:733-735
80. Manuck SB, Kaplan JR, Adams MR, Clarkson TB (1988) Effects of stress and the sympathetic nervous system on coronary artery atherosclerosis in the cynomolgus macaque. Am Heart J 116:328-333
81. Manuck SB, Kaplan JR, Clarkson TB (1983) Social instability and coronary artery atherosclerosis in cynomolgus monkeys. Neurosci Biobehav Rev 7:485-491
82. Kaplan JR, Manuck SB, Adams MR et al (1987) Inhibition of coronary atherosclerosis by propranolol in behaviorally predisposed monkeys fed an atherogenic diet. Circulation 76:1364-1372
83. Kaplan JR, Manuck SB (1989) The effect of propranolol on behavioral interactions among adult male cynomolgus monkeys (Macaca fascicularis) housed in disrupted social groupings. Psychosom Med 51:449-462
84. Rosenberg L, Hennekens CH, Rosner B et al (1981) Early menopause and the risk of myocardial infarction. Am J Obstet Gynecol 139:47-51
85. Kaplan JR, Manuck SB (2004) Ovarian dysfunction, stress, and disease: a primate continuum. ILAR 45:89-115
86. Hamm TB, Kaplan JR, Clarkson TB, Bullock BC (1983) Effects of gender and social behavior on the development of coronary artery atherosclerosis in cynomolgus macaques. Atherosclerosis 48:221-233
87. Kaplan JR, Adams MR, Clarkson TB, Koritnik DR (1984) Psychosocial influences on female "protection" among cynomolgus macaques. Atherosclerosis 53:283-295
88. Adams MR, Kaplan JR, Clarkson TB, Koritnik DR (1985) Ovariectomy, social status, and atherosclerosis in cynomolgus monkeys. Arteriosclerosis 5:192-200
89. Kaplan JR, Adams MR, Anthony MS et al (1995) Dominant social status and contraceptive hormone treatment inhibit atherogenesis in premenopausal monkeys. Arterioscler Thromb Vasc Biol 15:2094-2100
90. Kaplan JR, Manuck SB, Anthony MS, Clarkson TB (2002) Premenopausal social status and hormone exposure predict postmenopausal atherosclerosis in female monkeys. Obstet Gynecol 99:381-388

91. Sapolsky RM (2005) The influence of social hierarchy on primate health. Science 308: 648-652
92. Sapolsky RM (1993) The physiology f dominance in stable versus unstable social hierarchies. In: Mason WA, Mendoza SP (Eds) Primate social conflict. State University of New York Press, New York pp 171-204
93. Castles DL, Whiten A, Aureli F (1999) Social anxiety, relationships and self-directed behavior among wild female olive baboons. Animal Behav 58:1207-1215
94. Sapolsky RM, Alberts S, Altmann J (1997) Hypercortisolism associated with social subordinance or social isolation among wild baboons. Arch General Psychiat 54:1137-1143
95. Abbott DH, Keverne EB, Bercovitch FB et al (2003) Are subordinates always stressed? A comparative analysis of rank differences in cortisol levels among primates. Horm Behav 43:67-82
96. Carter CS, Lederhendler I, Kirkpatrick B (1997) The integrative neurobiology of affiliation. Introduction. Annals New York Academy Sciences 15:XIII-XVIII
97. Uchino BN (2004) Social support and physical health: Understanding the health consequences of relationships. University Press, Cambridge
98. Gallo LC, Matthews KA (2003) Understanding the association between socioeconomic status and physical health: do negative emotions play a role? Psychol Bull 129:10-51
99. Rozanski A, Blumenthal JA, Kaplan J (1999) Impact of psychological factors on the pathogenesis of cardiovascular disease and implications for therapy. Circulation 99:2192-2217
100. Houston BK, Babyak MA, Chesney MA et al (1997) Social dominance and 22-year all-cause mortality in men. Psychosom Med 59:5-12
101. Whiteman MC, Deary IJ, Lee AJ, Fowkes FGR (1997) Submissiveness and protection from coronary heart disease in the general population: Edinburgh artery study. Lancet 350:541-545
102. Siegman AW, Kubzansky LD, Kawachi I et al (2000) A prospective study of dominance and coronary heart disease in the normative aging study. Am J Cardiol 86:145-149
103. Greene RE Jr, Houston BK, Holleran SA (1995) Aggressiveness, dominance, developmental factors, and serum cholesterol level in college males. J Behav Med 18:569-580
104. Kop WJ (1999) Chronic and acute psychological risk factors for clinical manifestations of coronary artery disease. Psychosom Med 61:476-487
105. Rozanski A (1998) Laboratory techniques for assessing the presence and magnitude of mental stress-induced myocardial ischemia in patients with coronary artery disease. In: Krantz DS, Baum A (Eds) Technology and methods in behavioral medicine. Lawrence Erlbaum Associates, Mahwah, NJ pp 47-68
106. Smith TW, Baldwin M, Christensen AJ (1990) Interpersonal influence as active coping: effects of task difficulty on cardiovascular reactivity. Psychophysiol 27:429-437
107. Smith TW, Limon JP, Gallo LC, Ngu LQ (1996) Interpersonal control and cardiovascular reactivity: goals, behavioral expression, and the moderating effects of sex. J Pers Soc Psychol 70:1012-1024
108. Smith TW, Allred KD, Morrison CA, Carlson SD (1989) Cardiovascular reactivity

and interpersonal influence: active coping in a social context. J Pers Soc Psychol 56:209-218

109. Smith TW, Nealey JB, Kircher JC, Limon JP (1997) Social determinants of cardiovascular reactivity: effects of incentive to exert influence and evaluative threat. Psychophysiol 34:65-73

110. Brown PC, Smith TW (1992) Social influence, marriage, and the heart: cardiovascular consequences of interpersonal control in husbands and wives. Health Psychol 11:88-96

111. Engebretson TO, Matthews KA, Scheier MF (1989) Relations between anger expression and cardiovascular reactivity: reconciling inconsistent findings through a matching hypothesis. J Pers Soc Psychol 57:513-521

112. Davis MC, Matthews KA (1996) Do gender relevant characteristics determine cardiovascular reactivity? Match versus mismatch of traits and situation. J Pers Soc Psychol 71:527-535

113. Frankish CJ, Linden W (1996) Spouse-pair risk factors and cardiovascular reactivity. J Psychosom Res 40:37-51

114. Brown PC, Smith TW, Benjamin LS (1998) Perceptions of spouse dominance predict blood pressure reactivity during marital interaction. Ann Behav Med 20:294-301

115. Sussman RW, Garber PA, Cheverud JM. Importance of cooperation and affiliation in the evolution of primate sociality. Am J Anthropol, in press

116. Cooper MA, Bernstein IS (2000) Social grooming in assamese macaques (Macaca assamensis). Am J Primatol 50:77-85

117. de Waal FB, Luttrell LM (1986) The similarity principle underlying social bonding among female rhesus monkeys. Folia Primatol 46:215-234

118. Matheson MD, Bernstein IS (2000) Grooming, social bonding, and agonistic aiding in rhesus monkeys. Am J Primatol 51:177-186

119. Carter CS (1998) Neuroendocrine perspectives on social attachments and love. Psychoneuroendocrinology 23:779-818

120. Mendoza SP, Mason WA (1999) Attachment relationships in new world primates. In: Carter CS, Lederhendler II, Kirkpatrick B (Eds) The integrative neurobiology of affiliatio. The MIT Press, Cambridge pp 93-99

121. Seyfarth RM (1976) Social relationships among adult female baboons. Animal Behav 24:917-938

122. Seyfarth RM, Cheney DL (1984) Grooming, alliances and reciprocal altruism in vervet monkeys. Nature 308:541-543

123. Fuentes A, Malone N, Sanz C et al (2002) Conflict and post-conflict behavior in a small group of chimpanzees. Primates 43:223-235

124. Gruter CC (2004) Conflict and postconflict behavior in captive black-and-white snub-nosed monkeys (Rhinopithecus bieti). Primates 45:197-200

125. Manson JH, Perry S, Stahl D (2005) Reconciliation in wild white-faced capuchins (Cebus capucinus). Am J Primatol 65:205-219

126. Pereira ME, Schill JL, Charles EP (2000) Reconciliation in captive Guyanese squirrel monkeys (Saimiri sciureus). Am J Primatol 50:159-167

127. Silk JB, Alberts SC, Altmann J (2003) Social bonds of female baboons enhance infant survival. Science 302:1231-1234

128. Gust DA, Gordon T P, Brodie AR, McClure HM (1994) Effect of a preferred companion in modulating stress in adult female rhesus monkeys. Physiol Biol 55:681-684
129. Kutsukake N, Castles DL (2004) Reconciliation and post-conflict third-party affiliation among wild chimpanzees in the Mahale Mountains, Tanzania. Primates 45:157-165
130. Insel TR (1997) A neurobiological basis of social attachment. Am J Psychiat 154:726-735
131. Insel TR, Winslow JT, Wang Z, Young LJ (1998) Oxytocin, vasopressin, and the neuroendocrine basis of pair bond formation. Adv Exper Med Biol 449:215-224
132. Insel TR, Young LJ (2000) Neuropeptides and the evolution of social behavior. Cur Opin Neurobiol 10:784-789
133. Snowdon CT, Ziegler TE (2000) Reproductive hormones. In: Cacioppo JT, Tassinary LG, Berntson GG (Eds) Handbook of psychophysiology, 2 edn. Cambridge University Press, New York
134. Winslow JT, Noble PL, Lyons CK et al (2003) Rearing effects on cerebrospinal fluid oxytocin concentration and social buffering in rhesus monkeys. Neuropsychopharmacology 28:910-918
135. Petersson M, Alster P, Lundeberg T, Uvnas-Moberg K (1996) Oxytocin causes a long-term decrease of blood pressure in female and male rats. Physiol Behav 60:1311-1315
136. Petersson M, Hulting AL, Uvnas-Moberg K (1999) Oxytocin causes a sustained decrease in plasma levels of corticosterone in rats. Neurosci Lett 255:115-118
137. Windle RJ, Kershaw YM, Shanks N et al (2004) Oxytocin attenuates stress-induced c-fos mRNA expression in specific forebrain regions associated with modulation of hypothalamo-pituitary-adrenal-activity. J Neurosci 24:2974-2982
138. Carter CS, Altemus M (1997) Integrative functions of lactational hormones in social behavior and stress management. Ann NY Acad Sci 807:164-174
139. Volpi S, Rabadan-Diehl C, Aguilera G (2004) Vasopressinergic regulation of the hypothalamic pituitary adrenal axis and stress adaptation. Stress 7:75-83
140. Anderson NB, Armstead CA (1995) Toward understanding the association of socioeconomic status and health: a new challenge for the biopsychosocial approach. Psychosom Med 57:213-225
141. Kaplan GA, Kiel JE (1993) Socioeconomic factors and cardiovascular disease: a review of the literature. Circulation 88:1973-1998
142. Powell LH, Hoffman A, Shahabi L (2001) Socioeconomic differential in health and disease: let's take the next step. Psychosom Med 63:722-723
143. Reiff M, Schwartz S, Northridge M (2001) Relationship of depressive symptoms to hypertension in a household survey in Harlem. Psychosom Med 63:711-721
144. Kawachi I (1999) Social capital and community effects on population and individual health. Ann NY Acad Sci 896:120-130
145. Kawachi I, Kennedy BP, Lochner K, Prothrow-Stith D (1997) Social capital, income inequality, and mortality. Am J Public Health 89:1187-1193
146. Piferi RL, Lawler KA (2000) Hostility and the cardiovascular reactivity of women during interpersonal confrontation. Women Health 30:111-129.
147. Suarez EC, Harlan E, Peoples MC, Williams RB Jr (1993) Cardiovascular and emotional responses in women: the role of hostility and harassment. Health Psychol 12:459-468

148. Gallo LC, Smith TW, Kircher JC (2000) Cardiovascular and electrodermal respons-es to support and provocation: interpersonal methods in the study of psy-chophysiological reactivity. Psychophysiol 37:289-301

149. Lepore SJ (1998) Problems and prospects for the social support-reactivity hypoth-esis. Ann Behav Med 20:257-269

150. Uchino BN, Cacioppo JR, Kiecolt-Glaser JK (1996) The relationship between social support and physiological processes: a review with emphasis on underlying mech-anisms and implications for health. Psycholog Bull 119:488-531

151. Light KC, Grewen KM, Amico JA (2005) More frequent partner hugs and higher oxytocin levels are linked to lower blood pressure and heart rate in premenopausal women. Biol Psychol 69:5-21

152. Light KC, Grewen KM, Amico JA et al (2005) Oxytocinergic activity is linked to lower blood pressure and vascular resistance during stress in postmenopausal women on estrogen replacement. Horm Behav 47:540-548

153. Gerin W, Pieper C, Levy R, Pickering TG (1992) Social support in social interac-tion: a moderator of cardiovascular reactivity. Psychosom Med 54:324-336

154. Sheffield D, Carroll D (1996) Task-induced cardiovascular activity and the pres-ence of a supportive or undermining other. Psychol Health 11:583-591

155. Gerin W, Milner D, Chawla S, Pickering TG (1995) Social support as a moderator of cardiovascular reactivity in women: a test of the direct effects and buffering hypothe-ses. Psychosom Med 57:16-22

156. Kamarck TW, Manuck SB, Jennings RJ (1990) Social support reduces cardiovascular reactivity to psychological challenge: a laboratory model. Psychosom Med 52:42-58

157. Grewen KM, Anderson BJ, Girdler SS, Light KC (2003) Warm partner contact is related to lower cardiovascular reactivity. Behav Med 29:123-130

158. Allen KM, Blascovich J, Tomaka J, Kelsey RM (1991) Presence of human friends and pet dogs as moderators of autonomic responses to stress in women. J Pers Soc Psychol 61:582-589

159. Friedmann E, Thomas SA (1995) Pet ownership, social support, and one-year sur-vival after acute myocardial infarction in the cardiac arrhythmia suppression trial (CAST). Am J Cardiol 76:1213-1217

160. Bloor LE, Uchino BN, Hicks A, Smith TW (2004) Social relationships and physio-logical function: the effects of recalling social relationships on cardiovascular reac-tivity. Ann Behav Med 28:29-38

161. Smith TW, Ruiz JM, Uchino BN (2004) Mental activation of supportive ties, hostil-ity, and cardiovascular reactivity to laboratory stress in young men and women. Health Psychol 23:476-485

162. Lepore SJ, Allen KA, Evans GW (1993) Social support lowers cardiovascular reac-tivity to an acute stressor. Psychosom Med 55:518-524

163. Christenfeld N, Gerin W, Linden W et al (1997) Social support effects on cardio-vascular reactivity: is a stranger as effective as a friend? Psychosom Med 59:388-398

164. Fontana AM, Diegman T, Villeneuve A, Lepore SJ (1999) Nonevaluative social sup-port reduces cardiovascular reactivity in young women during acutely stressful performance situations. J Behav Med 22:75-91

165. Uno D, Uchino BN, Smith TW (2002) Relationship quality moderates the effect of

social support given by close friends on cardiovascular reactivity in women. Int J Behav Med 9:243-262

166. Heffner KL, Kiecolt-Glaser JK, Loving TJ (2004) Spousal support satisfaction as a modifier of physiological responses to marital conflict in younger and older couples. J Behav Med 27:233-254

167. Kiecolt-Glaser JK, Glaser R, Cacioppo JT, Malarkey WB (1998) Marital stress: immunologic, neuroendocrine, and autonomic correlates. Ann NY Acad Sci 840:656-663

168. Kiecolt-Glaser JK, Fisher L, Ogrocki P et al (1987) Marital quality, marital disruption, and immune function. Psychosom Med 49:13-34

169. Kiecolt-Glaser JK, Kennedy S, Malkoff S et al (1988) Marital discord and immunity in males. Psychosom Med 50:213-229

170. Kiecolt-Glaser JK, Malarkey WB, Chee M et al (1993) Negative behavior during marital conflict is associated with immunological down-regulation. Psychosom Med 55:395-409

171. Kiecolt-Glaser JK, Laser R, Cacioppo JT et al (1997) Marital conflict in older adults: endocrinological and immunological correlates. Psychosom Med 59:339-349

172. Fritz HL, Nagurney AJ, Helgeson VS (2003) Social interactions and cardiovascular reactivity during problem disclosure among friends. Pers Soc Psychol Bull 29:713-725

173. Kors DJ, Linden W, Gerin W (1997) Evaluation interferes with social support: effects on cardiovascular stress reactivity in women. J Soc Clin Psychol 16:1-23

174. Smith TW (1992) Hostility and health: current status of a psychosomatic hypothesis. Health Psychol 11:139-150

175. Smith W, Glazer K, Ruiz JM, Gallo LC (2004) Hostility, anger, aggressiveness and coronary heart disease: an interpersonal perspective on personality, emotion, and health. J Pers 72:1217-1270

176. Chen YY, Gilligan S, Coups EJ, Contrada RJ (2005) Hostility and perceived social support: interactive effects on cardiovascular reactivity to laboratory stressors. Ann Behav Med 29:37-43

177. Lepore SJ (1995) Cynicism, social support, and cardiovascular reactivity. Health Psychol 14:210-216

178. Coyne JC, DeLongis AM (1986) Going beyond social support: the role of social relationships in adaptation. J Cons Clin Psychol 54:454-460

179. Ewart CK, Taylor CB, Kraemer HC, Agras WS (1991) High blood pressure and marital discord: not being nasty matters more than being nice. Health Psychol 10:155-163

180. Benazon NR, Foster MD, Coyne JC. Expressed emotion, adaptation and patient survival among couples coping with chronic heart failure. J Fam Psychol, in press

181. Kaplan GA, Salonen JT, Cohen RD et al (1988) Social connections and mortality from all causes and from cardiovascular disease: prospective evidence from eastern Finland. Am J Epidemiol 128:370-380

182. Kaplan GA, Wilson TW, Cohen RD et al (1994) Social functioning and overall mortality: prospective evidence from the Kuopio ischemic heart disease risk factor study. Epidemiol 5:495-500

183. Orth-Gomer K, Johnson JV (1987) Social network interaction and mortality: a six year follow-up study of a random sample of the Swedish population. J Chronic Dis 40:949-957

184. Orth-GomerK, Rosengren A, Wilhelmsen L (1993) Lack of social support and incidence of contrary heart disease in middle-aged Swedish men. Psychosom Med 55: 37-43
185. O'Shea JC, Wilcox RB, Skene AM et al (2002) Comparison of outcomes of patients with myocardial infarction when living alone versus those not living alone. Am J Cardiol 90:1374-1377
186. Reed D, McGee D, Yano K, Feinleib M (1983) Social networks and coronary heart disease among Japanese men in Hawaii. Am J Epidemiol 117:384-396
187. Coyne JC, Ellard JH, Smith DA (1990) Unsupportive relationships, interdependence, and unhelpful exchanges. In: Sarason IG, Sarason BR, Pierce G (Eds) Social support: an interactional view. Wiley, New York
188. Lyons R, Ritvo P, Sullivan M, Coyne J (1995) Close relationships through chronic health and illness. Sage, New York
189. Dickens CM, McGowan L, Percival C et al (2004) Lack of a close confidant, but not depression predicts further cardiac events after myocardial infarction. Heart 90:518-522
190. Chandra V (1983) The impact of marital status on survival after an acute myocardial infarction: a population-based study. Am J Epidemiol 117:320-325
191. Eaker ED, Pinsky J, Castelli WP (1992) Myocardial infarction and coronary death among women: psychosocial predictors from a 20-year follow-up of women in the Framingham study. Am J Epidemiol 135:854-864
192. Beach EK, Maloney BH, Plocica AR et al (1992) The spouse: a factor in recovery after acute myocardial infarction. Heart Lung 21:30-38
193. Coyne JC, Rohrbaugh MJ, Shoham V et al (in press) Prognostic importance of marital quality for survival of congestive heart failure. Am J Cardiol, in press
194. Gallo LC, Troxel WM, Kuller LH et al (2003) Marital status, marital quality, and atherosclerotic burden in postmenopausal women. Psychosom Med 65:952-962
195. Gallo LC, Troxel WM, Matthews KA, Kuller LH (2003) Marital status and quality in middle-aged women: associations with levels and trajectories of cardiovascular risk factors. Health Psychol 22:453-463
196. Orth-Gomer K, Wamala SP, Horsten M et al (2000) Marital stress worsens prognosis in women with coronary heart disease: the Stockholm female coronary risk study. JAMA 284:3008-3014
197. Case RB, Moss AJ, Case N et al (1992) Living alone after myocardial infarction: impact on prognosis. JAMA 267:515-519
198. Surtees PG, Miller PM (1994) Partners in adversity III. Mood status after the event. Europ Arch Psychiat Clin Neurosci 243:311-318
199. Artinian NT (1991) Stress experience of spouses of patients having coronary artery bypass during hospitalization and 6 weeks after discharge. Heart Lung 20:52-59
200. Delon M (1996) The patient in the CCU waiting room: in-hospital treatment of the cardiac spouse. In: Allan R, Scheidt S (Eds) Heart and mind: the practice of cardiac psychology. American Psychological Association, Washington, DC pp 421-432
201. Han B, Haley WE (1999) Family caregiving for patients with stroke. Review and analysis. Stroke 30:1478-1485
202. Langeluddecke P, Tennant C, Fulcher G et al (1989) Coronary artery bypass surgery: impact upon the patient's spouse. J Psychosom Res 33:155-159

203. Rohrbaugh MJ, Cranford J, Shoham V et al (2002) Couples coping with congestive heart failure: role and gender differences in psychological distress. J Fam Psychol 16:3-13

204. Stanley MJB, Frantz RA (1988) Adjustment problems of spouses of patients undergoing coronary artery bypass graft surgery during early convalescence. Heart Lung 17:677-682

205. Kettunen S, Solovieva S, Laamanen R, Santavirta N (1999) Myocardial infarction, spouses' reactions and their need of support. J Adv Nursing 30:479-488

206. Bengtson A, Karlsson T, Wahrborg P, Hjalmarson A, Herlitz J (1996) Cardiovascular and psychosomatic symptoms among relatives of patients of patients waiting for possible coronary revascularization. Heart Lung 25:438-443

207. O'Farrell P, Murray J, Hotz SB (2000) Psychologic distress among spouses of patients undergoing cardiac rehabilitation. Heart and Lung 29:97-104

208. Artinian NT (1992) Spouse adaptation to mate's CABG surgery: 1 year follow-up. Am J Critical Care 1:36-42

209. Arefjord K, Hallaraker E, Havik OE, Maeland JG (1998) Life after a myocardial infarction - the wives' point of view. Psychol Rep 83:1203-1216

210. Helgeson VS (1993) Implications of agency and communion for patient and spouse adjustment to a first coronary event. J Pers Soc Psychol 64:807-816

211. Hilbert GA (1993) Family satisfaction and affect of men and their wives after myocardial infarction. Heart Lung 22:200-205

212. Moore SM (1994) Psychologic distress of patients and their spouses after coronary artery bypass surgery. AACN Clin Iss Critical Care Nursing 5:59-65

213. Moser DK, Dracup K (2004) Role of spousal anxiety and depression in patients' psychosocial recovery after a cardiac event. Psychosom Med 66:527-532

214. Hagedoorn M, Buunk BP, Kuijer RG (2000) Couples dealing with cancer: Role and gender differences regarding psychological distress and quality of life. Psycho-Oncology 9:232-242

215. Hagedoorn M, Sanderman R, Ranchor AV et al (2001) Chronic disease in elderly couples: are women more responsive to spouses' health condition then men? J Psychosom Res 51:693-696

216. Hagedoorn M, Sanderman R, Buunk BP, Wobbes T (2002) Failing in spousal caregiving: the "identity-relevant stress" hypothesis explain sex differences in caregiver distress. Bri J Health Psychol 7:481-494

217. Tuinstra J, Hagedoorn M, Van Sonderen E et al (2004) Psychological distress in couples dealing with colorectal cancer: gender role differences and intracouple correspondence. Bri J Health Psychol 9:465-478

218. Kim Y, Duberstein PR, Sorensen S, Larson MR (2005) Levels of depressive symptoms in spouses of people with lung cancer: effects of personality, social support, and caregiving burden. Psychosom J Cons Liaison Psychiat 46:123-130

219. Bookwala J, Schulz R (1998) The role of neuroticism and mastery in spouse caregivers' assessment of and response to a contextual stressor. J Gerontol Series B Psychol Sci Soc Sciences 53:155-164

220. Hooker K, Monahan D, Shifren K, Hutchinson C (1992) Mental and physical health of spouse caregivers: the role of personality. Psychol Aging 7:367-375

221. Nijboer C, Tempelaar R, Triemstra M et al (2001) The role of social and psychologic resources in caregiving of cancer patients. Cancer 91:1029-1039
222. Vedhara K, Shanks N, Wilcock G, Lightman SL (2001) Correlates and predictors of self-reported psychological and physical morbidity in chronic caregiver stress. J Health Psychol 6:101-119
223. Given CW, Stommel M, Given B et al (1993) The influence of cancer patients' symptoms and functional states on patients' depression and family caregivers' reaction and depression. Health Psychol 12:277-285
224. Kurtz ME, Kurtz JC, Given CW, Given B (1997) Predictors of post-bereavement depressive symptomatology among family caregivers of cancer patients. Supportive Care in Cancer 5:53-60
225. Schulz R, Beach SR (1999) Caregiving as a risk factor for mortality: the caregiver health effects study. JAMA 282:2215-2219
226. Vitaliano PP, Zhang J, Scanlan JM (2003) Is caregiving hazardous to one's physical health? A meta-analysis. Psycholog Bull 129:946-972
227. Vitaliano PP, Young HM, Zhang J (2004) Is caregiving a risk factor for illness? Cur Direc Psychol Sci 13:13-16
228. Dyck DG, Short R, Vitaliano PP (1999) Predictors of burden and infectious illness in schizophrenia caregivers. Psychosom Med 61:411-419
229. Fang CY, Manne SL, Pape SJ (2001) Functional impairment, marital quality, and patient psychological distress as predictors of psychological distress among cancer patients' spouses. Health Psychol 20:452-457
230. Northouse LL, Templin T, Mood D (2000) Couples' adjustment to breast disease during the first year following diagnosis. J Behav Med 24:115-136
231. Scholte op Reimer WJ, de Haan RJ, Rijnders PT et al (1998) The burden of caregiving in partners of long-term stroke survivors. Stroke 29:1605-1611
232. Ruiz JM, Matthews KA, Scheier MF, Schulz R (2003) Does whom you marry matter? Effects of spouse traits on psychosocial adjustment following coronary artery bypass surgery. Citation poster presented at the Annual Meeting of the American Psychosomatic Society, Phoenix, AZ
233. Kulik JA, Mahler HI (1989) Social support and recovery from surgery. Health Psychol 8:221-238
234. Owens SI, Qualls SJJ (2002) Family involvement during geropsychiatry hospitalization. J Clin Geropsychol 8:87-99
235. Baker B, Szalai JP, Paquette M, Tobe S (2003) Marital support, spousal contact, and the course of mild hypertension. J Psychosom Res 55:229-232
236. Kulik JA, Mahler HI (1993) Emotional support as a moderator of adjustment and compliance after coronary artery bypass surgery: a longitudinal study. J Behav Med 16:45-63
237. Berkman LF, Leo-Summers L, Horowitz RI (1992) Emotional support and survival after myocardial infarction. A prospective, population-based study of the elderly. Ann Int Med 117:1003-1009
238. Newsom JT, Schulz R (1998) Caregiving from the recipient's perspective: negative reactions to being helped. Health Psychol 17:172-181
239. Manne S, Zautra (1989) Spouse criticism and support: their association with cop-

ing and psychological distress among women with rheumatoid arthritis. J Pers Soc Psychol 56:608-617

240. Manne SL (1999) Intrusive thoughts and psychological distress among cancer patients: the role of spouse avoidance and criticism. J Cons Clin Psychol 67: 539-546

241. Manne SL, Taylor KL, Dougherty J, Kemeny N (1997) Supportive and negative responses in the partner relationship: their association with psychological adjustment among individuals with cancer. J Behav Med 20:101-125

242. Manne S, Ostroff J, Rini C et al. The interpersonal process model of intimacy: the role of self-disclosure, partner disclosure and partner responsiveness in interactions between breast cancer patients and their partners. J Fam Psychol, in press

243. Manne S, Ostroff J, Sherman M et al. Couples' support-related communication, psychological distress and marital satisfaction among women with early stage breast cancer. J Cons Clin Psychol, in press

244. Ben-Zur H, Gilbar O, Lev S (2001) Coping with breast cancer: patient, spouse, and dyad models. Psychosom Med 63:32-39

245. Duits AA, Boeke S, Taams MA et al (1997) Prediction of quality of life after coronary artery bypass graft surgery: a review and evaluation of multiple, recent studies. Psychosom Med 59:257-268

246. Perski A, Feleke E, Anderson G et al (1998) Emotional distress before coronary bypass grafting limits the benefits of surgery. Am Heart J 136:510-517

247. Rumsfeld JS, MaWhinney S, McCarthy M Jr et al (1999) Health-related quality of life as a pedictor of mortality following coronary artery bypass graft surgery. JAMA 281:1298-1303

248. Soderman E, Lisspeers J, Sundin O (2003) Depression as a predictor of return to work in patients with coronary artery disease. Soc Sci Med 56:193-202

249. Bush DE, Ziegelstein RC, Tayback M et al (2001) Even minimal symptoms of depression increase mortality risk after acute myocardial infarction. Am J Cardiol 88:337-341

250. Carney RM, Blumenthal JA, Freedland KE et al, for the ENRICHD investigators (2004) Depression and late mortality after myocardial infarction in the enhancing recovery in coronary heart disease (ENRICHD) Study. Psychosom Med 66: 466-474

251. Frasure-Smith N, Lesperance F, Talajic M (1993) Depression following myocardial infarction: impact on 6 month survival. JAMA 270:1819-1825

252. Ladwig KH, Kieser M, Konig J et al (1991) Affective disorders and survival after acute myocardial infarction. Eur Heart J 12:959-964

253. Holmberg SK, Scott LL, Alexy W, Fife BL (2001) Relationship issues of women with breast cancer. Cancer Nursing 24:53-60

254. Manne SL (1998) Cancer in the marital context: a review of the literature. Cancer Investig 16:188-202

255. VessJD Jr, Moreland JR, Schwebel AI, Krau E (1989) Psychosocial needs of cancer patients: learning from patients and their spouses. J Psychosocial Oncol 6:31-51

256. Wimberly SR, Carver CS, Laurenceau JP et al (2005) Perceived partner reactions to diagnosis and treatment of breast cancer: impact on psychosocial and psychosexual adjustment. J Cons Clin Psychol 73:300-311

257. Zunkel G (2002) Relational coping processes: couples' response to a diagnosis of early stage breast cancer. J Psychosocial Oncol 20:39-55

258. Skelton M, Dominian J (1973) Psychological stress in wives of patients with myocardial infarction. Bri Med J 2:101-103

259. Stern MJ, Pascale L (1979) Psychosocial adaptation post-myocardial infarction: the spouse's dilemma. J Psychosom Res 23:83-87

260. Carver CS, Scheier MF (2000) Scaling back goals and recalibration of the affect system are processes in normal adaptive self-regulation: understanding 'response shift' phenomena. Soc Sci Med 50:1715-1722

261. Coyne JC, Smith DAF (1994) Couples coping with a myocardial infarction; contextual perspective on patient self-efficacy. J Fam Psychol 8:43-51

262. Suls J, Green P, Rose G et al (1997) Hiding worries from one's spouse: associations between coping via protective buffering and distress in male post-myocardial infarction patients and their wives. J Behav Med 20:333-349

263. Berkhuysen MA, Nieuwland W, Buunk BP et al (1999) Change in self-efficacy during cardiac rehabilitation and the role of perceived overprotectiveness. Patient Educ Counsel 38:21-32

264. Clarke DE, Walker JR, Cuddy TE (1996) The role of perceived overprotectiveness in recovery 3 months after myocardial infarction. J Cardiopul Rehab 16:372-377

265. Wicklund I, Sanne H, Vedin A, Wilhelmsson C (1984) Psychosocial outcome one year after a first myocardial infarction. J Psychosom Res 28:309-321

266. Fiske V, Coyne JC, Smith DA (1991) Couples coping with myocardial infarction: an empirical reconsideration of the role of overprotectiveness. J Fam Psychol 5:4-24

267. Riegel BJ, Dracup KA (1992) Does overprotection cause cardiac invalidism after acute myocardial infarction? Heart Lung 21:529-535

268. Skerrett K (1998) Couple adjustment to the experience of breast cancer. Fam System Health 16:281-298

269. Manne S, Ostroff J, Sherman M et al (2003) Buffering effects for family and friend support on associations between partner unsupportive behaviors and coping among women with breast cancer. J Soc Pers Rel 20:771-792

270. Karney BR, Bradbury TN (1997) Neuroticism, marital interaction, and the trajectory of marital satisfaction. J Pers Soc Psychol 72:1075-1092

271. Kiecolt-Glaser JK, Newton TL (2001) Marriage and health: his and hers. Psychol Bull 127:472-503

272. American Heart Association (2005) Heart disease and stroke statistics - 2005 update. American Heart Association, Dallas, Texas

273. Hoyert DL, Kung HC, Smith BL (2005) Deaths: preliminary data for 2003. National vital statistics reports, 53, no. 15. Hyattsville, MD, National Center for Health Statistics

274. Keppel KG, Pearcy JN, Wagener DK (2002) Trends in racial and ethnic-specific rates for the health status indicators: United States, 1990-1998. Healthy people statistical notes, no 23. Hyattsville, MD, National Center for Health Statistics

275. Schnittker J, McLeod JD (2005) The social psychology of health disparities. Ann Rev Sociol 31:75-103

276. Hochstim JR, Athanasopoulos DA, Larkins JH (1968) Poverty area under the microscope. Am J Public Health 58:1815-1827

277. Marmot M, Ryff CD, Bumpass LL et al (1997) Social inequalities in health: next questions and converging evidence. Soc Sci Med 44:901-910

278. Sorlie PD, Backlund E, Keller JB (1995) US mortality by economic, demographic, and social characteristics: the national longitudinal mortality study. Am J Public Health 85:949-957

279. Gump BB, Matthews KA, Raikkonen K (1999) Modeling relationships among socioeconomic status, hostility, cardiovascular reactivity, and left ventricular mass in African American and White children. Health Psychol 18:140-150

280. Haukkala A, Uutela A (2000) Cynical hostility, depression, and obesity: the moderating role of education and gender. Int J Eating Disord 27:106-109

281. Lantz PM, House JS, Lepkowski JM et al (1998) Socioeconomic factors, health behaviors, and mortality. JAMA 279:1703-1708

282. Lynch JW, Kaplan GA, Salonen JT (1997) Why do poor people behave poorly? Variation in adult health behaviours and psychosocial characteristics by stages of the socioeconomic lifecourse. Soc Sci Med 44:809-819

283. Clark R, Anderson NB, Clark VR, Williams DR (1999) Racism as a stressor for African Americans: a biopsychosocial model. Am Psychol 54:805-816

284. Harrell JP, Hall S, Taliaferro J (2003) Physiological responses to racism and discrimination: an assessment of the evidence. Am J Public Health 93:243-248

285. Krieger N (1999) Embodying inequality: a review of concepts, measures, and methods for studying health consequences of discrimination. Int J Health Serv 29:295-352

286. Brondolo E, Rieppi R, Kelley KP, Gerin W (2003) Perceived racism and blood pressure: a review of the literature and conceptual and methodological critique. Ann Behav Med 25:55-65

287. James K, Lovato C, Khoo G (1994) Social identity correlates of minority workers' health. Acad Manag J 37:383-396

288. Krieger N, Sidney S (1996) Racial Discrimination and blood pressure: the CARDIA study of young black and white adults. Am J Public Health 86:1370-1378

289. TroxelWM, Matthews KA, Bromberger JT, Sutton-Tyrrell K (2003) Chronic stress burden, discrimination, and subclinical carotid artery disease in African American and Caucasian women. Health Psychol 22:300-309

290. Pinel EC (1999) Stigma consciousness: the psychological legacy of social stereotypes. J Pers Soc Psychol 76:114-128

291. Pinel EC (2002) Stigma consciousness in intergroup contexts: the power of conviction. J Exper Soc Psychol 38:178-185

292. Hebl MR, Tickle J, Heatherton TF (2000) Awkward moments in interactions between nonstigmatized and stigmatized individuals. In: Heatherton TF, Kleck RE, Hebl MR, Hull JG (Eds) The social psychology of stigma. Guilford, New York pp 273-306

293. Major B, Quinton WJ, Schmader T (2003) Attributions to discrimination and self-esteem: impact of group identification and situational ambiguity. J Exper Soc Psychol 39:220-231

294. Blascovich J, Mendes W, Hunter SB et al (2001) Perceiver threat in social interactions with stigmatized others. J Per Soc Psychol 80:253-267

295. Abraido-Lanza AF, Dohrenwend BP, Ng-Mak DS, Turner JB (1999) The Latino mortality paradox: a test of the "Salmon bias" and healthy migrant hypotheses. Am J Public Health 89:1543-1548

296. Abraido-Lanza AF, Chao MT, Florez KR (2005) Do healthy behaviors decline with greater acculturation? Implications for the Latino mortality paradox. Soc Sci Med 61:1243-1255
297. Hunt LM, Schneider S, Comer B (2004) Should "acculturation" be a variable in health research? A critical review of research on US Hispanics. Soc Sci Med 59: 973-986
298. Sorlie PD, Backlund E, Johnson NJ, Rogot E (1993) Mortality by Hispanic status in the United States. JAMA 270:2464-2468
299. Carlson M, Earls F (1997) Psychological and neuroendocrinological sequelae of early social deprivation in institutionalized children in Romania. Ann NY Acad Sci 807:419-428
300. Clarke AS, Kraemer GW, Kupfer DJ (1998) Effects of rearing condition on HPA axis response to fluoxetine and desipramine treatment over repeated social separations in young rhesus monkeys. Psychiat Res 79:91-104
301. Coe CL, Lubach G, Ershler WB (1989) Immunological consequences of maternal separation in infant primates. New Dir Child Developm 45:65-91
302. Levine S, Weiner SG (1988) Psychoendocrine aspects of mother-infant relationships in non-human primates. Psychoneuroendocrinology 13:143-154
303. Sanchez MM, Ladd CO, Plotsky PM (2001) Early adverse experience as a developmental risk factor for later psychopathology: evidence from rodent and primate models. Developm Psychopathol 13:419-449
304. Repetti RL, Taylor SE, Seeman TE (2002) Risky families: family social environments and the mental and physical health of offspring. Psycholog Bull 128:330-366
305. Russek LG, Schwartz GE (1997) Perceptions of parental caring predict health status in midlife: a 35-year follow-up of the Harvard mastery of stress study. Psychosom Med 59:144-149
306. Meaney MJ (2001) Maternal care, gene expression, and the transmission of individual differences in stress reactivity across generations. Ann Rev Neurosci 24:1161-1192
307. Liu D, Diorio J, Tannenbaum B et al (1997) Maternal care, hippocampal glucocorticoid receptors, and hypothalamic-pituitary-adrenal responses to stress. Science 277:1659-1662

Chapter 14

Psychological Stress in Women: the Stockholm Female Coronary Risk Study

K. ORTH-GOMÈR

Although it is well known that women are victims of coronary disease almost as frequently as men are, it is also well known that women coronary patients tend to be poorly rehabilitated after an acute heart attack, compared to men.

Recent studies from both the US [1] and Europe [2] have confirmed that mortality rates in women patients exceed those in men, even after taking age and comorbidity into account.

Studies sensitive to risk factors associated with gender differences have thus far not offered plausible explanations for the higher female mortality. The higher mortality rates are mostly confined to younger women, i.e., women who acquire the disease before age 60, and, in the case of Swedish women, before they retire from employment outside home. Unfortunately, previous research on standard coronary risk has been largely focused on men, leaving many research questions about women unanswered. This is equally true for social and psychological risk factors, both as concerns primary and secondary risk.

In the early 1990s, as a result of powerful lobbying by many influential women in the US Congress, the female coronary situation seemed to brighten; a beneficial effect of hormone replacement therapy (HRT) was reported in reliable population-based cohorts, such as the Nurses Health Study in Boston.

These findings highlighted the need for powerful clinical trials, and, shortly afterward, the Women's Health Initiative - a multicenter, randomized clinical trial, comprising 16,000 women - was launched. This trial, however, had to be stopped because the hypothesized cardio-protection by HRT seemed to result in an increased coronary risk among women taking HRT (estrogen was given in combination with progesterone to counteract the increased risk of cancer of the uterus, caused by unopposed estrogen use) [3]. Thus, the beliefs and hopes that primary and secondary prevention in women could be achieved through the use of a pill were determined to be false.

Given this situation, the Stockholm Female Coronary Risk Study, set out to accomplish two goals: to assess risk factors known to be relevant in men; and to test new hypotheses derived from the specific situations of women.

The FemCorRisk study was initiated as a community-based, case-control study of Stockholm women in active ages (younger than age 65) that were admitted with an acute coronary syndrome (acute myocardial infarction and unstable angina pectoris) during a three-year period. Around 300 women, aged 30 to 65, were identified and compared to an equal number of age-matched, healthy women obtained from the Stockholm census registry.

We found that lipoprotein (a) put women at increased risk of similar magnitude to that previously found in studies of men [4].

We also found that diabetes type II increased the risk of developing, as well as worsening, coronary disease among women [5].

Among psychosocial factors, we found that low SES was a significant coronary risk factor in these women of productive ages. Table 1 shows the results concerning work stress and marital stress in relation to depressive symptoms.

Women with mandatory education (7-9 years) had twice the risk, and women with an unskilled manual job four times the risk, of academic women for heart attack - i.e., hospitalization for an acute coronary syndrome [6].

We also found that women who were depressed and women who were socially isolated, lacking emotional, informational and tangible support, had an increased risk of developing coronary disease, as well as an increased risk of a recurrent attack once they had acquired the disease [7] and [8]. The depressive symptoms seemed to result not only from the presence of a life-threatening illness, such as coronary disease, but also from stresses in their family situation. For the latter, we developed an interview instrument to assess the level of self-rated stress from the family domain (the Stockholm Marital Stress scale - see Table 1).

Table 1. The Stockholm Marital Stress Scale

1. Is the relationship with your spouse loving?
2. Is the relationship with your spouse friendly?
3. Is the relationship with your spouse routine-like?
4. Is the relationship with your spouse problematic?
5. Do you engage in leisure activities with your spouse?
6. Do you have your own private life outside the relationship with your spouse?
7. Is your spouse your closest confidant?
8. Does your spouse consider you his closest confidant?
9. Are there things you can't talk openly about with each other?
10. Have you had serious problems in the relationship with your spouse previously?
11. Do you have serious problems in the relationship with your spouse currently?
12. Have you had serious crises in your relationship?
13. Have you solved problems actively together?
14. Do you have a sexual relationship with your spouse?
15. Do you find the sexual relationship satisfactory?
16. Has your sexual relationship been affected by your heart disease?
17. Has your sexual relationship ceased due to your heart disease?

*A marital stress score of 1 was assigned if the respondent answered "no" to items 1,2,5,7,8,13,14, and 15, and "yes" to the remaining items. Another score of 1 was assigned for each problem (infidelity, substance use/abuse, economic problems, health problems, or other unspecified problems, as shown by answers to question 10 and 11). Total scores were obtained by summing all scores.

Both in case-control comparisons and in long-term followups, family stresses, as well as work stress, were found to be important as cardiovascular risk factors (Figg. 1, 2). We felt that this comparison was warranted in the Stockholm women, as almost all of them were professionally involved. At the onset of the study, only two of 600 women said that they were housewives. Those women

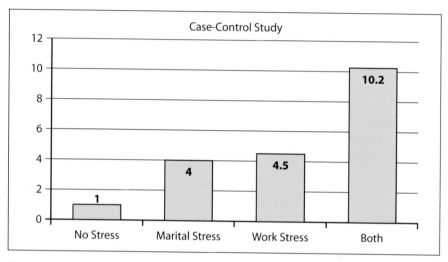

Fig. 1. Marital and work stress and CHD. Odds ratio: OR. Multivariate adjusted for age, education, smoking, BMI, SBP, cholesterol, triglycerides, HDL

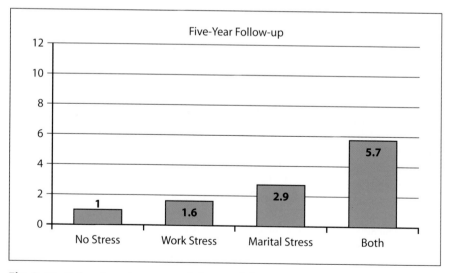

Fig. 2. Marital and work stress, and CHD at follow-up. Odds ratio: OR. Multivariate adjusted for age, education, smoking, BMI, SBP, cholesterol, triglycerides, HDL, diabetes and left ventricular dysfunction

who reported both marital and work stress had the greater risk and the worst prognosis over 5 years of follow-up [9].

The findings of depressive symptoms were closely correlated to the level of marital stress in all women. The higher and more severe the marital stress, the more likely the report of depressive symptoms. This graded response was found in healthy women, as well as women patients. But the latter group had about twice the levels of depression as the group of healthy women. In women with coronary disease, work stress did not appear to be related to the depressive symptoms, nor to the prognosis [10]. Table 2 shows the results concerning work stress and marital stress in relation to depressive symptoms. Whether these are unspecific pathogenic effects, which might accompany and be caused by the disease process, or whether they are directly conducive to atherosclerotic change, is the focus of ongoing studies. These studies involve effects on standard behavioral risk factors, as well as direct neuro-endocrine and metabolic changes, and how these processes relate to the progression of atherosclerotic disease in the coronary arteries.

Table 2. Type of stress and depressive symptoms

Depressive symptoms	Work stress				Marital stress			
	Low	Medium	High	p	Low	Medium	High	p
Age adjusted	3.5	3.8	3.2	n.s.	2.3	3.3	4.7	.000
Multivariate adjusted	2.5	3.6	3.3	n.s.	2.1	2.8	4.4	.000

Balog P, Janszky I, Leineweber C, Orth-Gomèr K; APS 2002

References

1. Vaccarino V, Berkman LF, Krumholz HM (2000) Long-term outcome of myocardial infarction in women and men: a population perspective. Am J Epidemiol 152: 965-973
2. Marrugat J, Sala J, Masià R et al (1998) Mortality differences between men and women following first myocardial infarction. JAMA 280:1405-1409
3. Manson J, Hsia J, Johnson K et al (2003) Estrogen plus progestin and the risk of coronary heart disease. Women's Health Initiative Investigators. N Engl J Med 349:523-534
4. Orth-Gomèr K, Mittleman M, Schenck- Gustafsson K et al (1997) Lipoprotein (a) as a determinant of coronary disease in young women. Circulation 95:329-334
5. Al-Khalili F, Svane B, Janszky I et al (2002) Significant predictors of poor prognosis in women aged </=65 years hospitalized for an acute coronary event. J Intern Med 252:561-569
6. Wamala SP, Mittleman MA, Schenck-Gustafsson K, Orth-Gomèr K (1999) Potential explanations for the educational gradient in coronary heart disease: A population based case-control study of Swedish women. Am J Public Health 89:67-72
7. Orth-Gomèr K, Horsten M, Schenck-Gustafsson K et al (1998) Social relations and extent and severity of coronary artery disease. Eur Heart J 19:1648-1656

8. Horsten M, Mittleman M, Wamala SP et al (2000) Social isolation and depression in relation to prognosis of coronary heart disease in women. Eur Heart J 21:1072-1080
9. Orth-Gomèr K, Wamala SP, Horsten M et al (2000) Marital stress worsens prognosis in women with coronary heart disease. JAMA 284:3008-3014
10. Balog P, Janszky I, Leineweber C et al (2003) Depressive symptoms in relation to marital and work stress in women with and without coronary heart disease. The Stockholm Female Coronary Risk Study. J Psychosom Res 54:113-119

Advanced Statistical Tools for the Study of Psychological Risks Aspects

Chapter 15

Application of Neural Networks and Other Artificial Adaptive Systems in Prediction and Data Mining of Risk Psychological Profile for CHD

E. Grossi ▪ A. Compare

▪ Introduction

Current and consolidated data suggest that cardiac rehabilitation (CR) may help reduce standard cardiac risk factors [1] in patients with coronary heart disease (CHD) by increasing functional capacity [2]. Cardiac performance in exercise training is the acknowledged endpoint of CR [3, 4]. Metabolic equivalents (MET) and heart rate recovery (HRR) are measures of cardiac performance in exercise training; and, during the past two decades, they have become well-established predictors of cardiovascular and overall mortality [5-7].

The MET is defined as the amount of oxygen consumed while sitting at rest and provides a convenient method for describing the functional capacity or exercise tolerance of an individual as determined from progressive exercise testing; it is also used to define a repertoire of physical activities in which a person may participate safely, without exceeding a prescribed intensity level [8]. Researchers [3, 9, 10] have pointed out that when MET is used to determine improvement after exercise training - which is also strongly influenced by age, activity status and gender [11] - the predictive power of the risk of death among both normal subjects and those with cardiovascular disease seems to be independent of the use or non-use of beta-blockers [7, 12, 13]. A recent large study [7] of 6213 subjects showed that each 1-MET increase in exercise capacity conferred a 12% improvement in survival.

The HRR is defined as the decrease in the heart rate (HR) from peak exercise to one minute after the cessation of exercise. A delayed decrease in the HR during the first minute after graded exercise, which may be a reflection of decreased vagal activity, is a powerful predictor of overall mortality, independent of workload, the presence or absence of myocardial perfusion defects, and changes in HR during exercise [14-17]. The increase in HR that accompanies exercise is due in part to a reduction in vagal tone; moreover, exercise training in a cardiac rehabilitation program usually results in HRR improvement [18].

Recovery of the HR immediately after exercise is a function of vagal reactivation. Because a generalized decrease in vagal activity is known to be a risk factor for death, it has been hypothesized that a delayed fall in the HR after exercise might be an important prognostic marker [17].

Cardiac rehabilitation can be expected to increase exercise capacity and reduce the myocardial oxygen requirement for submaximal tasks. Most patients who participate in CR programs improve their aerobic capacity [1, 19-21]. However, some patients fail to show an increase in maximal exercise capacity [22, 23]. Previous attempts to identify patient characteristics that predict the effect of exercise training on cardiac patients have had limited success [3, 24-28]. Some previous studies have suggested that CR training effect may be impaired by gender [29, 30].

The importance of psychosocial factors in the development and expression of coronary artery disease (CAD) has been much debated; however, an extensive recent literature now establishes that psychosocial factors contribute significantly to the pathogenesis of CAD. Despite research that has pointed out the impact of psychological factors such as anxiety, depression and personality on the pathogenesis of cardiovascular disease and the underlying pathophysiological mechanisms [31], only two studies have analysed the effect of psychological factors on the change of exercise capacity consequent to CR. Glazer et al. [32] - whose research is consistent with previous research in CR populations [33] - pointed out that, because depression at baseline accounts for 9.2% of the variance in improvement of oxygen consumption, it represents an indirect measure of exercise tolerance, after controlling for age and gender. The absence of a prospective on the psychological comorbidity conditions that takes into account the *psychological risk profile (PRP)* is regarded as a weakness of this study. The reason for this weakness is methodological and results from the use of linear statistical analysis.

Advanced, non-linear statistical tools based on neural networks are now able to include the psychological profile linked to CAD risk and CR outcome [34] from a bio-psychosocial prospective that takes into account psychological comorbidity. Despite this capability, however, only two studies have investigated the role of psychological factors on cardiac disease using Artificial Neural Network (ANN) tools: [35], who developed and validated a model that predicts the length of hospital stay, and [36], whose findings pointed out that ANN classifications of cardiac time-series data with enhanced ultradian variations and cardiac data recorded around the interval when a person was in bed were useful in differentiating clinically meaningful subgroups with and without depression. There are no specific studies on psychological CAD risk factors and rehabilitation outcomes.

The purpose of the current study is to evaluate the advantages of a non-linear prospective, based on ANN tools and other artificial adaptive systems, compared with a conventional linear statistic prospective for determining the patient's psychological profile 1) linked to CAD risk and 2) predictive of CR outcomes in a group of patients with ischemic heart disease and hypertension. According to Cole et al. [17], Myers et al. [7] and Gulati et al. [11], CAD risk is evaluated in terms of METs, HRR and diagnosis (ischemic heart disease and hypertension), while CR outcomes are evaluated in terms of METs and HRR. For this article, artificial adaptive systems relate to ANN and Evolutionary Algorithms (EA).

ANNs and EA are adaptive models for analyzing data inspired by the functioning processes of the human brain and evolution, respectively. They are systems that are able to modify their internal structure in relation to a functional objective. They are particularly suited for solving problems of the non-linear type, either because they are able to reconstruct the approximate rules that associate a certain set of data (which describes the problem being considered) with another set of data that provides the solution (ANNs), or because they are able to reconstruct the optimal data for a given set of rules or constraints (EA). For a detailed description of these models and tools we refer the reader to the recent reviews of Buscema [37, 38].

◼ Rationale for the Use of ANNs: Becoming Aware of the Non-Linearity of Clinical Data

We are aware of the fact that the most powerful and well-established statistical methods were developed in the first half of the last century when the amount and comprehension of information from clinical observations was rather limited and almost negligible in comparison with today. The same methods used then are well established today for analyzing medical data, and they are considered by regulatory agencies to be standard tests. All of these methods rely on the assumption that medical variables are linear in nature. The explanation of this phenomenon is quite easy:

- Firstly, linear models are undoubtedly user-friendly in comparison with non-linear ones, which require stronger theoretical assumptions in the pre-analysis phase;
- Secondly, the limited historical exposure to medical data has resulted in an assumption by physicians that biological phenomena could easily share the linear mechanics of physical systems going back to Newtonian mechanics.

The potential for the actual non-linearity of medical data, as an issue or as a problem, has very rarely been raised in medical literature. Epidemiologists and statisticians specializing in the medical field were obviously happy with their techniques, having initially been trained with them. Physicians and other health professionals were also happy, provided that statisticians and the relevant regulatory body did not think differently, resulting in a classical "transfer of technology" syndrome and/or a "business as usual" tradition.

The history of data processing may have started with linear analysis. This long overdue reality must be revisited. Important theoretical and applied breakthroughs have been made in mathematics, physics, and in economics and medicine, and these breakthroughs are relevant to contemporary medicine in terms of prevention, diagnostics, treatment, research and educational needs and mandates. The dynamic multidimensionality of networks, their mapping and their hubs, nodes and linkages are one current example.

It is not difficult to understand, in hindsight, why linear analysis was used for revealing mechanisms and making predictions. Simple systems or small-intensity effects may well remain linear; or, due to the fact that the calculations are to be done by hand, linearity may be forced upon the systems and effects. Alternatively, missed correlations and dependencies may leave room for linear analysis. This, however, is no longer acceptable. Moreover, exercising in linearity is not without its dangers. If, for example, two variables are measured and a correlation coefficient of, say, 0.018 is calculated under a linear hypothesis, and if a P-value of, say, 0.80, is added, then the resulting relation of the two is discarded.

It seems important to ask the fundamental question: *is the mathematics in medicine what it can be*? In medicine, we study systems that are far from simple or static. Medicinal or treatment "doses" can hardly be kept within the limits of the linear. Omitting (or playing down) correlations is unthinkable. And, of course, calculations by hand are in the past. Inventing mathematics, in and of itself, has never been a problem. Actually, what mathematics serves has existed for many decades now, and is increasingly available and accessible for helping us to map what we need to understand, and to understand what we already know in order to make new connections.

It is useful to remember that research - and teaching and practicing medicine, diagnosis and therapy - are formidable, largely due to the increasing presence of physics and the need to take into account the contributions of mathematics. Assuming linearity for certain conditions and phenomena means simplifying processes that may be more complex and, thus, distorting reality. A moment of reflection is in order.

The actual data collected in contemporary medical research needs to be analysed and communicated (i.e., transformed) into information, knowledge and, at times, even into wisdom, so that the appropriate intervention can be planned, implemented, followed-up and learned from. The advancement of knowledge and the progress of understanding the nature of bodily rhythms and processes have shown that complexity (hence, non-linearity) is ubiquitous in living organisms. The rhythms arise from stochastic, nonlinear, biological mechanisms interacting with fluctuating environments. Non-linear dynamics force us to rethink our ideas about causation, risk assessment and intervention. Can one attribute "cause" to effects when influences are multifactorial, contextual and non-linear? Interventions could be directed at multiple contributing factors in order to reduce non-linear interaction effects, and occasionally this may be necessary. For example, lowering cholesterol below a desired threshold should reduce the amplification effect of high Lp(a), a risk factor that is not easily dealt with. The prevention, cure or more effective treatment of cancer may reside in multiple smaller inputs at critical points. Small, appropriately selected, changes may yield disproportionate social and cultural benefits that impact health, disease and prevention.

General Characteristics of Artificial Adaptive Systems

Artificial Adaptive Systems (AAS) are able to simultaneously handle a very high number of variables notwithstanding their underlying non-linearity. This results in a tremendous advantage over classical statistical models in a situation in which the *quantity* of available information is enormously increased and non-linearity dominates. With AAS, one is neither concerned about the actual number of variables, nor their nature. Due to their particular mathematic infrastructure, AAS have no limits in handling increasing amounts of variables that constitute the input vector for the recursive algorithms.

When a single-factor approach is applied to the analysis of multifactor data, only one factor is varied at a time, and the others are held constant. This is the case with classical multivariable statistical techniques. With these techniques the combined interpretations of a given set of potential predictors with respect to individual patients has been difficult, due to the limitations imposed by the underlying non-linear links and the complex interactions between the factors being studied. There are many unanswered questions about the dynamics of these rhythmic processes:

- For example, how do the rhythms interact with each other and the external environment?
- Can we decode the fluctuations in physiological rhythms to better diagnose human disease?

Mathematical and physical techniques, combined with physiological and medical studies, are addressing these questions and transforming our understanding of the rhythms of life. Mathematical analyses of physiological rhythms show that non-linear equations are necessary to describe physiological systems.

The physiological variation of blood glucose, for example, has traditionally been considered linear. Recently, however, a chaotic component has been described both in diabetic patients and in normal subjects. This chaotic dynamic is also common in other physiologic systems. These ideas represent a fundamental change in our world-view and provide a previously unavailable scientific model for interpreting observed variation and irregular, uncertain and unpredictable events.

Neural networks can receive multiple inputs simultaneously, combining and recombining them in different ways according to specific (generally non-linear) equations. The difference, in terms of predictive values and in the number of predictive parameters modeled, can be explained by the fact that conventional statistics reveal only parameters that are *significant for the entire population*, whereas neural networks include parameters that might not reach significance for the entire population, but are *highly significant within subgroups*.

AAS differ from normal digital computer programs because of their ability to classify and analyze problems:

- that are inherently complex and large in size;
- that have many data input points;
- for which hard-and-fast rules cannot be easily applied; and
- that excel at repetitive tasks.

ANNs have good pattern recognition abilities, which are needed for decision-making. They are also robust classifiers with the ability to generalize and make decisions from large and somewhat fuzzy input data.

ANNs provide better solutions than linear discriminant analysis (LDA) for classification and estimation problems involving a large number of non-homogeneous (categorical and metric) variables.

■ Comparison Between Non-Linear and Linear Conventional Statistic Prospective on a Cardiac In-Patient Sample Study

Sample
The sample is composed of 149 inpatients (62 women, 87 men) admitted to the Unity of Cardiac Rehabilitation of S. Giuseppe Hospital (Verbania, Italy) for heart disease. Table 1 describes the cardiac diagnoses of the sample. The average entry age was 59.4 years (SD = 7.82). The average hospitalization was 24.2 days (SD = 4.07).

Table 1. Cardiac diagnoses of the sample

Ischemic heart disease		Hypertension	
n	(%)	n	(%)
77	(51.7)	110	(73.8)

All patients underwent a cardiovascular rehabilitation program (CRP) following the indications of international guidelines [39], consisting of aerobic physical activity individualized on the basis of the results of an exercise test at admission, and all patients had a balanced, moderately hypocaloric diet, as well as patient education and counselling. Criteria for exclusion included: schizophrenia and others psychotic disorders (DSM-IV-R), illiteracy or pathologies that prevent the compilation of the questionnaires (myopia, etc.).

Data Collection and Measures

Baseline Measures
Baseline data collection took place using standardized protocols during the first week of the hospital stay and before the CRP. Psychological variables were assessed by trained psychologists, and measurements pertaining to cardiac risk were evaluated by trained cardiologists. Table 2 describes the baseline cardiac and psychological variables.

Table 2. Descriptive of baseline cardiac and psychological variables

Variables	Mean	SD	Range
Cardiac variables			
ABP (mmHg)	125.72	18.30	(90-180)
HR (bpm)	73.11	13.13	(46-110)
METs (ml/kg/min)	55.18	21.89	(3-119)
HRR (bpm)	18.54	8.91	(45-2)
Psychological variables			
Anxiety			
STAI-S	38.93	10.12	(20-67)
STAI-T	42.04	10.45	(22-69)
Personality profile			
EPQ-E	8.51	3.13	(0-12)
EPQ-N	4.96	3.31	(0-12)
EPQ-P	2.55	1.49	(0-6)
Psychophysiological profile			
QPF	48.87	9.63	(33-89)
Fear and phobia profile			
IP-F	61.04	30.29	(0-147)
IP-PH	18.48	22.38	(0-116)
IP-1	16.79	8.46	(0-37)
IP-2	18.85	9.34	(0-42)
IP-3	8.46	7.36	(0-29)
IP-4	4.52	4.78	(0-23)
IP-5	6.08	4.38	(0-22)
Depression			
QD	6.85	4.47	(0-17)
Obsessive/compulsive profile			
MOCQ-R	6.86	4.22	(0-18)
MOCQ-1	3.63	2.55	(0-9)
MOCQ-2	2.55	1.69	(0-7)
MOCQ-3	1.10	1.20	(0-4)

SD standard deviation; *Cardiac Variables:* ABP arterial blood pressure (mmHg), HR heart rate (beats/min), METs metabolic equivalent (ml/kg/min), HRR Heart Rate Recovery, HR decrease during 1 minute recovery after the effort test. *Psychological Variables:* Anxiety: STAI (State-Trait Anxiety Inventory), S state anxiety, T trait anxiety; *Personality profile:* EPQ (Eysenck Personality Questionnaire), E extroversion, N neuroticism, P maladjustment and anti-sociality; *Psychophysiological profile:* QPF (Psychophysiological Profile Questionnaire); *Fear and phobia profile:* F fear, PH phobia, 1 disaster, 2 social rejection, 3 animal, 4 dismissal, 5 blood and physician; *Depression:* QD (Depression Questionnaire); *Obsessive/Compulsive profile:* MOCQ (Maudsley Obsessional-Compulsive Questionnaire), R global subscale , 1 checking, 2 cleaning, 3 doubting/ruminating

Psychological Variables

- *Anxiety (STAI, State-Trait personality Inventory).* Anxiety was measured with the State-Trait Anxiety Inventory (STAI [40]). The STAI clearly differentiates between the temporary condition of "state anxiety" and the more general and long-standing quality of "trait anxiety." The instrument assesses feelings of apprehension, tension, nervousness, and worry as the feelings are experienced.

- *Personality Profile (EPI, Eysenck Personality Inventory* [41]*)*. Eysenck's theory is based primarily on physiology and genetics. Extroversion is characterized as being outgoing, talkative, high on positive affect (feeling good), and in need of external stimulation. According to Eysenck's arousal theory of extroversion, there is an optimal level of cortical arousal, and performance deteriorates as one becomes more or less aroused than this optimal level. Arousal can be measured by skin conductance, brain waves or sweating. At very low and very high levels of arousal, performance is low, and at a more optimal mid-level of arousal, performance is maximized. Extroverts, according to Eysenck's theory, are chronically under-aroused and bored and therefore in need of external stimulation to bring them up to an optimal level of performance. Introverts, on the other hand, are chronically over-aroused and jittery and therefore in need of peace and quiet to bring them up to an optimal level of performance. Neuroticism or emotionality is characterized by high levels of negative affect, such as depression or anxiety. Neuroticism, according to Eysenck's theory, is based on activation thresholds in the sympathetic nervous system or visceral brain. This is the part of the brain that is responsible for the fight-or-flight response in the face of danger. Activation can be measured by heart rate, blood pressure, cold hands, and by sweating and muscular tension (especially in the forehead). Neurotic people, who have low activation thresholds and therefore are unable to inhibit or control their emotional reactions, experience negative affect (fight-or-flight) in the face of very minor stressors – i.e., they become nervous or upset easily. Emotionally stable people, who have high activation thresholds and therefore good emotional control, experience negative affect only in the face of very major stressors, and they tend to remain calm and collected under pressure. Psychotic behavior is rooted in the characteristics of tough-mindedness, non-conformity, inconsideration, recklessness, hostility, anger and impulsiveness.
- *Psychopysiological Profile (QPF* [42]*)*. This profile consists of a list of psychophysiological symptoms that can be obtained from the patient. It contains 30 questions, which ask about the frequency of different psychophysiological reactions. The analyzed construct is the somatic complaint.
- *Fear and Phobia Profile (IP, Phobia Inventory* [42]*)*. This inventory lists different stimuli that can produce fear as assessed by Likert measurements. The general indexes measure the number and the intensity of the fears. Patients are presented with five classes for analysis: disaster, social rejection, animal, dismissal, blood and physician.
- *Depression (QD, Depression Questionnaire* [42]*)*. This questionnaire allows the physician to individualize the presence of a depressive condition and to quantify it using 5 factors that engender feelings related to: relationship of the subject with his/her usual activities, relationship of the subject with others, oral troubles, fatigue and suicidal thoughts. The patient is invited to consider and respond to each question concerning whether the affir-

mations that you/they read describe his or her "actual condition of life."
- *Obsessive/Compulsive Profile (MOCQ, Maudsley Obsessional-Compulsive Questionnaire).* The DSM-IV (APA, 1994) [43] describes OCD according to five diagnostic criteria. The main features of the disorder are: a) recurrent thoughts or images (termed 'obsessions') that are considered intrusive and that cause significant distress; and b) ritualistic behaviors (termed 'compulsions'), typically engaged in to rid or neutralise obsessive thoughts. Although it may be difficult to ascertain the degree of distress, the DSM-IV maintains that an individual must experience a significant disturbance in normal functioning, or engage in obsessive-compulsive activity for at least one hour/day, to be given a diagnosis of OCD. Further, the individual must, at some point during the course of the disorder, recognise the irrationality of his/her thoughts and behavior. A specification of poor insight may be added to the diagnosis of OCD when an individual does not currently recognise that the obsessions and compulsions are excessive or unreasonable. The Maudsley Obsessional Compulsive Inventory (MOCQ [44]) is able to determine a total score for OCD symptomatology, as well as scores on the subscales washing, checking, slowness and doubting.

Cardiac Variables
- *Heart Rate.* HR was sampled continuously for 1 minute as the patient lay in a hospital bed and was subsequently recorded in the patient's medical record as beats per minute. To increase the reliability of indexing resting HR, three 1-minute periods were sampled at 6-hourly periods, and the average of these three measures was calculated to obtain mean resting HR values.
- *Arterial Blood Pressure (ABP).* Blood pressure measurements were made using auscultatory methods with mercury sphygmomanometers. Three blood pressure readings were taken and the final measure consisted of the average of the three. ECG was recorded at rest in the upright position, before exercise stress test.

Cardiac Risk and CR Outcomes Variables
- *METs.* Exercise capacity is expressed in units of metabolic equivalents (MET) and is an estimate of the maximal oxygen uptake for a given workload [45]. A MET is a measure of ventilatory oxygen consumption expressed as multiples of basal resting requirements, where 1 MET is 1 unit of basal oxygen consumption, which equals 3.5 mL oxygen consumption per kilogram of body weight per minute for an average adult. The exercise capacity (in MET) is estimated by the speed and grade of the treadmill [46]. The exercise stress test is done on a treadmill (Marquette series 2000). We utilized a ramp protocol [47] that has small increments in workload. Initial speed is 1.5 km/h with 0% inclination; by the end of the second minute of exercise, a speed of 1.8 km/h and an inclination of 2.0% is reached. Upon completion of the second minute of exercise the treadmill speed increases by 0.075 km/h and the incli-

nation by 0.25% every 15 seconds. With this type of exercise protocol most patients exercise for 6-12 minutes, reaching the suggested test duration [48, 49]. During the test, cardiac rhythm is monitored. The test has a mean duration of 9.44 minutes (SD = 2.48), according to the guidelines that suggest a 10 minute duration for functional evaluation. HR was continuously monitored. Criteria for test interruption were dyspnea or fatigue, excessive HR or ABP increase, non-sustained, ventricular tachycardia or symptoms. Exercise capacity was assessed at baseline (before the CR program) and at end (after CR program) time. An increase of 10% of METs value after the CR was considered a good outcome.

- *HRR (Heart Rate Recovery).* After achieving peak workload, all the patients spent at least two minutes in a cool-down period during treadmill testing at a speed of 2.4 km (1.5 mi) per hour and a grade of 2.5 percent. This period was considered the recovery period. The value for the recovery of heart rate was defined as the reduction in the heart rate from the rate at peak exercise to the rate one minute after the cessation of exercise. HRR was assessed at baseline (before the CR program) and at end time (after the CR program). An increase in 10% of the HRR value after the CR was considered a good outcome.

Cardiac Risk Condition

- *METs.* Exercise capacity (in MET) was modelled as a continuous variable and as a categorical variable. Exercise capacity was stratified in:
  - 2 categories - the cut-off value is 6 (in absolute terms): a greater or equal value is considered high risk (METs-HO), while a smaller value is considered low risk (METs-LO) [50].
  - 3 categories - as < 5 MET, 5-8 MET, or >8 MET. This categorization is based on prior studies that show decreased survival among those who achieve <5 MET and increased survival among those who are able to achieve >8 MET when estimated either from exercise activities or a stress test [7, 51, 52].
- *HRR.* Heart rate recovery was modelled as a continuous variable and as a categorical variable using the cut-off value 12 (in absolute terms): an abnormal value for heart-rate recovery is < or = 12 beats per minute; a greater or equal value is considered high risk (HRR-HO), while a smaller value is considered low risk (HRR-LO)[17].

For descriptive purposes, the patients were divided into groups on the basis of the values for the HRR and METs. Continuous variables were presented (see Table 3) as mean ±SD. Differences between groups were compared using the Student's t-test, Wilcoxon's rank-sum test, and the chi-square test, as appropriate.

Cardiac Recovery Outcomes

The METs and HRR were considered CR outcome of the CRP. They were determined by finding the difference between the final measure (i.e., the day before hospital discharge) and the baseline cardiovascular measure (final – baseline). In accordance with recent articles on outcome of cardiac rehabilitation, and in order to facilitate the statistic analysis, we have dichotomized the outcome values using the cutoff value of 10% for METs increase and HRR increase.

Patients' Characteristics at Baseline and Cardiac Risk Condition: Linear Conventional Statistic Prospective

METs

The mean value for METs was 55.18 beats per minute, with a range from 119-3 (ml/kg/min). An abnormal value for METs was found in 81 patients (54.4%). The baseline characteristics of patients with respect to whether their heart-rate recovery was normal or abnormal are summarized in Table 3. Compared with the patients with normal values for METs, those with abnormal values (<6) were hypertensive. Patients with abnormal METs had higher obsessive/compulsive symptoms than those with normal METs (6.26±4.24 vs. 7.62±4.12; p=.03). Psychological symptoms linked to cardiac risk were obsessive/compulsive behaviors, with a focus on cleaning (2.28±1.66 vs. 2.81±1.65; p=.04) and doubting/ruminating (.90±1.13 vs. 1.33 ±1.27; p=.03).

The three risk categories of METs included low: <5; medium: 5-8; and high: >8. Twenty-six were found to have low risk (17.4%), 63 were found to have medium risk (42.3%) and 60 were found to have high risk (40.3%). The baseline characteristics of the patients according to whether their heart-rate recovery was normal or abnormal are summarized in Table 3. Patients with medium or high risk had ischemic heart disease. Psychological symptoms linked to cardiac risk conditions were:
- *anxiety*: high risk was linked with high trait anxiety (37.58±8.81 vs. 42.33±11.07 vs. 44.45 ±9.77; p=.02).
- *psychophysiological profile*: high risk was linked with high psychophysiological reactions (44.23 ±7.51 vs. 48.40 ±8.27 vs. 51.53 ±10.58; p=.01)
- *fear and phobia*: high risk was linked with high fear (46.96 ±28.82 vs. 62.75 ±29.07 vs. 65.57 ±31.26; p=.05) and phobia (9.38 ±13.62 vs. 18.67 ±20.47 vs. 21.47 ±25.74; p=.04) symptoms.
- *depression*: high risk was linked with high depressive symptoms (4.92 ±4.84 vs. 7.14 ±4.66 vs. 7.82 ±4.06; p=.01).
- *obsessive/compulsive*: high risk was linked with high obsessive/compulsive symptoms (5.27 ±4.45 vs. 7.37 ±4.08 vs. 7.37 ±4.13; p=.05), with a focus on cleaning (1.85 ±1.62 vs. 2.75 ±1.63 vs. 2.70 ±1.69; p=.05) and doubting/ruminating (.65 ±1.20 vs. 1.22 ±1.21 vs. 1.25 ±1.23; p=.02).

HRR

The mean value for HHR was 18.54 beats per minute, with a range from 45-2 beats per minute. An abnormal value for HRR was found in 39 patients (26.2%). The baseline characteristics of the patients according to whether their heart-rate recovery was normal or abnormal are summarized in Table 3. As compared with the patients with normal values for HRR, those with abnormal values (<12 beats per minute) were older. Psychological symptoms did not appear to be linked to cardiac risk condition.

Table 3. Baseline characteristics of the patients according to the value for the HRR and METs*

Variables	HRR			METs-2		
	Normal (>12 bpm)	Abnormal (≤12 bpm)	P value	Normal (>6 bpm)	Abnormal (≤6 bpm)	P value
Age – yr	58.72 ±7.91	61.29 ±7.33	.042	58.46 ±7.85	60.18 ±7.75	ns
Female sex – no (%)	46 (30.9)	16 (10.7)	ns	27 (18.1)	35 (23.5)	ns
Cardiac disorders						
HY diagnosis – yes (%)	84 (56.44)	26 (17.4)	ns	45 (30.2)	65 (43.6)	.04
IHD diagnosis – yes (%)	61 (40.9)	16 (10.7)	ns	40 (26.8)	37 (24.8)	ns
Psychological variables						
Anxiety						
STAI-S	38.71 ±10.10	40.62 ±10.25	ns	38.13 ±9.42	40.11 ±10.68	ns
STAI-T	42.03 ±10.76	43.28 ±9.39	ns	40.65 ±10.17	43.79 ±10.44	ns
Personality profile						
EPQ-E	8.46 ±3.24	8.72 ±3.10	ns	8.44 ±3.32	8.60 ±3.11	ns
EPQ-N	5.19 ±3.38	4.72 ±3.03	ns	5.00 ±3.35	5.12 ±3.25	ns
EPQ-P	2.49 ±1.51	2.64 ±1.51	ns	2.31 ±1.35	2.72 ±1.61	ns
Psychophysiological profile						
QPF	48.66 ±9.12	49.69 ±10.44	ns	47.72 ±7.95	49.95 ±10.51	ns
Fear and phobia profile						
IP-F	60.20 ±29.03	63.74 ±34.46	ns	59.49 ±31.77	62.51 ±29.45	ns
IP-PH	17.24 ±20.33	20.82 ±26.65	ns	15.94 ±20.19	20.05 ±23.58	ns
IP-1	16.36 ±8.15	17.79 ±9.45	ns	16.53 ±8.79	16.91 ±8.30	ns
IP-2	19.02 ±9.50	19.10 ±9.31	ns	19.29 ±10.36	18.83 ±8.61	ns
IP-3	8.44 ±7.19	8.59 ±7.92	ns	8.15 ±7.45	8.75 ±7.32	ns
IP-4	4.30 ±4.29	5.08 ±5.81	ns	3.87 ±4.33	5.04 ±5.00	ns
IP-5	5.88 ±4.32	6.38 ±4.65	ns	5.65 ±4.11	6.32 ±4.63	ns
Depression						
QD	6.95 ±4.80	7.23 ±3.79	ns	6.38 ±4.77	7.57 ±4.31	ns
Obsessive/compulsive profile						
MOCQ-R	6.76 ±4.27	7.67 ±4.02	ns	6.26 ±4.24	7.62 ±4.12	.03
MOCQ-1	3.61 ±2.56	4.05 ±2.55	ns	3.40 ±2.61	4.00 ±2.49	ns
MOCQ-2	2.53 ±1.73	2.69 ±1.51	ns	2.28 ±1.66	2.81 ±1.65	.04
MOCQ-3	1.03 ±1.18	1.44 ±1.31	ns	.90 ±1.13	1.33 ±1.27	.03

*Plus–minus values are mean ±SD (SD = standard deviation). METs = metabolic equivalent (ml/kg/min); HRR = Heart Rate Recovery; HR decrease during 1 minute recovery after the effort test. *Psychological Variables:* Anxiety - STAI (State-Trait Anxiety Inventory), where S= state anxiety and T = trait anxiety; Personality profile: EPQ (Eysenck Personality Questionnaire), where E = extroversion, N = neuroticism, P = maladjustment and antisociality; Psychophysiological profile as determined by the QPF (Psy-

▓ Patients' Characteristics at Baseline and Cardiac Risk Condition: Application of Non-Linear Mapping of Descriptors Through "Evolutionary" Algorithms

Traditional statistical techniques cannot easily project onto two-dimensional space a high number of variables according to the matrix of their reciprocal distances since the computational time tends toward infinitum. Non-linearity is also burdened with inherent difficulties.

	METs-3			
	>8	5-8	<5	P value
Age – yr	57.43 ±8.17	59.42 ±7.44	60.23 ±8.03	ns
Female sex – no (%)	4 (2.7)	29 (19.5)	29 (19.5)	ns
Cardiac disorders				
HY diagnosis – yes (%)	16 (10.7)	45 (30.2)	49 (32.9)	ns
IHD diagnosis – yes (%)	16 (10.7)	39 (26.1)	22 (14.7)	.01
Psychological variables				
Anxiety				
STAI-S	35.38 ±8.94	39.65 ±10.15	40.40 ±10.38	ns
STAI-T	37.58 ±8.81	42.33 ±11.07	44.45 ±9.77	.02
Personality profile				
EPQ-E	8.42 ±3.51	8.32 ±3.06	8.80 ±3.23	ns
EPQ-N	4.50 ±3.47	5.22 ±3.35	5.15 ±3.17	ns
EPQ-P	2.69 ±1.32	2.38 ±1.47	2.62 ±1.63	ns
Psychophysiological profile				
QPF	44.23 ±7.51	48.40 ±8.27	51.53 ±10.58	.01
Fear and phobia profile				
IP-F	46.96 ±28.82	62.75 ±29.07	65.57 ±31.26	.05
IP-PH	9.38 ±13.62	18.67 ±20.47	21.47 ±25.74	.04
IP-1	13.12 ±8.64	17.57 ±8.06	17.43 ±8.61	ns
IP-2	15.92 ±9.66	20.22 ±9.64	19.15 ±8.91	ns
IP-3	5.31 ±5.61	8.81 ±7.43	9.50 ±7.68	ns
IP-4	3.38 ±4.94	4.40 ±4.03	5.10 ±5.26	ns
IP-5	4.54 ±3.71	5.79 ±4.00	6.88 ±4.91	ns
Depression				
QD	4.92 ±4.84	7.14 ±4.66	7.82 ±4.06	.01
Obsessive/compulsive profile				
MOCQ-R	5.27 ±4.45	7.37 ±4.08	7.37 ±4.13	.05
MOCQ-1	2.92 ±2.54	3.87 ±2.65	3.92 ±2.44	ns
MOCQ-2	1.85 ±1.62	2.75 ±1.63	2.70 ±1.69	.05
MOCQ-3	.65 ±1.20	1.22 ±1.21	1.25 ±1.23	.02

chophysiological Profile Questionnaire); Fear and phobia profile, where F = fear, PH = phobia, 1 = disaster, 2= social rejection, 3 = animal, 4 = dismissal, 5 = blood and physician; Depression profile as determined by the QD (Depression Questionnaire); Obsessive/Compulsive profile, as determined by the MOCQ (Maudsley Obsessional-Compulsive Questionnaire), R = global subscale , 1 = checking, 2 = cleaning, 3 = doubting/ruminating

A new mathematical approach consists in measuring the general dependence of random variables related to a group of subjects, without making any assumption about the nature of their underlying relationships, and finding their optimal spatial distribution through the use of a special kind of evolutionary algorithm belonging to the family of unsupervised artificial adaptive systems.

The mathematical system is called PST, and it was conceived by M. Buscema at the Semeion Research Center in 1999. The system is able to determine the spatial distribution of N points, which ideally respects their reciprocal Euclidean distances without exploring all possible combinations, by "evolving" adaptively toward the best solution. In other words, given the reciprocal distances of the variables, this adaptive system identifies the emerging natural clusters. In this manner, PST makes it possible to observe hidden "connections" or "associations" between descriptors that would be overlooked relying only on their linear correlation.

Description of the Evolutionary Algorithm

PST is designed to determine the factors that constitute the base structure of the observed data, and to place all points of the dataset onto a 2D space while minimizing the distortion of the original distances between points [53]. PST approximates the solution, without knowing if it exists and without *a priori* knowledge of the research space structure. PST enables us to project any matrix consisting of vectorial distances onto a 2-dimensional map.

The problem: defining a Map Distance: $Md_{ij} = \sqrt[2]{(Px_i - Px_j)^2 + (Py_i - Py_j)^2}$

and a Vector Distance: $Vd_{ij} = \sum\limits_{k=1}^{L} |Pv_{ik} - Pv_{jk}|$

We can set up the optimization problem:

min E; $E = \dfrac{1}{C} \cdot \sum\limits_{i=1}^{N-1} \sum\limits_{j=i+1}^{N} |Md_{ij} - Vd_{ij}|$; $C = \dfrac{N \cdot (N-1)}{2}$

We define:

State (S) as a configuration of points on a plane with known distances between them, despite the rotation of the configuration

Angle of tolerance (a) as the angle defining an arc on the circumference where two points are not distinct:

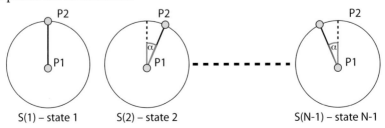

S(1) – state 1   S(2) – state 2   S(N-1) – state N-1

The number of possible states starting from the distances among N points is:
$$S = \alpha^{(N-2)}$$
P is defined as the number of tests necessary to verify the distances between N points in one state:
$$P = \frac{M \cdot (M-1)}{2} \quad M = N-2$$
Total number of tests in all possible states: $Q = S \cdot P$

The mapping problem we have presented is an NP problem, highly complex when the angle of tolerance, expressed in radians, increases.

An Example

	LA	NY	BOSTON	DETROIT	BUFFALO	PITTSBURG	CHICAGO	SAINT LOUIS	CINCINNATI	DALLAS	ATLANTA	MEMPHIS
LA	0											
NY	5600	0										
BOSTON	6109	509	0									
DETROIT	4532	1145	1527	0								
BUFFALO	5091	764	1018	209	0							
PITTSBURG	4838	764	1145	509	382	0						
CHICAGO	4073	1655	2038	509	1018	891	0					
SAINT LOUIS	3564	2038	2418	1018	1527	1273	638	0				
CINCINNATI	4327	1273	1655	382	764	509	509	764	0			
DALLAS	2800	2927	3436	2038	2545	2291	1655	1018	1782	0		
ATLANTA	4327	1527	2038	1145	1400	1018	1145	1018	764	1527	0	
MEMPHIS	3564	2164	2545	1273	1782	1400	1018	382	891	891	764	0

Flight Distances between 12 USA Cities (in miles) in a geographic space
Every air route has three types of alteration in 2D Euclidean space:
1) Longitudinal alteration,
2) Altitude alteration and
3) Structural alteration.

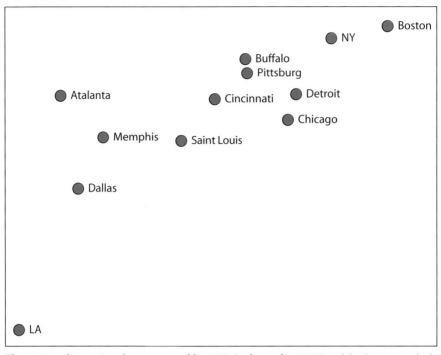

Fig. 1. Two-dimensional map created by PST: it places the 12 USA cities in a very similar way to how they actually appear on physical maps

Application of PST to Psychological Variables

In Table 4 the variables assessed with the use of PST are shown.

Table 4. Variables assessed with the use of PST

Outcome variables	
METs = metabolic equivalent (ml/kg/min)	
METS-LO	Low risk
METS-HO	High risk
HRR = Heart Rate Recovery	
HRR-LO	Low risk
HRR-HO	High risk
Psychological variables	
Anxiety State-Trait Anxiety Inventory	
STAI-S	State anxiety
STAI-T	Trait anxiety
Personality profile Eysenck Personality Questionnaire	
EPQ-E	Extroversion
EPQ-N	Neuroticism
EPQ-P	maladjustment and antisociality
Psychophysiological profile Psychophysiological Profile Questionnaire	
QPF	

Fear and Phobia Profile Psychophysiological Profile Questionnaire

IP-F	Fear
IP-PH	Phobia
IP-1	Disaster
IP-2	Social rejection
IP-3	Animal
IP-4	Dismissal
IP-5	Blood and physician

Depression Questionnaire

QD	

Obsessive/Compulsive profile Maudsley Obsessional-Compulsive Questionnaire

MOCQ-R	Global subscale
MOCQ-1	Checking
MOCQ-2	Cleaning
MOCQ-3	Doubting/ruminating

Figures 2 and 3 show the matrix of the correlation indexes among the 20 variables in the study. Figure 2 presents the results for METs risk, while Figure 3 presents the risks for HRR risk.

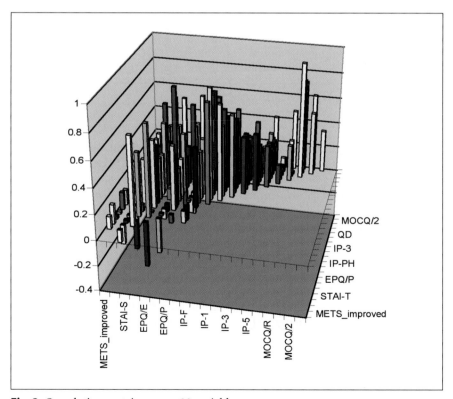

Fig. 2. Correlation matrix among 20 variables

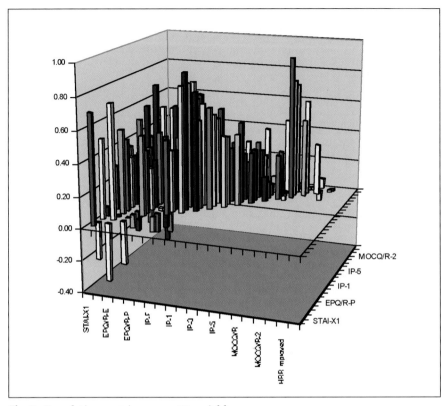

Fig. 3. Correlation matrix among 20 variables

As expected, high linear correlation values were observed among subgroups of variables related to a common dominion such as STAI-S and STAI-T (r = 0.69), IP-F and IP-PH (0.79), MOCQ/1 and MOCQ/R (0.91).

The improvement or non-improvement in METs was poorly correlated to the psychological variables (see Fig. 4). The higher values were observed for MOCQ dominion (positive correlation with METs-HO and negative correlation with METs-LO).

For HRR outcome the risk condition was poorly correlated to the psychological variables and, in particular, with the personality profile of extroversion (r= 0.23) (see Fig. 5).

Figure 6 shows the variable map obtained with the PST system, taking the METs risk into account. Figure 7 shows the variable map obtained with the PST system, taking the HRR risk into account.

Regarding the METs risk, interesting clusters of variables were seen between EPQ/P, IP-1, IP-2 & STAI-S, between STAI-T, QD & MOCQ/1, and between IP-4, QPF, MOCQ/2 & MOCQ/3. These clusters would have been missed using a linear approach, such as Principal Component Analysis.

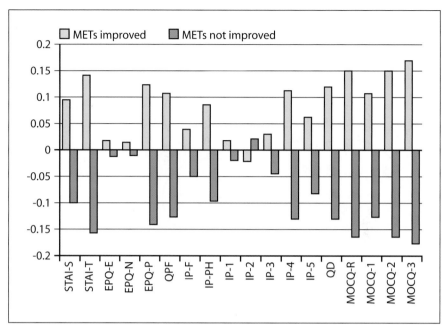

Fig. 4. Correlation between METs outcome and psychological variables

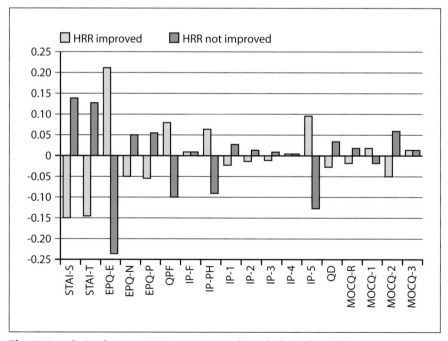

Fig. 5. Correlation between HRR outcome and psychological variables

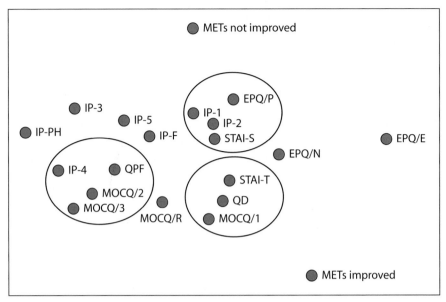

Fig. 6. Variable map obtained with PST (METs risk)

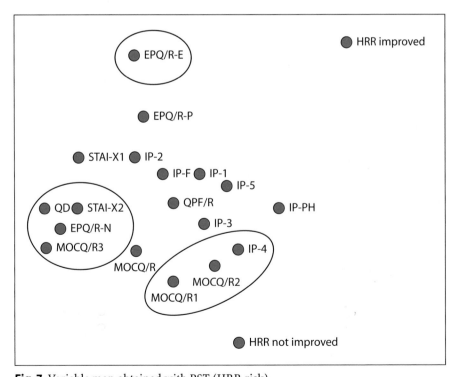

Fig. 7. Variable map obtained with PST (HRR risk)

Regarding the HRR risk, interesting clusters of variables were seen between QD, MOCQ/R-3, EPQ/R-N & STAI-X2, and between IP-4, MOCQ/R-2 & MOCQ/R-1. EPQ/R-E was associated with HRR-LO, while IP-4, MOCQ/R-2 & MOCQ/R-1 were associated with HRR-HO.

It is interesting that PCA (Principal Component Analysis) projects points with a *linear transformation*; axes of new space (factors) are linear combinations of original variables. For a complex dataset, one would need more than two factors to explain all the information in the dataset, and you don't know how many. The advantage of the PST system is that it "places" each point onto the 2D space using a non-linear evolutionary approach, minimizing the global error of projection. In this way, a new space is defined with minimal distortion of the original distances, providing a simple but powerful visual data analysis.

Non-Linear Clustering of Records through Special Kinds of Unsupervised Neural Networks: Self-Organising Maps (SOMs)

Data-clustering tasks performed by traditional statistic methods suffer from the inherent non-linearity of descriptive variables; furthermore, the need to establish an *a priori* number of "to be defined clusters" introduces a potential bias. Advanced statistical techniques, such as K-means, also have some limitation, being unable to perform a feature mapping on data.

Self organising maps (SOMs), one of the most popular architectures of unsupervised artificial neural networks (ANNs), are a powerful tool for examining multidimensional data spaces having a large number of variables. By projecting the large, multidimensional dataset onto a bi-dimensional map that preserves the local topological ordering between variables and allows their complex, non-linear relationships to be displayed, SOMs accomplish two tasks: they reduce data dimensionality and they display similarities by clustering. One of the most important characteristics of SOM networks is that they can organize and cluster data in a map without any supervision, using only the "fuzzy" similarity of the independent variables of each record (a record is a single case in the dataset).

As noted above, SOMs are one of the most popular neural networks. They were developed mainly by Kohonen between 1979-1982. Kohonen's more recent research (1995) [54] has been motivated by the possibility of representing knowledge of specific categories as geometrically organized feature maps.

The main task of SOM networks is to run a self-organizing process that, through mathematical algorithms, creates maps similar to those created by the brain. These tools have almost never been employed in the field of medicine. SOMs are a special kind of neural networks consisting of two layers of interconnected artificial neurons (nodes):
- the input layer, formed by N nodes, each processing an input signal and connected to each node of the output layer;
- the output layer, known as the Kohonen layer, whose nodes form a matrix M=MR x MC, with MR= row and MC=column.

The weights of the connections from each input node to a single node of the Kohonen layer define a model vector mi (mi1, min), where n denotes the number of elements, the same as the input vectors. Together, the model vectors form a codebook. The neurons of the Kohonen layer are connected to adjacent neurons by a neighbourhood relationship that specifies a precise organization in space. That is, each neuron has its physical location, which dictates the topology of the two-dimensional map.

These networks are trained with an unsupervised learning process called "Competitive Learning." The main advantage of using ANNs with an unsupervised learning process is that they do not require target values for their outputs; consequently, there are no examples with reliable target output. Competitive Learning is an adaptive process in which various artificial neurons specialize to represent different input types. When an input is presented to the ANN, the node (of the output layer) best able to represent it, i.e., the node whose model vector is closest to the input, is determined the winner unit (WU), and its weights are adjusted, bringing them closer to the input vector. The metric most often used to calculate the distance between the input vector (x) and the model vectors (y) is the Euclidean one:

$$d = \sqrt{\sum_{i=1}^{N} (x_i - y_i)^2}$$

where n = number of input variables, xj = j[th] variable of input vector, yj = j[th] variable of model vector.

The updating of the connection weights takes place not only on the WU; during the learning process, the weight of all the output neurons that lie within a certain radius around the WU are changed. As a result, all neighbouring neurons on the matrix can learn by virtue of the input signals, becoming gradually specialized to represent similar inputs. Since the neurons are located in a topologically ordered matrix, their input representations also then become ordered on a "map" (Fig. 1).

The number of neighbourhood weights are modified depending on the neighborhood relationship defined by a decreasing function of the distance of the neurons from the WU.

The function width defines the neighbourhood dimension and is wide at the beginning of the learning processes to obtain a global ordering of the map. During learning, both function width and height are decreased until only the WU model vector is changed ("Mexican hat," Gaussian or sine functions). In other words, during this ordering phase when a new input vector is processed, the learning rate (i.e., the amount of weight changes) decreases, and the neighborhood radius also decreases. At the beginning of the learning process, the training weight vectors are initialized with small random values, and input vectors are visible to the network randomly. After the training is over, the network reaches a more or less stable state, in which the weight changes almost cease; in this convergence phase, the neurons get more "specialized" to respond to specific input patterns.

In other words, SOMs learn to recognize different emergent patterns of input data. The output of a SOM network is an array of "classification bin" nodes, each representing a specific pattern of input data. Bins are spatially arranged in an ordered way so that near neighbours represent very similar patterns and distant neighbours represent dissimilar patterns. SOMs provide a means of visualising multifactorial data in two-dimensional space. Their key feature is that they preserve the distance between clusters emerging in data space and represent it as a topographic map (also called a Feature Map).

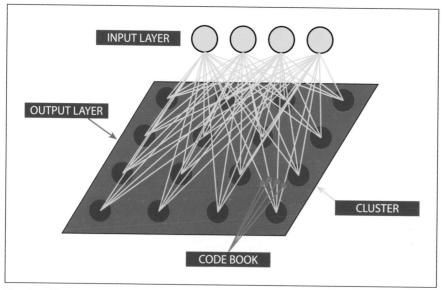

Fig. 8. Self-organizing maps (SOMs)
SOMs are neural networks composed by
- A single input unit level (Input layer)
- A single output unit level organised in a (n X m) matrix
- An initial set of random "weights" connecting input and output layers, which, during the training phase, is updated according to a specific learning law.
All the weights connecting an input vector (single patient) with any output unit are referred to as the codebook. A codebook represents the prototype for all the input vectors close to it. This enables the SOM to generate a spontaneous clustering of the records onto the map according to a complex density function distribution.

We have assessed the natural clustering of the subjects using SOM projection. Input data consisted of 18 variables (see Table 3). Dataset analysis performed by the SOM network was carried out using a square 5x5 output matrix. The software employed for the analyses was conceived and developed by the Semeion Research Centre. The map resulting from the SOM elaborations was analysed using the matrix codebook neighbourhoods. The subject's distribution on the matrix is shown in Figure 9.

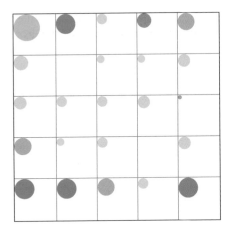

Fig. 9. Distribution of study population on the SOM matrix according to frequency - each spot size is proportional to the number of records represented

The dimension of each circle corresponds to the number of subjects assigned to the cluster. The results show that most of the variables distributed quite homogeneously throughout the matrix. The psychological variables considered in the SOM analysis are shown in Table 3.

The distribution of male and female subjects, assessed *a posteriori*, produced results that are markedly different, as shown in Figure 10, below.

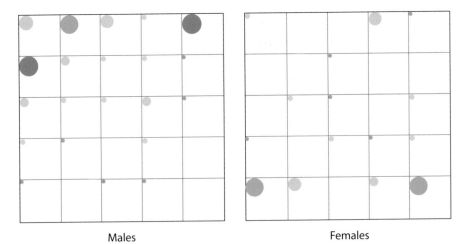

Males   Females

Fig. 10. Distribution of subjects according to gender

This is the first time in the literature in which auto-clustering of cardiopathic patients according to a multidimensional, non-linear projection has been attempted. The feasibility of using SOM networks as a robust alternative to factor analysis and clustering for data mining applications has been evaluated, comparing their performance to factor analytic and K-Means clustering solutions. In general, the comparisons indicate that the SOM networks provide solutions superior to unrotated factor solutions, and that they also provide more accurate recovery of underlying cluster structures when the input data are skewed. It is interesting to note that the descriptive statistics of the variables under study for the two genders didn't reveal any significant differences in their mean values or distributions. As a result, neural network analysis seems to identify a complex matrix of non-linear multifactorial interactions among psychological descriptors that appear to be dominated by gender. This pattern inevitably would have been missed by traditional statistic analysis. We can infer that during the training phase, the SOM network has dynamically removed from the other variables relevant information used to distinguish gender. In other words, the other variables contain information related to the gender.

Prediction of Cardiac Rehabilitation Outcomes: Linear Conventional Statistic Prospective

Patient's Psychological Profile and Cardiac Rehabilitation Outcomes

METs
Viewing the METs variation as a continuous variable, the multiple regression revealed that the psychological predictors included psychophysiological reactions (beta= -0.222; t=-2.12; F=1.59; p=0.04) and disaster phobia (beta= -0.539; t=-2.37; F=1.59; p=0.02).

Using the cutoff value of 10% of METs increase to maximize the log-rank test statistic, the analysis revealed that the extroverted personality characteristic (relative risk = 1.205; 95% CI= 1.058-1.371; p=0.005) and fear symptom (relative risk = 1.112; 95% CI= 1.010-1.225; p=0.03) were predictive of the CR outcome for METs. Figure 1 shows the relative likelihood of a good METs outcome as extroversion and fear symptoms increase.

HRR
Viewing the HRR variation as a continuous variable, the multiple regression showed that the psychophysiological reactions were predictors (beta= -0.228; t=2.11; F=1.11; p=0.04).

Using the cutoff value of 10% of HRR increase to maximize the log-rank test statistic, the analysis indicated that an extroverted personality characteristic (relative risk = 1.165; 95% CI= 1.024-1.32; p=0.02) and phobia symptom (relative risk = 1.034; 95% CI= 1.0-1.069; p=0.05) were predictive of a CR outcome for HRR. Figure 2 shows the relative likelihood of a good outcome as extroversion and phobia symptoms increase.

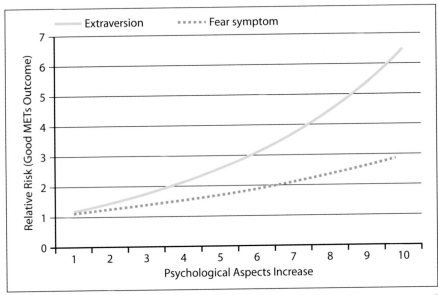

Fig. 11. Estimates of the Relative Risk of a good outcome for METs as extroversion and fear symptoms increase

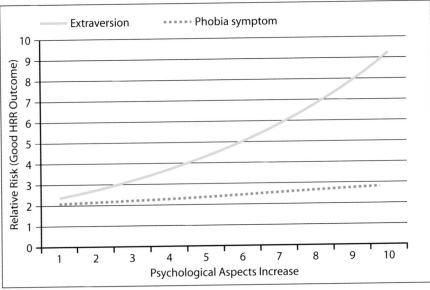

Fig. 12. Estimates of the Relative Risk of good outcome for HRR as extroversion and phobia symptoms increase

◼ Prediction of Cardiac Rehabilitation Outcomes Using a Non-Linear Prospective: Artificial Neural Networks

Again, ANNs are adaptive models for the analysis of data, inspired by the functioning processes of the human brain. They are systems that are able to modify their internal structure in relation to a functional objective. They are particularly suited for solving problems of the non-linear type, being able to reconstruct the approximate rules that put a certain set of data - which describes the problem being considered - with a set of data that provides the solution.

In this study, we applied supervised ANNs, networks in which the result of the processing (the output desired) is already defined. Supervised ANNs calculate an error function that measures the distance between the desired fixed output (target) and their own output, and adjust the connection strengths during the training process to minimize the result of the error function.

The learning constraint on the supervised ANNs requires having their own output coincide with the determined target. The general form of these ANNs is: $y = f(x, w^*)$, where w^* constitutes the set of parameters which best approximate the function. The ANNs used in the study are characterized by the laws of learning and topology. The laws of learning identify equations that translate the ANNs' inputs into outputs, and they identify rules by which the weights are modified to minimize the error or the internal energy of the ANNs.

The topology identifies the structure of the nodes of the ANNs' connections and the signal's flow within them. ANNs can be further distinguished by two broad categories:

- Feedforward ANNs (FF): the signal proceeds from the input to the output of the ANNs, crossing all of the nodes only once;
- Recurring ANNs: the signal is subject to specific feedback, determined beforehand, or tied to the occurrence of particular conditions.

The experiments carried out anticipate the use of both ANNs and Artificial Organisms, i.e., complex combinations of multiple networks. Supervised software (Semeion©), which allows the combination of each law of learning with each type of topology, was used for all the testing.

Law of learning:
Bp = Back Propagation (standard)
SN = Sine Net (Semeion©)
BM = Bi-Modal Network (Semeion©)
Topology:
FF = Feed Forward (standard)
Self = Self Recurrent Network (Semeion©)
Tasm = Temporal Associative Subjective Memory (Semeion©)
Order:
DA = Dynamic and Adaptive Recurrency (Semeion©)
SA = Static and Adaptive Recurrency (Semeion©)
SMDA = SoftMax Discriminant Analysis

The Validation Protocol

The validation protocol is a fundamental procedure for verifying a model's ability to generalize the results ascertained in the testing phase. Among the different protocols reported in the literature, the preferred protocol is that with the greatest capacity for generalization with respect to data unknown to the model. The procedural steps in developing a validation protocol are:

- Subdividing the dataset randomly into two sub-samples: the first called Training Set, and the second called Testing Set; choosing a fixed ANN (and/or Organism) which is trained on the Training Set. In this phase, the ANN learns to associate the input variables with those that are indicated as targets; saving the weight matrix produced by the ANNs at the end of the training phase, and freezing it with all of the parameters used for the training. This involves showing the Testing Set to the ANN, so that in each case, the ANN can express an evaluation based on the training just performed. This procedure takes place for each input vector but not every result (output vector) is communicated to the ANN; in this manner, the ANN is evaluated only in reference to the generalization ability that it has acquired during the Training phase;
- Constructing a new ANN with an architecture that is identical to the previous one, and repeating the procedure described above.

This training plan has been further developed to increase the level of reliability of the generalization of the processing models. The experiments have been done using a random criterion of distribution of the samples. We have employed the so-called "5x2 cross-validation protocol" [55], which produces 10 elaborations for every sample. It consists of dividing the sample five times into two specular sub-samples, each containing a similar distribution of cases and controls.

Artificial neural networks were employed in order to understand the role played by psychological profile variables in influencing the outcome of rehabilitation. The input variables for the neural networks analysis are shown in Table 2.

The outcome variable considered in this analysis was HRR. Two target outcomes were established (HHR-improved; HRR-not improved); and a critical improvement of the heart rate recovery was modelled using the cutoff value of 10% of HRR increase.

The ANN was trained using half of the original data set and validated on the remaining half, to which the network had not been previously exposed. This ensured an unbiased validation. Thus, the sample of 145 patients was randomly subdivided into two equal and balanced sub-samples: one for the training phase (Training) and one for the prediction phase (Testing). In the training phase, different ANNs, including the simple "Free-Forward with Back-Up Propagation to the Complex Recurrent," were trained to discriminate between different outcomes. All the customised software used for the ANN analysis was developed by the Semeion Research Center of Rome.

To reduce the number of input variables and select those with the lowest value of linear correlation with dependent variables, the 'Training and Testing' (T&T)

model associated with the Input Selection (IS) system, both originally developed by the Semeion, was used. The T&T algorithm is a population of ANNs managed by an evolutionary system, where a separate ANN represents a model of distribution for the complete dataset in a training-and-testing set. The score that each ANN achieves in the testing phase represents how good its fit is, and, consequently, its probability of evolution. The evolutionary algorithm, at each generation, combines the different hypothesis of distribution of every ANN according to the goodness of fit criterion. In this way, the best distribution of the whole data set, in the training set and in the testing set, is achieved after a finite number of generations. The evolutionary algorithm controlling the process, referred to as the 'Genetic Doping Algorithm' (GenD), was also developed by the Semeion Research Center. The IS system becomes operative on a population of ANNs, each of which has a capability of selecting independent variables for the validation set. In other words, each ANN learns from the training set and is evaluated on the testing set. Through the GenD evolutionary algorithm, different hypotheses with respect to each ANN change over time, generation after generation. When the evolutionary algorithm no longer improves, the process stops, and the best hypothesis of the input variables is selected and employed on the Validation subset. The goodness-of-fit rule of GenD promotes, at each generation, the best testing performance with the minimal number of inputs.

Input Selection system selected 16 variables and, according to this data input, the dynamic self-recurrent neural network was able to reach the following predictive performance: 70.0% sensitivity and 66.7% specificity, with an overall accuracy of 68.33%. Figure 13 shows the architecture of the dynamic self- recurrent neural network that achieved the best performance.

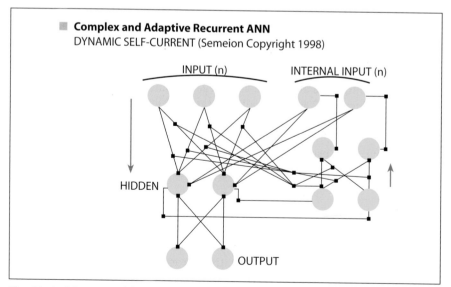

Fig. 13. Architecture of the best performance ANN

Figure 14 shows the relative importance of each single variable in the complex model build by the artificial neural network during the training phase.

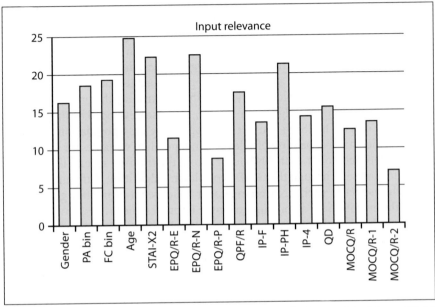

Fig. 14. Input relevance of variables selected in the predictive model of the artificial neural network

A logistic regression was also performed on the same data set to analyse the predictive performance of conventional statistics. The conventional statistical analysis used, even though advanced, was based on the assumption of linear correlations, and revealed a limited capacity for discriminating between patients with positive outcomes and those with negative outcomes. In fact, the logistic regression achieved 52% of overall accuracy. Table 5 shows the comparison between ANN and logistic regression.

Table 5. Comparative performance of ANN and logistic regression in predicting HRR

Model	Sensitivity	Specificity	Overall accuracy
ANN	70%	66.7%	68.3%
Logistic regression	54%	50%	52%

These results confirm the power of artificial neural networks in overcoming the limitations of classical statistics tools. They also underscore the importance of psychological variables in influencing the outcome of cardiac rehabilitation.

Discussion

To recap, the application of non-linear statistical methods allows us to detect aspects that traditional linear statistical analysis cannot. In particular, the application of ANN seems to be effective in fields where the application of a biopsychosocial model is necessary, such as psycho-cardiology. The bio-psychosocial paradigm tries to overcome the traditional reductionist medical model, which considers pathology merely from a biologic-organic perspective. It emphasizes that individuals, with their pathology, are the outcome of complex dynamic and circular interactions that involve biological aspects, psychological variables and their social environment [56]. It is currently acknowledged that psychosocial risk factors have a significant impact on the onset and course of cardiac pathology. Therefore, it is necessary that the rehabilitation process incorporate multi-level interventions that take into consideration not only the medical condition but also the mental and emotional one [57].

The application of ANN, and, in particular, PST, shows that the psychological profile of cardiac patients, when risk is determined based on METs, is characterized by the trait of anxiety, depression and obsessive-compulsive behaviors. As far as HRR-determined risk is concerned, the psychological profile is characterized by obsessive-compulsive personality traits and social anxiety (above all in terms of fearing rejection from other people).

Trait anxiety is described as a general trend to perceive stressors as extremely dangerous and threatening. It is distinguished from state anxiety, which is mainly a feeling of insecurity and powerlessness that emerges when facing a specific event perceived as stressful. Both are characterized by a significant activation of the sympathetic nervous system [58-62]. Trait anxiety is a relevant risk factor, both because the individual continuously experiences a generalized physiological activation that, in the long run, may damage the cardiovascular system, and because the continuous strain may lead the person to adopt risk behaviors (such as smoking, an unbalanced diet, compulsive behaviors, etc.) aimed at reducing the emotional charge.

Based on DSM-IV, depression can be defined as a change of mood. Its development can be related to an experience of loss. A depressive condition is strongly associated with the decrease of functional abilities, fear of death and feelings of hopelessness. In cardiac patients this can be tied to the awareness of a medical condition that has a high mortality rate [63, 64]. Depression can also influence cardiac rehabilitation because it may deter the adoption of healthy behaviors (diet, not smoking, exercise) [64-69].

According to DSM-IV's description, the essential features of obsessive-compulsive personality disorder are concern for order, perfectionism, and mental and interpersonal control that results in a loss as far as flexibility, or being open to new perspectives or ways of doing things, is concerned. This personality profile appears within adult age and is pervasive. Other salient characteristics of the obsessive-compulsive personality are the need to maintain control over the environment, and an excessive attention to rules, futile details and lists. Obsessive-compulsive individuals are excessively accurate and prone to repetitive behaviors: their extraordinary attention for details and procedures often causes them to miss the point of the activity they are engaged in, or to fail to complete the activity or project [70, 71]. People with an obsessive-compulsive personality disorder are excessively devoted to work and the idea of productivity, and they sometimes end up excluding leisure activities and social life. This last feature of obsessive-compulsive personality disorder is strongly reminiscent of Type A personality characteristics (in particular, hostility, competitiveness and time urgency).

There can also be an association between obsessive-compulsive personality disorder and anxiety disorders [72]. In particular, social phobia should be mentioned; according to DSM-IV, this is a "prominent and persistent fear of social or performance situations that can create embarrassment." The fear of being judged and/or rejected can strongly interfere with everyday life and may lead the individual to experience significant distress due to the self-imposed limitations that are aimed at avoiding situations that trigger anxiety. Individuals with social phobia are worried about feeling embarrassment, and about other people considering them anxious, weak, "crazy" or stupid. They almost always report anxiety symptoms (palpitations, tremors, perspiration, gastro-intestinal discomfort, muscular tension, face rash or confusion) in feared social settings. In some cases, all this may result in panic attacks. Avoiding social environments may negatively influence cardiac patients' quality of life and the cardiac condition itself. As a matter of fact, it has been shown that social support (or its perception) plays a significant role in improving treatment compliance, promoting a sense of general well being and increasing coping skills [73, 74].

In summary, ANN investigations incorporating METs as a parameter for cardiac risks indicate that patients who present a very anxious personality and worry excessively about minor things are storing up a significant charge of emotional tension. According to DSM-IV, compulsive behaviors are aimed at decreasing the anxiety load resulting from obsessive thoughts. The tendency to worry excessively, intensified by anxiety traits, can result in a need to maintain complete control over everything in the environment in order to appease anxiety. It can also be associated with feelings of powerlessness. Every time the individual is exposed to a new situation that is out of his/her control, anxiety becomes overwhelming and compulsive behaviors are enacted to restore control. Moreover, patients experience a depressive condition, which could also be associated with feeling powerless in the face of life events.

Risk factors to the recovery of cardiac patients include the fear of social rejection and obsessive-compulsive traits. These factors could be related in that compulsive behaviors momentarily help manage the anxiety load.

Extroversion seems to have a protective role, since it is not associated with cardiac risk.

Traditional linear statistical analysis is not able to identify psychological characteristics connected to HRR cardiac risk. Another important application of ANNs concerns gender influence. Other studies have shown that there are significant gender differences in cardiovascular disease, as far as incidence and mortality rates are concerned, as well as causes, symptoms, and treatments and outcomes [75, 76]. These differences are extremely complex. In contrast to traditional statistical analysis, the use of SOMs might enable us to determine the underlying mechanisms (or psychological profile) responsible for the fact that cardiac risk is significantly different in men than in women. Moreover, because the data suggest that different underlying psychological traits are involved, there is a strong need for research that looks at men and women separately [77, 78].

Thus, the application of ANNs to the study of cardiac rehabilitation outcomes identifies a psychological profile characterized by trait anxiety, obsessive-compulsive personality, social phobia and depression. ANNs also point out other variables that are relevant in cardiac rehabilitation outcomes, such as age and gender, and physiological variables (blood pressure, heart rate). Linear statistical analysis has revealed the predictive power of extroversion on HRR consequent to cardiac rehabilitation program.

Conclusion

The main advantage in applying non-linear statistical methods in psycho-cardiology relates to the possibility of detecting the complexity of phenomena involved in cardiac disease, which include the simultaneous presence of various psychological and social variables. Results have also demonstrated that ANNs have a higher predictive power, even when compared with advanced statistical techniques (such as logistic regression).

References

1. Wenger NK, Froehlicher ES, Smith LK et al (1995) Cardiac rehabilitation clinical practice guidelines. Agency for Health Care Policy and Research and the National Heart, Lung, and Blood Institute, Rockville, MD
2. Maines TY, Lavie CJ, Milani RV, Cassidy MM et al (1997) Effects of CR and exercise programs on exercise capacity, coronary risk factors, behavior, and quality of life in patients with coronary heart disease. South Med J 90:43-49
3. Shiran A, Kornfeld S, Zur S, Laor A et al (1997) Determinants of improvement in exercise capacity in patients undergoing cardiac rehabilitation. Cardiology 88:207-213
4. Pierson LM, Miller LE, Herbert WG (2004) Predicting exercise training outcome from cardiac rehabilitation. J Cardiopulm Rehabil 24:113-118; quiz 119-120
5. Chang JA, Froelicher VF (1994) Clinical and exercise test markers of prognosis in patients with stable coronary artery disease. Curr Probl Cardiol 19:533-587
6. Pate RR, Pratt M, Blair SN et al (1995) Physical activity and public health: a recommendation from the centers for disease control and prevention and the american college of sports medicine. JAMA 273:402-407

7. Myers J, Prakash M, Froelicher V, Do D et al (2002) Exercise capacity and mortality among men referred for exercise testing. N Engl J Med 346:793-801

8. Jette M, Sidney K, Blumchen G (1990) Metabolic equivalents (METS) in exercise testing, exercise prescription, and evaluation of functional capacity. Clin Cardiol 13:555-565

9. Balady GJ, Jette D, Scheer J, Downing J (1996) Changes in exercise capacity following cardiac rehabilitation in patients stratified according to age and gender: results of the Massachusetts Association of Cardiovascular and Pulmonary Rehabilitation Multicenter Database. J Cardiopulm Rehabil 16:38-46

10. Taylor A (1999) Physiological response to a short period of exercise training in patients with chronic heart failure. Physiother Res Int 4:237-249

11. Gulati M, Pandey DK, Arnsdorf MF, Lauderdale DS et al (2003) Exercise capacity and the risk of death in women: the St James women take heart project. Circulation 108:1554-1559

12. Murray DP, Tan LB, Salih M, Weissberg P et al (1988) Does beta adrenergic blockade influence the prognostic implications of post-myocardial infarction exercise testing? Br Heart J 60:474-479

13. Ronnevik RK, von der Lippe G (1992) Prognostic importance of pre-discharge exercise capacity for long-term mortality and non-fatal myocardial infarction in patients admitted for suspected acute myocardial infarction and treated with metoprolol. Eur Heart J 13:1468-1472

14. Aktas MK, Ozduran V, Pothier CE et al (2004) Global risk scores and exercise testing for predicting all-cause mortality in a preventive medicine program. JAMA 292:1462-1468

15. Vivekananthan DP, Blackstone EH, Pothier CE, Lauer MS (2003) Heart rate recovery after exercise is a predictor of mortality, independent of the angiographic severity of coronary disease. J Am Coll Cardiol 42:831-838

16. Nishime EO, Cole CR, Blackstone EH et al (2000) Heart rate recovery and treadmill exercise score as predictors of mortality in patients referred for exercise ECG. JAMA 284:1392-1398

17. Cole CR, Blackstone EH, Pashkow FJ et al (1999) Heart-rate recovery immediately after exercise as a predictor of mortality. N Engl J Med 341:1351-1357

18. Tiukinhoy S, Beohar N, Hsie M (2003) Improvement in heart rate recovery after cardiac rehabilitation. J Cardiopulm Rehabil 23:84-87

19. Redwood DR, Rosing DR, Epstein SE (1972) Circulatory and symptomatic effects of physical training in patients with coronary artery disease and angina pectoris. N Engl J Med 286:959-965

20. May GA, Nagle FJ (1984) Changes in rate-pressure product with physical training of individuals with coronary artery disease. Phys Ther 64:1361-1366

21. Fletcher GF, Balady GJ, Amsterdam EA et al (2001) Exercise standards for testing and training: a statement for healthcare professionals from the American Heart Association. Circulation 104:1694-1740

22. Froelicher VF, Jensen D, Genter F et al (1984) A randomized trial of exercise training in patients with coronary heart disease. JAMA 252:1291-1297

23. Myers J, Froelicher VF (1990) Predicting outcome in cardiac rehabilitation. Am J Cardiol 15:983–985

24. Hammond HK, Kelly TL, Froelicher VF, Pewen W (1985) Use of clinical data in predicting improvement in exercise capacity after cardiac rehabilitation. J Am Coll Cardiol 6:19-26
25. Fioretti P, Simoons ML, Zwiers G et al (1987) Value of pre-discharge data for the prediction of exercise capacity after cardiac rehabilitation in patients with recent myocardial infarction. Eur Heart J 8(Suppl G):33-38
26. Van Dixhoorn J, Duivenvoorden HJ, Pool J (1990) Success and failure of exercise training after myocardial infarction: is the outcome predictable? J Am Coll Cardiol 15:974-982
27. Heldal M, Sire S, Sandvik L, Dale J (1996) Simple clinical data are useful in predicting effect of exercise training after myocardial infarction. Eur Heart J 17:1821-1827
28. Digenio AG, Noakes TD, Cantor A et al (1997) Predictors of exercise capacity and adaptability to training in patients with coronary artery disease. J Cardiopulm Rehabil 17:110-120
29. Con AH, Linden W, Thompson JM, Ignaszewski A (1999), The psychology of men and women recovering from coronary artery bypass surgery. J Cardiopulmon Rehabil 19:152-161
30. Brezinka V, Dusseldorp E, Maes S (1998), Gender differences in psychosocial profile at entry into cardiac rehabilitation. J Cardiopulmon Rehabil 18:445-449
31. Rozanski A, Blumenthal JA, Kaplan J (1999) Impact of psychological factors on the pathogenesis of cardiovascular disease and implications for therapy. Circulation 99:2192-2217
32. Glazer KM, Emery CF, Frid DJ, Banyasz RE (2002) Psychological predictors of adherence and outcomes among patients in cardiac rehabilitation. J Cardiopulm Rehabil 22:40-46
33. Ades P, Maloney A, Savage P, Carhart RL (1999) Determinants of physical functioning in coronary patients. Arch Int Med 159:2357-2360
34. Lisboa PJG (2002) A review of evidence of health benefit from artificial neural networks in medical intervention. Neural Network 15:11-39
35. Mobley BA, Leasure R, Davidson L (1995) Artificial neural network predictions of lengths of stay on a post-coronary care unit. Heart Lung J Acute Critical Care 24:251-256
36. Gaetz M, Iverson GL, Rzempoluck EJ, Remick R et al (2004) Self-organizing neural network analyses of cardiac data in depression. Neuropsychobiology 49:30-37
37. Buscema M (2002) A brief overview and introduction to artificial neural networks. Subst Use Misuse 37:1093-1148
38. Buscema M (2004) Genetic doping algorithm (GenD): theory and applications. Expert Systems 21: 63-80
39. Tietz NW (1997) Practice guideline for cardiac profiling. Am J Clin Pathol 108:696-699
40. Spielberger CD, Gorusch RL, Lushene R (1983) Manual for the State-Trait Anxiety Inventory (STAI). Consulting Psychologists Palo Alto, California
41. Eysenck, HJ, Eysenck SBG (1975) Manual of the Eysenck personality questionnaire. Hodder & Stoughton, London
42. Sanavio E, Bertolotti G, Michielin P et al (1986) CBA-2.0 scale primarie, una batteria a vasto spettro per l'assessment psicologico. Organizzazioni Speciali, Firenze
43. American Psychiatric Association (1994) Diagnostic and statistical manual of mental disorders. 4th ed DSM-IV. APA Press, Washington

44. Hodgson RJ, Rachman S (1977) Obsessional-compulsive complaints. Behav Res Ther 15:389-395
45. Bruce RA, Kusumi F, Hosmer D (1973) Maximal oxygen intake and nomographic assessment of functional aerobic impairment in cardiovascular disease. Am Heart J 85:546-562
46. American College of Sports Medicine (2000) ACMS's Guidelines for exercise testing and prescription, Baltimore, Md. Lippincott Williams & Wilkins 368
47. Fleg JL, Pina IL, Balady GJ et al (2000) Assessment of functional capacity in clinical and research applications: an advisory from the committee on exercise, rehabilitation, and prevention; council on clinical cardiology, American Heart Association. Circulation 102:1591-1597
48. Kaminsky LA, Whaley MH (1998) Evaluation of new standardized ramp protocol: the BSU/Bruce ramp protocol. J Cardiopulm Rehab 18:434-438
49. Ashley EA, Myers J, Froelicher V (2000) Exercise testing in clinical medicine. Lancet 356:1592-1597
50. Myers J, Buchanan N, Walsh D et al (1991) Comparison of the ramp versus standard exercise protocols. J Am Coll Cardiol 17:1334-1342
51. Roger VL, Jacobsen SJ, Pellikka PA et al (1998) Prognostic value of treadmill exercise testing: a population-based study in Olmsted County, Minnesota. Circulation 98:2836-2841
52. Mark DB, Shaw L, Harrell FE Jr et al (1991) Prognostic value of a treadmill exercise score in outpatients with suspected coronary artery disease. N Engl J Med 325:849-853
53. Buscema M and the Semeion Group (1999) Artificial neural networks and complex social systems. Franco Angeli, Milan
54. Kohonen T (1999) Comparison of SOM point densities based on different criteria. neural computation. 11:2081-2095
55. Dietterich TG (1998) Approximate statistical tests for comparing supervised classification learning algorithms. Neural Computation 10:1895-1923
56. Gatchel RJ (2004) Comorbidity of chronic pain and mental health disorders: the biopsychosocial perspective. Am Psychol 59:795-805
57. Blumenthal JA, Lett HS, Babyak MA et al (2003) Depression as a risk factor for mortality after coronary artery bypass surgery. Lancet 362:604-609
58. Spielberger CD (1972) Anxiety: current trends in theory and research. Academic Press, New York, NY
59. Spielberger CD (1980) Test anxiety inventory. Preliminary professional manual. Consulting Psychologists Press, Palo Alto, CA
60. Spielberger CD (1983) Manual for the State-Trait Anxiety Inventory (STAI). Consulting Psychologists Press, Palo Alto, CA
61. Spielberger CD, Rickman RL (1990) Assessment of state and trait anxiety in cardiovascular disorders. In: Byrne DG, Rosenman RH (Eds) Anxiety and the heart. Hemisphere Publishing Corporation, New York pp 73-92
62. Spielberger CD, Gorsuch RL, Lushene RD (1970) Manual for the State-Trait Anxiety Inventory. Consulting Psychologists Press, Palo Alto, CA
63. Carney RM, Blumenthal JA, Catellier D et al (2003) Depression as a risk factor for mortality after acute myocardial infarction. Am J Cardiol 92:1277-1281

64. Frasure-Smith N, Lesperance F, Talajic M (1995) Depression and 18-month prognosis after myocardial infarction. Circulation 91:999-1005

65. Frasure-Smith N, Lesperance F, Juneau M et al (1999) Gender, depression, and one-year prognosis after myocardial infarction. Psychosom Med 61:26-37

66. Frasure-Smith N, Lesperance F, Talajic M (1994) Depression following myocardial infarction. Impact on 6-month survival. JAMA 271:1082

67. Frasure-Smith N, Lespérance F (2003) Depression and other psychological risk factors following myocardial infarction. Arch Gen Psychiatry 60:627-636

68. Frasure-Smith N, Lesperance F (2005) Reflections on depression as a cardiac risk factor. Psychosom Med 67(Suppl 1):S19-S25

69. Frasure-Smith N, Lesperance F, Talajic M (1995) Depression and 18-month prognosis after myocardial infarction. Circulation 91:999-1005

70. Parmet S, Glass TJ, Glass RM (2004) Obsessive-compulsive disorder. JAMA 292:2040

71. Summerfeldt LJ, Kloosterman PH, Antony MM et al (2004) The relationship between miscellaneous symptoms and major symptom factors in obsessive-compulsive disorder. Behav Res Ther 42:1453-1467

72. Diaferia G, Bianchi I, Bianchi ML et al (1997) Relationship between obsessive-compulsive personality disorder and obsessive-compulsive disorder. Compr Psychiat 38:38-42

73. Cottraux J, Bouvard MA, Milliery M (2005) Combining Pharmacotherapy with cognitive-behavioral interventions for obsessive-compulsive disorder. Cogn Behav Ther 34:185-192

74. Westenberg HG, Liebowitz MR (2004) Overview of panic and social anxiety disorders. J Clin Psychiat 65(Suppl 14):22-26

75. Glazer KM, Eurery CF, Frid DJ, Branyasz RE (2002) Psychological predictors of adherence and outcomes among patients in cardiac rehabilitation. J Cardiopulm Rehabil 22:40-46

76. Marrugat J, Sala J, Masià R, et al (1998) Mortality differences between men and women following first myocardial infarction. JAMA 280:1405-1409

77. Vaccarino V, Berkman LF, Krumholz HM (2000) Long-term outcome of myocardial infarction in women and men: a population perspactive. Am J Epidemiol 152:965-973

78. Wulsin LR, Singal BM (2003) Do depressive symptoms increase the risk for the onset of coronary disease? A systematic quantitative review. Psychosom Med 65:201-210

Chapter 16

Person Measurement and Rehabilitation Outcome: the New Perspective of Rasch Analysis

L. Tesio

Disability, Rehabilitation, Measurement

Disability as Whole Person Malfunctioning

According to the World Health Organization (WHO) 1980 definition, disability consists in any restriction or lack of ability (resulting from impairment) to perform an activity in the manner or within the range considered normal for a human being [1]. The new WHO model (2001) gives to the term *disability* a broader, more general connotation, but nonetheless confirms the importance of "activities" as the constitutive elements of a person's "functioning" [2]. *Disability* and *activity* are viewed in relation to the person as a whole. For example, a heart condition (according to the 1980 WHO model) might be defined as a lessening (or malfunctioning) of one body part. Difficulty going up stairs likewise represents a deficit with respect to an activity (since a whole person, only, can climb stairs). A deficit in one or more activities defines a malfunctioning of the whole person and is therefore called a disability. Usually, the definition of "function" is misunderstood. In the context of rehabilitative medicine, a recent definition [3, 4] – namely, energy or information exchange – is useful. For although this definition is general, it makes an important distinction between physiologic functions (breathing, nerve conduction, etc.), and functions that take place between the person and environment - in other words, "activities."

Rehabilitation as a System of Interventions Designed to Recover "Ability"

Rehabilitation leads to the restoration of damaged or lost activities, as far as this is possible for the person involved. The recovery of an "ability" can be accomplished by an intervention focused on part of the person (i.e., passive movement), on the whole person (speech therapy), or on the environment-person (for example, providing aids, removing architectural barriers, and so forth).

Sometimes "contextual" interventions that would not by themselves be considered rehabilitative may make the rehabilitative intervention possible. Examples include medications, functional surgery, and environmental adaptation (hospital transportation, subvention, laws, etc.).

Measurement of Rehabilitation Outcomes and Measuring the Person

Regardless of the level of intervention, the long-term consequence for the person involved can be included under the category of "outcomes" - i.e., the final change(s) after the various processes and/or actions as they affect the person as a whole. The process (action) must have an effect on the interaction between the person and environment, and it must be perceptible to the person involved.

The short-term result is called the output. For example, after hospital admission for heart infarct, the increase of the ventricular ejection fraction can be observed as output. Later on, an outcome can be returning to work, the reduction of anxiety and stren or dyspnoea, or a decrease in mortality risk.

The outcome cannot be deducted from the output (as represented by measurements of "bodily functions"). A reduction in cardiac power can result in the loss of self-sufficiency, but many other conditions (for example, paralysis) can result in the same negative outcome. Conversely, an elevator can produce the positive outcome desired independently of the degree of heart power.

Indicators of rehabilitative outcome must be behavioral measures, like those for knowledges or attitudes. Questionnaires are the basic tools used to measure these indicators.

Biometry and Person-Metric

Specificity of the Medical-Rehabilitative Model in Comparison with the Biomedical and Epidemiologic Model

Some specificities esist that make the medical-rehabilitative field distinct from the health sector defined as biomedical [5, 6]. The term *biomedical* reminds the strong link with the chemical-physical and biological sciences (see for example endocrinology or immunology).

First, the relationship with the social aspect is inextricable: a non-medical context is a necessary condition for the medical-rehabilitative intervention. For example, although a diabetic person can find an almost complete therapeutic answer within the clinical context, the interventions required for a patient who experiences a brain stroke and loses self-sufficiency are not geared specifically toward mobility. These interventions would also consist in, for example, providing daily care or social assistance.

Second, the outcome measures are psychometric, i.e., they are based on the subjective assessment by an observer (sometimes the subject himself) who evaluates the behavior or psychic state of the whole person (depression, knowledges, attitudes, pain, and so on). The indicators on a self-administered depression questionnaire evaluate personal behaviors (crying, isolation, etc.) or perceptions (sadness, suicidal tendencies, etc.). Of note is the fact that an observable motor behavior is necessary (lethargy, crying, etc.) in order to infer a psychic state. Because the variables inferred through the questionnaire may seem impalpable compared with motor actions that are not "pure" psychic states such as walking, dressing, etc., the term "psycho-metric" may appear somewhat reductive. However, given that the aim is to observe and to measure a variable in relation to the *whole person*, it seems more opportune, as it has been suggested [7], to speak of *person-metric* rather than *psychometric*.

Organisms, Persons, Populations: a Fit Measurement Model for Every Concept

A biomedical area pertains to epidemiology. The name clearly derives from the Greek word *démos:* population. Population can be viewed both as an organism and a as person. To the population-organism one can apply most of the biomedical measurement techniques usually applied to the single individual: incidences, probabilities of a certain event, etc. The measurement approach is, in any event, deterministic, and the phenomenon itself is a given. The uncertainty depends only on factors pertaining to the precision of the measurement technique and – as is typically the case for epidemiology – to the interferences between the available sample and the real population.

On the other side, population can be seen also as a sort of macro-person, if the variable to be investigated is one of the person. This approach, although rare in medicine (the recent success of satisfaction questionnaires in hospitals being an exception), is frequent in social sciences. Opinion surveys – in which what a single person thinks is used to estimate what the whole population "thinks" – are a well-known example. Apart from the uncertainty of the relationship between the sample and the population, there is the intrinsic indeterminacy of the single person answers. Indeed, if the variety of the sample is operating to reduce the differences among individual answers ("people in general think that…"), the more accurate is the expectation with respect to the population (lower general variance compared to the average), the more deviating will be the real single person's answers compared to the "abstract" mean. If we accept the idea that the individual variance does not reflect just random error, but an intrinsic impredictability in the answers instead, there remains a problem in recognizing and emphasizing the systematic and structural components lying behind sub-groups or individuals. Therefore, a specific statistical and experimental paradigm should be adapted. Otherwise, the epidemiologist's conclusions will turn into in a Procustean bed, with the outcome representing (statistical) dictatorship of the majority. Medicine will be dulled by health service. These considerations suggest that not only should the term *psycho-metric* be replaced by *person-metric* but, also, that the term *biometric* should mean both *biomedical and epidemiologic*, a convention that will be followed henceforth in this investigation to generally indicate the measurement of variables originating in the biomedical world (both chemical-physical and epidemiologic), a practice that is more familiar to physicians and biomedical technicians (Table 1).

Table 1. Minimum glossary of measurement models

Measurement	Bio-metric		Person-metric
	Bio-medical	**Epidemiologic**	
	Measurement of the chemical-physical variables (length, temperature, voltage, etc.)	Measurement of the population variables (incidence, prevalence, risk, etc.)	Measurements of variables that refer only to the single and indivisible person (pain, independence, satisfaction, depression, knowledge, fatigue, preferences, etc.)

Consequences of the Rehabilitative Specificity on Measurement Methodology: Evident and Latent Variables

Medical indicators are still very much based on chemical-physical measures (arterial pressure, glycemia, body temperature) or, conversely, on epidemiologic measurements (mortality, relapse probability etc.). In fact, measurements associated with populations (or part of the person) are prevailing in the literature [8]. Both biomedical and epidemiologic measurements can be directly observed and hence (apart from error coming from the measurement instrument itself) provide a high degree of certainty. Taking the thermometer as an example, it is possible to mention a mistake linked to the intrinsic precision of the instrument (temperature modifies, for example, not only the mercury volume but also the volume of the glass envelope). In the case of epidemiology, errors resulting from sampling estimates can occur (due to the fact that percentage calculations based on samples that by definition do not perfectly represent the whole population). If, however, we accept a certain degree of imprecision, the observed value can reasonably be thought of as "true" (or "deterministic" in the language of statistics): the thermometer indicates 37.1°C; the percentage of teenagers in a certain sample of people is 20.2%, etc.

The same reasoning does not apply, however, to the gap left between the measurement of parts of a *single and unique* person and the measurement of populations [7]. This is because the person generates variables (objects that can be measured) that are not entirely (or directly) *observable*. It is better to call them, as is done in statistics, "latent" variables. In fact, the person has the ability to generate spontaneous behaviors (not only deterministic answers to external stimuli) and, hence, intrinsically unforeseeable behaviors, irrespective of the accuracy of the observation [9]. The evaluation of a gym performance, for instance, can be very precise: seven judges agree with score "8." But the day after, in a non-agonistic contest, the athlete might be less motivated and the score might change. This is because the person's property *is intrinsically variable*.

"Gymnastic ability" is not immediately apparent in the gymnast but shows itself through behaviors (the performances during the competition) that *represent* in some way, yet *are not* the latent variable. Different gymnastic trials can represent the "gymnastic ability," even if none in particular *is* itself the gymnastic ability. In contrast, the temperature *is* the object's temperature; the percentage of teenagers *is* the percentage of teenagers within that given sample of people.

From *How* to Measure to *What* to Measure

Choosing the variables is, in the end, a problem of expert agreement. The first step is to decide if and when are we going to use "person" variables. The second step consists in finding the variables to measure.

Which Program: Cardiac Function Rehabilitation or Cardiac Patient Rehabilitation?

The choice to measure not only biomedical but even person-metric aspects reflects the aim of the intervention. In the cardiovascular sciences, the theme has a political importance if we give to Cardiology a rehabilitative role. We one should not speak of cardiologic rehabilitation but of the rehabilitation of cardiac patients instead. The functional recovery of a damaged heart is the domain of biomedicine, even when therapeutic exercise is used as an adjuvant. The some does not hold for the disability of the cardiac patient. For, psychological and educational interventions need specific methods and skills. Even therapeutic exercises inside a secondary prevention program can require non cardiologic competencies (e.g., physiatry or sports sciences).

While functional recovery (ventricular ejection fraction first) can be monitored through the use of biomedical indicators, the strictly rehabilitative parts of a clinical program must rely upon valid person-metric measurements. It would be ingenuous to think that biomedical variables could replace the person-metric ones. The relationship between the recovery of an organ and the rehabilitation of a person is not strictly predictable because there is no direct causality as the "deterministic-reductionist" scientific model postulates [5, 6].

If the heart works better, it does not necessarily mean that the patient will be able to perform all of the activities he or she was precluded from performing (walking, communicating, etc.). The nature of this relationship is not so evident in cardiology: if the heart works better, surely there is no reason to think that the patient should not *feel better*. As a result, cardiology is thought to be always implicitly rehabilitating. This is only partially true, however. The predictability is higher if the damaged organ or its functions are a) not substituted for by other organs or functions, and b) not substituted for by adaptations either of the subject and/or of the environment.

As an example, let's consider the case of an elderly person who underwent the amputation of a lower limb, replaced by a prosthesis. While wearing the prosthesis, he/she may or may not be able to walk outside his house anymore. In the outcome the conditions of the contralateral lower limb will intervene, as well as patient's motivations, architectural barriers, etc. Now, let's consider the case of a patient just over a myocardial infarction, with an ejection fraction raising from 20% to 50%. This in itself seems sufficient to guarantee that the patient could get back to walking outside his house. However in this case, there is uncertainty on the individual outcome. The patient could be suffering from a severe depressive syndrome, or, due to a weight increase, he could be afraid of being seized by another heart attack, due to the fact that the stairs at entrance has so many steps, etc. These examples illustrate that the outcome must be directly measured, and cannot be deducted from biomedical observations.

The relationship between personal variables and the theme of pain deserves separate consideration. The attempt to measure pain through body parameters is very ancient. It is true that pain reduction can have marked objective consequences. The resolution of lumbar-sciatic pain, for instance, results in the normalization of lower limb tendon reflexes and electric somato-sensorial evoked potentials. Even if pain is not, broadly speaking, an "activity," nevertheless, it remains whole person variable. It is not reducible to neurophysical mechanisms, although these are implied.

No "biological equivalent" of pain can effectively replace the direct measure of a person's experience. Evidence comes from the fact that, no indirect measurement, considered separately, is sufficiently related to the subjective judgment of "feeling better" after an analgesic treatment. It therefore becomes necessary to observe variables directly in the form of questionnaires on pain intensity, disability induced by pain, loss of working ability induced by pain, etc. It is not surprising that a questionnaire specifically aiming to assess the interaction between pain and disability has become be an "outcome" measurement much more suitable in quantifying the overall assessment of subjective improvement [10].

Which Variables are Necessary to Supervise the Rehabilitation Program?

If the methodological context of the outcome measurement in rehabilitation is accepted as being the same as that of person measurement in general, it will be necessary to define which variables are critical for the measurement of improvement of rehabilitative procedures. Biomedical researchers seldom give decisive importance to the choice of person-metric instruments. They usually accept without particular criticisms the instruments already sanctioned by prestigious journals. The metric validity of most of these instruments is often completely insufficient. One critical point (among others) concerns the cross-cultural validity of instruments assumed to be valid in international studies. Much attention has been focussed on the techniques used to assess linguistic translations. Almost always, however, it is forgotten that a good linguistic translation in itself does not guarantee two things: a) that the original questionnaire has good metric features; and b) that the "value" of the items stays same across different cultures.

In a famous questionnaire on disability, the items concerning "eating" or "bathtub/shower transfer" (and related scoring) were perfectly translated from English to Japanese. Nevertheless they suggest very different ability levels when one considers the decreased difficulty involved in using a spoon versus oriental chopsticks, or shower plates or a horizontal bathtub versus the vertical showers that have difficult access rather common in Japan [11].

The success of a measurement depends on several unpredictable factors, such as the ability of foreseeing important events, the simplicity of its application, practical utility, etc. The "success" of both biometric and person-metric measures often has little to do with their complexity. In cardiac electrophysiology, the old- fashioned electrocardiogram has always outweighted vector-cardiography. In determining the extent of dyspnoea, the old-fashioned, straightforward NYHA classification (with only 4 degrees) for heart failure still prevails despite much more sophisticated questionnaires [12, 13]. This explains the impossibility of defining a valid standard set of rehabilitation indicators without considering the culture and technology providing the backbone of modern questionnaires for person measurement.

Person Measurement: the Proposal from the Georg Rasch Model

Why is an Original Statistic Model Necessary?
"Individual measurements," as pointed out above, concretely are questionnaires spawning cumulative scores. The questionnaire's limits are well known. For example, a questionnaire's score shows floor-ceiling effects (it extends from fixed minimum and maximum values); the balance between score and implied "real quantity" is difficult to achieve (i.e., 3-2 *does not mean the same thing as* 4-3); between any given score and the following one there is a discontinuity whose extent is unknown; the different items in a questionnaire can represent "apples and oranges" (in effect, making it impossible to sum them up); score criteria must be subjectively interpreted; etc. All statistical-psychometric traditions dating back to the second half of 19th century produced remarkable mathematical methods and philosophical theories for assigning metric validity to rough scores [14]. Nevertheless, the validity of these measurements is still considered minor (or "subjective"), compared with chemical-physical measurements (which are considered, often optimistically, to be "objective"). The advantage of measurements from statistical-psychometric traditions when applied to the rehabilitation field is the fact that they are the only valid means available for accessing the "latent" variables of an individual. In other words, a person's latent variables can be measured only by assigning scores to observations of individual activities (such as walking, getting dressed, etc.). The statistical model that, since 1960, has made it possible for questionnaire measurements to approximate the validity of chemical-physical measurements results from the contributions of Georg Rasch (for an overview of the statistical movement inspired by him, visit the website *www.rasch.org*). The validity of his model is definitively demonstrated by a theorem that, in summary, proves that if (and only if) the questionnaire presents properties complying with the Rasch model, the measurement obtained is objective in the sense that it is not dependent on the particular set of items, persons or raters interucting in the misurement process.

No real dataset perfectly respects the model's expectations. The differences between observed data and expected data therefore result in a worthy guide for identifying the questionnaire's imperfections or unexpected answers from a single subject or from groups of subjects. The result is the possibility of a semiology of unexpected answers. This makes it possible to assess whether, for example:

a) the questionnaire has an intrinsic heterogeneity (its items consist of "apples and oranges") or is formulated ambiguously;
b) there may be an incorrect survey due to a lack of preparation or distractions of the surveyors taking measurements;
c) there may be opportunistic behavior from surveyors;
d) there may be particular subgroup characteristics that systematically interfere with the subjects' answers.

Today, there are techniques that allow us to *estimate* (absolute exactness is unattainable) the presence and seriousness of each one of the above flaws. The control on data quality, therefore, may go well beyond the classic controls related to congruence and completeness, and it can reach the intrinsic likelihood level of the scoring profile [15].

■ The Rasch Model: an Overview

When evaluating a score obtained from a questionnaire, it is necessary to answer at least three questions.

1. Does the same increase in score always indicate an equal increase of the amount of the variable measured at all the levels of the variable? In geometry, for example, when talking about length, it is claimed that the difference between 2 and 1 meters is equal to the difference between 102 and 101 meters.
2. If so, which substantial increase (in terms of self-sufficiency, pain, dyspnoea, etc.) is represented by the numerical increase? Do not forget that the number of items in a scale and the score levels of each item may be very different and are arbitrarily prefixed.
3. What is the reliability/reproducibility with respect to which scoring provides a measure? The reliability concept is wider than the reproducibility one. A subject passing difficult items and failing easy ones could maintain this unexpected behavior in different situations. The scale itself, however, would not have an intrinsic reliability, as it assumes a different meaning for different subjects (i.e., "what is measured" is different among subjects: numbers can be reproducible, meanings are not).

It is necessary to have a model that provides a joint but independent assessment of subjects' abilities and item difficulties. It is also necessary that the measurements be reproducible. The model must dictate:
- the existing relationship between the observed frequency of answers (general) and the answer probability;

- the existing relationship between probability of observed answer and expected probability on the basis of items difficulty; and
- the error surrounding the estimates.

A model is an equation that fixes the rules of interaction among the magnitudes that come into play - namely, the parameters. The first model satisfying the requirements of a real measurement was the one conceived by Georg Rasch in 1960 for dichotomous answers (no/yes) [16]. Subsequently, other Rasch-compatible models were developed, and these were suitable for the construction of "polytomous" scales ("rating-scales" with item levels such as no/sometimes/always=0/1/2; no/light/moderate/severe=0/1/2/3, etc.). They were also suitable for the study of severity and consistency from different observers (i.e., the "many-facet" models, which jointly evaluate items, subjects and surveyors) [17].

The original Rasch dichotomous model refers to scales in which the only possible answers are 0 or 1. The real ability of a subject's scoring "0" or "1" on a certain item is computable with an intermediate value, if intended as the probability of event "1." The leading equation is expressed as:

$$P = P_{(x=1|0,1)} = \left(\frac{e^{\beta-\delta}}{1+e^{\beta-\delta}} \right) \qquad [1]$$

It is read as follows: "the probability P that the observed answer X is equal to 1, given that the answer can only be 0 or 1, is given by… (see the function in brackets).

The equation can be rewritten, to evidence linearity, as:

$$\log\left(\frac{P}{1-P} \right) = \beta-\delta \qquad [2]$$

where:
P = P(1) = probability of observing answer "1"
1-P = probability of occurrence of the alternative answer "0"
X is the observable answer (0 or 1)
e = 2.718…, base of natural logarithms
β = is the subject's "ability" parameter
δ = is the item's "difficulty" parameter

Now it is even more evident that the model foresees that the probability of observing "1" depends on the difference between the two, and only the two parameters (hence, the model's linearity). Rasch measures are really "intervals," because a numerical distance (e.g., between 3 and 2, between 103 and 102) always maintains the same qualitative meaning. There is only one evident complication, and this is due to the fact that, on the left of Eq. [2], the probability has been replaced by an unfamiliar term for the medical field.

The term log [P/(1-P)] (odd ratio logarithm, log-odd) is defined logit. The term *logistic*, assigned to the Rasch model and similar models, derives from this term. The logistic transformation of probability P has several advantages.

One is that, unlike P, the logit is not confined to 0 or 1; in fact the difference between ability and difficulty conceptually has no limits. All it is necessary to understand at this point, nonetheless, is that the logit grows as the value of P grows. This model is defined "1-parameter," as it exclusively considers the subject's *ability* (by convention, the parameter of "difficulty" is not taken into account).

It can also be demonstrated in a formal way (the Rasch theorem of "separability") that only the "1-parameter" logistic model can estimate the subject's relative ability independently of the difficulties of the particular items examined, and, furthermore, only this parameter assesses the item difficulties independently of the ability of the particular sample of subjects examined. This independence is a fundamental requisite for any measure. Using an analogy with physical measures, 1 meter has to represent the same heigth on any subject, and also the measurement of a subject's height has to remain the same, no matter which instrument of measurement is used. Further considerations that make the Rasch model the only valid solution from a theoretical standpoint are contained in Appendix 1.

Application Backgrounds

There is an extensive literature available for obtaining a practical understanding of Rasch analysis [18-22]. A simplified list of the advantages of this technique, as applied to a person's variables, both psychological and physical, is provided below.

a. The Rasch analysis on existing ordinal scales, which reveals modest interval properties, allows improving the scales, removing inconsistent items or redefining the score category (what is meant by 0/1/2, etc.). It is also possible to change scores in to measures with interval characteristics. This transformation makes all conventional parametric statistics appropriate.

b. The construction of new scales, already bound to item-answer techniques, and, in particular, to Rasch analysis, helps with the construction of instruments having excellent internal coherence features (uni-dimensionality) and ordinal scores already close to real interval measures, thereby making their Rasch transformation unnecessary for common clinical applications.

c. The availability of scales whose item metric properties are known allows the study not only of ability but also the extent of inconsistency in the answer profile of the subjects, with respect to the different difficulties of items (so-called *misfit*). Unexpected answers (e.q. an easy item failed by an able subject) may reveal inaccurate or opportunistic distorted measures, or they may point out clinical peculiarities, unsuspected in a particular subject. Moreover, the availability of such scales makes it possible to perform a sophisticate quality control on the questionnaire in the context of econometric and epidemiologic studies [15].

d. The independence of item difficulty parameters from a particular examined sample of subjects points out possible variations in the "behavior profiles" of subpopulations. As an example, Appendix 2 shows how a variation in the hierarchy of *difficulty* between admission and discharge items in a disability scale (FIM™) may reveal inappropriate admissions, where the total score would have rather suggested the opposite.

e. Generally, a scale producing "real measurements" applied to a sample of subjects not showing a severe misfit makes appropriate the correlation between continuous variables (biomedical, econometric and so on) and behavioral variables. This opens the way to the study of person outcome induced by biomedical procedures [11, 22].

f. Knowing the intinsic/objective difficulty of an item paves the way for international multicentric studies, where the same items may have different quantitative "meaning" across Countries, despite a correct linguistic translation [23].

▩ Appendix 1 – Why just the Rasch Model?

In the Rasch model, the parameters β and δ in Equation 2 have been "estracted" through "maximum likelihood" procedures. In simplistic terms, they are the parameters originating in a model pursuant to Equation 2 in relation to which the matrix of the actually observed answers in the sample of examined subjects has the maximum probability of occurring. Despite its formal simplicity (and elegance) the equation has several distinctive strong points.

The more the subject is skilled in a certain item, the greater the likelihood of observing the answer "1." Every β and δ value, therefore, corresponds to one unique value in terms of the answer's probability. The relationship between P e (β-δ) is monotonically increasing: on the same item, more skilled subjects always have a greater probability of a certain answer. How much greater? The function follows an "s-shaped" trend typical of these "logistic" equations, while the ratio between logit and dependent variable remains proportional. The unit of measurement ("logit"), although it may seem awkward, is particularly useful in correcting the "floor effect" (and the ceiling effect), determined by the confinement of possible answers between 0 and 1. In other words, the logit units prevents subjects with different skills from "crowding" around similar probabilities. For example, a subject whose probability for passing an item improves from 50 to 75% will have gained around 1 logit. The same applies to a subject who seemingly improves his probabilities by much less, say, from 75 to 90%, or from 90 to 95%. Only ability and difficulty are determining factors for the probability of the answer (and therefore the logit measurement). Conventionally, the parameter "difficulty" will not be counted, and therefore it is said that the Rasch model is "1-parameter". This characteristic radically differentiates it from the so-called models "with more than one parameter" (n-pl models or n-parameters logistic models). In these models, parameters are introduced that make the matrix of the observed answers even "more likely." For example, it has to be taken into account that a proportion of "1" may come from random answers. Therefore, the model will assign a minimum probability of answers "1" not only to subjects who demonstrate improvement, but also to those subjects who may be infinitely less skilled than required for passing a certain item. It is also possible to take into account other factors that influence the answers such as gender, age, diagnostic class, and so on. Although this may seem appealing, including these considerations distorts the purpose of the analysis. This must remain transforming dichotomons answers, subjected to either random or systematic interferences, into strong interval measurements. By introducing other *ad hoc* parameters, the measurements of ability and difficulty become dependent on the particular sample of subjects (or on the particular set of items) being examined. For example, the tendency to answer at random might be expected specifically from less skilled or slower subjects (in the case of a time-limited tests). Specifically, the items more affected by random answers might be the most difficult ones, or simply, the last items in a long list. If the day after the same subjects face a measurement scale with easier items, or the same test with the same items in a different order, the rating associated with their "ability," in comparison with that on the previous day, changes. Similarly, if the same test is presented to more skilled subjects, or faster subjects, the item difficulty measures change.

So, the 2-pl model (ability and "random answer percentage") measures not only a combination of examined and unknown variables, it measures them *in a way* that cannot be generalized to another group of subjects or items involved in the same measure mentprocess. As a consequence, the Rasch model can lead to the finding that some subjects are inconsistent ("misfitting") regarding the demanding expectations of the model itself, such as, for instance, unexpectedly passing items very much beyond their overall ability.

This leads to important diagnostic considerations. Did the subjects answer at random or in an opportunist way [15]? Alternatively, one might wonder whether there are items that do not reflect the examined variable and therefore result in answers that are not true measures of the subjects' abilities with respect to that variable. The removal of "misfitting" subjects can help in determining the ability of the remaining ones, and the removal of "misfitting" items can help improve the measurement scale, making it conceptually more homogeneous and therefore more capable of reproducible measurements in future samples.

Appendix 2 - Example of Application of Rasch Analysis to a Measurement Scale

FIM™ Disability Scale

Figure 1 shows the Functional Independence Measure - FIM™ (© UB Foundation Inc., State University of New York, Buffalo NY). The FIM probably is the most widely used questionnaire for measuring disability. It is an international standard for measurements of effectiveness, efficiency, pertinence and costs associated with the rehabilitating intervention [24]. The Italian version has been available since 1992 (*www.so-ge-com.it*) [25]. The total score from the different items can vary from 18 (total dependence) to 126 (total self-sufficiency). It is also possible to use the "motor" scale (item 1-13, score from 13-91) and the "cognitive" scale (item 14-18, score from 5-35) distinctly.

Personal care	**Communication**
1. Eating	14. Comprehension
2. Grooming	15. Expression
3. Bathing	
4. Dressing, upper body	**Cognitive-relation capacities**
5. Dressing, lower body	16. Social interaction
6. Toileting	17. Problem solving
	18. Memory
Sphincter management	**LEVELS**
7. Bladder management	7. Complete independence
8. Bowel management	6. Modified independence
	5. Supervision
Mobility (Transfers)	4. Minimal assistance
9. Bed-chair-wheelchair	3. Moderate assistance
10. Toilet	2. Maximal assistance
11. Tub, shower	1. Total assistance
Mobility (indoors and outdoors)	
12. Walking-wheelchair	
13. Stairs	

Fig. 1. FIM™ Scale-Functional Independence Measure. Dedicated courses teach proper scoring procedures

Starting from raw scores, Rasch analysis estimates a linear measure for item difficulty and subject ability, making it possible to represent the relationship between the measurement scale and the subjects measured, a relationship that is analogous to that of the familiar "ruler." The ruler associated with the FIM scale is shown in Figure 2. The graphical representation was produced by a widely used Rasch Analysis software (Winsteps.com, Chicago 2002; slightly modified image). The vertical line represents the "independence" variable (increasing upward), along which, on the right side, the items of the FIM scale are lined up.

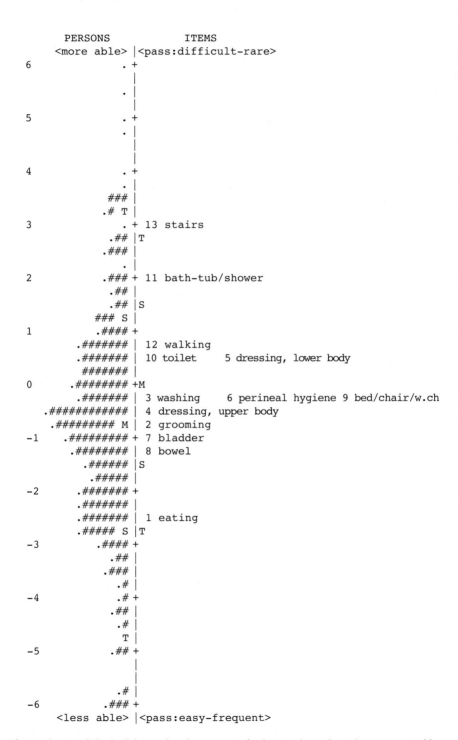

Fig. 2. The Rasch "ruler" shows the alignement of subjects along the ticks represented by the difficulties of the various items on the FIM™ scale

There is a strong analogy with the ticks of a ruler, which is why this graphical representation has been called "Rasch ruler" or "items/persons map." The distances between items are actual interval distances (that is, they are proportional to the quantities the variables are meant to represent). The measurement units (log-odd units, or "logit"), when necessary, can be transformed into more familiar units, such as 0-100 1-step grades. To interpret the picture, it is sufficient to consider the distance between 2 and 1 as equal to the distance between 1 and 0, etc. Each symbol "#" represents the "ability" of the subject (or subjects, in the case of numerous samples; in which case, single subjects are represented by a dot). In this instance, the subjects consist of about 200 patients at discharge from a post-acute inpatient rehabilitation unit (kind permission of So.ge.com srl - Milano, *www.so-ge-com.it*). Conventionally, the measurement scale is centered on "0," which corresponds to the average difficulty across the items. If a subject is located at the same height as an item, this means that the subject's probability of passing the item is 50% [see (Eq. 1)]. To convert logit units to units easier to understand, it is enough to remember that if, for example, the ability measurement of a subject is 0, 1, 2 or 3 logits higher than the difficulty of a certain item is, the probabilities associated with passing that same item are, respectively, 50%, 73%, 88% and 95% (M = average; S = 1 SD; T = 2 SD from the difficulty of the item - shown on the right - or of the ability of subjects, shown on the left).

This representation makes it easy to appreciate at a glance the metric properties of the scale. For example, the scale is "centered" on the ability of the subjects (the indicators of the rules are particularly dense where the ability measurements of the subjects are also dense). The accuracy of the scale is higher for subjects with high and medium-high ability levels (dense "indicators") in comparison to subjects with low ability (rare indicators). There is a certain redundancy of the intermediate difficulty items (e.g., different items with the same difficulty), etc.

Figure 3 illustrates a management application of FIM measurements. Each frame indicates (with full dots) the Rasch difficulty measurement of the 13 FIM-motor items (the other 5, not shown, are cognitive). The measure is estimated starting from the same sample of 200 patients. Shown in Figure 1, for the left panel, and from 200 patient sample from another unit, for the right panel.

The values (linear logit units) on admission and at discharge are given on the ordinate and on the abscissa, respectively. If a measurement tool is stable, then, for any subpopulation, its "indicators" (the items) must remain unchanged in time with respect to their reciprocal difficulty (e.g., "walking" must be permanently more difficult than "eating," etc.). As a result, it is expected that the different values (full dots) stay on the identity line - i.e., within the surrounding 95% confidence levels (continuous lines). The values shown to the right of the identity line indicate greater difficulties at admission, compared with discharge. The names of the items are indicated only if they fall outside the confidence limits. The left panel refers to a rehabilitation inside a rehab-only center (rehab "free-standing facility"). The right panel refers to a unit inside a general hospital. In both cases, it is evident that "walking" seems more difficult on admission to the unit than at discharge. This reflects the fact that on admission, often the raters defer the assessment of walking (to which the minimum score is therefore assigned). Nevertheless, in the in-hospital structure, the phenomenon is much more evident and also involves the item, "transfer bed-chair-wheelchair." This profile seems to be a typical feature of units that admit emergency cases and/or patients from Surgical units of the same hospital, forced to maintain a high turnover. As a result, once in the rehab ward the patient is "forced" to stay in bed at first, not because of his or her intrinsic level of disability, but a) because of clinical instability or b) in order to wait until diagnostic and surgical procedures (blood parameters, wound, healing, X-ray controls) have been completed. Therefore, a low FIM score at admission does not suggest that this unit typically accepts patients with more serious disabilities. It suggests a "cort shifting" process from acute to rehab units.

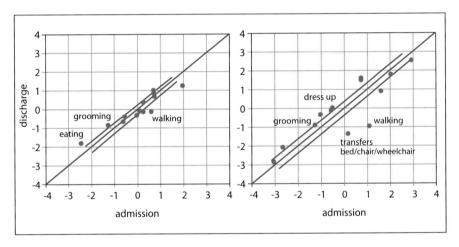

Fig. 3. Application of FIM scale to the study, of appropriateness of admission to neuro-motor rehab units

References

1. WHO (1980) International classification of impairments, disability, and handicaps
2. WHO (2001) International classification of functioning, disability and health, ICF
3. Tesio L (2006) Functional assessment in rehabilitation medicine. Principles methods (in italian). Encycl Med Chir I-26-030-B-10, pp 1-6
4. Tesio L (2003) Functional measures in rehabilitation medicine. Principles and methods (in italian). Giorn Ital Med Riabil 3:25-31
5. Tesio L (1995) Biomedicine between science and assistance. Rehabilitation medicine: the science of assistance (in italian). Il Nuovo areopago 2:80-105
6. Wade DT, Halligan PW (2004) Do biomedical models of illness make for good health care systems? BMJ 329:1398-1401
7. Tesio L (2004) Measurement in clinical vs. biological medicine: the Rasch model as a bridge on a widening gap. J Appl Meas 4:362-366
8. Feinstein AR (1987) Clinimatrics. University Press, Yale
9. Tesio L (2003) Outcome research in rehabilitation: variable construction, trial design and statistical inference. In: Soroker N, Ring H (Eds) Advances in physical and rehabilitation medicine. Monduzzi Editore, Bologna, pp 449-505
10. Tesio L, Granger CV, Fiedler R (1997) A unidimensional pain-disability scale for low back pain syndromes. Pain 69:269-278
11. Tsuji T, Sonoda S, Domen K et al (1995) ADL structure for stroke patients in Japan based on the functional independence measure. Am J Phys Med Rehabil 6:432-438
12. Hajiro T, Nishimura K, Tsukino M et al (1998) Analysis of clinical methods used to evaluate dyspnoea in patients with chronic obstructive pulmonary disease. Am J Respir Crit Care Med 4:1185-1189
13. Criteria Committee NYHA (1964) In: diseases of the heart and blood vessels: nomenclature and criteria for diagnosis. Little Brosn & Co Inc, Boston, MA, p 114
14. Tesio L (2003) Measuring a person's behaviors and perceptions: rasch analysis as a tool for rehabilitation research. J Rehabil Med 35:1-11
15. Tesio L, Franchignoni FP, Battaglia MA, Perucca L (1997) Quality assessment of FIM (functional independence measure) ratings through rasch analysis. Eur Med Phys 33:69-78
16. Rasch G (1960) Probabilistic models for some intelligence and attainment tests. University of Chicago Press
17. Bond TG, Fox CM (2001) Applying the Rasch model: Fundamental measurement in the human sciences. Erlbaum, Mahwah, NJ
18. Wright BD, Stone MH (1979) Best test design. Rasch measurement. MESA Press, Chicago
19. Wright BD, Masters GN (1982) Rating scale analysis. Rasch measurement. MESA Press, Chicago
20. Andrich D (1998) Rasch models for measurement. Sage Publications, Newbury Park, CA
21. Penta M, Arnould C, Decrunayère C (2005) Développer et interpréter une échelle de mesure. Applications du modèle de Rasch. Pierre Margada éditeur, Liège
22. Tesio L, Valsecchi MR, Sala M et al (2002) Level of activity in profound/severe mental retardation (LAPMER): a rasch-derived scale of disability. J Appl Meas 1:50-84

23. Tennant A, Penta M, Tesio L et al (2004) Assessing and adjusting for cross-cultural validity of impairment and activity limitation scales through differential item functioning within the framework of the rasch model: the PRO-ESOR project. Med Care 42:I37-I48
24. Franchignoni FP, Tesio L, Martino MT et al (1998) Length of stay of stroke rehabilitation inpatients: prediction through the functional independence measure. Ann Ist Sup San 4:463-467
25. Tesio L, Granger CV, Perucca L et al (2002) The FIM™ instrument in the United States and Italy: a comparative study. Am J Phys Med Rehabil 81:168-176

Interlude

The "Heart" of Cardiology: an Imaginary Conversation with Bernard Lown*

E. Molinari

While I was preparing this volume with Angelo Compare and Gianfranco Parati and I was also asking some major international experts for a collaboration with several chapters which make up this book, I felt the need to include the human dimension, some relational and emotive aspects in the treatment of the cardiac patient, together with the technical-scientific dimension, produced by research in psycho-cardiology.

My fear was the one expressed by Doris Lessing in "*The four gated city*": "In every situation there is always a key fact, the essence. But generally, it is always another fact, hundreds of facts, to which we pay attention to, those which we examine and discuss. The central fact is generally ignored, or else it is not seen". The joyful encounter with Bernard Lown, has satisfied my need to look for the "key fact", the "heart" of psycho-cardiology.

In this chapter I will introduce an ideal conversation between Bernard Lown and myself, but it can be considered to be real since the answers are derived from his works.

Bernard Lown was born in Lithuania on the 7ᵗʰ of June 1921, and he emigrated with his family in the United States in 1935, avoiding the holocaust (his father was a rabbi). He studied medicine in the University of Maine and after that in the Johns Hopkins University School of Medicine in Baltimore, where he completed his doctorate in 1945 under the supervision of Samuel Levine. After a practicum which was carried out in several hospitals, he worked as a researcher in cardiology, in the Peter Bent Brigham Hospital in Boston, from 1950 to 1953.

---

* Comment by E. Molinari: Bernard Lown has carefully read this interview and he has expressed his kind approval. He acknowledges that it was able to capture the essence of his thinking with regard to medical practice. We both agree that the current focus in the medical field is on providing care and trying "to fix" organs that do not function properly. We also both wish that future efforts will be directed toward patients' healing, and we agree that it requires a psychologically artistic enterprise.

He finished his military service, and he proceeded with his work in the Peter Bent Brigham Hospital and within the Harvard Medical School. From 1956 to 1980, Lown was the director of the Samuel A. Levine Cardiovascular Research Laboratory, from 1956 to 1980, he also formed part of the staff of the Peter Bent Brigham Hospital. Besides he was an assistant within the Harvard School of Public Health, between 1961 and 1967, and he then became an associate professor in the same university. In those years, he coordinated a joint study between the United States and the Soviet Union on sudden death caused by cardiac problems.

Presently, Bernard Lown is a professor emeritus in cardiology in the Harvard School of Public Health, and a senior doctor in the Brigham and Women's Hospital in Boston.

Besides being a doctor who is really dedicated to his patients, he is also interested in health and politics, and he founded the International Physicians for the Prevention of Nuclear War (IPPNW), Amongst his scientific merits, the ones which especially deserve of being mentioned are the introduction of lidocaine as an antiarrhythmic drug and the development of the continuous current defibrillator. Lown has discovered that ventricular fibrillation can be prevented, by regulating the electric shock in order to avoid the vulnerable period in the cardiac cycle, offering a secure method to invert tachycardia; he called this method "cardioversion". His most recent works demonstrate the role of the psychological factors and behaviors in heart regulation.

Dr. Lown was awarded several degrees *ad honorem* and other awards, both in the United States and also abroad; a few of these which are worth mentioning are the George F. Kennan Award, and the Pioneer in Cardiac Pacing and Electrophysiology Award awarded by the North American Society of Pacing and Electrophysiology (nowadays called the Heart Rhythm Society).

■ Conversation:

Molinari - Prof. Lown, you have always paid a lot of attention to your patients' psychological aspects and their influence on the heart. According to you, how important is the psychological dimension in cardiac pathology?

Lown - I believe that the psyche has a great influence on the body and on the heart in particular. This relationship has always been recognised; in fact we can find many expressions which include the heart, such as "to die from a broken heart", "from the bottom of one's heart", "to take something at heart" "to have one's heart in one's mouth". A disturbed psyche can create heart problems, especially through stress. Even experiments which I conducted on animals demonstrate this relationship between stress and cardiac disease... the problems of at least half of my patients are due to stress, not due to organic reasons.

M - Besides stress, which is quite a generic term, what would you consider as being risk factors for cardiac illnesses?

L - Negative emotional states such as anger, fear and resentment can be risk factors for cardiac diseases. In fact these emotional states not only influence the appearance of cardiac illness, but they can make the symptoms worse, decrease the probability of a good prognosis and hinder the healing process. Interpersonal conflicts, public humiliation, threats of separation from the spouse, mourning, failures at work, and sometimes even nightmares… all these are situations which generate psychological tension, which effects the heart.

M - I couldn't agree more! I believe that these repercussions are even more evident in the more serious cases, for example depression…

L - Depression plays a very important role in cardiac illnesses. This is even more evident in the elderly, but it is not limited to them only. Depression alters the body state: it doesn't slow down the rhythms of the organism, but it increases them very much, with devastating effects on the cardiovascular system. One of the causes of depression is a lack of appreciation of one's work, or its loss. Even a carrier which does not progress as one expects or retrocession because of age, can be physiologically and psychologically destructive. Besides, when someone is depressed, they don't feel the necessity to keep fit, and they let themselves go physically (for example by not doing any sport), and this leads to dramatic results on the physique. As we said, in the elderly depression is very widespread, it takes the form of a "subtle boredom" towards life, but it is often difficult to perceive, because of the constant presence of a mask of socialisation. In the case of depression, pleasant activities do not give any joy, not even the contact with the grandchildren.

M - I personally believe that wellbeing cannot only be personal, but it also has to do with the relational dimension; if there isn't a good relationship in the family, for example.

L - Certainly. Dissatisfaction at work, with the spouse or with the children is often expressed physically. I would distinguish between two categories of psychological tension: those provoked by objective conditions, and those which are auto-generated, connected to embedded behavioral models, which sometimes have a genetic basis. An excessive social tension can be the cause of sudden death, as much as smoking and obesity. Obviously, family and work don't only have a negative influence. United families and interesting occupations reduce cardiac risk. Would you like to know another element which diminishes these risks? The presence of domestic animals!

M - What is the influence of getting old, with the end of an occupational activity and the possible condition of solitude?

L - Well, the majority of my patients are quite elderly with a clear physical and quite often psychological deterioration. Many elderly people are overwhelmed by solitude, also because in most cases the persons of their same age are dead.

Pearson observed, to remain in this theme, that wives and husbands tend to die a year from their partner's death. Going to the doctor is also a way to deal with solitude. We often witness excessive medical treatments in the case of the elderly; sometimes this is wanted by their children, who feel guilty for having neglected the elderly parent and who fear his or her death. But the elderly are not scared of dying in itself, as much as the long process of dying.

M - In fact, according to many psychologists the fear of death can be considered to be the basis of all human anguish…

L - In any way, I believe that the thought of dying, of an "external assistance" terrorizes everyone, even religious people. Death is scary also because of the idea of having to deal with the "unknown" completely alone.
For many people, a sudden death is the best way of dying, but I don't agree; a death like this leaves life incomplete, making it more difficult for the people who care for you to adapt to the situation. A sudden death removes the emotive space necessary to come to terms with the loss and the detachment from life; I believe that the most serious aspect is that there is no possibility of putting in order the relationships with others. Nevertheless, in the cases of a "slow" death one struggles most of all to remain attached to one's own identity. I believe, as I have written in many of my works, that dying in little steps, when one is still conscious and lively, gives rise to a trembling anger, which remains unexpressed.

M - Could one summarise what you are saying with the phrase "a good death is facilitated by a good life"?

L - Precisely. Unfortunately, I believe that scientific medicine, with all its depersonalisation, and its therapeutic tenacity, often lengthens and improves life, but it worsens death, taking away the person's dignity.

M - How can the psychological dimension be paid attention to, in a hospital or in a clinic? My impression is that there is a lot of attention on the body of the patients, but that their most intimate needs are not considered.

L - There are many forethoughts, which can be small or big, which can help to take into consideration the psychological factors of the person, facilitating his/her healing process. A good example of this is, is the following consideration; following the suggestions of my mentor, doctor Sameul A. Levine, I started to allocate patients who had suffered from a heart attack, on comfortable armchairs, instead of the usual beds, with real benefits on their health. Cardiac attacks cause thoughts on death, or on invalidity: by forcing someone in bed for long periods of time, as was done in the past, the patients are taken into a situation in which they lose control on the environment, reinforcing the perception of the seriousness of their condition. The use of an armchair allows an active and informed participation of the patient and it takes away the negative signals associated with staying in bed, which in our culture, is the place where we die. When I obtained the funds to create the coronary unit of the Peter Bent Brigham, I made sure that it would be constructed with attention in order to limit factors of psychological stress: lighting which doesn't blind the patients, the radio has to be listened to with the earphones, signs with "do not disturb" on the door during the visits... It was important that it would be a peaceful environment in half-light, in order not to disturb the patients and to help then to relax.

Obviously, the moment in which the psychological aspects are mostly considered, the one regarding the whole person and not only those linked to the illness, is during the medical visit. The interview, and building up the clinical case history are fundamental instruments to carry out the medical profession.

M - Can you tell me something more about why the interview and building up a clinical case history are so important?

L - I am convinced that medicine requires that the most personal details of the emotional life of the patients are known, they have to feel comfortable with the doctor, as if he/she were a close friend.

Even Paracelso, the most important German doctor in the XVI century, used to say that doctors have to use intuition, sensibility and empathy.

By listening carefully to patients from the first visit one can guarantee a correct treatment. During the first visit I spend at least one hour with the patient until I catch a glimpse of the human being who is behind the medical symptoms. I am strongly against the conception of the human being as a machine to repair, which is unfortunately very widespread between doctors nowadays.

The complaints which the patient refers to the doctor, even if they are referred to a specific organ, have a functional aspect and they essentially come from some difficulties in life, which often originate from a tormented heart which a modern instrument cannot pick up, whereas they can be noticed by someone who is used to perceive the subtle signals of a person who is suffering.

An accurate construction of a case history enables to formulate a correct diagnosis in 70% of the cases, and it is the most simple way (but not for this reason a less useful way) amongst all the exams and technologies available.

I believe that a doctor who is moved by the desire to cure and heal, needs to research all the particulars of the emotive life of the person, even those which close friends don't know. An empathic comprehension of the unknown parts of the person don't take away the past's wounds, but they make them more tolerable, and they enable to understand the framework of the pathological situation. The doctors' wisdom is shown when they understand that the origin of the clinical problem, is not in an organ, but in a human being. Doctors don't have to take care only of the symptoms, but also of the difficult aspects of their patients' life. Drugs can only eliminate a symptom, but this can represent itself in a different way; in order to cure and heal someone is necessary to understand their underlying difficulties. As a cardiologist, I would summarise what I have just said in the following phrase: we don't have to try to heal a heart, but a human being who has a heart.

M - As a psychologist I couldn't agree more with you. The relationship with the doctor could be considered as the "first drug" which is given to the patient; the doctor-patient relationship can become the foundation in the treatment process. For this reason, it is very important not to use this relationship badly, by giving the impression that one is in a hurry, or by using superficial and aggressive words.

L - The doctor's words can be a source of great hope and healing but when they are inappropriate, they can harm as much as a physical wound. Illness humiliates one's sense of self, making patients more vulnerable to the doctor's words. An inappropriate word can push patients to desperation and make them imagine the worst; for example a diagnosis which is communicated tactlessly, can cause a tachycardia, or worst. Doctors shouldn't instil uncertainty or fear, but they should explain things properly and reassure. Unfortunately, often doctors use gloomy tones to communicate with patients; sometimes this comes from a wrong preconception according to which in order to be listened to, one has to be unpleasant; at other times, there is the fear of a contention, for which the patient is prepared to the worst; besides if a doctor says that the case is very serious, the majority of the people don't call into question his opinion, the patient and his family become remissive and yielding; on the other hand, if the diagnosis is favourable, the doctor is bombarded with questions.
However the doctors' words have a big potential to cure and heal. In order to heal, they have to mobilize the patients' positive expectations and their trust. Listening to the patients' story is already therapeutic in itself. Even when the pathology is so embedded to make the cure difficult, the doctor's words can help the patients by offering them support; the doctor's attentions help to ease suffering making life more acceptable.

M - But according to you, what are the characteristics, the attitudes and behaviors of a good doctor?

L - I believe that a good doctor cannot do without listening. Listening to the patients carefully from the first time you see them is a guarantee to a correct treatment. It seems banal, but I have the impression that few doctors really listen, also because listening takes time and therefore it costs money. Listening to patients is not only done by using words, but one should also pay attention to the words which are not uttered, those communicated by body language (especially by mimics). As regard to this, one way to establish a different relationship is through touching; therefore a good handshake, before and after the first visit are very important.
The doctor does not have to take away the hope which the patient hangs on to. I always try to keep an optimistic attitude, which communicates trust. People don't only expect words of optimism only with regard to their medical problems, but also to improve their life in general. Doctors' words should be authoritative, but not dogmatic because the patients need certainties; which are not conveyed only by words but also by prescribing many changes in the patients'

lifestyle. Personally I try not to impose any categorical restrictions, I prefer flexibility and moderation because I think that, despite the illness, patients should be pushed to live fully according to their inclinations or predispositions. Once I even gave my consent to one of my patients with serious cardiac problems to go on a fishing holiday in Alaska! And he came back on the ball!

In my opinion, an element which characterises smart doctors is the capacity to recognise their own mistakes, and eventually the availability to apologize with patients who suffered from harm because of them. They shouldn't be oppressed with the idea of being charged; who fears to be charged so much, will be in the end. "Defensive medicine" with the consequent utilisation of a lot of complicated and useless analyses in order not to be accused of negligence, can make patients perceive themselves as a potential enemy. I am convinced that who listens to patients and does not put into practise a depersonalising medicine, is never, or nearly never charged, because negligence is avoided when patients are put in the first place.

I believe that good doctors should establish a good relationship with patients, allowing them to speak about tabooed arguments, which scare them, but which are part of their story, including sex, family problems, fear of death…sometimes, little lies can give great relief and help patients. It isn't always necessary to communicate dramatic news, especially when they are not useful, or when they can worsen the situation!

M - And what about the seriously ill patients, who will inevitably pass away?

L - None of the patients, even if they are dying, should be neglected with more superficial treatments. In the case of chronic and incurable illness, it is often better not to try to prevent death with extraordinary heroic acts, but to prepare for its arrival with good sense and compassion. One does not always have to fix something which is broken!

When I visit terminal patients in hospital, and there is nothing left to do, I turn their pillow on the side which is not humid, so that their head can lie on a fresh and smooth fabric. I always keep in mind the words of a Siberian doctor: "Every time a doctor sees a patient, he/she should feel better after". Sometimes little effort is necessary to make someone feel better.

M - What do you think about the evolution in medicine nowadays?

L - My mentor, Levine, once told me that the golden age in medicine was finishing, because the concern for ill people was being substituted by the concern for illness. In fact, nowadays medicine is very depersonalising, entrenched in the technology of extremely new machines, with the risk of losing the contact with the patient. Medicine is based both on taking care of people and on science. If one takes care of the other without science, there might be good intention, but it is certainly not medicine. On the other hand, if there is science, but one does not take care of patients, medicine is emptied of its thaumaturgical aspect, making it similar to other sciences, such as physics, engineering…these two aspects, taking care of others, and science, complete one another and are essential in medicine. I would like to add that taking care of people is different from healing them; in the first case, one has to do with organs which don't function well, and in the second case with a human being who suffers. I believe that medicine should orient itself towards healing.

Part II
Psychological Treatments in Cardiac Rehabilitation

Chapter 17

The Art of Listening to Cardiac Patient and his Family: the Meanings of Suffering Along Temporal Dimension

A. COMPARE ▪ M. SIMIONI

> "*We never stay within the limits of the present time. We antic-
> ipate what is to come as if it were too slow to arrive, nearly
> to rush it; or else we evoke the past to stop it; it is too much
> in a rush; we are so imprudent to frolic in times which do
> not belong to us and not to think of the only time which
> belongs to us; we are so fatuous to dream about times that
> don't exist any more and to escape the only one which real-
> ly exists without thinking about it. Because usually the pres-
> ent torments us*".
>
> B. Pascal, *Thoughts 1670*

▓ Premise

The word "clinical" origins in ancient epoch: the Greek word klinē. By this was
pointed out the stretched out position of the sick and the lowered physician
to his bedside. Such representation contains the essence of the "clinical method":
the relationship with the patient. This relationship, considered the tools and
the knowledges of the ancient medicine, was personalized, prolonged in the
time, careful and intimate. The whole history of life of a person and the family context in which lived had to be known to take care of the patient. The recent
success of the evidence based treatments in clinical psychology [1] has induced
to minimize the qualitative and clinical aspects of the clinician-patient relationship [2].

The psychological suffering is a way to recover the subjective narrative truths
into the clinical relationship that is the essence of the "clinical method".

Psychological pain is considered to be universal experience. But is it really
true? What is universal, surely, when it comes to pain, is harm – for example,
illness – i.e., the way in which the harm is experienced. But even if universal,
the harm can be interpreted in various ways. This being the case, it would seem
that the experience of suffering results from the circularity between harm and

one's sense of it, or, more precisely, between one's ordinary sense of things and the non-sense which pain causes. Pain in fact defies reason, forcing man to question himself about himself. *Why did this happen to me? What have I done to deserve this?* When we suffer we are strongly induced to look for words that can transform something that does not make sense into something that makes sense to us. We are born into contexts of sense which precede us and give us the language and the terms we need to become interpreters, more or less capable of making sense of our experience and suffering.

We all try to communicate about and take care of our suffering and the suffering of others, but no one can ever relieve one of one's own suffering. In fact, there is nothing that reveals our fragility as individuals, and our uniqueness, as much as pain. Nothing more than pain exposes us to the unpredictability of personal experience. This precisely is the difficulty that we have when we grapple with the concept of pain: it alters the meaning that each one of us attributes to our existence, to our very identity.

Psychological pain, which can affect the cardiac patient following, for example, a heart attack, is often thought to be the result of a *communication disturbance*, i.e., an impossibility patients encounter in expressing what they are going through [3]. In extreme cases, words may be felt to be insufficient for expressing pain [4]. Those who suffer to this extreme degree must consequently do so in silence. It is no coincidence that one is often said to be "paralysed by fear". On the other hand, patients may not be capable of expressing pain because (for example they are delirious, and the words they speak are consequently incapable of conveying the experience of suffering which their pain causes. "Listening to others" is an expression that reminds us of an active attention, in which through listening we try to make out the meaning which unites itself with language and flows from one discourse to another. What kind of listening allows the practitioner to comprehended the sense of the suffering that the patient expresses? How can we develop a relationship that is characterised by trust and provides a therapeutic alliance with patients within the context in which they find themselves [5]? In this chapter we attempt to answer these questions by carefully analysing a crucial aspect of the psychological exchange with the patients who present with psychological suffering, the crucial aspect being: our ability to *listen to pain*. We attempt to accomplish this by exploring two dimensions of listening: the patient's narration and the temporal dimension of time in their accounts.

▪ Listening to the Patient

During sessions with patients who present psychological suffering, there is the *possibility* of an *authentic encounter*. The nature of the authenticity of the encounter lies in the capacity of accepting the "otherness" [6], in the capacity to perceive other persons as they really are, and in the acceptance and confirmation of the other person being *"that specific person, in his or her way of being like that,"* without any limitations. The term "possibility" was highlighted to emphasise the fact that the possibility of an authentic encounter during a session is not to be taken for granted. The encounter with the practitioner can occur in a technical way, with the sheer passage of information, or in a monologue where false conversations take place. These modalities of communication do not utilise fully our aptitude with respect to relationships, and we remain in a stage where the exchange is simulated rather than spontaneous.

The information contained in the patient's medical and clinical case histories is the initial reference from which the "emotive prelude" of the practitioner towards the encounter with the patient is developed. The need to understand, to situate, and also the desire to verify a theoretical and clinical hypothesis, are sometimes present in the practitioner's mind (often, also due to institutional needs), and this can become an obstacle to the relationship. In fact, knowledge in itself, rather than being an instrument of psychological enlightenment, can be applied to a patient's reality without any consideration of its authenticity, becoming in this manner a defence for the practitioner, like a bulwark erected to defend oneself against the unknown [7]. In this case, one might say that the illusion of understanding replaces real comprehension, even though, often, the practitioner experiences a sense of satisfaction. This urgency, which can be a source of reassurance in one confronted with the suffering of others, clashes with the necessity of spontaneous listening, which welcomes the patient's account and embodies a willingness to construct new meanings with him or her. Trying to let go, being active and being receptive constitute a psychological stratagem for the practitioner that is temporal and rhythmic, and within which the relationship between the practitioner and patient can unfold. In order to understand and to create an authentic listening it is necessary to know how to tolerate the frustration and the distress of not knowing something: this involves the possibility of being able to withstand doubts and of being able to wait, without rushing in to find premature answers. Getting to know something does not mean having all the answers beforehand, but "becoming" something different as a consequence of the encounter with the other [8-10].

The mindset that serves as the foundation for creating an authentic encounter [6] views the patient as someone who could *bestow on us something of himself or herself,* which for us would contain the elements of novelty and surprise, i.e., with respect to the ideas, the psychopathological theories and the emotions that characterise our encounter with the patient. The essence of the gift lies, on the one hand, in the fact that it is free, or rather, in the absence of an obligation to reciprocate what has been received, and, on the other hand, in the creation of a relational bond [11]. The experience of having received a gift connects to our nature as social animals, since through giving we create the possibility of establishing a bond with other people. The effect the act of giving has on the relationship has been confirmed by studies of the psychotherapeutic process, which show that *self-disclosure* highly correlates with the therapeutic alliance [12, 13].

The creation of authentic listening, therefore, requires that one be predisposed to the surprise of the unexpected, maintain a curiosity when it comes to things that one does not know, and be able to tolerate the edginess that results from experiencing an absence of certainty and the ensuing disorientation. In the words of the musician, C. Rosen [14], listening to others means keeping oneself on the *"edge of sense, on the edge of the sound of the words"*.

As Rosen's words imply, art overlaps the dimension of authentic listening [15]. Broadly speaking, through their works, artists have always demonstrated an innate aptitude for "exposing themselves at the edge of sense." When Stravinskij was six years old, he encountered a mute peasant who was capable of expressing himself by producing sounds with his arm; he had found a voice that did not involve the vocal cords or mouth, using sound not to create meaning through words, but in a different way. One could say that he attempted to find a sense at the limits and at the edge of sense. Listening authentically to the patient and his pain implies at least the availability, or the desire to experience, listen to and comprehend something new, something unknown. If "understanding" entails comprehending a sense, listening[1] entails being open to a *possible sense*, one that may not be immediately accessible.

Concerning this border zone, between the said and the not-yet-said, Rober [16] focuses on patient's hesitation and proposes to use it as a metaphor to give meaning to some nonverbal utterances of patients in such a way that spaces is opened up in a respectful way for as yet-untold stories.

By considering the authentic encounter with the patient as a moment in which he or she can bestow upon us something of theirs, we are encouraged to consider the theme of care in the act of giving. An exploration of this theme emphasises the importance of the dimension of silence and the creative dimension that is part of the act of self-expression.

Patient's and Clinician's Silences

During sessions with patients, it is important that practitioners predispose themselves to listening to the act of giving. The dimension of care is inseparable from listening and is conveyed through the ability to understand and welcome what the patient has to say. This is also expressed in the etymology of the term care - còera, còira, quia cor urat: warmth, stimulation of the heart. Authentic listening warms the heart and stimulates the act of giving, thereby also stimulating the growth of a relationship. This has to do with recognizing the internal rhythm in one's encounters with patients, the "weaving" between the sounds and the intervals, and it involves training our listening to apprehend what sometimes words cannot convey but which interludes of silence can reveal.

Although silence is often defined negatively, as emptiness or the absence of something, or a gap that needs to be filled [17], from another point of view, silence, both on the part of the patient and the practitioner, is an integral part of the dialogue; it represents another modality of expression, capable of conveying rich, underlying meaning [18]. The following clinical report of Stephan's case demonstrates the specific qualities silence conveys.

---

[1] Listening means, "lending one's ear." The verb *to listen* implies both the use of a sensory organ, the ear, *auris* - a word that forms the first part of the verb, *auscultare* or "lending one's ear" - and also one's intention and attention

Stephan entered the room and quickly went toward the chair after a quick handshake while looking downward. His clinical file was in front of me: he was 42 years old and he had had a heart attack. He was in the intensive therapy unit after having received urgent medical aid. He was married and had an eight-year-old daughter. A session with a practitioner had been requested by the cardiologist in charge of the rehabilitation unit; with the following indication, "Routine psychological visit. Possible altered moods".

Stephan had his arms crossed. *"Why am I here?"* *"Why do I have to be visited?"* Stephan greeted me with these questions. The tone of his voice was firm, decisive, and I could see resentment in his eyes.
"When will they discharge me? Do you know anything about this?"
"Who is waiting for you at home?" I asked him.
"My life. The life which this illness wants to take away from me", he answered. There was silence. Stephan looked away, staring out the window. Outside was a typical wintry scene, branches covered in snow, which had just fallen. Stephan's hands were clutching his forearms, as if he were looking for a hug or grasping to contain his emotions which otherwise might soon pour out and overwhelm him. His eyes began to water and with a trembling voice he said, *"Its not right! I don't deserve this"*.
The silence of his voice was substituted by other words, his tears. Stephan was a company director. He had reached this position only after a great deal of effort and sacrifice in terms of quality time with his wife and daughter. He had started his career with only a secondary school diploma.
"Do you understand that I will be downgraded? What will they think of me?" he added in tears.
The pain overtook him, and, during the remainder of the session, he continued to cry. He was in pain and disoriented as a result of the rage and resentment he felt toward the "broken up time" and his own "impotence" in the face of an event he wanted to get rid of. The patient's face and the his stare struck me: there was an intense sadness and emptiness in his light blue eyes, which had changed from being transparent and lively, to being flooded with tears. His eyes and his tears marked his words, accompanying the memories from which Stephan's narration had started. This first impression was very intense and it immediately qualified the emotive tone of my listening.

Paying attention to the undertones of the discourse allows us to appreciate the power that the practitioner's silence can have in the encounter with the patient [7, 15]:
- Listening as an effort to *understand:* according to this perspective, silence is not a passive attitude, a *giving up of words*. Instead, it makes itself felt as a tension with respect to understanding the interlocutor. This "tension" results from the attitude intrinsic to authentic listening, which makes itself felt as an attempt to overcome the natural extraneousness the interlocutor provokes.

- Listening as a *"sound box"*: the practitioner's silence can become a "sound box" of the patient's words. It is a silence that first of all predisposes the patient to a dialogue with himself or herself, and secondly predisposes the patient to a dialogue with the practitioner.
- Listening to *countertransference:* the patient's comprehension not only occurs through listening to his or her words and silences, but also from the emotive reactions of the practitioner. Anger, scepticism, detachment, compassion, tenderness are all emotions which can reveal things about the patient's way of being.

Silence can be utilised by patients to represent and express pain. The patient's silence manifests itself in different ways. Tears are one way of talking in silence; however, unlike words, crying is distinguished by its "eruptiveness, violence, being unarticulated" [19], and for this reason, it seems far removed from reason. Since tears are words of silence, they are able to communicate what cannot be said using words. As the musician and art historian, Jean-Loup Charvet [20], stated: *"Tears reveal what man is silent about, they are the words of silence"*. As can be seen in Stephan's case, crying represents a liberating moment for someone closed up inside himself, who cannot find a way in words of communicating the experience of distress. The patient's tears reveal to the practitioner the patient's authentic emotions, which are offered in what might otherwise appear to be a desert in the communicative context [21]. If shedding tears is a way of creating a dialogue in moments of silence, the absence of tears might appear to be, within the context of suffering, a clear signal of the drama occurring inside the patient of the impossibility of communicating. In some conditions of psychological suffering, expressing oneself by crying appears to be nearly impossible. For example, in depression one is often confronted with the experience of "not being able to cry" [22]: a downright silence of the body.

The Inherent Acknowledgement in Listening

The term *acknowledgement* signifies "according/conceding a determined status" to something or someone. According to the "subjective idealism" postulated by George Berkeley [23], the existence of objects is subordinate to their being perceived. As Hillman [24] affirms, man always asks the same question: "Here I am, right in front of your eyes, can't you see me?" Patients are, in fact, always "other" from the practitioner: because of the difference in age, social condition, education, gender and the way in which they express themselves, and experience their emotions and life events. As Taylor [25] states, an adequate acknowledgment is an essential human need. *Everyone* needs to be acknowledged for his or her *identity*, which is unique. The process of acknowledgment might therefore be considered as being a differentiation of the capacity to "give meaning" which is highly specialized.

Acknowledging oneself and having others acknowledge one's identity is a need that easily can be fulfilled under conditions of well-being and health. In illness and suffering, however, there is a sort of "absence of acknowledgement" of one's body and of oneself: what the person once was in a way does not exist anymore, and the sick individual does not recognise his or her new identity. This difficulty in recognising oneself also prevents being oneself both with respect to oneself and others. Consequently, there is the experience of the absence of acknowledgment, which results in a weakened self and a weakened possibility of expressing one's suffering.

The encounter with the practitioner nonetheless presents itself as a space in which the "dialogical risk" [6] can be present. In other words, the psychological session can still create a space where an authentic encounter takes place, thereby transcending the conventions of day-to-day conversations. Alternatively, it can be the place par excellence for a dialogic checkmate, where patient and practitioner do not manage to establish a therapeutic alliance. This barbed wire separating the patient from the practitioner often is created because the professional adopts a language that is too technical, reacts in ways that undermine the trust of the patient, and/or because the practitioner fails to convey a willingness to accompany the patient in the exploration and understanding of his/her emotions.

▪ Listening to the Semantic Dimension in Narratives

When we talk about ourselves, or narrate our psychological suffering, we have to invent ourselves. Since pain, even in its essential need to be expressed, does not find a specific and subjective correspondence in the words that represent it [4], it is necessary to create a new language. At the foundation of this act of creation, in the narration of one's suffering, there is a mysterious interplay between discovery and invention, which also characterises artistic creation. In a manner similar to artistic creation, providing a narrative about oneself answers the need of being reborn [26]. Emotions trigger and colour discourse, and they "thaw" concepts. Discourse is the context within which the narration is realised, the progress, or rather, movement, from one word to the other that characterises the act of providing a narrative about oneself.

In order to comprehend why "narrating oneself," i.e., the act of narrating one's own story, which is a creative act, it is helpful to consider the reflections of great artists. In the view of Mikhail Bulgakov, for example, art and narration have always tried to *"inscribe in the world of awareness their shadows and their mysteries, in this world of light which is so pure to be blinding at times"* [27]. In order to represent the world with all its shadows, the artist has to expose himself or herself, as Baudelaire, affirms, in a *"proud ostentation of themsel[ves]"* [28]. Kafka's [29] narration transforms reality into a "dreamy interior life" of the writer, in which the narration exists as an "assault to limitation" and, consequently, does not tend to confirm the facts. By utilising the artistic metaphor, one could say that patients, similar to artists in relation to their need to express their own suffering, also render a proud presentation of themselves in which their narrative exists as an "assault to limitation" – one that goes beyond the existing categories to try to find new ones in an effort to reveal the internal experience.

The capacity and the inclination to construct a story about one's life is a necessity that characterises the human being [30]. The creation of maps of knowledge and the construction of models are both expressions of this necessity, and attempts to fill with meaning the life experiences which, because of their dramatic nature – as, for example, in a sudden illness – result in confusion and mystery [31, 32].

Through the personal narration, the story of the patient's suffering comes to life. The body and history, in art as in life, are related in an indissoluble and multiform reality. As exemplified by some artistic references, every story embodies something and every body has its own story. Usually in literature, the bodies are *inside* the stories. Walt Whitman, the body poet, invites his readers to come close to him: *"Touch me, rest the palm of your hand on my body while I pass by. Do not be scared of my body"* [33]. Every novel tells a story, and, in the figurative arts, the story is suggested by a body. The story is *in the body*. In a painting, or sculpture, the opposite occurs, as intimated by Francis Bacon, who said *"I would like that my paintings appeared to be as if human beings had passed over them, leaving a trail of mnemonic traces of past events"* [34]. Thus, there are bodies in stories and stories in bodies. One of the greatest writers of the 1900s, Kundera [35], pointed out that the great knowledge of modernity, that which gives rise to its multifaceted interweaving, can be found precisely in narration. According to Kundera, narration represents the way in which the truth is expressed: like art, it does not give any certainties. The truth, he states, has *"ruffled borders"*, and just as *"nobody can say where a colour starts and where it finishes in the iris,"* so, too, *"nobody can say, in our life interwoven with shadow, where the light ends and where darkness begins"* [35]. Narration is the knowledge of uncertainty, given in a language composed of forms and figures that have an interrogative format. There is an intense bond between narration and narrator expressed in a story. This is hardly surprising given that a story is susceptible to different narrative forms: comedy or tragedy, subtle humor or drama, all represent different ways in which a story can develop. As W. Allen points out in one of his recent films [36], the narrative form of a story depends on the perspective of the narrator.

Semantics and Narrative

The coordinates of the meaning of psychological pain consequent to a serious and sudden illness, such as a heart attack, can be traced back to the patient's narrative [31, 37]. By analyzing the patient's narrative about his or her illness, it is possible to reconstruct the salient semantic dimensions through which the patient structures his or her personal identity, beginning with the context in which the patient belongs [38]. Inside this point of view, the constructivist perspective [39] which represents a recent evolution of the Milan Approach in the family therapy field [40], offers a useful contribution in the comprehension of the semantics of psychological suffering. Constructionism emphasises the analysis of the relational context and the position the patient has adopted. Within this epistemology, much importance has been given the semantic aspects as conceptualised by Ugazio [41] in his theoretical model of "semantic polarities". According to this model, individuals establish a relationship with others and define themselves on the basis of the particular meanings found within their context of reference. Within the model, the analysis of the position adopted by patient holds a central role: the family does not exist if not as a com-position of individuals. Indeed, the clinical observation of the family reveals how everyone, including patients, view positions and relational modalities, which are very different for each member of their family. Birth in a particular family and in a particular culture, like stories, which are also "com-positions", delimits the possible roles individuals can play.

A semantic analysis of the narrative of patients with a Type-A personality, for example, might reveal these patients to be identified with what has been characterised as the "semantic of power" [41]. That is, in the patient's relationships there is an emphasis on the "winner/loser" semantic dimension, according to which the winners have control over themselves and others, whereas the losers are passive and at the mercy of the tyranny of others.

The authentic encounter with the practitioner can therefore be seen as the start of a relationship that can help the patient to tell another story. In the hermeneutic perspective, therapeutic change is represented by the diologic creation through dialog of a new narrative. Throughout the evolution of the conversation between patient and practitioner, a new narrative, characterised by "stories-which-haven't-yet-been-told" is mutually created. Whereas the experience cannot be modified, the response to the drama and the tragedy in the story can be adapted by a reinterpretation of the meaning of the events [39] and by the reconstruction of a new story [42].

Relational Semantics and Psychological Suffering

Cardiac illness is a test for the people who are affected with it and also for the people who "embody" their context: their partners and relatives. It affects the relationships within the family system and tests the family's adaptive processes. As demonstrated by a study of a 54-year-old male heart attack victim (utilising Olson's [43] Circumflex Model of Systems), the family, which, in this case, included a wife and children, is subjected to changes along the dimensions both of cohesion and flexibility (Fig. 1). During the first weeks following the cardiac event the family relationships can become chaotically enmeshed, due to an elevated emotional involvement and a relaxed definition of rules.

Within this perspective the concept of *patient* expands and contracts. Because individuals belong to a network of relationships (family, friends and community), they do not have clear and rigid boundaries making interpersonal relationships impermeable to their health status. For this reason, the patient is not the only one who suffers from the illness and pain connected to the illness. The entire system of relationships belonging to the patient is affected. Moreover recently results from

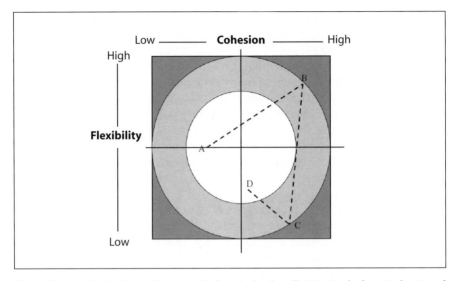

Fig. 1. Changes in the family before and after the husband's IMA (A: before; B: the 1st and 2nd weeks; C: the 8th week; D: the family at present)

a series of published studies suggest there may be links between self reported coping styles and physical health; in detail repressive coping style seems to be linked with adult attachment style and physical health. The implications of these findings for family relationships and clinical practice are been explored [44].

Can a relationship, be it in a family or in a couple, be a resource in the care giving of seriously ill patients? By paying attention to the narrations the patients provide about themselves and their illness, practitioners can gain access to the meaning that the pathology has within the context where the patients belong [31, 37]. In particular, when we listen without "anticipating" with theoretical models of reference, the families' own model of significance relative to the nature of health and the relationship between health and illness emerges. The patients and their families are themselves models relative to how to deal with treatment and illness, and these models guide them in understanding why they got sick, what they have to do to heal and what their roles - and the roles of their families and professional caretakers - are in the process of healing. Patients' queries about their illness, especially if it is sudden, as in the case of a heart attack, allow them to express what has been defined as the "family myth" [45] - that is, the narrative structure in which the family tries to give an answer the fundamental questions about life and death. Therefore the myth defines the sexual roles, and the affective, social and psychological functions that each member of the family carries out. The myth about health, which collectively the family constructs and they all share, helps us understand how the family deals with health/illness. It also helps us understand the relational modalities enacted between the family members who are taking care of the patient.

Clinical work with the families of heart attack patients has identified three typical modalities in the narratives: *sharing, adhesion* and *tragedy* [46]. The need to share the sorrow, the pain and the same illness transforms the illness into a challenge, which demonstrates how important a resource the family can be a resource in the treatment. In families where the sharing modality prevails, there is the possibility of "shifting" part of the sorrow and pain the patients feel onto those close to them, so that the patients feel that they are also experiencing the sorrow and pain.[2] A second modality is the adhesion to common values, for example, faith or other values that bind the family members either to one another, or to the value given to life. In these families, those who suffer feel and know (even though they may not feel it in their body or in their mind) that they believe in the same values. A metaphor that can be used for such families is one in which they are holding out their hands to the same point. In other families, the illness is experienced as a tragedy: it does not connect in the least bit to health but it is totally divided from it. Two different scenarios can develop as a consequence: the absence of sorrow and pain on the one hand; and the damnation of pain on the other. The feeling is catastrophic and nothing manages to heal the relationships between the family members. In these families, the mental pain connected to the cardiac illness becomes unmentionable and impossible to face.

A familial micro-context relevant to the adult patient is represented by the couple relationship, which, as seen in the work John Ruiz and colleagues [47], can exert a significant influence on the psychological condition of the cardiac patient. In order to understand whether the couple relationship of the couple can be a resource in the patient's treatment, it is important to identify the thematic nuclei around which the representations of the couple are organised. According to some authors [46, 48], three thematic nuclei can be identified: *normalisation, disablement* and *nemesis*. The normalisation of an illness can be expressed through a form of denial. This prevents the patient from integrating the illness present in his or her body into the relationship with others and, consequently, it prevents the suffering from being expressed in the form of a dialogue. The body is viewed as a machine, in which everything worked efficiently previously, irrespective of any effort or challenge. This is why the discovery of an illness is accompanied by the feeling of disbelief and panic. One views oneself as a "machine that has broken down," leaving one "half human". Finally, the cardiac illness can been viewed as a "nemesis," as in the olden times, requiring penance and resulting in feelings of guilt.

In a nutshell, taking care of the medical and the psychological aspects of cardiac illness also entails listening to the manner in which the patients represent their illness, as given by their family's point of view with respect to illness, and, in particular, by the conjugal couple's point of view. This is necessary in order to understand whether (and how) the bond that exists among family members supports the healing process or colludes with denial and avoidance.

---

[2] This could be defined as being an experience that is "common" to others, in which there is a shared boundary that creates the possibility of sympathizing with others

Semantics of Suffering and the Relationship with the Practitioner

Families develop mythical representations of health/illness, and these representations also involve professionals, who are viewed by the family in a particular manner [46]. The family can establish with the professional an *exclusively exploitive relationship,* in which the family takes charge of the healing process, and the doctor or practitioner are considered "bureaucratic objects". Alternatively, a member of the family can form a "coalition" with the professional in charge and integrate with the care-providing team, establishing the central role in the treatment. A third type of exploitive relationship takes place when the doctor or the practitioner is looked upon as a saviour, who is available and welcoming in every circumstance. In this case, the relationship with the caregiver serves as a surrogate for what is missing in the family relationships.

The relationship established between the patient, the family and the caregiver affects the temporal dimension the illness adopts. In the narration the family provides about the relationship with the caregivers, temporality can be represented in one of two different ways: either as an *impeding past,* laden with unresolved problems and personal resentment; or as a *desperate focus on the present and on everyday life,* in which the loss of what is familiar is unthinkable. In the first temporal form, the family transfers onto the caregiver the denial of memory: memories are held back because they are too dangerous and painful. In this manner the exploitive relationship is characterised by indifference-distance toward the caregiver. As a result, professional caregivers and the services they provide, quite apart from the competencies of the caregivers, become part of the family's logic and serve only to periodically remove the heaviness that the illness entails. With the second form of temporality (*desperate focus on the present and on everyday life*), the family transfers onto professionals and the services they provide a feeling of anguish-ruin, in which there is no hope and no future. The family becomes obsessed with the daily tasks required by the illness and asks the caregivers to participate in this obsessive ceremony. The caregivers are invested with feelings of belittling, and they are perceived as not being competent in their handling of the illness. They are also often viewed as dangerous and intolerable (just as the family views the possibility of death).

◼ Listening to the Temporal Dimension

Subjective Time and Existential Time

The experience that is created in the moment in which there is the encounter between practitioners and their patients occurs inside a dimension that represents the necessary framework within which the narration and the welcoming of the patients' stories takes place: the temporal dimension.

From the psychological point of view, the perception of time is a subjective phenomenon, strictly dependent on factors such as the culture of the subjects, their personality and also their psychological condition. In fact, every psychopathological condition has its specific temporal characterisation, which is more or less impaired, depending on the severity of the clinical condition. For example, depressed patients live in suspended and dilated time, which never passes; they expect something vaguely and at the same time they are incapable of waiting, which serves as the source of their sense of emptiness and distress [22, 49, 50]. In the case of the psychosis, on the other hand, there is a total alienation from the temporal dimension, which does not allow the representation of time in a continuous and unitary manner as the framework of thoughts and memories. Psychotic patients are trapped in fragmented time, and, since they do not project towards the future, they remain fixated in a circular and repetitive movement of the present moment [51].

The capacity to perceive and represent the passing of time is strictly linked to the possibility of individuals to comprehend and narrate (to themselves and to others) their own story. The development of a unique sense of self that is continuous and long-lasting, and the construction of an identity capable of situating itself in the present, are indispensable for human beings if they are to attribute meaning to time in their lives. The meaning that is conferred by patients to their own subjective time (on the basis of their story, their expectations, the significant relationships they have established and all their significant life events) can be considered the outcome of a complex psychological elaboration. The effort of this elaboration enriches subjective time with existential and deep relational aspects [52]. The character of the subjectivity given to time is therefore not only an expression of the human capacity to perceive and represent an "objective" physical time, it is an expression of an aspect that permits individuals to comprehend in which moments of their own story they can place themselves and enter into a relationship with the time of other people. If subjects acknowledge that there is a time to study, to work, to get married and to have children, and that there is also a time to get older and to die, it is reasonable to assume that these same subjects construct part of their identity on the basis of the perception of *adequacy* with respect to these dimensions. Living in synchrony with others, representing oneself and telling a life story that is integrated with that of other people, provides the basis for the construction of a relational identity.

The plasticity of subjective time enables healthy individuals to feel that they are within a present time that is coherent with their expectations, a time which can go by slowly or quickly, but which guarantees continuity with respect to the perception of their existence. A historical identity is constructed within this continuity, and is made up of past times and future times, which can be described or imagined, and it is also made up of times lived and perceived within significant relationships. In the words of Ugazio [40], a story that is told, which is a narration within a temporal and relational framework of the story that is lived, represents the pivotal point of the construction of personal identity.

The *Temporal Breakdown*: when Pathology Causes Discontinuity in the Existential Temporal Dimension

Temporal perception is at risk of being profoundly altered in people who have to deal with events that partially or completely modify their perspective of life. Sudden cardiac illness, as well as some other pathologies which can put an individual's sense of continuity at risk, confront the subjects with the necessity of redefining the meaning of their present time, as well as their past and future times. When one is healthy, the present time remains mostly implicit, experienced and understood between a past and a future time; however, when one is ill, the present time becomes the predominant focus. The transition from something conceptualised implicitly to that which is explicit is problematic, because it is in the nature of the present to be a boundary that cannot extend beyond the two temporal dimensions of past and future, which last for specific periods. When someone discovers that he or she is ill, suddenly time is experienced predominantly in the present, subjectively and existentially, and the person is forced to rethink and reposition him or herself along the temporal axis. Finding oneself in a situation in which the prevalent perception is that of not having more time at one's disposal, but having less time than one had imagined, creates a great deal of distress, in which time, like a thread which suddenly gets all tangled up, appears to be uncertain and forced, or worse, interrupted.

The concept of *"temporal breakdown"* is a metaphor that symbolises what patients talk about when they try to express their feelings about their illness and the loss of their future prospects. Especially if the subjects are young, the thought of a sudden shortening of their lifetime becomes extremely heavy and burdensome. This can result in a complete halt in thoughts about their future, and a reorganisation of their existence based on the present moment, which appears to be decontestualised with respect to their subjective story. Time breaks down because the thoughts projected into the future are replaced by ones linked to the illness and to the limitations it entails, forcing the subjects to focus on the present and depriving them of their temporality. In the moment of the diagnosis, or during the beginning of the illness, when the first symptoms appear, the mind becomes rigid and bi-dimensional, like a canvas on which only one photo of the life of the patient can be projected: the one which represents actual time.

The overlap of present and alleged future times (growing old and dying) to time perceived as current (being healthy, alive and fertile) breaks the rules which lie at the basis of temporal chronology, compromising the possibility of sharing these times. Subjective times, constructed by individuals within interpersonal relationships, are in fact modified by illness, generating in them a sense of suddenly having found themselves "outside of time," in a condition of solitude which cannot be communicated. This temporal displacement is expressed by the difficulty in sharing feelings and emotions. The temporal breakdown forces individuals into "another time," characterised by solitude and uncertainty, as though they were suspended in a life that cannot be "lived" or shared because it is devoid of any dimensionality.

Finding oneself with an uncertain future and one which is potentially much shorter that one had imagined, also conditions the perception of past times, making them more or less significant on the basis of the story of the individual. In fact, an increase in the awareness of the subjective perception of time passing by causes the memories and past experiences to become more vivid, as if to try and balance out the presumed loss of future time with an increased awareness of the time which has passed. Conversely, the distress associated with the temporal breakdown can be so overwhelming that it obscures the entire existential temporal dimension, preventing individuals from perceiving their pasts as well as their futures. In this situation, life experiences are often judged to be useless and incapable of informing the present moment, which appears devoid of meaning.

The temporal discontinuity the subject feels, brought about by the sudden pathology, makes it difficult to rally the resources necessary for dealing with the distress and sense of loss linked to the illness. The paradox represented by the fact that the present time is also the only one void of duration forces both the sick individual and the caregiver into a highly ambivalent position: while the resources of the subject must be fortified within this time which is in continuous movement, it is also within this time that the individual is the most aware of the changes and limitations imposed by the illness.

The Present Time as a Resource in the Psychological Session

Working with patients who are affected by a severe and/or chronic organic pathology often entails that the practitioner works in a context where there is not an explicit request for help. Even though the psychological repercussions of the illness are extensive, they remain in the background, or they tend to be underestimated, because the risk of losing one's life occupies the center of the patient's attention. The fear of dying or of being disabled puts the individual in a situation of extreme emotional vulnerability, and amplifies the sensation of extraneousness with respect to one's story. Experiencing the precariousness of one's existence and marking one's rhythm of life according to the outcome of the treatment and interventions forces the subject always to remain fixated on the present time, that is a sickness time, and unable to extend themselves.

The ability to define this emotional vulnerability in nonclinical or technical language, without mentioning mood or anxiety disorders, which add another pathology to a clinical picture already heavily laden, requires a good relationship with the patient, who as a result, has positive feelings about the psychological intervention. By focusing on existential time and working on the meaning that the present time acquires, the practitioner helps the patient share feelings and feel less overwhelmed by the discontinuity and alienation of his or her condition.

The metaphor that portrays listening as an artistic form can help us understand the value of focusing on the meaning of the present time. Artistic geniuses often express a paradoxical essence: while they "paint" nothingness and death with great precision, their representation has something lively in it, something which tones and cheers up the soul. What is the origin of this paradox? If we think of life as an unstoppable flow that is constantly changing, it is very hard to conceptualise it using logical and theoretical language. The life that is experienced, which always risks escaping into nothingness, is grasped by artists in present time. They express themselves in a complex way, in an intrigue of differences and in a richness which also contains our weakness and our incapacity to say everything or to put the fragments of our experience of reality together to form a totality. We are aware that we must die: we get to know about it habitually, but not through our experience and consciousness. When do we gain a real awareness about death, or rather *our* death? When it barges in on our lives in the form of an illness, which always follows us, like an "absurd habit," as Cesare Pavese [53] would say. Art proposes this encounter with death, and does so very intensely, with freely expressed authentic emotion. For example, every novel, every poem starts with an inexorable measure of time: "when" proposes in this way a temporality which includes becoming and the end, not as abstract terms, but as something that is interwoven in life itself and which makes us ask ourselves what sense and what meaning the present time has for us [54].

The psychological work with the cardiac patient takes place when the present moment, which was previously implicit and contained between past and future, becomes explicit. Being in the present, commonly perceived as something negative during illness, can be transformed into a dimension that is more acceptable, thanks to the philosopher E. Bloch's conceptualization of the present as "not-yet-come-into-being" [55]. What has not yet come into being, the anticipation of the future, and the movement towards it, represents the starting point of any possibility. In the "not" there is a concentration of hope, which cannot be precisely defined. The impulse toward change can be found in the experience of time, which results in being "not past and not future." To be able to view present time not only as a time during which one is ill, and, consequently, suspended and disconnected from one's own story, but as a time in which "healing has not yet taken place," which can be examined and modified, permits the creation of the space necessary for the recovery of a thought process that exists in developmental time. The psychological session, which occurs during the present and in limited time, offers the possibility of dealing with the same type of temporal experience as occurs in illness, only in a shared and structured environment. In the same type of temporal experience as that which the patient encounters in his or her illness, i.e., during the counseling session, which is present and limited, the patient's past stories and fantasies with respect to the future can be listened to. In the present - which is devoid of extensions - the means of disentangling the thread of time experienced by the ill patient can be found; and the wound caused by the experience of discontinuity, which the psychological pain connected to the illness provoked, can be healed.

The capacity of the therapist to work in "ambiguous" and undetermined time, while also realizing logical leaps in another temporal dimension, provides the patient with the possibility of sharing the experience of the "temporal breakdown" he or she is going through. Stephan's session with the practitioner discussed previously in this chapter provides a good illustration of the various phases that can occur during a psychological intervention with a cardiac patient.

Typically, the patient poses questions about the present time ("Why am I here? Why do I have to be visited? When are they going to discharge me? Do you know anything about this?"), and he or she maintains an attitude of coyness and anger toward whomever presents themselves. The practitioner helps create a shift in the temporal dimension that enables the patient to reconnect the present time - that dominated by illness - which up until now has been devoid of ties to the past and future. This unexpected shift from meaning strictly linked to the illness ("Who is waiting for you at home?") communicates the availability on the part of the practitioner to listen to the patient's suffering, because it offers the possibility of returning to the network of relationships in which the patient belonged before the illness. The exit from present time forces the patient's narration to develop and connects it with the patient's emotions. The element of surprise introduced by the question, which does not seem connected with the conversational context and is far removed from the request of the diagnostic evaluation, opens the flow of emotions in an individual whose identity was deeply altered as a result of seeing time "break down" as a result of illness.

A complex and creative operation takes place when the link to the present time is transformed into a resource, and the psychological work with the cardiac patient plays an important role in this process. The *possibility* of a therapeutic relationship based on *authentic listening* can unlock the different meanings the present time can take on. Time can be recreated, shared and divided, within the context of the psychological session, in a present time that reconnects past and future in a new narrative plot – one which welcomes the new meaning of psychological suffering.

■ Conclusion

In the spirit of the artistic and clinical essence which inspired this chapter, one can say that, similarly to what Gregory Bateson, an anthropologist deeply interested in the nature of man has said, and similar also to what philosopher and literary critic Michail Bachtin has said, that the authentic listening to a patient's suffering requires an "ecologic" [56] and "polyphonic" [57] point of view if one is to figure out the temporal and semantic aspects of its narration.

In order to create an authentic listening of patients and their suffering, practitioners are therefore required to move from a simple system to a complex system considering the relationship context where the psychological pain is expressed [58] (Tabella 1). In this more complex system, authentic listening is: a) *dynamic*, based on the plurality of perspectives (vs. static, based on a single perspective); b) *active*, based on the construction of reality (vs. passive, based on the mirroring of reality); c) *approximate*, entailing that unexpected events be evaluated positively (vs. "in control," where unexpected events are evaluated negatively), d) *have as their purpose the goal of exploring possible worlds* (vs. objective); and, finally, e) entail that *emotions play a central role* (vs. requiring that emotions be neutralised).

Table 1. Simple system vs Complex system

The simple system	The complex system
a. The same things have the same meaning	a. The same things have different meanings
b. Similar implicit premises	b. Different implicit premises
c. What we take for granted (framework) helps us to communicate	c. What we take for granted (framework) does not allow us to communicate
d. First degree control: knowing how to predict possible reactions	d. Second degree control: knowing how to transform unexpected reactions into knowledge
e. Neutralization of emotions	e. Emotions play a central part

We would like to conclude with the musical image of Vladimir Jankélévitch, according to which authentic listening is "…what allows us to listen to another voice, which is spoken in another language: a voice which comes from somewhere else… to discover *the most secret music out of all music*" [59].

■ References

1. Sanderson WC (2003) Why empirically supported psychological treatments are important. Behav Modif 27:290-299
2. Herbert JD (2003) The science and practice of empirically supported treatments. Behav Modif 27:412-430
3. Borgna E (2000) Noi siamo un colloquio. Feltrinelli, Milan [trad. We are a conversation]
4. Balsamo M (2000) Soggetti al delirio. Elaborazioni del dolore e percorsi della cura. Franco Angeli, Milan [trad. Subjects to the delirium. Elaborations of the pain and path of the care]
5. Horvarth A, Luborsky L (1993) The role of the therapeutic alliance in psychotherapy. J Consult Clin Psychol 61:561-573
6. Buber M (2002) Between man and man. Routledge, London, New York
7. Doherty WJ (1995) Soul-searching: why psychotherapy must promote moral responsibility. Basic Book, New York
8. Bollas C (1995) Cracking up. Routledge, London
9. Ceruti M, Preta L (1990) Che cos'è la conoscenza. Laterza, Bari [trad. What the knowledge is]
10. Ceruti M (1994) Constraint and possibilities: The evolution of knowledge and knowledge of evolution. Gordon and Breach Publishers, Amsterdam
11. Godbout JT, Caillé A (1998) The world of the gift. Mc Gill-Queen's Up, Montreal
12. Safran JD, Muran JC (2000) Negotiating the therapeutic alliance: A relational treatment guide. Guilford Press, New York
13. Derlega VJ, Mettz S, Petronio S, Margulls ST (1993) Self-disclosure. Sage, Newbury Park, CA
14. Rosen C (1998) Aux confins du sens - Propos sur la musique. Seuil, Paris [trad. At the edge of the sense-intention on the music]

15. Nancy JL (2002) Listening. Éditions Galilée, Paris
16. Rober P (2002) Some hypothesis about hesitation and their nonverbal expression in family therapy practice. J Fam Ther 4:187-204
17. Dentone A, Bracco M (2000) Dialogo, silenzio e empatia. Bastoni, Foggia [trad. Dialogue, silence and empathy]
18. Zeligs MA (1960) The psychology of silence. Its role in transference, counter transference and the psychanalytic process. J Am Psychoanal Ass 9:7-43
19. Plessner H (1979) Laughing and crying: a study of the limits of human behavior. Northwestern University Press, Northwestern
20. Charvet JL (2001) The eloquence of the tears. Medusa, Milan
21. Herbette G, Rimé B (2004) Verbalization of emotion in chronic pain: patients and their psychological adjustment. J Health Psychol 9:661-676
22. Bschor T (2004) Time experience and time judgement in major depression, mania and healthy subjects. A controlled study of 93 subjects. Acta Psychiatr Scand 109:222-229
23. Pappas GS (2000) Berkeley's Thought. Cornell University Press, Ithaca, New York
24. Hillman J (1996) The soul's character, calling and fate. Random House, New York
25. Taylor C (1992) Multiculturalism and politics of recognition. Princeton University Press, Princeton, NJ
26. Semi AA (1995) Tecnica del colloquio. Raffaello Cortina Editore, Milan [trad. Tecnique of the interview]
27. Haber EC (1998) Mikhail Bulgakov: the early years. Harvard University Press, Harvard
28. Baudelaire C (1981) Selected writings on art and artist. Cambridge University Press, Cambridge
29. Kafka F (1972) The metamorphosis. Bantam Press, New York
30. Becker G et al (1998) Knowledge and care of chronic illness in three ethnic minority groups. Fam Med 30:173-178
31. Kleinman A (1988) The illness narratives: suffering, healing and the human condition. Basic Books, New York
32. Brody H (1987) Stories of sickness. Yale University Press, New Haven
33. LeMaster JR, Kummings DD (1998) Walt Whitman: an encyclopedia. Garland Publishing, New York
34. Zagorin P (1999) Francis Bacon. Princeton University Press, Princeton
35. Kundera M (1988) The art of the novel. Faber and Faber, London
36. Woody A (2004) Melinda and Melinda, A. Woody, Editor, 20th Century Fox
37. Radley A (1994) Making sense of illness: the social psychology of health and disease. Sage Publications, London
38. Neimeyer RA (2000) Narrative disruptions in the construction of the self. In: Neimeyer RA, Raskin JD (eds) Constructions of disorder. APA, Washington, DC
39. Kelly GA (1995) The psychology of personal constructs. Norton, New York
40. Campbell D (1999) Family therapy and beyund: where is the Milan systemic approach today? Child Psychology & Psychiatry Review 4:76-84
41. Ugazio V (1998) Storie permesse storie proibite. Bollati Boringhieri, Torino [trad. Permitted histories and prohibited histories]
42. Monk G et al (1997) Narrative therapy in practice. Jossey-Bass, San Francisco
43. Thompson SC, Medvene LJ, Freedman D (1995) Caregiving in the close relationships

of cardiac patients: exchange, power, and attributional perspectives on caregiver resentment. Personal Relationships 2:125-142

44. Vetere A, Myers LB (2002) Repressive coping style and adult romantic attachment style: is there a relationship? Personality and individual differences 32:799-807

45. Ferreira A (1963) Family myth and homeostasis. Gen Arch Psychiat 9:457-463

46. Rolland JS (1994) Families, illness and disability: an integrative treatment model. Basic Books, New York

47. Ruiz JM, Hamann HA, Coyne JC, Compare A (2006) In sickness and in health: interpersonal risk and resilience in cardiovascular disease. In: Molinari E, Compare A, Parati G (eds) Clinical psychology and heart disease. Springer, New York

48. Cigoli V (1992) Il corpo familiare. L'anziano, la malattia, l'intreccio generazionale. Franco Angeli, Milan [trad. The family body. The elderly one, the illness, the generational interlacement]

49. Hellstrom C, Carlsoon SG (1996) The long-lasting now: disorganization in subjective time in long-standing pain. Scand J Psychol 37:416-423

50. Kitamura T, Kumar R (1982) Time passes slowly for patients with depression. Acta Psychiatr Scand 65:415-420

51. Ladame F (1992) Treatment of psychotic adolescents: difficulties and pitfalls. In: Schwartzberg A (ed) International annals of adolescent psychiatry. University of Chicago Press, Chicago, pp 221-228

52. Charles STIE (1999) The role of time in the setting of social goals across the life span. In: Hess TM, Blanchard F (eds) Social cognition and aging. Academic Press, San Diego, CA, pp 319-342

53. Lajolo D (1978) An absurd vice: a biography of Cesare Pavese. New Directions Publishing Corporation, New York

54. Ricourer P (1970) Time and narrative. University of Chicago Press, Chicago

55. Bloch E (1967) The principle of hope. MIT Press, Cambridge

56. Bateson G (1972) Steps to an ecology of mind. Chandler Press, San Francisco, CA

57. Bachtin M (1979) Estetica e romanzo. Einaudi, Torino [trad. Aesthetics and novel]

58. Vetere A, Myers L (2005) Families, coping styles and physical health. In Crane R, Marshall E (eds) Handbook of families and health. Sage, Thousand Oaks, CA

59. Jankélévitch V (1998) Music and the ineffable. Princeton University Press, Princeton

Chapter 18

Interpersonal Psychotherapy for Depression in Patients with Coronary Heart Disease

D. KOSZYCKI

▇ Introduction

Depression is common in patients with coronary heart disease. It is estimated that 15-20% of post-myocardial infarction (MI), unstable angina, congestive heart failure and post-bypass surgery patients meet diagnostic criteria for major depression during hospitalization, with another 15-25% experiencing mild forms of depression [1-4]. Although there are relatively few longitudinal studies of depression in patients with coronary artery disease available, data indicate that it tends to follow a chronic course, resulting in significant disability and psychosocial impairment [5, 6]. In a substantial number of patients, moderate-to-severe depression has been reported one-year post-MI [7]. Moreover, one third of patients recovering from MI show substantial depressed mood three years later [8] and one fifth fail to achieve emotional adjustment 5 years later [9]. It has also been reported that a significant proportion of coronary patients with minor depression at index progress to major depression over the course of 12 months [6].

One of the most serious consequences of depression in cardiac patients is cardiac mortality. Major depression following MI is associated with a fourfold increased risk of cardiac mortality during the first year, and there is risk with minor forms of depression as well [1, 10-11]. Further, the prognostic impact of depression is as large as, and independent of, other major prognostic factors, including ventricular dysfunction and the severity of coronary atherosclerosis. Frasure-Smith and Lespérance [12] reported that depressive symptoms predicted 5-year cardiac mortality in a large post-MI sample, and Barefoot et al. [13] found that even after 10 years of a cardiac event, depressed patients have a greater risk of cardiac death than non-depressed patients. The mechanism by which depression increases cardiac morbidity and mortality is not well understood. Decreased compliance with medication and lifestyle changes, such as smoking cessation, diet, and regular exercise, are possible mechanisms [14].

Pathophysiological alterations associated with depression, including decreased platelet activity, decreased heart rate variability, and altered HPA axis activity, have also been implicated [15]. However, many cardiologists are not convinced of the negative prognostic impact of depressive disorders on cardiac morbidity and mortality, and despite strong epidemiological evidence linking the two, this has had little impact on cardiologic practice [16].

The finding that depression in patients with cardiac disease is consequential highlights the need for early recognition and optimal treatment of depressive symptoms. Therapeutic options for the treatment of depression in non-medically ill patients include depression-focused psychotherapies, antidepressant drugs, and a combination of the two. Among the psychotherapies, cognitive behavior therapy (CBT) and interpersonal psychotherapy (IPT) have demonstrated both acute and maintenance efficacy [17]. However, the efficacy of these evidence-based psychotherapies in depressed cardiac patients is unknown and their widespread use is limited by the lack of mental health professionals with specialized training in these therapies. Pharmacotherapy is universally available through primary care physicians and, for many, represents the first choice of treatment. Unfortunately, well-designed placebo-controlled trials focused on pharmacological treatments for depressed cardiac patients are lacking. This is due to the fact that medically ill patients are typically excluded from drug trials. As a result, we cannot assure patients that they will experience the same levels of efficacy and tolerability as medically healthy patients who are depressed. Given the high lifetime rate of depression in cardiac patients and its serious impact on morbidity and mortality, appreciable efforts need to be devoted to evaluating the safety, efficacy, and acceptability of different treatment modalities in this population, and to developing guidelines for helping clinicians choose optimal treatments.

One treatment that may be particularly suited for depressed cardiac patients is IPT. The purpose of this chapter is to acquaint the reader with this depression-focused psychotherapy and its usefulness in treating depressed patients with cardiac disease.

◾ Overview of Interpersonal Psychotherapy for Depression

Background

IPT is a time-limited (12-16 weekly 1-hour sessions) manualized psychotherapy that was developed in the early 1970's by Gerald Klerman and Myrna Weissman and colleagues as an intervention for outpatients with unipolar major depression [18]. The historical roots of IPT include Myers's biopsychosocial model of psychopathology, Sullivan's interpersonal paradigm and Bowlby's attachment theory, as well as other interpersonal psychotherapies that emerged in the 1940's and 1950's emphasizing the potent role of environmental events, versus strictly intrapsychic conflicts, in the genesis of psychopathology [18-20]. IPT was further influenced by empirical research demonstrating a link between disturbed mood and adverse life events, such as death of a loved one, marital disharmony, and loneliness and social isolation, and the protective effect of interpersonal resources against depression [18, 21-23].

IPT makes no assumptions about the etiology of depression but emphasizes the current social and interpersonal context associated with disturbed mood [18]. It is based on the presumption that interpersonal issues affect mood and mood impairs interpersonal functioning. IPT conceptualizes clinical depression as having three component processes: symptom formation caused by biological and/or psychological mechanisms; social functioning (involving, obviously, social interactions with others); and enduring personality traits. IPT intervenes in symptom formation and social dysfunction but does not address enduring personality traits in view of the time limits of treatment, the relatively low level of psychotherapeutic intensity, the emphasis of treatment on the current depressive episode, and the difficulty in accurately evaluating personality in the midst of an Axis I disorder [18, 20, 24].

Characteristics of IPT

The following summarizes some of the main features of IPT [18, 24-27]:

i)   IPT is time-limited. The acute phase of treatment is typically 12-16 weekly sessions and is discussed with patient at the outset of treatment. The brevity of the treatment imposes a structure that pressures the patient and therapist to work quickly to alleviate depressive symptoms and resolve the current interpersonal crisis linked with the depression, thus discouraging the patient becoming dependent on the therapist.

ii) IPT is a focal intervention. For each patient, therapy focuses on one or, at most, two interpersonal problem areas that are identified as precursors of the current depressive episode. These problem areas were derived from extensive research on the role of environmental influences on mood and are characterized as unresolved grief following the death of a loved one, role transitions (difficulty adjusting to changed life circumstances), interpersonal role disputes (conflicts with a significant other) and interpersonal deficits (impoverished social networks). Maintaining the focus of treatment on a problematic interpersonal issue prevents the therapy from becoming too diffuse and forces the therapist and patient to discuss material that is relevant to the focal area and treatment objectives.

iii) IPT focuses on the "here and now," that is, on current problematic interpersonal issues that are amenable to change, rather than on reconciling unresolved interpersonal problems having to do with the past. The focus on resolving current interpersonal problems and developing strategies for warding off future problems helps reduce the depressed patient's tendency to ruminate about past events and experiences that cannot be changed and which only serve to reinforce the patient's already low sense of self-esteem and dysphoria.

iv) IPT uses a medical model. IPT defines depression as a medical illness, which allows the patient to assume the "sick role" in need of treatment. The medically oriented approach of IPT helps the patient see his or her depressive symptoms as ego-dystonic, rather than as aspects of personality, and facilitates combining psychotherapy and pharmacotherapy, if medication is necessary.

vi) IPT targets the current depressive episode. The primary goal of IPT is to obtain the remission of depressive symptoms by facilitating resolution of a current interpersonal crisis. The narrow treatment goals of IPT are explained to patients at the outset of treatment. Although IPT recognizes the role of personality in mediating a person's response to interpersonal experiences, personality change is not a therapeutic focus given the time constraints of treatment. Nevertheless, as treatment progresses, many patients acquire new interpersonal skills that may help compensate for characterological problems.

Therapist's Stance

As with any form of psychotherapy, IPT seeks to engender an ambiance of warmth, trust and understanding, thereby establishing and maintaining a therapeutic alliance. While the IPT therapist shares many characteristics with those who practice CBT or other solution-focused therapies, he or she differs considerably from psychodynamically oriented therapists [30]. The IPT therapist has an active stance and guides the patient in the discussion of relevant material during the therapeutic session, explores options that exist for change, provides clarification, promotes problem solving, and helps the patient feel more competent in managing life. The therapist is not neutral but actively works with the patient to relieve depression by conveying a hopeful attitude that treatment goals can be achieved, by being supportive, and by reassuring the patient and providing direct advice when appropriate [24]. Transference is not emphasized in IPT unless it jeopardizes treatment. IPT focuses on the patient's interpersonal environment outside the office rather than on the therapeutic relationship or transference. Negative transference is addressed by discussing the way the patient is behaving toward the therapist and exploring how similar behaviors contribute to problematic interpersonal relationships outside of therapy. From an IPT perspective, the patient's disruptive behavior is often attributed to indirect and ineffective communication of negative feelings. For example, research has shown that depressed women are fearful that voicing opposition or anger will be met with negative consequences [28]. The therapist helps the patient find more adaptive ways of communicating oppositional feelings, which helps resolve possible conflict not only with the therapist, but also significant others in the patient's life [24, 29].

Psychotherapeutic Techniques

The therapeutic strategies and techniques of IPT are designed to help the patient master the interpersonal problem area associated with depression. These techniques are similar to those used in other psychotherapies and include exploratory techniques (nondirective exploration and direct elicitation of material), encouragement of affect, clarification, communication analysis, and the use of the therapeutic relationship and various behavioral change techniques (role playing, decision analysis, directive techniques). IPT does not use interventions such as interpretation, dream analysis, focus on transferential themes, or monitoring or challenging distorted cognitions [24, 30]. The reader should refer to the IPT manuals of Weissman et al. [24] and Stuart and Robertson [31] for a full description of IPT techniques.

Outcome Research with IPT

IPT has been extensively researched and shown to be effective as acute and maintenance treatment for major depressive disorder. IPT's efficacy as an acute treatment for major depression was initially established in a 16-week trial comparing IPT and amitriptyline, alone or in combination [32]. IPT and amitriptyline were equally effective in decreasing depressive symptoms at endpoint, although amitriptyline engendered improvements more rapidly than IPT. The combined IPT and amitriptyline treatment produced a greater reduction in depressive symptoms than either treatment alone. At one-year follow-up, patients who received IPT had better psychosocial functioning than those who did not receive this treatment [33].

The National Institute of Mental Health Treatment of Depression Collaborative Research Program (NIMH TDCRP) is the largest study to date that has evaluated the efficacy of acute IPT in depressed patients [34]. Two hundred and fifty patients who met DSM-III criteria for major depression were randomly assigned to 16 weeks of IPT, CBT, imipramine or placebo. The results revealed that IPT was superior to placebo and equivalent to imipramine and CBT in treating mild to moderate depression (defined as a score of <20 on the Hamilton Depression Rating Scale (HDRS)). IPT was found to be somewhat better than CBT in treating severe depression (HDRS score >20); however, neither psychosocial treatment was as effective as imipramine. Nevertheless, at endpoint, the recovery rate for IPT was similar to that of imipramine (43% and 42%, respectively) and better than that of placebo (21%). The study concluded that, in general, IPT is an effective monotherapy for patients with mild to moderate depression, but that antidepressant medication should be used as a first line treatment for severely ill patients.

Since publication of the NIMH TDCRP study, IPT has been adapted and shown to be effective in treating other depressed populations, such as those afflicted with dysthymia [25, 35] and antenatal and post-partum depression [36, 37]. IPT has shown been shown to be effective in treating depressed HIV patients [38], depressed adolescents [39, 40], late-life depression [41], depression in primary care settings [42], and bipolar disorder [43]. Although studies on the combination of IPT and antidepressants are limited, there is evidence that a combined approach is more effective than monotherapy in treating depressed elderly patients and patients with bereavement-related major depression [41]. The combined approach is also more effective in enhancing psychosocial functioning [44]. In dysthymic patients, the combined approach enhances interpersonal and social functioning [45] and significantly decreases utilization of health and social services, suggesting that IPT is a cost-effective treatment [35]. In addition, IPT has recently been adapted for group settings [29, 46, 47], which provides a perfect forum for role-playing and practicing interpersonal skills.

Frank and colleagues, from the University of Pittsburgh, have adapted IPT as a maintenance treatment for patients with recurrent depression [48, 49]. Their research showed that the mean depression-free survival time was significantly longer for patients who receive monthly IPT, versus placebo, over a three-year period. However, patients who received medication, with or without monthly IPT, had the longest depression-free survival time, suggesting that patients with a recurring illness benefit most from maintenance medication. Nevertheless, the data indicate that maintenance IPT may be an effective alternative for patients who do not want to take medication or who cannot tolerate its side effects.

Interpersonal Psychotherapy for Coronary Heart Disease Patients with Co-Morbid Depression

Rationale

Prospective epidemiological data strongly indicate that social ties and relationships are important determinants of health status and risk for mortality in the general population [50]. Among patients with cardiac disease, interpersonal supports mediate adaptive coping with disease, as well as the outcome of illness. Patients with poor interpersonal supports are more likely to become depressed, are more impaired by their illness, and have a worse outcome [51]. Low levels of interpersonal support have also been linked to increased mortality in several epidemiological studies of patients with coronary artery disease [52-54]. For example, living alone after MI is an independent risk factor for cardiac death within the first 6 months [52]. The pathways by which interpersonal supports influence cardiac prognosis are complex and not fully understood. One potential mechanism is that the presence of a good support structure alters the cardiovascular risk factors, by helping the patient to quit smoking, for example, or to control hypertension [55-57].

Interpersonal supports can be conceptualized as having three main components: the interpersonal network; the type and amount of support provided by the network; and the adequacy of the support [58]. The interpersonal network includes family, friends, co-workers, the medical system and community resources. Total network size and network characteristics (e.g., having a spouse) have not been found to be associated with mental and physical outcome in patients with cardiac disease [51, 59]. In fact, some characteristics of the support network, such as marital status, can have either a positive or negative influence on the patient [60]. However, the number of emotionally close network members seen regularly has been shown to have beneficial effects [51]. The types of interpersonal support include emotional-affectional (providing empathy, caring, and love), educational (offering information and advice for dealing with the illness) and tangible (providing financial and physical help) [61]. The type of support needed depends on the course of the disease and the individual [62]. For example, tangible support may be more important for an elderly cardiac patient who is functionally impaired and who requires assistance with daily care and transportation to medical appointments. However, tangible support can be problematic, as it may engender feelings of dependency. Adequacy of support refers to the availability and effectiveness of social supports for dealing with specific problems [51]. The perceived adequacy of support is strongly associated with improved physical and emotional well-being, and it is influenced by the number of network members seen regularly and the type and amount of support provided.

IPT may be ideally suited for the treatment of depressed cardiac patients because it deals with issues that are common to patients with coronary heart disease: including social isolation; conflicts with members of the patient's social network that can lead to hostility, anger, and distress; difficulty adjusting to changes in social roles brought about by the disease or other life circumstances; and the loss of network supports and attachments due to death. In addition to the role of interpersonal stressors in precipitating a depressive episode, IPT also recognizes the adverse effects of depression itself on interpersonal functioning and relationships. Indeed, the interpersonal consequences of depression, such as social withdrawal, rejection by others, and increased interpersonal conflict, are well established [23, 63], and they can have a negative prognostic impact on cardiac morbidity and mortality.

Recently, our group conducted an open-label pilot study to evaluate the efficacy and acceptability of IPT for patients with stable coronary heart disease who met DSM-IV criteria for major depression [64]. IPT was delivered over 12 weekly sessions, each lasting 45-50 minutes, by therapists trained in IPT who had extensive experience treating patients with cardiac disease. Therapy followed the treatment manual of Weissman and colleagues [24], with slight modifications specifically relevant to cardiac patients. IPT produced a significant reduction in depressive symptoms, with over half of the subjects meeting stringent criteria for remission (i.e., a score of <8 on the HDRS and a score of <14 on the Beck Depression Inventory-II). Only one patient dropped out of the study because of poor treatment response. Unmedicated and medicated patients responded similarly to IPT, suggesting that IPT alone could be an alternative treatment for patients who prefer a nonpharmacological approach, or who may be particularly sensitive to the adverse effects of antidepressant drugs. The study also revealed that IPT requires minimal adaptation for depressed cardiac patients, and that it is well accepted and tolerated by patients. A 12-week dose of IPT appears to be sufficient to alleviate depressive symptoms in a substantial number of patients experiencing moderate-to-severe depression. Currently, our group is conducting a randomized trial to determine the efficacy of IPT, alone or in combination with an antidepressant, in depressed patients with stable coronary heart disease [65]. The results of this study will provide a more definitive evaluation of the usefulness IPT for the treatment of depression in coronary heart disease.

Applying IPT for Depressed Cardiac Patients

As noted above, the pilot study has shown that IPT requires minimal adaptation for patients with stable coronary heart disease. The following briefly describes a 12-week treatment adapted from Weissman et al. [24] for depressed patients with comorbid cardiac disease. The reader should refer to the treatment manual developed by Klerman et al. [18], and recently updated by Weissman et al. [24], which provides an overall approach to treatment, as well as specific techniques and guidelines for their application. In our adaptation of IPT for coronary patients [64,65], therapy is delivered over 12 weekly session, each lasting 45-50 minutes. Although, originally, the intention was to provide IPT in 16 weekly, one-hour sessions, it was felt that a shorter duration of treatment would be better suited for depressed medical patients who may have difficulty sustaining an hour-long session. An allowance is made to conduct some of the sessions by telephone, especially if the patient is too ill to come to the therapist's office or requires hospitalization. This helpes maintain continuity in the treatment.

Therapy is divided into 3 phases: the initial phase (sessions 1-3), the middle phase (sessions 4-9) and the termination phase (sessions 10-12). Each of these phases has specific goals and strategies. The goals and strategies of the middle and termination phases of therapy are essentially the same as those described in the IPT manual for depression by Weissman et al. [24].

The Initial Phase

The initial phase of treatment includes a diagnostic evaluation and psychiatric and medical history and sets that framework for treatment. The therapist conducts a comprehensive evaluation of the depressive's symptoms, elicits information about life events associated with the onset and course of depression, elicits information about the cardiac event and the patient's reaction to it, and establishes a diagnosis of major depression according to established criteria (e.g., DSM-IV or ICD-10). If warranted, a medical assessment should be conducted to rule out medical problems that mimic mood symptoms. The use of standardized rating scales such as the HDRS or BDI ensures a thorough review of symptoms and provides the therapist and patient with an index of illness severity. These scales can be administered weekly or biweekly during the course of treatment for clinical monitoring of progress. Patients are explicitly told that they have two medical conditions: cardiac disease and major depression, and thus are given the "sick role" [66]. The patient's mood disorder is defined as a medical illness that is not the patient's fault, and it is compared to other medical conditions, such as hypertension, that respond to psychological and pharmacological interventions. The purpose of this strategy is to mitigate self-criticism by helping the depressed patient blame the depression rather than himself/herself, and to instill a sense of hope that the depressive disorder is treatable. The sick role associated with cardiac disease includes becoming educated about cardiac disease, following through on cardiac rehabilitation, and engaging in health-promoting behaviors. The sick role temporarily excuses the patient from certain social obligations but also requires that he or she work in treatment to recover.

The psychiatric history includes an interpersonal inventory, consisting of a systematic review of the strengths and weakness of the patient's interpersonal world, focusing on the current milieu. The therapist gathers information about important relationships, including specifics about the interactions (e.g., frequency of contact, activities shared, etc.), mutual expectations and whether these expectations are fulfilled, positive and negative aspects of the relationship, and desired changes in relationships. In reviewing the patient's interpersonal inventory, a history of significant others who have died should also be obtained, including the circumstances of the person's death and the patient's reaction to it. The therapist utilizes the interpersonal inventory to identify social and interpersonal events that are linked to the onset of the current depressive episode. Examples may include the death of a loved one, a deteriorating relationship with a significant other, relinquishing valued activities because of changing circumstances in life, and loss of important social supports and attachments. The therapist also specifically inquires about changes in interpersonal and role functioning following the diagnosis of cardiac disease and the emergence of depressive symptoms.

The overall goal of the interpersonal inventory is to determine which of the four interpersonal domains (pathological grief, role disputes, role transitions, or interpersonal deficits) is the critical precursor to the depressive episode and, therefore, should be the focus of the remainder of treatment. In our pilot study with depressed coronary patients, the most common foci of treatment were role transitions and role disputes. These problem areas will be discussed in the ensuing section. The interpersonal inventory also provides the therapist with a rich source of data on the patient's attachment style (i.e., secure, anxious ambivalent, or anxious avoidant) and communication patterns [31], which have important implications for subjective well being and coping with interpersonal or major life stressors [67]. Additionally, the interpersonal inventory provides important details about the type, quality and utilization of interpersonal supports (including the medical system), perceived availability of support, and barriers to receiving the kind of support the patient needs. This additional information helps the therapist develop a more comprehensive formulation of the patient's interpersonal issues, and can be used to define goals for change and guide the treatment plan.

In this phase of treatment, a considerable part of the discussion is devoted to educating the patient about the nature and treatment of depression and correcting misperceptions about the disorder. For example, the therapist may need to correct the perception that depression is a normal reaction to cardiac disease that does not require help, rather than an illness requiring medical care [68]. Furthermore, psychoeducation is extended to cardiac disease and the negative prognostic impact of untreated depression on cardiac disease. The therapist should demonstrate expertise about depression and knowledge about cardiac disease. The provision of psychoeducation should also be extended to the patient's family, emphasizing that depression is an illness and not a weakness in character and that it is not something that will go away with positive thinking or maintaining a "stiff upper lip." Patients and their families should be encouraged to access other sources for information about depression and cardiac disease and become "experts" on these illnesses.

The therapist must evaluate the need for medication and determine whether IPT is appropriate for the patient. The decision to prescribe medication should be based on the severity of illness, degree of impairment, suicidality and the patient's preference [24]. Because therapists are dealing with a population with a comorbid cardiac condition (and possibly other medical conditions), regular monitoring of medication side effects and clinically significant worsening of both psychiatric and cardiac status, including cardiac symptoms, ECG changes and orthostatic blood pressure decreases, is necessary. Consultation with the patient's cardiologist before and during antidepressant treatment may be advisable [69]. Many cardiac patients are reluctant to accept adjunctive pharmacotherapy because of concerns about taking yet another medication. For these patients, a time-limited depression-focused psychotherapy may be more appealing. In general, IPT is best suited for patients whose depressive episode is clearly linked to a current psychosocial crisis, such as a role transition, a dispute with a significant other, or the death of a loved one. Depression that occurs in the absence of a life event and that is primarily associated with chronic social dysfunction (i.e. interpersonal deficits) has been reported to be less responsive to IPT [70]. Apart from interpersonal deficits, little is known about which patients are best suited for IPT versus other forms of therapy [31].

The information gathered in the initial IPT sessions allows the therapists to develop a case formulation. A case formulation consists of a model of the cause of the patient's problems and a plan for overcoming them. The IPT formulation attempts to explain the cause of depression within an interpersonal context. This formulation is reflected back to the patient and the therapist and patient collaboratively establish treatment goals that are meaningfully linked to the problematic interpersonal area. In some instances, the patient may present with multiple interpersonal problem areas. In this case, the therapist and patient must decide which area is most relevant to the depression and which is most amenable to change in the context of a brief intervention. Once the therapist and patient agree on the focus and goals of therapy, the therapist explains the treatment process, including the "here and now" focus, the social and interpersonal context of the intervention, the emphasis on solving a current problematic interpersonal issues rather than solving life problems, expectations for the type and level of patient involvement in the treatment process, and treatment arrangements such as the length of sessions, handling of missed appointments and so forth [24].

Case Vignette:
Mr. H is a 59 year old, married Caucasian male who works as a tax accountant. His cardiologist referred him for assessment of depression. He was well until three months ago when he suffered a significant MI while attending a wedding of a relative. He was hospitalized at a university-affiliated heart institute for one week and underwent two angioplasties. After discharge he participated in a car-

diac rehabilitation program. However, he continued to complain of numerous unexplained symptoms and decreased energy. He was referred to the psychologist at the cardiac rehabilitation center, where he was diagnosed with major depression. His symptoms included persistent depressed mood, frequent crying spells, loss of interest in his job, hypersomnia, decreased energy, poor appetite, feelings of worthlessness, poor concentration and suicidal ideation. His 17-item HDRS score of 20 indicated that he was moderately depressed. There is no previous history of depression or other psychiatric illness. In addition to cardiac disease, Mr. H has a 10-year history of diabetes and arthritis. Both of these illnesses are well controlled and have never impaired the patient's functioning.

A review of the patient's interpersonal inventory revealed that he has a good relationship with his wife of 25 years and his three children. He also reports having satisfying relationships with his extended family and friends and has been very active in his community. There were no recent deaths of relatives or close friends. Both of his parents died several years ago, but there was no evidence of pathological grief. Mr. H reported that in the year prior to his MI there were many changes at work and he began to feel increasingly dissatisfied with his job. He has been employed as a tax accountant for a large and prestigious accounting firm for the past 12 years. He has been successful in his career and, until recently, derived a great deal of satisfaction from his job. His relationships with his colleagues have been good and he had expected to remain with his company until his retirement. However, his company underwent substantial organizational changes in the year prior to his MI, which included downsizing staff in his division. As a result, more demands were placed on him and he was often required to work evenings and on weekends, leaving him little time to engage in other activities he enjoyed. In addition to increased work demands, he was unhappy with the direction the firm was taking and he felt he had little control over his work environment. After considerable reflection and discussion with his wife, he decided that he would leave the company within the next year and start a small business of his own. However, after the MI, he felt vulnerable and scared about venturing out on his own. Given his multiple health issues and current financial situation, he felt that it would be more prudent to remain in a financially secure job until his retirement. However, he felt demoralized and trapped and worried that the stress at work would precipitate another MI. When the therapist inquired about how Mr. H reacted emotionally to the MI, he stated that he was traumatized by the experience and saw himself as an aging man whose health was beginning to fail him. Although he had a long history of diabetes and arthritis, he never felt that these illnesses impeded his life in any way and he considered himself to be relatively healthy. Following the MI, he felt a profound sense of loss of health and worried about his future.

The therapist informed him that he was going through a depressive episode, a common and treatable illness that was not his fault. He was thus given the "sick role" and provided with psychoeducation about depression and cardiac disease. The patient did not want to take medication because he was already taking several prescription drugs for his multiple medical conditions and preferred a nonpharmacological approach to treating his depression. After reviewing the interpersonal inventory, the therapist suggested that IPT might be a suitable treatment for his depression. The therapist provided the patient with an interpersonal formulation, which specifically linked his depressive episode to the difficulties he was having adapting to the changes both in his work environment and in his health status. The therapist optimistically conveyed to the patient that his depression would resolve if the therapy focused on exploring how he can make these transitions more manageable. The therapist and patient collaboratively set goals for therapy, which included helping the patient mourn the loss of health and a work environment he once enjoyed, explore the positive aspects of these role transitions (e.g., an opportunity for re-evaluating his life) and examine realistically employment options, including starting his own business and renegotiating his role at work in order to decrease his stress level and possible risk of another MI. The patient agreed with the interpersonal formulation and treatment goals, and the therapist proceeded to discuss the practical aspects of treatment.

Middle Sessions: Sessions 4-9
The middle phase of therapy begins once the therapist and patient agree on the treatment contract and identified problem area. The middle session focuses on the problem area identified in the initial phase of treatment. In this phase, the therapist must ensure that the patient remains focused on the identified problem area, gains a better understanding of it, and attempts to bring about resolution of the problem. To help keep the focus of therapy on the "here and now," therapy sessions typically begin with the question, "How have things been since we last met?" [26].

Interpersonal Role Disputes
An "interpersonal role dispute" is a situation in which the patient and at least one significant other have "nonreciprocal expectations about their relationship" [18]. It is chosen as the problem area when the patient describes his or her depression in relation to conflict with a significant relationship.

Cardiac disease may precipitate or exacerbate conflicts with significant others, including spouses, other family members, friends, and coworkers. Disputes may revolve around changes in dependence-independence levels, role function, decreased levels of involvement or loss of intimacy that can be burdensome to the patient and significant other. Coronary patients may also have difficulty communicating their need for help or support or renegotiating their roles and relationships with key individuals in their interpersonal environment [24]. While dysfunctional relationships can precipitate mood changes, depression itself can lead to problematic interactions and relationships with others. For example, depressed patients often withdraw socially and isolate themselves from important sources of emotional support that can ease the distress associated with cardiac disease. Depression can also have a negative impact on others [63]. Depressed individuals are less effective in enlisting support from others and often elicit eventual rejection because of irritability and negative affect. The outcome of this is a reduction of rewarding social interactions, increased social isolation and despair, and possible complication of the course and outcome of cardiac disease.

In treating role disputes, the IPT therapist helps the patient identify the issue(s) in the dispute, explore options for changing the relationship, and modify expectations of the relationship and maladaptive communication patterns. If the dispute is at an impasse and the relationship is irretrievably damaged, the therapist and patient may explore options of leaving the relationship. In the dissolution stage, the therapist helps the patient grieve the loss of the relationship and encourages the formation of new attachments. At this juncture, the interpersonal problem is reframed as a role transition. The dissolution of a dysfunctional relationship may not be a viable option for many cardiac patients, particularly for those who are elderly or severely ill or who have limited economic and interpersonal resources. In this circumstance, the therapist helps the patient tolerate unpleasant aspects of the relationship and focus more on positive aspects, while at the same time encouraging the patient to build and utilize his or her extended social network [24].

Case Vignette:
Mrs. A is a 52-year-old woman who lives with her 60-year-old husband and her 78-year-old widowed mother, who is afflicted with multiple sclerosis. The patient underwent bypass surgery several months ago after experiencing her first MI. After discharge from hospital she was enrolled in a cardiac rehabilitation program but was not compliant with treatment. She missed sessions and did not adhere to prescribed lifestyle changes, including weight reduction and regular exercise. The staff at the rehabilitation program felt that her lack of compliance was attributable, in part, to depression, and referred her to a psychiatrist for evaluation and treatment. At assessment, she complained of depressed mood, crying easily, irritability, preoccupation with her mother's health, early morning awakening, difficulty concentrating, lack of energy, feeling worthless and transient suicidal ideation. Her HDRS score was 25, suggesting that she was moderately depressed.

A review of the interpersonal inventory revealed a long-standing dispute with her husband that revolved around the care of her mother. Mrs. A is an only child and is very close to her mother, who has lived with her and her husband following the death of her father seven years earlier. Mrs. A felt that it was her duty to protect and care for her mother, and she found this role deeply satisfying. As her mother's health deteriorated in the last two years, Mrs. A gave up her job as a secretary to become a full time caregiver. Mrs. A's husband, on the other hand, wanted his mother-in-law admitted to a nursing home. He resented the financial burden and there were frequent arguments about money. In addition, he deeply resented the time his wife devoted to her mother and complained that his wife was neglecting him. Mrs. A felt torn between her mother and husband, and she resented her husband for withdrawing support when she desperately needed it. Following Mrs. A's cardiac event, the role of primary care giver was more difficult and she often felt exhausted both emotionally and physically. She began to neglect her health and had little time to follow through on prescribed lifestyle changes. While Mrs. A's husband agreed to help with some household tasks and run errands during her recovery period, he became more and more intolerant of the demands of his mother-in-law's illness and more insistent that she be admitted to a nursing home. Arguments about her mother became progressively more frequent and Mrs. A felt more hopeless and depressed.

After completing the interpersonal inventory, the therapist and the patient agreed that her depression was clearly linked to the dispute she was having with her husband about her role as the primary caregiver for her ill mother. The goals of therapy were 1) to clarify the nature of the dispute, 2) to appraise the expectations Mrs. A and her husband had of each other and determine whether they were realistic, 3) to review past strategies Mrs. A had used to resolve the dispute with her husband and generate potential solutions (which included identifying external support systems that could provide Mrs. A with some relief from caring for her mother), 4) to improve Mrs. A's ability to communicate her feelings to her husband effectively and facilitate a more productive dialogue with him about their respective needs and wishes, and 5) to develop social support resources, such as joining a support group for caregivers of patients with multiple sclerosis.

Role Transitions

A problem in role transition is defined as difficulty adjusting to a life change that requires a new or different role [18]. Difficulties in making the transition from one role to another can result in depression. These difficulties may arise because 1) the role is unexpected, 2) the role is undesired, 3) the person is not psychologically or emotionally prepared for the new role, or 4) the old role is missed [39]. The social impairment and sense of loss can contribute to feelings of depression. The diagnosis of cardiac disease can be conceptualized as a role transition, characterized by loss of the healthy self, uncertainty about the future and fear of death, and life changes the disease produces. Cardiac disease can result in alterations in everyday roles, such as financial provider, as well as loss of independence, productivity, valued activities, and social supports and attachments. Furthermore, a new role arises with loss of health which demands that the patient comply with disease-controlling or health-promoting behaviors [62]. While the burden and losses associated with cardiac disease can precipitate depression, the behavioral manifestations of depression can also undercut adaptive coping to life changes that arise because of cardiac diseases. For example, loss of interest and decreased energy can compromise a patient's ability to follow through on prescribed behaviors that elicit and maintain good cardiac health. Similarly, social withdrawal can interfere with the patient's ability to seek out and effectively utilize social support networks that enhance adherence to health-promoting behaviors and provide role models for effective coping.

In IPT, treatment for role transitions involves helping the patient mourn and accept the loss of the old role, adapt more effectively to life changes associated with coronary artery disease, find new life goals, restore a sense of self and integrity, create new social ties, and facilitate the acquisition of new skills necessary for the new role [24].

Case Vignette:
Mr. S is a 73-year-old married male, with a four-year history of coronary artery disease and postural hypertension. Until 6 months ago, he was going for a daily cardiac walk and playing golf two times a week. Although semi-retired, he worked 4 days a week as a salesman in a men's clothing store he built thirty-five years ago and which his older son has taken over. He was also active in his community and sat on the board of directors of a charitable organization. Six months ago, he suffered a second serious MI and required bypass surgery. He fully recovered from the surgery and was expected to resume many of his activities. However, he complained of feeling tired all the time, felt dizzy and light- headed and worried about his health. Because his cardiologist felt that there were no medical reasons for his physical complaints, he was referred to a psychiatrist for an evaluation. At the time of evaluation, the patient complained of frequent crying spells, lack of energy, social withdrawal, insomnia, decreased appetite, psychomotor retardation, and feelings of worthlessness. He met DSM-IV criteria for major depression and had a score of 23 on his HDRS. A review of his interpersonal inventory revealed that his symptoms of depression began shortly after his cardiac condition worsened. He experienced his MI as a major setback and was angry and bitter that his cardiac condition had deteriorated despite his diligence in maintaining a healthy lifestyle. In addition, his cardiologist had recommended that he slow down and reduce the number of hours he worked in his clothing store to two half days a week. When the therapist inquired how Mr. S felt about this change he became tearful and acknowledged that it was a great loss, as this role contributed to his sense of contribution, competence and mastery. The therapist linked the patient's depression to the difficulty he was having adjusting to the deterioration in his cardiac status and having to relinquish valued activities. The goals of therapy included helping him 1) mourn the further loss of health, 2) adjust to his new life circumstances, 3) develop new skills to meet the challenges of his deteriorating heart condition, 3) explore the positive aspects of the change, and 4) encourage him to find other meaningful activities that would not compromise his health.

Pathological Grief
Grief is considered the problem area when the onset of the patient's symptoms is associated with a death, either present or past [18]. Normal grief can resemble depression, except that in normal grief the depressive symptoms remit over time. In a pathological grief reaction, the usual depressive symptoms that accompany the grieving process develop into a profound, unremitting and severe depression [71]. This often occurs in the context of traumatic bereavement, conjugal bereavement or the death of a child [31]. For example, in the first year of conjugal bereavement, approximately 10-20% of persons develop clinically significant depression [72]. Pathological mourning can be due to a recent loss, as in a distorted or exaggerated grief response, or it can be of a long-standing nature, as in chron-

ic or delayed grief. Grief may be delayed either because the body of the deceased is lost, destroyed or was never viewed, causing the death to seem unreal, or because the survivor represses the grief-related affect, displays little affect, or largely denies the loss. Grief can also be distorted as a result of problematic aspects of the survivor's relationship with the deceased prior to the death, such as unresolved anger [71]. The survivor may therefore actually be relieved about the death but subsequently feel guilty and become depressed. Signs of pathological grief include a history of preserving the environment, anniversary reactions, ambivalence about the relationship, multiple deaths, fear of illness that caused the death and absence of supports during bereavement [24].

In IPT, the treatment goals of pathological grief are to facilitate the grieving process and help the patient re-establish interests and relationships, as well as new attachments that can substitute for what has been lost. The strategies employed in IPT include helping the patient discuss the loss and circumstances surrounding the death, reconstructing the relationship so that the patient can develop a clearer and more realistic picture of the relationship with the deceased, and reintegrating the patient into her or his social environment [24].

Case Vignette:
Mr. C is a 60-year-old married male who was referred by his family doctor for the treatment of depression. He had two MIs, the most recent one occurring three months ago. A comprehensive psychiatric assessment revealed that the patient met DSM-IV criteria for major depression, and his HDRS score of 25 indicated that he was moderately depressed. A review of his interpersonal inventory revealed that a year prior to the onset of his depression, his 27-year-old son had died of an inoperable brain tumor. While the death was anticipated, it was a severe blow to Mr. C, who had been estranged from his son for several years and had only begun to reconcile two months before his death. Mr. C struggled with the death of his son and experienced intense feelings of guilt and regret about their problematic relationship. He was angry and bitter about the fact that his son had died just as they were beginning to take steps toward reconciliation. Although he turned to his wife for emotional support, she told him the best thing to do was to try to forget. Other family members did not discuss the death out of fear that it might make him more susceptible to a fatal heart attack. Eventually, Mr. A became depressed and withdrawn, and avoided any discussion of his grieving with others.

After reviewing the interpersonal inventory, the therapist linked Mr. C's depression to the difficulty he had been having mourning the tragic death of his son and moving beyond suffering. The goals of therapy were 1) to help him mourn the loss of his son by describing his experience, including his emotional reactions to the death, 2) to help him accept the painful emotions he was experiencing, including intense guilt and regret about his estrangement from his son, 3) to explore his relationship with his son so that he could develop a more balanced view of their relationship, 4) to help him communicate his loss to others, and 5) to help him reconnect with others, especially his other children.

Interpersonal Deficits
Interpersonal deficits are a focus of treatment if the interpersonal inventory reveals a paucity of social relationships or a history of chronically unfulfilling relationships. Typically, patients with interpersonal deficits have lifelong personality problems and difficulty with loneliness and shyness [24, 26]. The category, interpersonal deficits, is the least developed of the IPT foci, and the one associated with the worst outcome [26, 66]. If possible, this problem area should not be the primary focus. Because medical conditions, such as cardiac disease, inherently provide a role transition, therapists are able to ignore the alternative interpersonal deficits. Nevertheless, helping the patient adapt to the role transition may be complicated by the presence of interpersonal deficits, particularly since a primary goal of IPT is to encourage the patient to establish or extend social networks. If working on interpersonal deficits is one focus of treatment, the goal of treatment is to reduce the patient's social isolation and improve or facilitate the development of interpersonal relationships. The IPT therapist uses various interventions, such as role playing to enact difficult social interactions, focusing on the therapeutic relationship as a model for developing other relationships and examining repetitive patterns in relationships [24].

Case Vignette:
Mr. D is a 42-year-old, self-employed carpenter, with a 2-year history of coronary artery disease. He lives alone in a rural area about 50km from the city. He suffered from angina and underwent bypass surgery 5 months ago. After discharge from hospital he was scheduled to attend a 12-week cardiac rehabilitation program but failed to attend the program. His family doctor referred him to a psychiatrist because the patient was having suicidal thoughts. A review of his symptoms revealed that the patient met DSM -IV criteria for major depression. His score on the HDRS was 30, suggesting that he was severely depressed. He had three previous episodes of depression that responded well to medication. Because of the severity of his current episode, the patient was prescribed an antidepressant. He also met criteria for avoidant personality disorder.

A review of the interpersonal inventory revealed that Mr. D has an impoverished social network. He had lived with his parents until they died 10 years ago and he had no siblings. He had some extended family in a nearby city but was rarely in contact with them. He had no intimate friends. He occasionally interacted with two of his neighbors and found these interactions enjoyable. In reviewing past relationships, Mr. D recalled having few friends at school and a tendency to keep to himself. He was very shy with girls and never dated. He had one girlfriend in his late twenties, whom he had met at a church event. However, the relationship ended when she moved to the city for a job and he lost contact with her. He felt very lonely and this feeling became more intense during the recovery period after his bypass surgery. The therapist linked Mr. D's depression to loneliness and social isolation, and to the difficulties he had had in establishing close relationships with other people. The patient and therapist agreed that the therapy should focus on decreasing the patient's social isolation by finding settings and activities where acquaintances and friendships could be easily formed (this included attending a cardiac rehabilitation group, volunteering at a local hospital, and participating in church activities) and by improving the patient's social skills in order to increase his comfort and sense of success in interpersonal exchanges.

Termination Phase: Sessions 10-12

Although the termination phase occurs in weeks 10 through 12, the therapist will have reminded the patient of the termination date throughout the course of therapy. The principle goal of this phase of treatment is to help the patient consolidate treatment gains made during the therapy and to help the patient establish independence from the therapist [24]. The therapist reviews with the patient the gains made during treatment and the extent to which the therapy goals were attained. The therapist ensures that the patient understands what they did to produce the treatment gains in order to enhance his or her sense of self-sufficiency and competence in dealing with future problems autonomously. Feelings of sadness and apprehension about ending therapy are normalized and distinguished from a return of clinical depression.

In this stage of therapy, the therapist provides additional psychoeducation about depression, focusing on the possible risk of recurrence, and developing a strategy for relapse prevention. Research in patients without cardiac disease indicates that the risk for recurrence is 50% after the first episode, 70% after two episodes and 90% after three or more episodes [73, 74]. Research in patients with coronary heart disease suggests that 20% of patients with major depression at index and who remitted relapsed at 12-month follow-up [6]. These findings underscore the importance of relapse prevention as a treatment component during the termination phase of therapy. In this regard, the therapist reviews the presenting symptom of the current depressive illness and alerts the patient to early warning signs of future depressive episodes and the therapeutic strategies that will help manage these symptoms and prevent a relapse. The termination phase is a time in which the therapist must decide whether further sessions are required. If the patient has not responded to treatment or has only partially responded, it is important to review other treatment options. The therapist must be careful to minimize the patient's tendency to self-blame for treatment failure and to highlight the patient's efforts and successes during the course of treatment [26].

Summary

IPT is an empirically supported psychotherapy that may be useful in the treatment of cardiac patients with co-existing depression. IPT has been found to be effective in a number of depressed populations; a preliminary uncontrolled pilot study suggests that depressed cardiac patients may benefit from this brief intervention, either alone or in combination with medication [64]. The results of large, ongoing, randomized clinical trials will determine more definitively whether IPT should be included in the treatment armamentarium for depressed cardiac patients [65].

■ References

1. Frasure-Smith N, Lespérance F, Talajic M (1995) Depression and 18-month prognosis after myocardial infarction. Circulation 91:999-1005
2. Lespérance F et al (2000) Depression and 1-year prognosis in unstable angina. Arch Intern Med 160:1354-1360
3. Jiang W et al (2001) Relationship of depression to increased risk of mortality and rehospitalization in patients with congestive heart failure. Arch Intern Med 161:1849-1856
4. Connerney I et al (2001) Relation between depression after coronary artery bypass surgery and 12-month outcome: a prospective study. Lancet 358:1766-1771
5. Lespérance F, Frasure-Smith N, Talajic M (1996) Major depression before and after myocardial infarction: its nature and consequences. Psychosom Med 58:99-100
6. Hance M et al (1996) Depression in patients with coronary heart disease: a 12 month follow-up. Gen Hospital Psychiat 18:61-65
7. Follick MJ et al (1988) Quality of life post-myocardial infarction: effects of a transtelephonic coronary intervention system. Health Psychol 7:169-182
8. Waltz M et al (1988) Marriage and the psychological consequences of a heart attack: a longitudinal study of adaptation to chronic illness after 3 years. Soc Sci Med 27:149-158
9. Havik OE, Maelands JG (1991) Patterns of emotional reactions after a myocardial infarction. J Psychosom Med 100:555-561
10. Frasure-Smith N, Lespérance F, Talajic M (1993) Depression following myocardial infarction: impact on 6-month survival. JAMA 270:1819-1825
11. Ladwig KH et al (1992) Factors which provoke post-infarction depression: results from the post-infarction late potential study (PILP). J Psychsom Res 36:723-729
12. Frasure-Smith N, Lespérance F (2003) Depression and other psychological risk factors following myocardial infarction. Arch Gen Psychiat 60:627-636
13. Barefoot JC, Helms MJ, Mark DB et al (1996) Depression and long-term mortality risk in patients with coronary artery disease. Am J Cardiol 78:613-617
14. Carney RM et al (1995) Major depression and medication adherence in elder patients with coronary artery disease. Health Psychol 14:88-90
15. Musselman DL, Evans DL, Nemeroff CB (1998) The relationship of depression to cardiac disease. Arch Gen Psychiat 55:580-592
16. Krishnan KRR (2002) Comorbidity of depression with other medical diseases in the elderly. Biol Psychiat 52:559-588
17. Hollon SD et al (2002) Psychosocial intervention development for the prevention and treatment of depression: promoting innovation and increasing access. Biol Psychiat 52:610-630
18. Klerman G et al (1984) Interpersonal psychotherapy of depression. Basic Books, New York
19. Markowitz JC, Swartz HA (1997) Case formulation in interpersonal psychotherapy

for depression. In: Eels TD (Ed) Handbook of psychotherapy case formulation. Guildford Press, New York pp 192-222

20. Weissman MM , Markowitz JC (2002) Interpersonal psychotherapy for depression. In: Gotlib IA, Hammen CL (Eds) Handbook of depression. Guildford Press, New York pp 404-421

21. Aneshensel CS, Stone JD (1982) Stress and depression: a test of the buffering model of social supports. Arch Gen Psychiat 39:1392-1396

22. Weissman MM et al (1974) Treatment effects of the social adjustment of depressed patients. Arch Gen Psychiat 30:771-788

23. Coyne JC (1976) Depression and the response of others. J Abnorm Psychol 85:186-193

24. Weissman MM, Markowitz JC, Klerman GL (2000) Comprehensive guide to interpersonal psychotherapy. Basic Books, New York

25. Markowitz JC (1998) Interpersonal Psychotherapy for Dysthymia. American Psychiatry Press, Washington DC

26. Markowitz JC, Weissman MM (1995) Interpersonal Psychotherapy. In: EBeckham EE, Leber WR (Eds) Handbook of depression. Guildford Press, New York pp 376-390

27. Swartz HA, Markowitz JC, Frank E (2002) Interpersonal psychotherapy for unipolar and bipolar disorders. In: Hofmann SG, Tompson, MC (Eds) Treating chronic and severe mental disorders: a handbook of empirically supported interventions. The Guildford Press, New York pp 131-158

28. Jack DC (1999) Silencing the self: inner dialogues and outer realities. In: Joiner T, Coyne JC (Eds) The interactional nature of depression. American Psychological Association, Washington, DC pp 221-246

29. Wilfley DE et al (2000) Interpersonal psychotherapy for groups. Basic Books, New York

30. Markowitz JC, Svartberg M, Swartz HA (1998) Is IPT time-limited psychotherapy? J Psychother Pract Res 7:198-195

31. Stuart S, Robertson M (2003) Interpersonal psychotherapy: a clinician's guide. Oxford University Press, New York

32. Weissman MM et al (1979) The efficacy of drugs and psychotherapy in the treatment of acute depressive episodes. Am J Psychiat 136:555-558

33. Weissman MM et al (1981) Depressed outpatients: results one year after treatment with drugs and/or interpersonal psychotherapy. Arch Gen Psychiat 38:51-55

34. Elkin J et al (1989) National Institute of Mental Health treatment of depression collaborative research program: general effectiveness of treatments. Arch Gen Psychiat 46:971-982

35. Brown G et al (2002) Sertraline and/or interpersonal psychotherapy for patients with dysthymic disorder in primary care: 6-month comparison with longitudinal 2-year follow-up of effectiveness and costs. J Aff Dis 68:317-330

36. Spinelli MG, Endicott J (2003) Controlled clinical trial of interpersonal psychotherapy versus parenting education for depressed pregnant women. Am J Psychiat 160:555-562

37. Stuart S, O'Hara MW (1995) IPT for postpartum depression. J Psychother Pract Res 4:18-29

38. Markowitz J et al (1998) Treatment of HIV-positive patients with depressive symptoms. Arch Gen Psychiat 55:452-457

39. Mufson L et al (1993) Interpersonal psychotherapy for depressed adolescents. The Guildford Press, New York

40. Mufson L et al (1999) Efficacy of interpersonal psychotherapy for depressed adolescents. Arch Gen Psychiat 56:573-579
41. Reynolds CF III et al (1999) Treatment of bereavement-related major depressive-episodes in later life: a controlled study of acute and continuation treatment with nortriptyline and interpersonal psychotherapy. Am J Psychiat 156:202-208
42. Schulberg H et al (1996) Treating major depression in primary care practice: eight month clinical outcomes. Arch Gen Psychiat 153:1293-1300
43. Frank E, Swartz HA, Kupfer DJ (2000) Interpersonal and social rhythms therapy: managing the chaos of bipolar disorder. Biol Psychiat 48:593-604
44. Lenze EJ, Dew MA, Mazumdar S (2002) Combined pharmacotherapy and psychotherapy as maintenance treatment for late-life depression: effects on social adjustment. Am J Psychiat 159:466-468
45. Hellerstein DJ et al (2001) Adding group psychotherapy to medication treatment in dysthymia: a randomized prospective pilot study. J Psychother Pract Res 10:93-103
46. Levkovitz Y et al (2000) Group interpersonal psychotherapy for patients with major depression disorder - pilot study. J Aff Dis 60:191-195
47. Scocco P, De Leo D, Frank E (2002) Is interpersonal psychotherapy in group format a therapeutic option in late-life depression? Clin Psychol Psychother 9:68-75
48. Frank E et al (1990) Three-year outcome for maintenance therapies in recurrent depression. Arch Gen Psychiat 47:1093-1099
49. Kupfer DJ, Frank E, Perel JM (1992) Five-year outcome for maintenance therapies in recurrent depression. Arch Gen Psychiat 49:769-773
50. Berkman LF, Syme SL (1979) Social networks, host resistance, and mortality: a nine-year follow-up study of Alameda county residents. Am J Epidemiol 79 109:186-204
51. Oxman TE, Hull JG (1997) Social support, depression, and activities of daily living in older heart surgery patients. J Gerontol 52B:1-14
52. Case RB et al (1992) Living alone after myocardial infarction: impact on prognosis. JAMA 515-519
53. Berkman LF, Leo-Summers L, Horwitz RI (1992) Emotional support and survival after myocardial infarction: a prospective population-based study of the elderly. Ann Intern Med 117:1003-1009
54. Williams RB et al (1992) Prognostic importance of social and economic resources among medically treated patients with angiographically documented coronary artery disease. JAMA 267:520-524
55. Wallerston BS et al (1983) Social support and physical health. Health Psychol 2:367-391
56. Gianetti VJ, Reynolds J, Rihn T (1985) Factors which differentiate smokers from ex-smokers among cardiovascular patients: a discriminant analysis. Soc Sci Med 20:241-245
57. Williams CA et al (1985) The Edgecombe County high blood pressure control program, III: social support, social stressors and treatment dropout. Am J Public Health 75:483-486
58. Oxman TE, Berkman LF (1990) Assessment of social relationships in elderly patients. Int J Psychiat Med 20:65-84
59. Oxman TE et al (1994) Social support and depression after cardiac surgery in elderly patients. Am J Geriatric Psychiat 2:309-323

60. Bramwell L (1990) Social support in cardiac rehabilitation. Can J Cardiovasc Nursing 1:7-13
61. Schaefer C, Coyne JC, Lazarus RS (1981) The health-related functions of social support. J Behav Med 4:381-406
62. Goodheart CD, Lansing MH (1997) Treating people with chronic disease: a psychological guide. American Psychological Association, Washington, DC
63. Segrin C (2001) Interpersonal processes in psychological problems. The Guildford Press, New York
64. Koszycki D et al (2004) Open trial and interpersonal psycotherapy, with or without medication, in depressed patients with coronary disease. Psychosomatics 45:319-324
65. Frasure-Smith N et al CREATE (Canadian Cardiac Randomized Evaluation of Antidepressant and Psycotherapy Efficacy) (2006) Design and rationale for a randomized controlled trial of interpersonal psycotherapy and citalopram for depression in coronary disease. Psychosom Med 68:87-93
66. Parsons T (1951) Illness and the role of the physician: a sociological perspective. Am J Orthopsychiat 21:452-460
67. Mikulincer M, Florian V, Wller A (1993) Attachment styles, coping strategies and posttraumatic psychological distress: the impact of the gulf war in Israel. J Pers Soc Psychol 64:817-826
68. Lespérance F, Frasure-Smith N (2000) Depression in patients with cardiac disease: a practical review. J Psychosomatic Res 48:379-391
69. American Psychiatry Association (1993) Practice guideline for major depressive disorder in adults. Am J Psychiat (Suppl 150):4
70. Sotsky SM et al (1991) Patient predictors of response to psychotherapy and pharmacotherapy: findings in the NIMH treatment of depression collaborative research program. Am J Psychiat 148:997-1008
71. Stoudemire A, Blazer DG (1985) Depression in the elderly. In: Beckham ER, Leber WR (Eds) Handbook of depression: treatment, assessment and research. The Dorsey Press, Illinois
72. Krause (1991) Stress and isolation from close ties in later life. J Gerontol 46:S183-194
73. Solomon DA et al (1997) Recovery from major depression: a 10-year prospective follow-up across multiple episodes. Arch Gen Psychiat 54:1001-1006
74. Keller MB et al (1983) Predictors of relapse in major depressive disorder. JAMA 250:3299-3304

Chapter 19

Hanging onto a Heartbeat: Emotionally Focused Therapy for Couples Dealing with the Trauma of Coronary Heart Disease

H.B. MacIntosh ▪ S.M. Johnson ▪ A. Lee

Introduction

Our understanding of trauma is expanding as clinical vignettes gradually flesh out the bones of the DSM-IV's narrow definition [1]. Threat of loss of life is central to all definitions of trauma and is a pivotal element to the experience of cardiac events such as myocardial infarctions (MI) in coronary heart disease (CHD). The threat of loss is not only experienced by patients but is also vividly and vigilantly lived by the partners who watch and wait in waiting rooms and by bedsides hanging onto the every heartbeat of the person with whom they share their life and love. The majority of patients who suffer myocardial infarctions are married men under the age of 70 [2]. CHD is the leading cause of death for men and women in the United States, with 14 million people living with CHD and 1.5 million new MIs each year [3].

Literature pertaining to stress and coping following major illness has focused primarily on the experience of the individual patient and his or her recovery without an inclusive understanding of the primacy of the couple relationship in enduring and adapting to this traumatic and life-threatening experience [4]. Relationships play a role at every level in the health and welfare of members of the couple. They play an element in causation, a key factor in coping and an important resource for future outcomes [5]. The partner is the most relevant and influential contributor to the creation of a supportive context during the acute phase following cardiac surgery [6]. At the same time, twenty percent of men in hospitals following a myocardial infarction (MI) attribute problems with their partner as an important cause of their cardiac problem.

It is the goal of this chapter to offer a conceptualization of CHD as a traumatic event and to integrate the partner into our understanding of the impact of and recovery from CHD. Emotionally focused therapy (EFT) for couples will be proffered as an example of a treatment modality for the psychological distress of CHD that uses the primacy of the couple relationship as a resource for healing and change. The term *patient* will be used to describe the member of the couple who has coronary heart disease. The term *partner* will be used to describe the partner of the patient with coronary heart disease.

The Couple Relationship and Physical Health

The couple relationship has consistently been associated with various measures of physical health. Two explanations have been offered to explain the health-enhancing properties of intimate relationships: selection and protection. The first explanation suggests that healthier people are more likely to be in and stay in intimate relationships. The second suggests that relationships act as protections, in that the individuals involved tend to take better care of themselves because, usually, they have more resources [7].

Couple conflict has been associated with high levels of catecholamines, and hormones related to stress and illness such as corticotropins and growth hormones [8]. Kiecolt-Glaser [9] examined the impact of the couple relationship on immune functioning. They consistently found that cortisol levels increased during conflict and decreased when partners were talking about the positive aspects of their relationship. These findings were more marked in women than men, with women demonstrating much higher increases in cortisol and slower and smaller decreases. Additional studies have confirmed these findings and linked relationship distress to depression and decreased immune system functioning [9-11]. House and coll. [12] emphasized in their research that being in a conflictual, unhappy relationship is more damaging to physical health than smoking cigarettes for many years.

The Couple Relationship and Coronary Heart Disease

Couple relationship stress has a direct and indirect relationship to cardiac problems. Indirectly, the couple relationship has been associated with the development of depressive symptoms, which are strongly associated with increases in cardiac problems. In an empirical study [13], found that 17-36 percent of individuals with chronic depression go on to develop cardiac problems. In a study of 1,151 individuals, Pratt [14] found a consistent relationship between depression and the risk for CHD, with increases in mortality, morbidity and longer hospital stays in response to cardiac events.

Couple conflict has also been associated with increased blood pressure, which is a risk factor for CHD [15]. Similarly, distress contributes to increases in morbidity and has been found to be a risk factor for future health complications and premature death in CHD patients [16]. Self-reported couple quality was found to moderate the relationship between stress and well-being, acting either as a protective factor, or increasing vulnerability, when patients were confronted with other risk factors [6].

Results of a study of 736 men with CHD followed over six years suggest that couple stress and conflict can trigger the onset of acute myocardial infarction (AMI), the progression of atherosclerosis, endothelial dysfunction and plaque instability. Being in an emotionally supportive, close relationship significantly decreases new cardiac events, while patients in relationships with a combination of low intimacy and high conflict experience more anxiety and depression [8, 17]. It therefore appears undeniable that the quality of the relationship impacts the likelihood of a recurrence of the disease.

Impact of Coronary Heart Disease on Partner

Partners of CHD patients have been described as "hidden patients" [18] and are at considerable risk for psychological distress following their partner's MI [19]. Partners have shown higher levels of psychological distress, including anxiety and depression, than patients during hospitalization for CHD [20-22]. Twenty-four to thirty-eight percent of partners evidence persistent psychological distress such as anxiety one year after their partner's MI [19, 23, 24].

Central to the well-being of the partner is the quality of the couple relationship and the ability of the patient to offer support to the partner [19, 25]. Pre-MI couple happiness is consistently associated with lower levels of stress in partners after MI [19, 26].

The level of physical health of the patient has been found to be directly associated both with the partners' coping ability and with the ability to effectively utilize family resources and support networks. Additionally, improvement in the health of the patient has a positive impact on the reported quality of life of the partner [27, 28].

Stressors that have a significant impact on the mental health of partners during the acute hospitalization phase of CHD include feeling a lack of control with respect to the hospital process and what is happening to their partner, feeling uninformed by hospital staff, lacking information about the safe resumption of sexual activity, having limited opportunities to express distress and fear about losing their spouse and the security of the relationship and, lastly, experiencing fears about changes in family roles. Additionally, self-blame has been identified as a significant stressor for partners - feeling that somehow they had a role in the illness of their partner. Some researchers envision the partner's ability to cope with the CHD of their partner as a series of critical tasks such as living with the fear of the death of their partner [29-31].

In a study of social support and wives of CHD patients, quantitative aspects of social support, e.g., the number of persons offering help, were unrelated to emotional adjustment and the utilization of healthcare services. However, qualitative aspects of social support, such as satisfaction with support from children, partners and partners' families, were associated with all outcomes [5]. Essentially, it is the experience of feeling supported rather than the actual number of casseroles brought to a partner's door that makes the difference with respect to coping ability.

Relationship Between Partner and Patient Distress in CHD

A significant relationship has been found between the psychological distress of each partner and their couple adjustment in dealing with CHD. As the patient's distress increases, so does that of the partner. Levels of psychological distress in both partners and patients have been identified as significant, with 57% of patients and 40% of partners meeting criteria for a psychiatric disorder following a major cardiac event. This distress also strongly correlates within the couple itself, with a higher level of distress in one member bringing about a higher level of distress in the other. Researchers have suggested that this is an expression of empathy as indicated by the fact that higher levels of personal distress in the couple are also associated with high levels of satisfaction with the couple relationship [4, 32]. Interestingly, the partners' level of distress can be predicted from retrospective reports of couple quality before the MI [4]. This information is crucial in our understanding of the need to include partners in the recovery process, especially given the finding that lower levels of psychological distress in partners has been found to predict higher self-efficacy in the patient after the MI [4].

Impact of CHD on Couple Relationship

Given the strong relationship between partners' distress in dealing with CHD it is inevitable that CHD will have an impact on the couple relationship. CHD illness has been associated with increases in couple closeness, but, at the same time, relationship problems that existed before a cardiac event tend to become worse after an episode [8, 33].

Relationship concerns reported by couples dealing with CHD include the return to sexual activity after coronary events, the potential impact of CHD on couple relationship satisfaction, worries about the health of the partner and, lastly, guilt and resentment about how the illness is affecting their lives [28]. In learning to cope with CHD, couples needed to respond and adapt to role reassignment, the redistribution of responsibilities, undertaking of illness-related tasks and dealing with the conflicting emotions that arise from these changes [6].

The Impact of Couple Relationship on CHD

Psychosocial factors have been found to be more powerful predictors of adjustment following AMI than physical health indicators [34-36]. Given the primacy of the couple relationship in the life of the patient, this has been an important area of study in research on factors related to recovery in CHD. The patient's relationship has been found to be a powerful predictor of recovery from a cardiac event; patients who were visited more often by their partners used less medication, had shorter stays in the intensive care unit and left the hospital earlier than their less-visited counterparts [37].

In several studies, support from a partner, relational cohesiveness and time together have been shown to influence recovery more than any other aspect of coping, and even to lead to a decreased risk of dying, as well as to an increase in psychological functioning during the recovery phase [6, 38, 39]. Intimacy leads to decreased worrying about symptoms and death, which has been shown to have an effect on cardiac symptoms such as dyspnea and angina [35]. Couples who feel that they can have open discussions about their feelings have also been found to display lower levels of chest pain post-MI and lower levels of rehospitalization in the year following the MI [40].

Chronic problems and difficulties in relationships increase the risk of further cardiac events over a 5-year period. Counter to early hypotheses, problems with work and other stressors did not contribute to the increase of cardiac risk [15]. Self-reported couple stress has been associated with poorer prognoses as measured by cardiac death, myocardial infarction and revascularization. Women patients who reported severe couple stress displayed three times the risk for a new coronary event following initial rehabilitation [8]. Poor couple communication has been found to predict mortality after an MI [4]. Couple conflict has been seen as a factor in the development of excessive cardiovascular reactivity to stress, which is a risk factor for the development of hypertension and CHD [7]. Conflictual marriages characterized by low cohesiveness have been associated with increased cardiovascular responses and higher blood pressure when patients have contact with their partners [41, 42].

In terms of the process of recovery, the active support of a partner leads to increases in compliance with medical regimens, decreases in patient anxiety and depression, and increased coping [43, 44]. Conversely, Ewart [42] suggests that the failure to resolve relational conflict contributes to enhanced sympathetic tone, which is believed to play an early role in hypertension and atherogenesis.

The couple relationship can make or break a recovery. A positive, intimate relationship can lead to greater self-efficacy in the patient, decreased symptoms and a lower risk of dying. A negative and conflictual relationship can lead to depression, increased cardiac symptoms and a greater risk of death by new cardiac event. It is essential that the couple relationship be seen as the resource that it is. Couples who are struggling will benefit from the relational enhancement of couple therapy and those who are thriving will benefit from the forum for sharing their feelings and fears about the CHD through learning how to be even closer and share their fears in the safe haven of their partner.

Coronary Heart Disease as a Trauma

The definition of trauma according to the diagnostic and statistical manual of mental disorders (DSM IV TR [1]) is the exposure to an event in which a person experiences, witnesses or is confronted by the threat of death or serious injury, and in which the person responds with intense fear, helplessness or horror. Responses to traumatic events are often experienced through intrusive thoughts about the event, a sense of reliving the experience, intense psychological distress at exposure to internal or external cues reminiscent of the traumatic event, or physiological reactivity on exposure to internal or external cues that symbolize or resemble an aspect of the traumatic event. This can result in persistently avoiding reminders of the trauma and, especially in the case of CHD, avoiding physical sensations reminiscent of the cardiac event, restricted range of affect (such as trying to control emotions about the cardiac event) and avoiding thoughts that give rise to fear of a foreshortened future. Increased arousal is often represented by hypervigilance and in the case of CHD this can be related to the awareness of the closeness that the patient came to death [1].

McCurry [43] in his qualitative study examined the effects of CHD on partners of patients awaiting heart transplant. Themes that continued to arise in his interviews with wives included hypervigilance, difficulties managing overwhelming emotions, anxiety and emotionally focusing on the partner. The potential for death arose as an ever-present theme in the experience of these partners, who reported being constantly aware and fearful of this reality. "It seems like there is a new time bomb starting up," said one partner. Other studies have found that couples dealing with severe physical health problems indicate that they have difficulties in coping as a result of their vigilance with respect to the health problems and symptoms of the afflicted spouse, and the uncertainty and unpredictability of his or her health [45, 46]. This vigilance is reported to be very difficult to let go of and very disruptive to the functioning of the couple [43]. These descriptions are evocative of our growing understanding of the effect of trauma, and they support the view that we need to expand the definition of trauma to cardiac events that are life- threatening, potentially recurrent and terrifying.

■ Why Couples Need Treatment

By enlisting the most important person in a patient's life, therapists can help minimize risk factors over time, thereby contributing to decreased mortality and morbidity and to an increased ability for the couple to support themselves and each other in dealing with the impact of CHD. For couples that report high satisfaction and relationship quality, therapy can offer support in adjustment to illness- related changes, grieving CHD-related losses and processing the traumatic event. In addition to this, for couples who report low satisfaction and relationship quality, therapy can offer a remedy to the relational elements, such as conflict, stress, low cohesiveness, disclosure and intimacy, and distressing interpersonal interactions - all of which are risk factors for future cardiac events.

Schmaling and Sher [47] emphasized the need to include partners in the therapy of individuals dealing with illness. They articulated four issues important for healthcare professionals to understand when offering support to couples. These included:
1. understanding the reciprocal relationship between health and relationship satisfaction;

2. understanding the benefits from including the partner in therapy so that both spouses can learn and implement change in the immediate environment of the patient;
3. understanding that an effective treatment considers the needs of the partner as well as the needs of the patient;
4. understanding that psychotherapy can help couples cope with the effects of the illness on themselves, each other and their relationship.

Psychotherapy for couples dealing with CHD has been found to decrease anxiety in both patient and partner [48]. Similarly, psychosocial interventions added to rehabilitation programs have been found to reduce cardiac mortality and recurrent MI by 40% over the first 2 years [49]. In another study, patients who reported feeling that their relationship was capable of changing in response to their illness and who felt supported by their partners showed resiliency and direction in their path to recovery [6]. Also, partners who reported lower levels of anxiety in response to the CHD tended to use less denial, were better able to make plans for the future and were better able to cope with the challenges related to the recovery of their spouse from cardiac events. Conversely, partners who avoided disclosing their feelings and who felt that they needed to protect the patient from their fears and upsetting feelings showed the highest levels of distress and the lowest couple relationship satisfaction [4, 40, 50].

Another reason to include partners in recovery programs and to offer couple interventions concerns the relationship between couple quality and behaviors associated with success in recovery. Couples therapy can contribute to individual behavioral change [51]. Partners play an important role in supporting patients in their recovery and rehabilitation programs. Patients in distressed relationships reported that their partners offered them less emotional support, emotional sharing and less help with behaviors associated with enhanced recovery, such as exercising and quitting smoking. Their relationships were also troubled by potentially harmful behaviors such as conflict and neglect [3]. Additionally, partners have been found to help patients maintain or continue with weight loss after treatment has ended [52-54].

Several empirically validated approaches to couples therapy are used with cardiac patients to treat spouses. Emotionally focused couples therapy (EFT) is also used for couples facing chronic illness [55]. Rankin-Esquer and colleagues [3] described the development of a relationship support program for enhancing the relationship between the patient and his/her partner. This program was modeled after cognitive behavioral couple therapy but focused on increasing the couple's ability to cope with stress, and create in the relationship a source of support. They describe three phases in their therapy:

1. focusing on processing the experience of the cardiac event;
2. exploring how relationship issues affect and are affected by the cardiac event;
3. increasing general relationship skills to help the couple support each other and function optimally.

Trauma and Attachment

Feeling secure with a loved one increases a person's ability to tolerate and cope with traumatic experiences. The attachment system is evolution's way of maximizing possibilities for survival in a dangerous world. Humans have survived throughout the millennia by being social beings that provide a safe haven and secure base for their loved ones from which to explore and learn about the world [56, 57]. Secure attachment creates resilience in the face of terror and helplessness and a natural arena for healing. Isolation and a lack of secure attachment add to our vulnerability, exacerbate traumatic events and are actually wounding in themselves. It is also hard to develop an integrated, confident sense of self without secure connections to significant others.

Attachment has also been described as a "theory of trauma" [58] to denote that isolation and separation are intense adverse experiences for humans, especially in times of vulnerability. Affect is the music of the attachment dance [59]. The loss of affect regulation as a result of trauma can be expected to play havoc with close relationships.

Supportive interpersonal relationships mediate both the immediate and long-term impact of trauma and may be important to resilience [60-62]. Those who evidenced secure attachments with a caregiver or in a supportive relationship report fewer problems than those who do not [61, 62].

Caring touch can soothe a person in distress, and CHD patients with satisfying couple relationships can rely on feeling safe in the comfort and support of an intimate partner or in the confiding that gives meaning and structure to difficult experiences [63, 64].

Emotionally Focused Therapy for Couples

EFT has been investigated extensively and has been found to be effective with diverse populations, including depressed women [65-67], and families experiencing chronic stress or coping with a chronically ill child [68]. The therapy has also been used with couples coping with a partner who has survived severe trauma and has symptoms of PTSD [57, 69]. The process of change in EFT can be divided into nine treatment steps and three stages (see Table 1). EFT is a short-term, structured approach that has proven reliable in the repair of distressed couple relationships. It has demonstrated both clinical effectiveness [51] and relatively high and stable treatment effects [70].

Proponents of EFT view attachment as a theory well suited to adult love relationships and as one that addresses the gaps in existing paradigms of adult love. Attachment theorists postulate that humans are innately driven to develop and maintain strong affectional bonds to significant others [71]. In couple relationships, secure attachments are represented by relationships that are reciprocal, affectionate and where both partners feel close, safe and nurtured [72]. Secure bonds are characterized by accessibility and by the responsiveness of each partner toward the other. These bonds allow couples to help each other with the regulation of the emotional distress that arises in the context of life-threatening illness [60].

EFT was developed in the early 1980s in response to an absence of standardized and tested non-behavioral approaches within the couple's therapy field. Primarily, the field focused on behavioral and cognitive change while leaving the role of emotion unexplored both in theory and practice. EFT has been empirically validated and presently is recognized as one of only two empirically validated extant couple interventions [51, 73]. Numerous studies have validated EFT through outcome-based research methods. Couple distress has been the primary focus of these studies as measured by the Dyadic Adjustment Scale (DAS) [74]. In a review of the EFT research, nine studies revealed significant improvement in DAS scores [75-78], compared both with waiting list controls and pretreatment DAS scores; and in 70-75% of the EFT-treated couples, the criteria for recovery were met - i.e., the couples were no longer relationally distressed [70]. These studies have added greatly to the body of clinical literature on couple therapy. EFT is on the cutting edge of couples' therapy. It integrates intrapersonal and interpersonal perspectives, experiential and systemic orientations, and it is collaborate, validated and uses emotion as a key resource for bringing about change [55].

EFT clinicians and researchers envision the couple relationship as an attachment bond [79] whereby distressed relationships are viewed as insecure bonds. From within these insecure bonds, attachment needs for comfort, security and closeness are not being met due to compelling negative emotional responses and constricted interactional patterns that arise and block emotional connection and engagement between partners. The main focus of the therapy is on reorganizing patterns of underlying emotional responses to relational interactions in order to reorient and transform negative interactional patterns, thereby fostering secure attachments between partners [57-80].

Johnson [57] hypothesized that relationship distress results from the failure of the attachment relationship to provide a secure base for one or both partners. When this secure base is not available there is an intensification of attachment behaviors such as protest and clinging, avoidance or withdrawal. This process degenerates until neither partner is able to be responsive or accessible to the other. This unresponsiveness continues to generate more and more insecurity until emotional engagement cannot be sustained and results in a complete lack of safe emotional attunement. Attunement in adult relationships is the sensitive moment-to-moment being with a partner as he/she experiences and expresses an emotion, as well as exhibiting behaviors that convey that one can empathically enter into and share the other's affective state. As insecure attachment responses become extreme and impermeable, they may render partners almost incapable of the open responsiveness that is the foundation of the secure bond with others. Avoidance makes modification of attachment style difficult until, eventually, both partners withdraw and the relationship is in jeopardy.

Understanding the pivotal role that attachment patterns can play in the maintenance of relationship satisfaction and how relationship distress arises when attachment relationships fail to provide a secure base for partners is important, and it behooves clinicians to integrate an awareness of attachment-related processes into any couples therapy process. Secure attachment is associated with happier and closer relationships [60].

Critical elements in couple distress are hypothesized to be the absorbing states of negative affect such as anger or fear [81]. Melding experiential (intrapsychic), systemic (interpersonal) and humanistic theoretical approaches, therapeutic interventions using EFT create relationship change events and processes [80]. EFT rests on the premise that it is the failure of the couple to express their underlying emotional needs that inhibits communication and the ability to resolve conflict. Through unveiling shrouded emotional needs and attachment longings, and identifying negative interactional cycles, unhealthy patterns can begin to change [67]. EFT not only facilitates the expression of needs, it helps create new responses in each partner.

The process of change requires a shift from a dysfunctional interactional cycle such as blame/defend to a more open responsiveness exemplified by a secure attachment bond. A central tenet of EFT for CHD couples is the notion that assisting the couple in the creation and/or maintenance of a secure attachment bond will assist the CHD patient and partner in dealing with their traumatic experience within the context of the relationship, thereby improving both their psychological functioning and the satisfaction and security they derive from their relationship.

As shown in the table below, the process of change in EFT is divided into three stages and nine treatment steps [55]. In the first stage, De-escalation, there are four steps. The first step includes an assessment of the core issues and conflict using an attachment perspective. The therapeutic alliance is developed and the unveiling process is begun. In the second step the interactional cycles that maintain attachment insecurity and relationship distress are identified. The third step involves delving into the unacknowledged emotions underlying these self-reinforcing interactional patterns. The fourth step involves reframing the problems in terms of the cycle, underlying emotions and attachment needs. The second stage is devoted to Changing Interactional Positions. Step 5 promotes an identification with disavowed needs and facets of the self that have been withheld in relationship interactions and integrating them. Step 6 involves the promotion of acceptance of the partner's new "construction of experience in the relationship and new responses." Step 7 involves the key change event of facilitating the expression of specific needs and wants and creating emotional engagement. In the third stage, Consolidation/Integration, step 8 develops new solutions to old problem relationship issues, and step 9 consolidates new positions and cycles of attachment behavior [80].

Stages of EFT

Stages of EFT	Step	Focus
1. De-escalation	i Assessment	Of core issues and conflicts from attachment perspective
	ii Identification	Of problem interactional cycle maintaining attachment insecurity and distress
	ii Emotions	Accessing unacknowledged emotions and underlying interactional patterns
	iv Reframing	Of problem in terms of cycle, underlying emotions and attachment
2. Changing	v Identification of interactional patterns	Of disowned needs and aspects of the self, and integrating this knowledge into relationship
	vi Deepening & expanding experience & creating new interactions	Involving a new construction of experience in relationship and responses
	vii Facilitation	Of expression of specific needs and wants, creating emotional engagement
3. Consolidation/ integration	viii New solutions	To old problematic relationship issues are facilitated
	ix Consolidation	Of new positions and cycles of attachment behavior

In a recent theoretical exploration of the topic of how EFT can be successfully applied to the treatment of couples where one partner is dealing with trauma, Johnson [57], using an example of childhood sexual abuse, clearly articulated the goals and process of change for this therapy. Johnson indicated that the therapeutic process creates a holding environment. The goal of therapy is to help clients increase the permeability and complexity of working models of attachment by revising them both cognitively and affectively on the basis of new information, which is carefully choreographed within the therapeutic milieu. A more secure bond with a partner creates a safe haven that helps the traumatized partner regulate grief, anger and fear in a positive self- and relationship-enhancing way. This safe haven helps the patient and partner deal with re-experiencing emotionally loaded symptoms, such as nightmares, intrusive thoughts and flashbacks, in a constructive way. Echoes of past attachment relationships that create specific sensitivities in a present relationship are acknowledged in therapy, but not viewed as limiting in the sense of deterministic; attachment styles, often learned in past relationships, can be modified in new relationships. Isolation minimizes our ability to deal with stress, fear and traumatic events. Being able to turn to one's partner for comfort begins to replace other negative affect-regulation strategies such as self-mutilation or dissociation. If assuaging fear is the primary goal in the treatment of trauma [82], the patient and partner are made aware of the fact that the natural inborn antidote to fear in primates is contact comfort. The availability of the spouse also lessens the need for numbing and dissociation, and allows fear to be confronted. Spouses then become allies against the incursions of trauma rather than cues for traumatic memories.

A safe relationship can harbor distress and renders emotions such as shame and grief endurable. Since empathy counteracts shame, the creation of empathy between partners allows the couple to deal positively with issues such as the need for high levels of control with respect to closeness and physical contact. Attachment relationships are physiological and emotional regulators that organize emotional life, and, in so doing, provide a safe attachment that allows patients and partners to grieve and come to terms with the losses associated with CHD; over time, this enables the loss to become ground rather than figure, periphery rather than center stage [83].

Through EFT, therapists can assist couples in creating corrective emotional experiences, where soothing, comfort and support are experienced and solidified. Once this safe base is established, the safety that has been achieved facilitates the continued reprocessing and integration of traumatic experience and increases the coping ability of both partners. Affective states can then be used as cues to attend to incoming information rather than alarm signals that prime hyper-arousal or numbing. "Fight or flight" responses are not acted on by the CHD patient, or his or her partner, and the couple becomes better able to confide in and receive comfort from each other. This powerful process uses partners as allies in the process of recovery and healing rather than leaving them on the sidelines or excluding them.

▦ Case History: Even Though and Especially Since

Jeanine Alberto and her husband Tony were referred for couple therapy by a psychologist who had been treating Jeanine for depression. The therapist noted that Jeanine, who had recently taken several weeks away from her office job because she felt unable to cope with a particular stressful situation at work, was also distressed about her couple relationship. Jeanine was in her mid-fifties, a petite French-Canadian woman, soft-spoken, pleasant and stylishly dressed. She sat neatly on the edge of her chair as the interview began. Tony was a jovial, plump, 57-year-old man. His eyes crinkled when he smiled and his cheeks were very red. He had emigrated from Italy at the age of 20, and had worked for many years in computer maintenance. He had been laid off from his job four years previously and was currently working as an insurance salesman.

In the first session the couple described numerous stressors. Precipitating Jeanine's depression was a situation at her office involving a dishonest and lazy colleague and a boss who did not support her. In addition to symptoms of depression, Jeanine also had numerous non-specific physical complaints, including stomach problems, a sore neck and backaches. Jeanine's mother, who was a difficult and hostile woman, was terminally ill with cancer, and the couple's younger daughter was thinking of leaving her husband. Tony expressed considerable concern over Jeanine's depression, and elaborated on the situation with her mother, saying that his mother-in-law had always been cruel to his wife. He added that he had also been giving Jeanine plenty of advice concerning her workplace situation. Jeanine offered that Tony, too, had had problems, including a heart attack three years previously (eleven months after he lost his job) which, within a year, was followed by quadruple by-pass surgery.

When asked about his cardiac experiences, Tony dismissed them, saying that he was doing very well now; but he did acknowledge distress related to finances and a deep regret that his wife would have to keep working for several more years. He told me he'd be willing to attend couple sessions, if they would help his wife. When asked whether he could he see any benefits for himself, he replied that if his wife were happier, he would be happier, too. Jeanine obtained a score on the Dyadic Adjustment Scale (DAS) [74] of 64. This score indicates significant couple distress, as a score of 70 is typical of divorcing couples [74]. Tony's non-distressed score of 98 suggested that he was not acknowledging his feelings or somehow not connecting with his wife's distress.

When I asked them about their relationship, Jeanine spoke up.

JEANNINE:	*"Tony shuts me out and I have no one to talk to. He's fantastic with my mother, he really helps me to cope with her - he has so much patience and I appreciate this. But he doesn't listen to me. He doesn't want to know".*
TONY:	*"That's not fair. I've given you plenty of help with Stella at work. I've helped a lot".*
JEANNINE:	*"Tony, when I'm upset at work you give me sermons on what to do and what not to do. You never listen to how I feel".*
TONY:	*"I do care how you feel. I brought home flowers for you last Friday".*
JEANNINE:	*"Yes, you buy me flowers. You buy me diamonds that we can't afford, too. You do it to shut me up so that you can watch television. It's not what I want, Tony. I want my partner to be part of my life, not to shut me out".*

The picture of the couple's current distress began to emerge as a pursue-and-criticize, followed by a defend-attack-then-withdraw cycle, with Jeanine beginning to "burn out" or "give up" on her pursuit for closeness with Tony. Apparently Tony had always had a tendency to withdraw temporarily when upset, but, since the heart attack, the situation had escalated, and, in addition to withdrawing, he had become short tempered and irritable. Jeanine, who longed to spend time with her husband doing simple things, such as walking the dog together or sitting and enjoying the garden at night, instead found herself quite wary of him and beginning to avoid him. In the context of her difficulties at work, she resented that she could not obtain comfort from him. She suspected that he worried about his cardiac health, as she did, but he always brushed her off when she broached the subject.

Overall, the therapeutic alliance developed easily and well in the first session. Jeanine clearly felt validated and seemed to trust that I understood that she was lonely in her relationship. Tony tended to smile or make little jokes when painful subjects came up, but, after a while, he, too, relaxed and seemed find the session "not too dangerous". In EFT an alliance is our most important tool, for when clients feel safe, understood and supported, they will take greater risks and share more intimate experiences than if they do not feel supported, or if they feel judged. In essence, we try to create a "safe haven" in therapy sessions where clients can take risks.

In our second session Jeanine told her husband: "You can be really nice to other people, but when it comes to me, you snap or are mean. I get meanness from my mother, and I get meanness from Stella at work. I don't want meanness in my marriage, too. It makes me feel I am worthless, nothing, not valued by anyone, and it hurts me. You buy me flowers, yes, but the same evening you snap at me. So your flowers mean nothing to me".

I asked Tony if he understood what his wife meant by "mean?" He blushed, laughed and nodded.

THERAPIST: *"So Tony, help me to understand the 'mean.' What is it that happens on the inside, or between you, that leads to 'mean'?"*

TONY: Grins at therapist sheepishly.

THERAPIST: Reflects body language
"Tony - your smile is grinning at me, but your eyes are brimming with sadness".

TONY: Looks at the floor, and swallows, looks back at the therapist with tears in his eyes.

THERAPIST: *"You look sad, Tony".*

TONY: *"I don't mean to hurt her... to be mean. It's just that I don't know what I do to make her upset. I - I feel I'm losing her. She's stressed now, with her work and her mom. I don't want to rock the boat".*

Jeanine: Interjects
"So, if you are so worried for me, why do you have to be so mean?"

Immediately Tony, who had been looking at the therapist, whirled around to face his wife and snapped at her loudly: "What do you want from me?" As an EFT therapist, I find an interaction like this extremely valuable. The couple were enacting the cycle that maintained their distress right before my eyes. I reflected this to Jeanine and Tony, telling them that this was a useful opportunity for us to sort out together the kind of conflict that happens at home.

THERAPIST: *"So, I guess I saw a 'snap' happen there. Is that the sort of thing that you describe as 'mean' Jeanine?"*

JEANINE: *"Yes. When he talks to me like that I feel just awful".*

THERAPIST: Empathically. *"The snap feels' mean' to you and you feel upset?"*

JEANINE: Looks down at her hands. *"That's when I feel he doesn't care for me... like nobody does... at work... my mother... even Tony..."* She looks very tearful.

THERAPIST: *"It feels then like Tony doesn't love you".*
Tracking the negative pattern between the couple.
"It must be really painful for you when you get that feeling. What do you do then, Jeanine?"

JEANINE:	*"That's when I go away and just stay by myself. I cry sometimes, but sometimes I'm really mad. Last summer I even hit him. I pounded on his chest. He just walked away, so I hit him in the back too. But I don't want to be violent... imagine hitting a heart patient? So what I do now is go up to my room or I walk Pierrot, my dog".*
THERAPIST:	*"Right! So now you stay away and try to soothe yourself".* Jeanine nods. Therapist turns to Tony. *"Sounds like these are pretty difficult times for you both. Tony, I noticed that back there, before the snap there, you seemed to be feeling a little bit emotional just now, feeling a little..."* pause
TONY:	*"Yes, yes, I was a little sad. She doesn't need to hear that it's too heavy, too much for her".*
THERAPIST:	*"So am I understanding you here, Tony? It's kind of like when you feel sad, you snap at her to kind of put some distance - keep her away because it might be too much for her?"*
TONY:	Laughs impishly *"Snap! Snap! Like an alligator! I'm bad. I'm a bad boy!"*
THERAPIST:	Leans forward, empathic and soft, responding to the sadness expressed. *"Yes, Tony, but I'm wondering if there is quite a painful, sad place inside you?"*
TONY:	Looking uncomfortable. *"Sometimes I'm sad, yes, a little".*
THERAPIST:	*"Sometimes you're sad inside, Tony, yes? And perhaps you keep an alligator at the door? So that when Jeanine gets too close to the sadness, the alligator goes 'snap.' Is that right?"*
TONY:	Looks down. His face is red. He nods. *"Right. I can't rock the boat".*
THERAPIST:	*"You can't rock the boat?"*
TONY:	nods
THERAPIST:	*"You can't rock her boat?"*
TONY:	Shakes his head. *"My boat! My boat! My next paycheck is as good as my mood is up. Can't let anyone get me down".*

In that session, I encouraged Tony to tell his wife about his feelings of shame and inadequacy around losing his job, and his concerns about his inability to accumulate adequate income for their retirement. I then encouraged him to share concerns about his health.

"I feel like I'm letting you down, I've blown it," Tony told his wife. His usual response to feelings of failure was to distance himself from Jeanine, and he was vigilant for signs from her that she was dissatisfied with him. When she reprimanded him for eating the wrong foods or not exercising adequately, he misread her concern for him as scorn of him. As she listened to him, Jeanine began to understand his avoidance of her in terms of how he felt he was letting her down, instead of how little he cared about her. By the end of this session we were able to identify the cycle that maintained their distress, along with some of the underlying emotions that primed the cycle. The couple was framed as victims of this cycle. Both Jeanine and Tony appeared greatly relieved, fully endorsing this formulation of their distress. At this point, they were finishing the first stage of EFT, that is, they were beginning to de-escalate.

As the couple felt more and more safe in our sessions, Tony continued to share more of his experience, and was able to tell his wife about his feelings of inadequacy, which had started in Italy when he was a little boy. He was exuberant and often naughty. His mother frequently locked him in a closet to prevent him from doing naughty things and on several occasions even tied him to his bed. These events had caused him to feel angry and mistrustful of himself. When, as an adult, he lost his job then developed cardiac problems, he saw these events as a confirmation his own failure. He felt he had let his wife down badly. Jeanine reached for him in the session as he shared this, and comforted him, and he acknowledged that it was good to feel that she still loved him. Jeanine shared that she loved him "even though and especially since" - that is, *even though* he felt small sometimes and *especially since* he took the risk of sharing such intimate material with her. "It makes me feel close and special to you," she told him.

Jeanine also shared her own feelings of shame and inadequacy. The eldest child in a large French-Canadian Catholic family, she had been taken out of school to earn money for the family. Her father, an alcoholic, did not have a job. Her mother was harsh and demanding, and Jeanine had felt worthless. She told Tony: "The woman I am today would not have married you. I need more than you give me, but not money, not flowers, not diamonds. What I need is, YOU. You are what I have needed and now I can't go on with you, if you keep up your mask and don't share your life with me." Tony leaned into his wife, took both of her hands and told her: "To me, my love, you are priceless - I will love you 'even though and especially since'".

As the couple were now able to share their experience on a new, more intimate level, they were encouraged to discuss Tony's heart attack, the cardiac surgery and its aftermath. The heart attack had occurred in the morning while Tony was drinking coffee and smoking a cigarette prior to rushing off to work. Jeanine described how he became pale and breathless and extremely agitated. He told her he had terrible indigestion and asked her to call his first client, to say that he'd be late for his appointment. She was in agony trying to decide whether to call 911 - she knew he'd be angry, but she was frightened this was a heart attack. When she finally made the call, she couldn't speak to the operator she was in so much distress.

JEANINE: Tearful. *"And the next year, when they took you to the operating room for the surgery, I saw the scared little boy in you as you said goodbye to me".*

TONY: *"I thought I was going to my death".*

JEANINE: *"And now when I drive up the street and your car isn't there..."* (she reaches for a Kleenex and cries quietly)

THERAPIST: *"You live in fear of losing him?"*

JEANINE: *"It haunts me everyday. I keep seeing him in the ambulance that day. Sitting up on the stretcher, white, with an oxygen mask on…the doors closing… taking you away… so alone, so scared. I'm so afraid of losing you".*

TONY: Openly crying. *"And all that time I thought you wished I had died! I thought you did".*

JEANINE: Looks at her husband in horror:
"Oh Tony. How can you say that? Of course I don't want you to die. I need you".

TONY: *"But you have been so angry with me. You even hit me last summer. All the time after my surgery you've been on my case. Criticizing what I eat, nagging, angry with me".*

JEANINE: *"Of course I've been angry with you. You eat McDonald's for lunch, for God's sake. You haven't cared about your health. You go out to the boulangerie and buy sugar pies. You have not been responsible for your health".*

THERAPIST: *"That must be hard for you Jeanine. Hard to understand?"*

JEANINE: *"I feel that I'm not important enough for him to stay alive to be with me".*

TONY: *"And I thought you'd be better off if I died. You've been so sad, and so unhappy with me… you'd get my life insurance… I thought I might as well eat whatever I want and let it happen…"*

THERAPIST: *"You must have been feeling pretty desperate, Tony".*

TONY: Wiping his eyes quietly, does not reply for a short while.
"It's been really hard. Hard… no… it's scary. I have nightmares about it. I wake up sweating and my heart is bumping and pounding in my chest. I lie there every night and wait and wonder… is this when the big one comes? What will it feel like… will it hurt much this time? What's it like to die?"

The therapy moved to helping Jeanine and Tony discuss how each one could get comfort from the other when distressed by fears concerning his health, her work-related situation or various other life events. Jeanine felt that Tony was finally dropping his mask and revealing himself to her in a way that brought them closer than she had ever dreamed possible. As we finished the third phase of treatment, Consolidation and Integration, they found new solutions to the way they had previously dealt not only with personal issues of identity and the need for self protection, but also with Tony's struggle to change his health-related behaviors. Jeanine learned to take a backseat and agreed not to check up on his medications or diet, and Tony took responsibility for changing his own diet. Sugar pies were relegated to the status of "annual treat". They kept the image of the alligator before them. While exploring what they would do if the old cycle returned, Tony said: "Remember that behind the alligator is a little guy who just needs to be loved", and Jeanine replied, "and let the alligator remember that when he snaps a little gal gets injured by his teeth".

Couple therapy was finished in fourteen sessions. By that time Jeanine was no longer depressed. I received a postcard from the couple several months later, letting me know that they were very happy. On the postcard, they had written: "We try everyday to love each other even though and especially since".

Conclusion

In this case example, the heart attack exacerbated Tony's existing problematic coping style of withdrawing in order to cope with emotional distress. This coping style actually pushed his wife away from him when he needed her most, and created a sense of hopelessness that resulted in negative health behaviors. Couple therapy helped to establish a safe place for this couple, where they were able to share their grief and fears about Tony's cardiac health in a way that not only was soothing to both, but also positive for Tony's recovery.

Couples therapy is going through a revolution and becoming more and more widely used to address "individual" issues related to mental and physical health problems [55, 83]. Couples therapy was able to provide this couple with a safe base from which to explore their grief and fear. Emotionally Focused Therapy for couples is the ideal modality for couples beginning the journey to recovery from the trauma of a life-threatening cardiac event. Regardless of the level of distress experienced prior to the cardiac health problem, all couples can benefit from the addition of couples therapy to their recovery program. EFT helps couples learn to articulate their deepest fears and face the future together.

References

1. American Psychiatric Association (2000) Diagnostic and statistical manual of mental disorders (4th edition text revision-TR ed). American Psychiatric Association, Washington, DC
2. Maeland JG, Havik OE (1989) After the myocardial infarction. Scand J Rehab Med (Suppl 22):1-87
3. Rankin-Esquer LA, Deeter A, Barr Taylor C (2000) Coronary heart disease and couples. In: Schmaling, Goldmother (Eds) The Psychology of Couples and Illness
4. Coyne JC, Smith DA (1994) Couples coping with a myocardial infarction: contextual perspective on patient self-efficacy. J Fam Psychol 8:43-54
5. Hallaraker E, Arefjord K, Havik OE, Gunnar Maeland J (2001) Social support and emotional adjustment during and after a severe life event: a study of wives of myocardial infarction patients. Psychol Health 16:343-355
6. Elizur Y, Hirsh E (1999) Psychosocial adjustment and mental health two month after coronary artery bypass surgery: a multisystemic analysis of patients' resources. J Behav Med 22:157-177
7. Kiecolt-Glaser JK, Newton TL (2001) Marriage and health: his and hers. Psychologic Bull 127:472-503

8. Orth-Gomer K, Wamala SP, Horsten M, Schenck-Gustafsson K (2000) Marital stress worsens prognosis in women with coronary heart disease: the Stockholm female coronary risk study. JAMA 284:3008-3014

9. Kiecolt-Glaser JK (1999) Stress, personal relationships, and immune function: health implications. Brain Behav Imm 13:61-72

10. Kiecolt-Glaser JK, Malarkey WB, Chee MA et al (1993) Negative behavior during marital conflict is associated with immunological down regulation. Psycosom Med 55:395-409

11. Loving TJ, Heffner KL, Kiecolt-Glaser JK et al (2004) Stress hormone changes and marital conflict: spouses' relative power makes a difference. J Marriage Fam 66:595-612

12. House JS, Landis KR, Umberson D (1988) Social relationships and health. Science 241:540-545

13. Koenig JG (1998) Depression in hospitalized older patients with congestive heart failure. Gen Hospital Psychiat 20:29-43

14. Pratt LA, Ford DE, Crum RM et al (1996) Depression, psychotropic medication, and risk of myocardial infarction. Prospective data from the Baltimore ECA follow-up. Circulation 94:3123-3129

15. Balog P, Janszky I, Leineweber C, Blom M et al (2003) Depressive symptoms in relation to marital and work stress in women with and without coronary heart disease. The Stockhom female coronary risk study. J Psychosom Res 54:113-119

16. Carney RM, Freedland KE, Rich MW, Jaffe AS (1995) Depression as a risk factor for cardiac events in established coronary heart disease. Ann Behav Med 17:142-149

17. Waltz M (1986) Marital context and post-infarction quality of life: is it social support or something more? Soc Sci Med 22:791-805

18. Fengler AP, Balady G, Froelicher VF et al (1995) Wives of elderly disabled men: the hidden patient. Gerontologist 19:175-183

19. Coyne JC, Smith DA (1991) Couples coping with a myocardial infarction: a contextual perspective on wives' distress. J Pers Soc Psychol 61:404-412

20. Mayou R, Foster A, Williamson R (1978) The psychological and social effects of myocardial infarcts on wives. Bri Med J 1:699-701

21. Michela JL (1987) Interpersonal and individual impacts of a husband's heart attack. In: Baum A, Singer J (Eds) Handbook of psychology and health. Erlbaum, Hillsdale, NJ pp 255-300

22. Speedling EF (1982) Heart attack: the family response at home and in the hospital. Tavistock, New York

23. Shanfield SB (1990) Myocardial infarction and patients' wives. Psychosomatics 31:138-145

24. Thompson DR, Meddis R (1990) Wives' responses to counseling early after myocardial infarction. J Psychosom Res 34:249-258

25. Kriegsman DMW, Penninx BWJH, van Eijk JT (1994) Chronic disease in the elderly and its impact on the family. Fam Syst Med 12:249-267

26. Croog SH, Fitzgeral EF (1978) Subjective stress and serious illness of a spouse: wives of heart patients. J Health Soc Behav 19:166-178

27. Collins EG, White-Williams C, Jalowiec A (1996) Spouse stressors while awaiting heart transplantation. Heart Lung 25:4-13

28. McSweeney JC, Richards R, Innerarity SA et al (1995) What about me? Spouses quality of life after heart transplantation. J Transplant Coord 5:59-64

29. Bramwell L (1986) Wives' experiences in the support role after husbands' first myocardial infarction. Heart Lung 15:578-584

30. Gillis CL (1984) Reducing family stress during and after coronary artery bypass surgery. Nursing Clin North Am 19:103-111

31. Thompson DR, Cordle CJ (1988) Support of wives of myocardial infarction patients. J Advanced Nursing 13:223-228

32. Rohrbaugh MJ, Cranford JA, Shoham V et al (2002) Couples coping with congestive heart failure role and gender differences in psychological distress. J Fam Psychol 16:3-13

33. Wishnie HA, Hackett TP, Cassem NH (1971) Psychological hazards of convalescence following myocardial infarction. JAMA 215:1292-1296

34. Allen JA, Becker DM, Swank RT (1990) Factors related to functional status after coronary artery bypass surgery. Heart Lung 19:337-343

35. Fontana AF, Kerns RD (1989) Support, stress, and recovery from coronary heart disease. Health Psychol 8:175-193

36. Trelawny-Ross C, Russell O (1987) Social and psychological responses to myocardial infarction: multiple determinants of outcome at six months. J Psychosom Res 31:125-130

37. Kulic JA, Mahler JLM (1989) Social support and recovery from surgery. Health Psychol 8:221-238

38. Ell KO, Haywood LJ (1984) Social support and recovery from myocardial infarction: a panel study. J Soc Ser Res 4:1-9

39. Hanson BS, Isacsson S, Janzon L, Lindell S (1989) Social network and social support influence mortality in elderly men. Am J Epidemiol 130:100-111

40. Helgeson VS (1991) The effects of masculinity and social support on recovery from myocardial infarction. Psychosom Med 53:621-633

41. Carels RA, Sherwood A, Blumenthal JA (1998) Psychosocial influences on blood pressure during daily life. Int J Psychophysiol 9:117-129

42. Ewart CK, Taylor CB, Kraemer HC, Agras WS (1991) High blood pressure and marital discord: not being nasty matters more than being nice. Health Psychol 10:155-163

43. McCurry A, Thomas S (2002) Spouses' experiences in heart transplantation. West J Nursing Res 24:180-194

44. Trevino DB, Young EH, Groff J, Jono RT (1990) The association between marital adjustment and compliance with antihypertension regimens. J Am Board Fam Pract 3:17-25

45. Buse S, Dew M, Davidson S (1996) Impact of cardiac transplantation on the spouse's life. Heart Lung 19:641-648

46. Mishel M, Murdaugh C (1987) Family adjustment to heart transplantation: redesigning the dream. Nursing Res 36:332-338

47. Schmaling KB, Sher TG (1997) Physical health and relationships. In: Halford WK, Morkman HJ (Eds) Clinical handbook of marriage and couples interventions. Wiley & Sons, New York pp 323-345

48. Johnston M, Foulkes JM, Johnston DW et al (1999) Impact on patients and partners

of inpatient and extended cardiac counseling and rehabilitation: a controlled trial. Psychosom Med 61:225-233

49. Linden W, Stossel C, Maurice J (1996) Psychosocial interventions for patients with coronary artery disease: a meta-analysis. Arch Int Med 156:745-752

50. Arefjord K, Hallarakeri E, Havik OE, Gunnar Maeland J (1998) Myocardial infarction-emotional consequences for the wife. Psychol Health 13:135-146

51. Baucom D, Shoham V, Mueser KT et al (1998) Empirically supported couple and family interventions for marital distress and adult mental health problems. J Cons Clin Psychol 66:53-88

52. Brownell KD, Heckerman CL, Westlake RJ et al (1978) The effect of couples training and partner cooperativeness in the behavioral treatment of obesity. Behav Res Ther 16:323-333

53. Israel A, Saccone A (1979) Follow-up of the effects of choice of mediator and target on reinforcement on weight loss. Behav Ther 10:260-265

54. Murphy JK, Williamson DA, Buxton AE et al (1982) The long-term effects of spouse involvement upon weight loss and maintenance. Behav Ther 13:681-693

55. Knowles J, Johnson S, Lee A (2003) Chronic illness in couples: a case for EFT. J Marital Fam Ther 29:299-310

56. Bowlby J (1969) Attachment and loss: vol. 1 - Attachment. Basic Books, New York

57. Johnson SM (2002) An antidote to posttraumatic stress disorder: the creation of secure attachment in couples therapy. In: Atkinson L (Ed) Attachment: risk, psychopathology and intervention. Cambridge University Press, Cambridge

58. Atkinson L (1997) Attachment and psychopathology: from laboratory to clinic. In: Atkinson L, Zucker KJ (Eds) Attachment and psychopathology. Guilford, New York pp 3-16

59. Johnson SM (1996) The practice of emotionally focused marital therapy: creating connection. Brunner/Mazel, New York

60. Johnson SM, Whiffen VE (2003) Attachment processes in couples and families. Guilford, New York

61. Lynskey M, Fergusson DM (1997) Factors protecting against the development of adjustment difficulties in young adults exposed to childhood sexual abuse. Child Abuse Neglect 21:1177-1190

62. Runtz M, Schallow J (1997) Social support and coping strategies as mediators of adult adjustment following childhood maltreatment. Child Abuse Neglect 21:211-226

63. Pennebaker JW (1985) Traumatic experience and psychosomatic disease: exploring the psychology of behavioural inhibition, obsession and confiding. Can Psychol 26:82-95

64. Schore AN (1994) Affect regulation and the organization of self. Erlbaum, Hillsdale, NJ

65. Dessaulles A, Johnson SM, Denton W (2003) The treatment of clinical depression in the context of marital distress. Am J Fam Ther 31:345-353

66. Johnson SM (1998). Emotionally focused couples therapy: straight to the heart. In: Donovan J (Ed) Short term couples therapy. Guilford, New York

67. Johnson SM (1998) Listening to the music: emotion as a natural part of systems. J Syst Ther (Special Edition on the Use of Emotion in Couples and Family Therapy) 17:1-17

68. Gordon-Walker J, Manion I (unpublished) Emotionally focused therapy for the parents of chronically ill children: a two-year follow-up study

69. Johnson SM, Williams-Keeler L (1998) Creating healing relationships for couples dealing with trauma: the use of emotionally focused marital therapy. J Marital Fam Ther 24:25-40
70. Johnson SM, Hunsley J, Greenberg LS, Schindler D (1999) The effects of emotionally focused marital therapy: a meta-analysis. Clin Psychol Sci Pract 6:67-79
71. Bowlby J (1988) A secure base: parent-child attachment and healthy human development. Basic Books, New York
72. Johnson SM, Makinen J, Millikin J (2001) Attachment injuries in couple relationships: a new perspective on impasses in couples therapy. J Marital Fam Ther 27:145-155
73. Alexander JF, Holtzworth-Munroe A, Jameson P (1994) The process and outcome of marital and family therapy: research review and evaluation. In: Bergin CSL (Ed) Handbook of psychotherapy and behavior change. Wiley, New York pp 595-612
74. Spanier G (1976) Measuring dyadic adjustment. J Marriage Fam 38:15-28
75. Gordon-Walker J, Johnson SM, Manion L, Cloutier P (1996) Emotionally focused marital interventions for couples with chronically ill children. J Cons Clin Psychol 64:1029-1036
76. Johnson SM, Greenberg LS (1985) Emotionally focused couples therapy: an outcome study. J Marital Fam Ther 11:313-317
77. Johnson SM, Greenberg LS (1985) The differential effects of experiential and problem solving interventions in resolving marital conflict. J Cons Clin Psychol 53:175-184
78. Johnson SM, Talitman E (1997) Predictors of success in emotionally focused marital therapy. J Marital Fam Ther 23:135-152
79. Cohen J (1992) A power primer. Psychologic Bull 112:155-159
80. Johnson SM (1996) The practice of emotionally focused marital therapy: creating connection. Taylor and Francis, New York
81. Johnson SM, Whiffen VE (1999) Made to measure: adapting emotionally focused couple therapy to partner's attachment styles. Clin Psychol Sci Pract 6:366-381
82. Foa EB, Hearst-Ikeda D, Perry KJ (1995) Evaluation of a brief behavioral program for the prevention of chronic PTSD in recent assault victims. J Cons Clin Psychol 63:948-955
83. Johnson SM (2003) The revolution in couple therapy: a practitioner-scientist perspective. J Marital Fam Ther 29:365-384

Chapter 20

Type A Behavior Pattern and Its Treatment

A.T. Möller

The Type A behavior pattern (TABP) was first described in 1959 by two cardiologists, Meyer Friedman and Ray Rosenman [1], as "an action-emotion complex that can be observed in any person who is aggressively involved in a chronic, incessant struggle to achieve more and more in less and less time, and if required to do so, against the opposing effects of other things or persons" (p. 67). More recently, Rosenman, Swan and Carmelli [2] summarized individuals with TABP in terms of:

- intense, sustained drive to achieve self-selected but often poorly defined goals;
- profound eagerness to compete and need to "win";
- persistent desire for recognition and advancement;
- continuous involvement in multiple and diverse activities under time constraints;
- habitual tendency to increase the rate of doing most physical and mental activities;
- extreme mental and physical alertness; and
- pervasive aggressive and hostile feelings.

The TABP, generally characterized by extremes of competitive striving for achievement, impatience, hostility, aggressiveness and an exaggerated sense of time urgency, has been associated with academic performance [3], work performance [4], job attitudes [5], escalation of commitment [6], short-term health outcomes ([3] and increased risk for traffic accidents [7]. However, over the past decades the TABP has been mostly investigated as a possible risk factor for coronary heart disease (CHD).

Type A Behavior and Coronary Heart Disease

Almost 30 years ago Friedman and colleagues published a series of reports showing an increased rate of ischemic heart disease among men exhibiting the TABP [8, 9]. The Western Collaborative Group study (WCGS) of 3524 men, involving 8.5 years of follow-up, found that men displaying the TABP had twice as much ischemic heart disease as those without it [9]. The Framingham Study yielded similar results, showing Type A behavior to be associated with a twofold increase in the development of CHD [10]. In the French-Belgian cooperative heart study, Type A scores on the Bortner Scale were found to be significant predictors of severe CHD [11]. Coelho, Ramos, Prata, Maciel, and Barros [12] showed that the TABP was a significant feature of patients with acute myocardial infarction. Consequently, in 1981 the Review Panel on Coronary Prone Behavior and Coronary Heart Disease [13] recognized TABP as a risk factor independent of, and equal in magnitude to, the standard risk factors for CHD (including age, hypertension, diabetes, smoking and elevated serum cholesterol). These early studies suggested that TABP is associated with a) higher levels of total serum cholesterol in the absence of any changes in diet, b) faster blood clotting, c) greater "sludging" of red blood cells after ingesting high-fat meals, and d) higher levels of norepinephrine and adrenocorticotrophin-releasing hormone [14].

However, repeated attempts to replicate the findings of the WCGS rendered conflicting results [15]. In addition, several epidemiological studies failed to find a clear link between TABP and CHD [16-18]. Meta-analyses by Booth-Kewley and Friedman [19] and Matthews [20] showed only a moderate relation between TABP and CHD. Watkins and colleagues [21] concluded that, "despite nearly three decades of research, the Type A behavior pattern's status as a risk factor for cardiovascular disease is still unclear" (p. 113). Similarly, the Expert Working Group of the National Heart Foundation of Australia concluded that there is no strong or consistent evidence of a causal association between the TABP and CHD [22].

These inconsistent findings have generated controversy over the TABP as a risk factor for CHD. A growing body of evidence suggests that not all components of the global TABP, as originally described by Friedman and Rosenman [1], are equally related to the development of CHD. This introduced a new era in Type A research, focusing on specific subcomponents of TABP that may be more sensitive predictors of CHD [23, 24].

Toxic Components of Type A: Hostility and Time Urgency
The realization that the TABP construct is multidimensional in nature led a number of researchers to emphasize the need to distinguish between its benign and pathogenic components [25]. This line of research seems to point to the emotional components, namely, anger, hostility and aggressiveness as the toxic element [20, 26-34]. Hostility, the tendency to behave antagonistically, think cynically and feel anger [35], are all significantly related to atherosclerosis [36] and unstable angina [37], and these characteristics independently predict CHD and mortality [38]. This evidence suggests that hostility may eventually be established as an independent CHD risk factor [31].

However, the Expert Working Group of the National Heart Foundation of Australia recently investigated all available reviews of prospective studies on the relationship between hostility and CHD [22]. One review [39] concluded that there was consistent positive evidence of such an association, while two others [31, 40] reported an almost equal number of positive and negative prospective studies in healthy populations. The most recent review [41] found no evidence of an association. As the latter review included larger studies, with better measures of hostility and more studies of the general population, the Working Group gave greater credence to this better quality review and concluded that hostility is not a risk factor for CHD.

Although the other components of TABP were largely neglected by researchers, there is a growing body of literature relating time urgency (the everlasting struggle to achieve a great many goals in a short period of time) to a variety of measures of ill health [3, 42-47]. A study by Friedman and Ghandour [48] showed time urgency to be a better predictor of coronary morbidity or mortality than hostility. They argued that one source of hostility may be the accumulation of years, sometimes decades, of frustrated time urgency, and that hostility may be the endpoint in the worsening of TAB and not the cause [49].

Does this emphasis on its toxic subcomponents imply that the TABP as a global construct is no longer in vogue? Several reasons may explain why global TABP has inconsistently predicted CHD, including conceptual, assessment and methodological problems. Researchers increasingly question the self-report measures used to assess TABP for their lack of construct validity. For example, Edwards, Baglioni and Cooper [50] examined three commonly used measures of the TABP: the Jenkins Activity Survey [51], the Framingham Scales [10], and the Bortner Scale [52]. They found that these measures assessed different underlying constructs and failed to recognize the multidimensional nature of the TABP. Friedman et al. [49] also ascribed the controversy surrounding global TABP to the reliance on questionnaires and strongly argued that "a correct diagnosis of TAB cannot be made unless, as in any other medical disorder, an examination is performed in which both the psychomotor signs are observed and the specific traits or symptoms of the behavior are elicited" (p. 180). To address this problem, they converted the Videotaped Structured Interview (VSI; [53]) into the Videotaped Clinical Examination for Type A Behavior, by adding four new psychomotor signs (eye bulge, inappropriate laughter, teeth grinding and shoulder tic) and six additional symptoms of TABP (feeling that one is not liked by others, sleeplessness, difficulty with children, marital difficulties or competition and easily provoked irritability).

Apart from problems regarding the assessment of TABP, previous studies are also criticised on methodological grounds such as small sample sizes, using only cardiac death as outcome and not cardiac morbidity, etc. Espnes and Opdahl [54] concluded that it certainly seems that scientists working with global TABP have a strong case and that a new era in Type A research connected to CHD has been introduced.

Conceptualizing the Type A Behavior Pattern

The literature on the TABP revealed that relatively little has been written on how to conceptualize this behavior pattern, thereby emphasizing the need for a comprehensive theoretical model of TABP. Such a model would not only provide a framework for integrating existing empirical data, it would also allow for more appropriate treatment to be developed.

Various theories explaining the origin of the TABP are described in the literature. Glass [55] suggested that the TABP represents an attempt to gain and maintain control over potentially uncontrollable events in the environment that are perceived as potentially harmful. When Type As are faced with a stressful event, they struggle to control it and consequently appear hard driving, aggressive and competitive. Type A behaviors thus reflect a specific way of coping with environmental stress.

Price [56], from a cognitive social learning perspective, argued that Type A behavior and hostility are due to low self-esteem, which is moderated by constant achievement. This model asserts that cognition forms the core of this pattern, in particular the following three deeply stored schemata about self and others: a) I must constantly prove by my accomplishments that I am successful (worthy of esteem, love and approval) – the fear of insufficient worth and disapproval. b) There is no universal moral principle, no predictable and orderly relationship between the intention of my actions and their consequences – the fear that right actions may produce negative consequences and vice versa. c) All resources are scarce; therefore, your win is my loss, and I must strive against everyone to get what I need – the fear of an insufficient supply of life's necessities, such as time, achievements and recognition. According to Price's model, TABP centers around the belief that one needs to prove oneself, and the fear of insufficient time, ability, achievements, recognition, and other resources exacerbate the person's seemingly relentless efforts to prove himself or herself. The Type A pattern therefore seems to function as a set of interrelated coping strategies for dealing with a variety of largely socially determined personal beliefs and fears. A number of studies have found correlations between self-endorsed dysfunctional beliefs and TABP [57, 58].

Matthews [59] suggested that Type A behavior is associated with a combination of a strong value on productivity and ambiguous standards for evaluating this productivity. This combination leads to a sense of time passing rapidly. Situations that do not yield clear standards for evaluating performance elicit chronic achievement striving.

According to Van Egeren [60], TABP is a culturally sanctioned "success trap" created by a classic approach-avoidance dilemma. The highly individualistic, hostile, and impatient thoughts and behaviors associated with TABP may produce positive results over the short-term, but the long-term consequences may be pervasively negative. The individual becomes trapped in an inconsistent system of rewards and disappointments, and enmeshed in a series of futile challenges and perceived threats, prompting hopeless and helpless feelings and promoting a deep resentment and pervasive hostility.

Friedman and Rosenman [61] conceptualized the TABP as a coping style in dealing with situations perceived as challenging to self-esteem. They believed that beneath the Type A's facade of competence and control is a profound inward sense of insecurity and deeply felt inadequacy. The chronic struggle to achieve therefore serves to avoid or reduce negative appraisals from others, as well as from oneself. Friedman et al. [49] called this insecurity the nucleus of the TABP. Insecurity and precarious self-esteem result from beliefs such as:

- My worth depends on the quantity, not the quality, of my achievements;
- I must constantly prove my worth again and again, because my past accomplishments do not count;
- I must do more than others to be worthy.

Time urgency results from this overt insecurity and unstable and inadequate level of self-esteem [62], while the excessive need for control is considered a misguided effort to raise esteem. Similarly, impatience often encourages Type As to view others as obstacles in their way, thus promoting hostile behavior. This hostility can erode or destroy relationships, depriving the individual of social support, a critical source of self-esteem. This vicious cycle is considered to be at the root of TABP and helps perpetuate it [14].

Strube [63] argued that the uncertainty about one's ability to succeed in situations perceived as important, yet at the same time confusing and uncontrollable, stimulates the TABP as a coping style, a view similar to that held by Friedman and Rosenman [61] and Matthews [59]. Strube proposed stable clusters or schemata in memory about past Type A-related behaviors, emotions and situations, which function to reinforce basic beliefs about oneself. These self-schemata may, for example, cluster in memory around how to focus one's attention on outcomes rather than on processes in work situations perceived as important. Or, another cluster may center on the perceived conflict between needing to depend on and trust others, yet resenting this dependence. TABP may be explained by how these self-schemata influence the way social cognitive processing goes on in specific life situations that, in turn, prompt certain social behaviors and physiological changes [64].

These different perspectives on the TABP emphasize the individual's self-esteem and underlying personal beliefs as likely variables for this behavior pattern. Studies on the early development of the TABP offer some support for this view.

Several researchers have investigated the role of parental attitudes and child rearing styles on the development of the TABP. The results of these investigations indicate that a number of parental attitudes and behaviors may be involved - e.g., disapproval [65-67], emphasis on achievement, setting high goals, perceptions that goals are not being met and exhortations to perform better [66-68], strict childrearing practices, including the use of severe and frequent physical punishment or other hostile methods of control [65, 67, 69, 70], and little respect and affection [65]. Children often felt rejected and reacted to these parenting styles in terms of resentment [69, 70].

Studies have shown that parental control and demands associated with rejection and hostility are related to characteristics such as low self-esteem, external locus of control [71, 72], and aggressiveness [73] in children. Several studies have also found a parental style characterized by rejection, lack of acceptance and support, and punitive measures of control to be related to anger and hostility in children [74, 75]. These results suggest that several Type A characteristics are related to certain aspects of child-rearing style, and they offer support for the view that reducing insecurity, enhancing self-esteem and changing the underlying dysfunctional beliefs associated with TABP are essential for effective treatment.

In conclusion, TABP is a complex and multidimensional phenomenon, and none of the existing theories has adequately explained it in a comprehensive manner. In addition to the methodological shortcomings of studies on TABP and the associated assessment issues, this lack of conceptual clarity is probably one of the main factors contributing to the current confusion regarding the TABP.

Consequently, Smith and Anderson [76] argued that most theoretical models of TABP have taken a mechanistic unidirectional approach characteristic of biomedical models, according to which certain classes of environmental stimuli were seen as eliciting the TABP, which in turn caused physiological reactivity, fostering the progression of atherosclerosis and eventually causing CHD. They proposed a transactional model that acknowledges the interdependence of factors and changes over time. Such a model implies that the TABP is influenced by, and influences, the environment in reciprocal interactions. According to Thoresen and Powell [64], a complete understanding of these transactions would require assessment of all components, including: a) basic beliefs and emotions about self and the world stored in memory and elicited by current transactions; b) types of environmental events that trigger physiological and behavioral reactivity; c) cognitive attributions about the cause of specific environmental events; d) emotional, behavioral and physiological responses to these attributions; e) environmental responses to personal reactions; and f) changes in these person-environment factors over time.

In addition, Thoresen and Powell [64] argued that personal and social cognitions, with their associated emotional states related to specific situations, should be a high priority in future theoretically focused TABP research. Self-evaluative processes are considered to be at the heart of the TABP (p. 596). Also, existing models of the TABP have ignored the social and cultural context which may influence the development and maintenance of this behavior pattern (e.g., the ethic of self-absorbed individualism guided by economic, political, and social self-interest, resulting in a highly competitive, self-indulgent, yet dissatisfying life, without a sense of shared community; or the cultural belief that affection is dependent on performance). Cultural values and beliefs such as these, according to Thoresen and Powell, need to be incorporated into future models of the TABP [64].

Treatment of the Type A Behavior Pattern

The few early intervention studies yielded either mixed results or provided moderate support for changing the TABP [77-83]. However, these studies were criticized for their small sample sizes and for using self-report measures in assessing TABP.

The Recurrent Coronary Prevention Project (RCPP; [84]), initiated by Friedman and colleagues in the late 1970s, was the first large-scale controlled intervention for TABP. One thousand thirteen post myocardial infarction patients were observed for 4.5 years to determine whether their Type A behavior could be altered and the effect such alteration might have on subsequent cardiac morbidity and mortality rates for these individuals. Eight hundred sixty-two of these individuals were randomly assigned either to a control section of 270 participants who received group cardiac counselling or an experimental section of 592 participants who received both group cardiac counselling and Type A behavioral counselling (raising awareness of the signs and symptoms of TABP and including an early form of cognitive-behavior therapy through which participants learn how to alter selected behaviors, attitudes and beliefs using self-management techniques). Treatment consisted of 28 sessions of 90 minutes each during the first year, and approximately monthly sessions thereafter for 3.5 years, for a total of 62 sessions. The remaining 151 patients, who served as a comparison group, did not receive group counselling of any kind. Results showed a marked reduction in Type A behavior at the end of 4.5 years in 35.2% of participants given cardiac and Type A behavior counselling, compared with 9.8% of participants given only cardiac counselling. The cumulative 4.5 year cardiac recurrence rate was 12.9% in the 592 participants in the experimental group that received Type A counselling. This was significantly less than the recurrence rates observed in the 270 participants in the control group (21.2%) or comparison group (28.2%). In other words, the Type A counselling patients had a 40% lower rate of recurrence than their randomized counterparts and a 54% lower rate than comparison patients who received no special treatment.

This was the first study to show, within a controlled experimental design, that altering Type A behavior reduces cardiac morbidity and mortality in post infarction patients. Three recent studies also provide evidence that reduction of TABP in high-risk coronary patients alters physiological status. Burell et al. [85] showed that a cognitive-behavioral treatment, similar to the RCPP, reduced global TABP (assessed by the VSI) and its components in 25 post-infarct men over a period of 12 months. These changes were maintained at follow-up after 12 months. Changes in TABP measures occurred before reductions in serum cholesterol, triglycerides and resting systolic blood pressure, suggesting that reduced TABP played a role in the outcome. Bennett, Wallace, Carroll, and Smith [86] compared cognitive-behavioral treatment with stress management and delayed treatment in mild hypertensives. The cognitive-behavioral condition resulted in reduced TABP at post-treatment after 8 weeks and at 6-month follow-up. These changes were associated with physiological changes (e.g., reduced systolic blood pressure). Scherwitz and Ornish [87] reported a significantly reduced global TABP (assessed by means of the VSI) in a 12-month treatment to reverse coronary artery occlusion.

A few studies showed changes in TABP in healthy individuals. Levenkron et al. [88] found significant changes in TABP after a 6-session cognitive-behavioral treatment for business managers. Although blood pressure and heart rate reactivity did not change, the cognitive-behavioral treatment was associated with reduced levels of free fatty acids. Gill et al. [89] found reductions in TABP (assessed by means of the VSI) in military officers after 21 sessions of cognitive-behavioral treatment, confirmed by independent spouse ratings. Similarly, Roskies et al. [90] demonstrated that TABP (assessed by the Structured Interview) could be reduced in male business managers in 20 sessions of cognitive-behavioral treatment. In addition, several studies have demonstrated that brief interventions (2-12 weeks) have reduced Type A behaviors as measured by self-reports [91] or the VSI [92].

There have been several reviews of TABP outcome studies [93-95]. In general, these reviews showed that, despite methodological shortcomings in some studies, reductions of TABP are associated with positive psychosocial or cardiovascular outcomes. The meta-analysis by Nunes et al. [94] of 18 studies related to CHD outcomes showed that, when combined, these studies yielded a standardized effect size of 0.61 (average change more than 0.5 of a standard deviation, compared with control conditions). In addition, two studies of post-coronary patients reduced coronary events by almost 50% compared with controls.

In summary, the results of TABP intervention studies, although limited in number and despite conceptual and methodological shortcomings, are highly encouraging. They show that TABP can be altered, particularly in White men, and that reduced TABP is related to improved physical and psychosocial health status [64].

What is the best treatment for the TABP? Only a few controlled outcome studies are available in which different treatment modalities have been compared. Ketterer [96] analyzed the effects of several cognitive-behavioral interventions for coronary patients. His analysis of interventions that focused on TABP showed that, on average, those treated had 39% fewer nonfatal recurrences and 33% fewer cardiac deaths than patients in the control group. In a meta-analysis by Nunes et al. [94] eight types of treatment were compared. The researchers concluded that the strongest relationship with changes in TABP was found in interventions that used several procedures, addressing a number of different facets of TABP. From a review of intervention studies, it appears that effective treatment at least includes an educational component, cognitive restructuring and behavioral assignments. In the next section, two treatment programs are outlined: an adapted version of the treatment originally used in the RCPP [14] and an example of a briefer intervention based on the treatment program described by Möller and Botha [92].

The Adapted RCPP Treatment Program

A modified version of the original RCPP intervention program [84] was used in a large, multi-year intervention study, the Coronary and Cancer Prevention Project, involving over 3000 asymptomatic participants [14]. The original treatment program had been adjusted for Type A intervention, primarily as a preventive measure, by a) incorporating an expanded cognitive-behavioral perspective, coupled with more emphasis on existential, spiritual and philosophical issues, and b) changing the format and shortening the duration of treatment from the original 4.5 years to between 9 months and 2 years.

The modified version of the original treatment program was designed to take place in groups of 10-12 participants during 1.5-2 hour sessions. The objectives were

a) to develop insight into and create self-awareness of the manifestation and consequences of TABP, b) to teach strategies for physical and psychological relaxation, c) to provide behavioral exercises for developing healthier Type B behaviors,
particularly with respect to hostility and time urgency, d) to help participants
recognize and modify Type A attitudes and beliefs, particularly regarding insecurity
and negative self-esteem, e) to help them improve interpersonal relationships,
and f) to assist participants in developing a healthier philosophy of living.

Developing Insight and Self-Awareness

During the initial sessions of treatment, information is provided on the TABP and
its consequences, then gradually the focus is shifted to the participants' own experiences of the TABP. According to Bracke and Thoresen [14], individuals with TABP
seem to have lost much of their ability to be subjectively aware of themselves. They
chronically ignore their feelings (e.g., exhaustion, insecurity and loneliness) in
order to strive aggressively for more professional status and economic gain, or to
direct their lives in mindless attempts to impress or protect themselves from others. They frequently appear numb to their feelings, and often, at the beginning of
treatment, they deny their own TABP status or seriously doubt its association to
CHD. To foster a greater awareness of the nature and consequences of TABP, the
acronym "AIAI" (anger, irritation, aggravation, impatience) was created [14]. To
counter the tendency of participants to deny their impatience and anger, the group
leader explains that these are natural emotional responses that impact negatively
on health and well-being when they are intense, prolonged and chronic.

To facilitate self-awareness, a Type A self-monitor procedure is introduced to
help participants detach from the personal distress associated with a particular
situation by refocusing their attention on the occurrence of distress itself, thereby developing a more objective "third-person" perspective, one that optimally
provides an intimate awareness of the participant's emotional responses, fears,
attitudes, beliefs, behaviors and rationalizations, and that generally chooses to
respond in a patient, calm and reassuring manner. For example, a participant
who gets caught in slow traffic and impatiently begins criticizing the driver in front
and the inefficiency of the traffic officer, ideally, at this point, would be able to activate the self-monitor or "third person" awareness, which would allow the person
to recognize the hypercritical thoughts and impatient feelings, and choose patience
as the more desirable response and "going slow" as an opportunity, for example,
to think of a fun activity for the upcoming weekend. Development of the self-
monitor begins with a discussion of examples given by participants, or from the
immediate feedback about specific Type A behaviors that participants receive
from others as they discuss provocative topics or examples.

Reducing Arousal

Once participants begin to develop self-awareness, the group leader starts introducing relaxation procedures to reduce the physical and emotional arousal associated with the TABP. The goal of this component of the intervention program
is to assist participants in developing a personal style of relaxation that can be

used in daily situations that provoke impatience and anger. A variety of relaxation procedures (e.g., progressive muscle relaxation, autogenic training, meditation, guided imagery or self-hypnosis) are presented to allow participants to select the procedure or combination of procedures that works best for them.

Group sessions begin with some form of relaxation, also to sensitize participants to the contrast between their usual state of arousal and responding in a calm, relaxed way. A relaxation procedure is demonstrated by the group leader and practiced in the session. Participants also practice relaxation procedures daily between sessions, and their experiences are discussed during the next session [14].

Practicing Type B Behaviors

Once participants start responding in a more relaxed manner, the emphasis is shifted towards changing specific Type A behaviors. A set of structured exercises developed to foster the development of healthier Type B behaviors is used. These exercises are designed to change behaviors and attitudes related to impatience (e.g., Eat more slowly); hostility (e.g., Purposely say: "Maybe I'm wrong"); and self-esteem (e.g., Contemplate your positive achievements for 10 minutes). They are also designed to help participants with their relationships (e.g., Ask a family member about his or her day's activities) [14, p. 273]. To enhance motivation, the group leader presents the rationale for the exercises and emphasizes the specific value attached to completing them. During the following session, participants' experiences with the exercises are discussed in order to share the positive effects members report, provide support, and share suggestions on how difficult exercises might be successfully accomplished.

Reducing Time Urgency

Initially, the nature, causes and consequences of time urgency are discussed, with an emphasis on how time urgency promotes hostility, which, in turn, damages or destroys relationships. Through self-observation, exercises and group discussions of specific impatient behaviors, participants are made aware of their idiosyncratic manifestations of time urgency. Cognitive restructuring is then introduced: exercises are used to expose, examine and modify the beliefs underlying impatience and time urgency, particularly those associated with low self-esteem. For example, participants are shown how their reluctance to delegate is often due to an excessive need to retain control in a misguided effort to raise self-esteem [14]. In addition, participants practice developing prioritizing skills by learning to distinguish tasks that are truly urgent from those that are only important.

Reducing Anger and Hostility

The focus on time urgency automatically leads to a greater awareness of anger and hostility. Groups begin by discussing the essential features of Type A anger and hostility (a hypercritical world view, cynicism, distrust, suspiciousness and attribution of malevolence to others). They then examine their own particular manifestations of anger and hostility, and develop an awareness of the more subtle manifestations of anger and hostility, such as sarcasm, facial grimacing, etc. [14]. Cognitive restructuring is used to identify, examine and modify the narcissistic beliefs underlying Type A anger and hostility (e.g., other people ought to have the same beliefs, values, and perceptions that I have; my anger is justified and caused by the ignorance and incompetence of others; giving and receiving love and affection are signs of weakness; unlike others, I don't deserve to suffer life's obstacles and inconveniences) [14].

Enhancing Self-Esteem and Reducing Insecurity

Enhancing participants' self-esteem is considered essential for effective treatment. According to Bracke and Thoresen [14, p. 280], self-esteem may comprise a) the perception of some degree of control, b) a general sense of self-efficacy or personal competence, and c) a positive perception of one's worth as a person. Improvements achieved through interventions earlier in the program, such as the development of healthier Type B behaviors, an increased ability to control arousal levels, improved relationships and changes in Type A beliefs, may indirectly contribute to improvements in self-esteem. In addition, self-worth is enhanced through a variety of exercises and assignments. Because the self-worth of Type As is excessively dependent on career achievement, participants are encouraged to identify and develop other sources of self-esteem (e.g., strengthening relationships, broadening esthetic and spiritual interests, etc.). Greater self-acceptance is also promoted through an active evaluation of achievements and performance expectations. Despite their accomplishments, the Type A individual's self-esteem receives little validation because of perfectionistic expectations and harsh self-criticism. Discussions are consequently focused on the influence of achievement and expectations on self-esteem and on reducing excessive expectations [14].

Developing a Healthier Philosophy of Living

A final goal of treatment is to help participants develop a healthy personal philosophy of living, one that will enable them to maintain and extend the progress made during treatment. Apart from helping participants develop and improve relationships with family and friends by focusing on the skills necessary to foster genuine and intimate relationships, thereby lessening their sense of loneliness and improving self-esteem, this part of the treatment encourages participants to consider the broader issues and values in their lives. Participants also explore basic spiritual questions such as - What is truly important to me, and why? To what have I committed myself? Do I believe in a higher power or force in the world? What are my responsibilities to others and to the earth? [14 p. 281].

According to Bracke and Thoresen [14], the spiritual dimension of treatment is explicitly acknowledged at the end of each session, as participants stand in a circle, holding hands, while the following closing statement is read by one of the group members: "We are here because we realize that we all need more help than we can give ourselves. We need each other. So may all our efforts be of benefit to each other. And may friendship and love bring enrichment to all our lives, and to all those whose lives are in our care. We acknowledge this gratefully. Amen" (p. 282).

The rate and process of change vary considerably among participants. Some individuals improve rapidly, others require repeated and intensive work and time to change their Type A behaviors, while others make no progress at all, due to their profound fear of relinquishing control and their inability to tolerate the anxiety inherent in change [14].

A Brief Cognitive Restructuring Intervention

As previously indicated, several brief intervention studies of the TABP have been reported in the literature. Although these studies generally demonstrated that TABP or its subcomponents may be significantly reduced through relatively brief treatments (10 or fewer sessions), outcome was mostly assessed by means of self-report measures.

Möller and Botha [92] investigated the outcome of cognitive restructuring based on Rational-Emotive Behavior Therapy (REBT) in a group of 44 healthy male Type A insurance representatives after 15 hours of group treatment. A blind rater assessed outcome by means of the VSI. Results showed significant reductions in intensity of Type A behavior and the time urgency component from pre- to posttreatment, which were maintained at follow-up after 10 weeks. However, no improvement was found on the hostility subscale of the VSI. A possible explanation for this negative result, according to Möller and Botha [92], may be the duration of the intervention, resulting in an insufficient focus on the hostility component and insufficient behavioral exercises to implement cognitive changes. Subsequently, the treatment was adjusted to eliminate these problems.

Cognitive restructuring was based on REBT principles for the following reasons. Firstly, the dysfunctional evaluative beliefs postulated by REBT were considered particularly appropriate in explaining the TABP. These are a) demandingness (for example, rigid non-negotiable demands for achievement, perfectionism, utilizing time, etc.), b) awfulizing (the tendency to overestimate the seriousness or consequences if these demands are not met, for example - It's horrible when things are not done on time, It's awful if I don't succeed as I should), c) low frustration tolerance (the tendency to underestimate one's ability to cope with negative events or outcomes, such as not succeeding, not meeting deadlines, etc.), and d) negative rating of self and others (e.g., not succeeding means I am not worthwhile (negative esteem), or individuals opposing or hindering me or not valuing achievement are worthless). Secondly, REBT aims at promoting a philosophical or attitudinal change by helping participants reassess their fundamental rules of living and evolve a non-dogmatic, non-absolutist philosophy of living. For example, REBT emphasizes global human worth, irrespective of achievements, status, etc. It also emphasizes self-acceptance and acceptance of others by encouraging individuals to discard unrealistic, dogmatic demands and all forms of negative rating of self and others, and it advocates acceptance of human fallibility, etc. [97].

The revised program (described below) entails 10 weekly group sessions of 1.5-2 hours each and consists of three components, designed to a) educate participants about the TABP and its consequences, as well as how our perceptions, beliefs and rules of living result in and maintain these Type A behaviors; b) assist participants in identifying and replacing their dysfunctional beliefs through cognitive restructuring, and c) to help them develop healthier behaviors through behavioral assignments and exercises.

Sessions 1-2

Session 1: Apart from a brief discussion of the goals of treatment, the expectations of participants, treatment adherence, and the collaborative nature of the treatment relationship, the first session is devoted to an interactive discussion of the TABP. The signs and symptoms of the TABP, as well as its consequences, particularly in terms of general well-being and interpersonal relationships, are presented by the group leader, while participants are encouraged to present and discuss concrete examples of their own Type A behaviors, so as to foster self-understanding and group cohesion. In particular, the typical concern of group members that a reduction in the TAPB may adversely affect job involvement and performance is discussed, and the leader shares the research evidence that Type A behavior is irrelevant to success [98].

At the end of the session, participants are requested to read a handout on the TABP during the coming week and, in order to help increase self-awareness, to keep a diary of their Type A behaviors and to bring it to the next session.

Session 2: This session starts with feedback and a discussion of the previous week's homework. The focus is then shifted to the role of cognitions in facilitating and maintaining emotions and behaviors. It is presented in terms of the ABC model, where A refers to activating events (including thoughts and images), B refers to beliefs, and C to the emotional and behavioral consequences. It is stressed that Type A behaviors and emotions are not so much a result of environmental circumstances as the way in which these circumstances are perceived. The dysfunctional evaluative beliefs and the criteria for functional/dysfunctional beliefs [97] are discussed, and the ABC model is demonstrated by means of recent examples of Type A behaviors provided by group members.

In addition to dysfunctional beliefs, Type As are prone to certain cognitive errors. These include all-or-nothing thinking (the tendency to evaluate things in absolutistic or dichotomous categories, as either black or white, win or lose, success or failure); selective attention (directing the attention toward select aspects of environmental information, e.g., liabilities and failures); personalization (consistently exaggerating one's own importance, e.g., attributing one's own views to others, without questioning whether they have their own frames of reference); and attributions of causality (because Type As are inclined to attribute their success to effort and trying hard, when they fail they are inclined to believe that they did not try hard enough and to fault themselves for not trying harder). In addition to discussing dysfunctional beliefs, the group leader will point out these cognitive errors and examine them throughout treatment.

Homework for the next week includes a) a behavioral exercise in which two

Type A behaviors are selected from the previous week's diary and replaced with Type B behaviors (e.g., walk/eat slower; remain at the dinner table longer; relax while waiting in a line or driving in traffic), b) reading a handout on the ABC model, dysfunctional evaluative beliefs and the criteria for dysfunctional beliefs, and c) keeping a diary of Type A behaviors and emotions that includes the circumstances under which they occur, i.e., the activating events (A), the automatic thoughts (or beliefs) accompanying these events (B), and the emotional and behavioral consequences (C).

Sessions 3-10
Sessions 3 through 8 examine the dysfunctional thinking associated with specific subcomponents of the TABP, and provide exercises for establishing alternative Type B behaviors. Sessions 9 and 10 deal with the consequences of Type A behavior on interpersonal relationships, and examine self-esteem as a core element in maintaining the TABP. The leader emphasizes that these components are not unrelated. For example, dealing with anger and hostility may uncover dysfunctional beliefs regarding interpersonal relationships, or competitive, hard-driving behavior may be related to a negative self-rating. More detailed agendas follow.

Sessions 3 and 4: Are devoted to the cluster of Type A behaviors characterized by excessive job involvement and hard-driving competitiveness. After dealing with the previous week's homework, the nature of this cluster of behaviors is explained briefly at the beginning of session 3, and participants are encouraged to provide recent examples of their own competitive behaviors (e.g., reluctance to delegate, inability to reduce workload, working long hours, inability to refuse requests to do extra work, etc.). The beliefs underlying these behaviors are identified and examined. Typical automatic thoughts are: I'd rather do it myself, then I know it has been properly done; I prefer to be in control when such an important issue is at stake; I am worried what a colleague, my spouse or friends may think if I don't succeed; I like being the best. These thoughts reflect rigid, underlying demands for perfection, achievement, status and success, demands that are viewed as non-negotiable prerequisites for maintaining self-esteem and "earning" acceptance from others (self-rating). Not meeting these demands or rules of living are experienced as "bad," "horrible," "personal failure" (awfulizing), "which I can't stand" (low frustration tolerance).

These beliefs are challenged by the group leader, who examines them from the perspective of whether they meet the criteria for functional thinking. Alternatively, a particular participant may be asked to examine the dysfunctional beliefs of another group member (role-reversal), or imagery may be used, where group members imagine themselves in familiar hard-driving and competitive situations, having more functional thoughts or beliefs and performing the appropriate behaviors. At the end of the session, each participant writes down two or three such situations, along with more functional beliefs and behaviors to practice during the coming week.

Sessions 5 and 6: The routine followed in the two previous sessions is repeated in sessions 5 and 6, except that the emphasis is now on the time urgency component. Typical examples of these behaviors include walking, eating and speaking rapidly, doing more than one thing at a time (e.g., reading while talking on the phone), punctuality, getting upset about having to wait in line, etc. Examples of underlying thoughts are: I hate being late (I should never be late – demand); It is horrible (awfulizing) to have to wait in a line (and I can't stand it – low frustration tolerance); I must be on time for meetings or finish work on time (demand for personal efficiency, together with positive self-rating and possible fear of negative rating by others).

Again, these beliefs are identified and examined in an interactive way, with individual participants at the end of each session developing two or three more functional ABC sequences regarding time urgency. Each participant adds these to his or her existing list of Type B beliefs and behaviors that was started at the end of the third session. During the next two weeks participants practice these functional beliefs and behaviors, along with those developed in sessions 3 and 4 for job involvement and competitiveness.

Sessions 7 and 8: A routine similar to that followed in previous sessions is repeated here, except that the emphasis is on hostility. The group leader explains the nature of impatience and anger and the subtle ways in which these feelings often manifest behaviorally. The leader then requests recent examples experienced by participants. Typical examples include: frequent loss of temper while driving; difficulty falling asleep due to upset about what someone has said or done; and irritation as a result of somebody expressing a different view or "unjustified" criticism. Often, rigid and non-negotiable beliefs underlie the Type As anger and hostility. Examples include: People ought to have the same beliefs, views and perceptions that I have (and if they don't, I don't like them, don't want to associate with them, etc." – negative rating of others); People have no right to question, challenge or criticize me; My anger is justified and caused by the ignorance and incompetence of others; etc. In examining these beliefs it is important to point out to participants how futile they are, because in fact all humans are fallible, and we have virtually very little control over the behavior of other people. It is also important to make participants aware of the fact that anger and hostility undermine our interpersonal relationships and contribute to personal isolation.

The beliefs underlying hostile behaviors are examined in an interactive way, using the Socratic method, role-reversal, imagery techniques, etc. Each participant identifies two or three hostile behaviors, examines the underlying beliefs, and develops more functional beliefs. These ABC sequences are then added to the participant's existing list of Type B behaviors for practice during the coming weeks.

Session 9: Apart from supposed physical consequences, often Type A behavior also has detrimental effects on the individual's interpersonal relationships. Hard-driving competitiveness, excessive job involvement and hostile behaviors may contribute to strained relationships, alienation from others and eventually a deep sense of isolation and loneliness. Moreover, this may represent a deep-seated philosophy of life where success and material wealth take precedence over people and relationships. In contrast, sound intimate relationships foster security, and contribute to healthier self-esteem and a more meaningful and satisfying life.

The group leader discusses these issues with group members, inviting them to share their experiences. In this manner, the underlying beliefs and assumptions about intimacy and relationships are elicited. Examples include: People can never be trusted; Giving and receiving love and affection are signs of weakness; People can/must be controlled (or blamed and punished) for not acting the way I want them to behave; People are obstacles to achieving my goals; and so on. These beliefs, as well as behaviors for improving interpersonal communication, are discussed. The latter may include, for example, active listening, asking about other people's views, deliberately planning to spend more time with family and friends, assisting colleagues where possible, etc. At the end of the session, each participant decides on particular behaviors of concern, according to his or her own circumstances, and these are added to the list of behavioral exercises to be implemented during the next week.

Session 10: As indicated previously, negative self-esteem and the associated beliefs are thought to be at the core of the TABP. Although it is expected that changes in Type A beliefs and behaviors that were facilitated in previous sessions will contribute to improved self-esteem, session 10 focuses specifically on self-esteem. It is pointed out that all Type A components and behaviors really represent efforts to enhance and maintain self-esteem and a sense of security. Typical Type A beliefs related to self-esteem are identified and questioned (for example: My worth depends on the quantity, not the quality of my achievements; I am only as good as my accomplishments; Winning or losing is a reflection of one's worth as a person; Non-achievement oriented activities are a waste of time; I must do more than others to be a worthy person; What will others think if I am not successful?)

Participants are urged to re-examine their beliefs concerning human value and to strive towards self-acceptance and acceptance of others by scaling down the excessive demands and accepting themselves and others as fallible human beings. In doing so, they have to reconsider their perfectionistic demands, harsh self-criticism and constant comparison of themselves to others, as well as their fear of negative evaluations by others, belief that success and accomplishments equal human value, etc. It is essential that participants understand that, in order to have a meaningful and healthier life, they must develop a different set of rules for living, particularly with regard to themselves, their relationships, and their work and accomplishments.

Follow-up Sessions
The Type A pattern is an entrenched way of life, with culturally sanctioned reinforcers and rewards. Participants may, therefore, despite their new insights and understanding of themselves, struggle to internalize the functional beliefs and maintain their Type B behaviors in daily life. They may even struggle to main-

tain their motivation for treatment. For these reasons the intervention program includes a series of follow-up sessions. Usually 10 sessions are scheduled, either on a monthly basis, or initially bi-weekly and later monthly, depending on the needs and progress of the group.

These sessions deal with the problems which participants experience in changing their Type A beliefs and maintaining their Type B behaviors. Particular beliefs may be re-examined, new Type B behaviors agreed upon, or philosophical issues discussed again. It is also important to focus on the progress that has been made, and individual members are given opportunities to discuss changes in their thinking and behaviors. This may serve as valuable support and encouragement for other members in continuing the process of changing their Type A lifestyle.

Conclusion

Enthusiasm for the Type A behavior construct, first described by Friedman and Rosenman in 1959 [1] began to wane during the 1980s, largely because some studies failed to demonstrate a relationship between the TABP and CHD.

Methodological shortcomings, particularly the reliance on self-report measures of Type A behaviors, are believed to be responsible for these negative findings. To see a renewed interest in the Type A construct, prospective and cross-sectional studies based on reliable and valid assessment of the TABP, particularly in women and different cultural groups, are needed. The future of the TABP construct also depends on the development of new conceptual models that take into account the multidimensionality of the construct and are supported by empirical studies. There is also a need for well-controlled outcome studies, particularly of briefer TABP interventions.

However, despite methodological shortcomings, earlier reviews did show a significant relationship between the TABP and CHD for White men, when the Type A pattern was carefully assessed in general population studies. In addition, the few controlled intervention studies of Type A behaviors have demonstrated promising results. Clearly, at this stage, it seems premature to abandon the Type A construct as a means of understanding behaviors that may have maladaptive physical consequences.

References

1. Friedman M, Rosenman RH (1959) Association of specific overt behavior pattern with blood and cardiovascular findings. JAMA 173:1320-1325
2. Rosenman RH, Swan GE, Carmelli D (1988) Definition, assessment, and evolution of the Type A behavior pattern. In: Houston BK, Snyder CR (Eds) Type A behavior pattern: research, theory and intervention. Wiley, New York, pp 8-31
3. Spence JT, Helmreich RL, Pred RS (1987) Impatience versus achievement striving in

the Type A pattern: differential effects on students' health and academic achievement. J Applied Psychol 72:522-528

4. Barling J, Kelloway EK, Cheung D (1996) Time management and achievement striving interact to predict car sales performance. J Applied Psychol 81:821-826

5. Menon S, Narayanan L, Spector PE (1996) The relation of time urgency to occupational stress and health outcomes for health care professionals. In: Spielberger CD, Sarason IG (Eds) Stress and emotion: anxiety, anger, and curiosity. Taylor & Francis, London pp 127-142

6. Schaubroeck J, Williams S (1993) Type A behavior and escalating commitment. J Applied Psychol 78:862-867

7. Magnavita N, Narda R, Sani L et al (1997) Type A behavior pattern and traffic accidents. Br J Med Psychol 70:103-107

8. Jenkins CD, Rosenman RH, Friedman M (1976) Development of an objective psychological test for the determination of the coronary-prone behavior in employed men. J Chronic Dis 20:372-379

9. Rosenman RH, Brand RJ, Jenkins CD et al (1975) Coronary heart disease in the Western Collaborative Group Study: final follow-up experience of 8.5 years. JAMA 233:872-877

10. Haynes SG, Feinleib M, Levine S et al (1978) The relationship of psychological factors to coronary heart disease in the Framingham Study: II. Prevalence of coronary heart disease. Am J Epidemiol 107:384-392

11. French-Belgian Collaborative Group (1982) Ischemic heart disease and psychological patterns: prevalence and incidence studies in Belgium and France. Adv Cardiol 29:25-30

12. Coelho R, Ramos E, Prata J et al (1999) Acute myocardial infarction: psychosocial and cardiovascular risk factors in men. J Cardiovasc Risk 6:157-162

13. Review Panel on Coronary Prone Behavior and Coronary Heart Disease (1981) Coronary-prone behavior and coronary heart disease: a critical review. Circulation 63:1199-1215

14. Bracke PE, Thoresen CE (1996) Reducing Type A behavior patterns: a structural group approach. In: Allan R, Scheidt S (Eds) Heart and mind. The practice of cardial psychology. American Psychological Association, Washington, DC pp 255-290

15. Dimsdale JE, Hackett TP, Hutter AM et al (1986) Type A personality and extent of coronary atherosclerois. Am J Cardiol 42:583-586

16. Case RB, Heller SS, Case NB, Moss AJ (1985) Type A behavior and survival after acute myocardial infarction. N Engl J Med 312:737-741

17. Shekelle RB, Gale M, Norusis M (1985) Type A score (Jenkins Activity Survey) and risk of recurrent coronary heart disease in the aspirin myocardial infarction study. Am J Cardiol 56:221-225

18. Shekelle RB, Hulley SB, Neaton JD et al (1985) The MRFIT behavior pattern study, II. Type A behavior and incidence of coronary heart disease. Am J Epidemiol 122:559-570

19. Booth-Kewley S, Friedman HS (1987) Psychological predictors of heart disease: a quantitative review. Psycholog Bull 101:343-362

20. Matthews K (1988) Coronary heart disease and Type A behaviors: update on and alternative to the Booth-Kewley and Friedman (1987) quantitative review. Psycholog Bull 104:373-380

21. Watkins PL, Fisher EB, Southard DR et al (1989) Assessing the relationship of Type A beliefs to cardiovascular disease risk and psychosocial distress. J Psychopathol Behav Assessm 11:113-125
22. Bunker SJ, Colquhoun DM, Esler MD et al (2003) Stress and coronary heart disease: psychosocial risk factors. Medical J Australia 178:272-276
23. Byrne DG (1996) Type A behavior, anxiety and neuroticism: reconceptualizing the pathophysiological paths and boundaries of coronary-prone behavior. Stress Med 12:222-238
24. Eason KE, Mâsse LC, Tortolero SR, Kelder SH (2002) Type A behavior and daily living activity among older minority women. J Women's Health Gender-based Med 11:137-146
25. Dembroski TM, Williams RB (1989) Definition and assessment of coronary-prone behavior. In: Schneiderman N, Kaufmann P, Weiss SM (Eds) Handbook of research methods in cardiovascular behavioral medicine. Plenum, New York pp 221-245
26. Dembroski TH, MacDougall JM, Costa PT, Grandits GA (1989) Components of hostility as predictors of sudden death and myocardial infarction in the multiple risk factors intervention trial. Psychosom Med 51:514-521
27. Ganster DC, Schaubroeck J, Sime WE, Mayes BT (1991) The nomological validity of the Type A personality among employed adults. J Applied Psychol 76:143-168
28. Greene RE, Houston BK, Holloran SA (1995) Aggressiveness, dominance, developmental factors, and serum level in college males. J Behav Med 18:569-580
29. Kaplan JR, Botchin MB, Manuck SB (1994) Animal models of aggression and cardio-vascular disease. In: Siegman AW, Smith TW (Eds) Anger, hostility and the heart. Erlbaum, Hillsdale, NJ pp 127-148
30. Markovitz JH, Matthews KA, Kiss J, Smitherman TC (1996) Effects of hostility on platelet reactivity to psychological stress in coronary heart disease patients and in healthy controls. Psychosom Med 58:143-149
31. Miller TQ, Smith TW, Turner CW et al (1996) A meta-analytic review of research on hostility and physical health. Psycholog Bull 119:322-348
32. Ravaja N, Keltikangas-Jarvinen L, Keskivaara P (1996) Type A factors as predictors of changes in the metabolic syndrome: precursors in adolescents and young adults. A 3-year follow-up study. Health Psychol 15:18-29
33. Siegman AW (1994) From Type A to hostility to anger: reflections on the history of coronary prone behavior. In: Siegman AW, Smith TW (Eds) Anger, hostility and the heart. Erlbaum, Hillsdale, NJ pp 1-21
34. Williams RB, Haney TL, Lee KL et al (2001) Type A behavior, hostility, and coronary atherosclerosis. Adv Mind-Body Med 17:54
35. Barefoot JC (1992) Developments in the measurement of hostility. In: Friedman HS (Ed) Hostility, coping and health. American Psychological Association, Washington, DC pp 13-31
36. MacDougall JM, Dembroski TM, Dimsdale JE, Hackett TP (1985) Components of Type A, hostility and anger-in: further relationships to angiographic findings. Health Psychol 4:137-152
37. Mendes De Leon CF (1992) Anger and impatience/irritability in patients of low socioeconomic status with acute coronary heart disease. J Behav Med 15:273-284
38. Kawachi I, Sparrow D, Spiro A et al (1996) A prostpective study of anger and coronary heart disease. The normative aging study. Circulation 94:2090-2095

39. Scheier MF, Bridges MW (1995) Person variables and health: personality predispositions and acute psychological states as shared determinants for disease. Psychosom Med 5:255-268
40. Rozanski A, Blumenthal JA, Kaplan J (1999) Impact of psychological factors on the pathogenesis of cardiovascular disease and implications for therapy. Circulation 99:2192-2217
41. Kuper H, Marmot M, Hemingway H (2002) Systematic review of prospective cohort studies of psychosocial factors in the aetiology and prognosis of coronary heart disease. Seminars Vascular Med 2:267-314
42. Chidester TR (1986) Mood, sleep and fatigue in flight operations. Unpublished doctoral dissertation, University of Texas at Austin
43. Cole SR, Kawachi I, Liu S et al (2001) Time urgency and risk of non-fatal myocardial infarction. Internat J Epidemiol 30:363-369
44. Edwards JR, Baglioni AJ (1991) Relationship between Type A behavior pattern and mental and physical symptoms: a comparison of global and component measures. J Applied Psychol 76:276-290
45. Hart KE (1997) A moratorium on research using the Jenkins activity survey for Type A behavior? J Clinical Psychol 53:905-907
46. Julkunen J, Idänpään-Heikkila U, Saarinen T (1993) Components of Type A behavior and the first year prognosis of myocardial infarction. J Psychosom Res 37:11-18
47. Suls J, Marco CA (1990) Relationship between JAS and FTAS Type A behavior and non-CHD illness. A prospective study controlling for negative affectivity. Health Psychol 9: 479-492
48. Friedman M, Ghandour G (1993) Medical diagnosis of Type A behavior. Am Heart J 126:607-618
49. Friedman M, Fleischmann N, Price VA (1996) Diagnosis of Type A behavior pattern. In: Allan R, Scheidt S (Eds) Heart and mind. The practice of cardiac psychology. American Psychological Association, Washington, DC pp 179-195
50. Edwards JR, Baglioni AJ, Cooper CL (1990) Examining relationships among self-report measures of Type A behavior pattern: the effects of dimensionality, measurement error, and differences in underlying constructs. J Applied Psychol 75:440-454
51. Jenkins CD, Zysanski SJ, Rosenman RH (1971) Progress toward validation of a computer-scored test for the Type A coronary-prone pattern. Psychosom Med 33:193-202
52. Bortner RW (1969) A short rating-scale as a potential measure of pattern A behavior. J Chronic Dis 22:87-91
53. Friedman M, Thoresen CE, Gill JJ et al (1982) Feasibility of altering Type A behavior pattern after myocardial infarction. Recurrent coronary prevention project study: methods, baseline results and preliminary findings. Circulation 66:83-92
54. Espnes GA, Opdahl A (1999) Associations among behavior, personality, and traditional risk factors for coronary heart disease: a study at a primary health care center in Mid-Norway. Psycholog Rep 85:505-517
55. Glass DC (1977) Behavior patterns, stress, and coronary disease. Earlbaum, Hillsdale, NJ
56. Price VA (1982) Type A behavior pattern: a model for research and practice. Academic Press, New York
57. Burke RJ (1985) Beliefs and fears underlying Type A behavior: correlates of time urgency and hostility. J General Psychol 112:133-145

58. Hamberger LK, Hastings JE (1986) Irrational beliefs and underlying Type A behavior: evidence for a cautious approach. Psycholog Rep 59:19-25
59. Matthews KA (1982) Psychological perspectives on the Type A behavior pattern. Psycholog Bull 91:293-323
60. Van Egeren LF (1991) A "Success Trap" theory of Type A behavior: Historical background. J Soc Behav Personal 5:45-58
61. Friedman M, Rosenman R (1974) Type A behavior and your heart. Knopf, New York
62. Friedman M, Ulmer DK (1984) Treating Type A behavior and your heart. Knopf, New York
63. Strube MJ (1987) A self-appraisal model of the Type A behavior pattern. Perspectives Personality 2:201-250
64. Thoresen CE, Powell LH (1992) Type A behavior pattern: new perspectives on theory, assessment and intervention. J Consult Clin Psychol 60:595-604
65. Burke RJ (1983) Early parental experiences, coping styles and type A behavior. J Psychol 113:161-170
66. Matthews KA (1977) Caregiver-child interactions and the Type A coronary-prone behavior pattern. Child Developm 48:1752-1756
67. McCranie EW, Simpson ME (1986) Parental child-rearing antecedents of Type A behavior. Personal Soc Psychol Bull 12:493-501
68. Kliewer W, Weidner G (1987) Type A behavior and aspirations: a study of parents' and children's goal setting. Developm Psychol 23:204-209
69. Emmelkamp PM, Karsdorp EP (1987) The effects of perceived parental rearing style on the development of Type A pattern. Eur J Personal 1:223-230
70. Waldron I, Hickey A, McPherson C et al (1989) Type A behavior pattern: relationship to variation in blood pressure, parental characteristics, and academic and social activities of students. J Hum Stress 6:16-27
71. Loeb RC (1975) Concommitants of boys' locus of control examined in parent-child interactions. Developm Psychol 11:353-358
72. Loeb RC, Horst L, Horton DJ (1980) Family interaction patterns associated with self-esteem in pre-adolescent girls and boys. Merrill-Palmer Quarterly 26:203-217
73. Patterson GR (1982) Coercive family process. Castalia Press, Eugene, OR
74. Houston BK, Vavak CR (1991) Cynical hostility: developmental factors, psychosocial correlates and health behaviors. Health Psychol 10:9-17
75. Matthews KA, Woodall KL, Kenyon K, Jacob T (1996) Negative family environment as a predictor of boys' future status on measures of hostile attitudes, interview behavior and anger expression. Health Psychol 15:30-37
76. Smith TW, Anderson NB (1986) Models of personality and disease: an interactional approach to Type A behavior and cardiovascular risk. J Personal Soc Psychol 50:1166-1173
77. Blumenthal JA, Williams RS, Williams RB, Wallace AG (1980) Effects of exercise on Type A (cornonary-prone) behavior pattern. Psychosom Med 42:289-296
78. Jenni MA, Wollersheim JP (1979) Cognitive therapy, stress management training, and the Type A behavior pattern. Cognit Ther Res 3:61-74
79. Roskies E, Kearney H, Spevack M et al (1979) Generalizability and durability of treatment effects in an intervention program for coronary prone (Type A) managers. J Behav Med 2:195-207

80. Roskies E, Spevack M, Surkis A et al (1978) Changing the coronary prone (Type A) behavior pattern in a non-clinical population. J Behav Med 1:201-216

81. Suin RM (1975) The cardiac stress management program for Type A patients. Cardiac Rehabilit 5:13-15

82. Suin RM, Bloom LJ (1978) Anxiety management for Type A persons. J Behav Med 1:25-35

83. Thurman WT (1983) Effects of a rational-emotive treatment program on Type A behavior among college students. J College Student Personnel 24:417-423

84. Friedman M, Thoresen CE, Gill JJ et al (1986) Alteration of Type A behavior and its effect on cardiac recurrences in post myocardial infarction patients: summary results of the recurrent coronary prevention project. Am Heart J 112:653-665

85. Burell G, Ohman A, Sundin O et al (1994) Modification of Type A behavior pattern in post-myocardial infarction patients: a route to cardiac rehabilitation. Internat J Behav Med 1:32-54

86. Bennett P, Wallace L, Carroll D, Smith N (1991) Treating Type A behaviors and mild hypertension in middle-aged men. J Psychosom Res 35:209-223

87. Scherwitz L, Ornish D (1994) The impact of major lifestyle changes on coronary stenosis, CHD risk factors, and psychological status: results from the San Francisco Lifestyle Heart Trial. Homeos Health Dis 35:190-197

88. Levenkron JC, Cohen JD, Mueller HS, Fisher EB (1983) Modifying the Type A coronary-prone behavior pattern. J Consult Clin Psychol 51:192-204

89. Gill JS, Price VA, Friedman M et al (1985) Reductions in Type A behavior in healthy middle-aged American military officers. Am Heart J 110:503-514

90. Roskies E, Seragian P, Oseasohn R et al (1986) The Montreal Type A intervention project: major findings. Health Psychol 5:45-69

91. Kelly KR, Stone GL (1987) Effects of three psychological treatments and self-monitoring on the reduction of Type A behavior. J Counsel Psychol 34:46-54

92. Möller AT, Botha HC (1996) Effects of a group rational-emotive behavior therapy program on the Type A behavior pattern. Psycholog Rep 78:947-961

93. Levenkron JC, Moore GL (1988) Type A behavior pattern: issues for intervention research. Ann Behav Med 10:78-83

94. Nunes EV, Frank KA, Kornfeld DS (1987) Psychologic treatment for Type A behavior pattern and for coronary heart disease: a meta-analysis of the literature. Psychosom Med 48:159-173

95. Price VA (1988) Research and clinical issues in treating Type A behavior. In: Houston BK, Snyder CR (Eds) Type A behavior pattern: research, theory and intervention. Wiley, New York pp 275-311

96. Ketterer M (1993) Secondary prevention of ischemic heart disease: the case for aggressive behavioral monitoring and intervention. Psychosomatics 34:478-484

97. Walen SR, DiGuiseppe R, Dryden W (1992) A practitioner's guide to rational-emotive therapy. Oxford University Press, New York

98. Woods PJ (1987) Reductions in Type A behavior, anxiety, anger, and physical illness as related to changes in irrational beliefs: results of a demonstration project in industry. J Rational-Emotive Ther 5:213-237

Chapter 21

Relaxation Techniques and Hypnosis in the Treatment of CHD Patients

L. Bellardita ▪ M. Cigada ▪ E. Molinari

Introduction

It is now generally acknowledged that the functioning of the cardiovascular system is determined in large part by attitudes, emotions, anxiety and distress [1]. Resulting clinical implications include the use of behavioral and psychological interventions during cardiac rehabilitation in order to achieve relaxation [2], which can be defined as a state of physiological distension aimed at re-balancing changes deriving from distressful conditions. Relaxation techniques and hypnosis have become particularly relevant in treatment programs aimed at stress management and homeostatic rebalancing, since a continuous state of arousal can, in the long run, result in damage or dysfunction cardiovascular system. Many authors, however, argue that techniques aimed at achieving a relaxation condition can be considered elective in the treatment of cardiovascular disease [3-6].

In cardiac rehabilitation, psychological interventions are frequently based on cognitive-behavioral models (which focus on "restructuring" negative thoughts about oneself and the environment that emerge when confronting stressful events) [7, 8]. Compared to this approach, relaxation training and hypnosis have a unique, distinctive feature: rather than promote critical analysis of reactions to psychological distress, they try to by-pass rational mental processing.

The aim of this chapter is to provide an overview of relaxation techniques and hypnosis. After discussing the hypothesis with respect to underlying psychobiological processes, which attempt to explain how relaxation training and hypnosis can produce a positive impact during cardiac rehabilitation and after treatment programs, we will focus on the more widely used relaxation techniques and hypnosis procedures. Clinical practice highlights and issues for treatment of cardiac patients will be addressed.

■ Psychobiological Aspects

Autonomic Nervous System and the Relaxation Response

The role of the sympathetic nervous system has become increasingly important in cardiovascular medicine, in particular with respect to the therapeutic value of sympathetic nervous inhibition, which is under continuing investigation in regard to the pathogenesis of heart failure, essential hypertension and psychosomatic heart disease [9]. A decrease in the activity of the ortho-sympathetic branch of the autonomic nervous system (ANS) can be attained not only by pharmacological therapy, but also by inducing a relaxation response, a phenomenon that Benson and colleagues define as an integrated physiological response associated with decreased ortho-sympathetic activity [10-12]. These authors base their arguments upon early studies that showed the existence of a hypothalamic area that, when stimulated, determines the "trophotropic" response [13], a condition opposite that of the "fight-or-flight" response, which will be described below [14]. Physiological variations related to trophotropic response are:

- Decreased oxygen consumption
- Decreased blood pressure
- Decreased respiratory and heart rates

When facing a dangerous situation, the ortho-sympathetic branch of the ANS is activated with a consequent increase of cardiovascular activity in order to allow the organism to defend itself through either fight behavior or an escape reaction. Under normal conditions, once the danger is past, the parasympathetic branch "kicks in" in order to re-establish the homeostatic condition that preceded the "fight-or-flight" response. If the latter does not occur, the excessive activation of the hypothalamic-pituitary axis results in an increased blood level of cortical-adrenal steroid hormones. If this condition becomes chronic, a number of vital organs may be damaged and a significant reduction of physical well-being may occur [15]. As previously described in this book (Parati et al.), the prolonged activation of the ortho-sympathetic branch of the ANS by psychosocial stress has been recognized as responsible for increased heart rate and blood pressure, arrhythmia, myocardial ischaemia, pro-coagulation activity and endothelial dysfunction, all of which contribute to coronary artery disease.

It has been argued that the trophotropic response may constitute a protective mechanism against stress overload [16]. Relaxation techniques and hypnosis have proven to activate the trophotropic response by modulating autonomic arousal [17, 18].

One way of assessing autonomic functioning is to measure the spontaneous variability of heart rate. Heart rate variability (HRV) can be detected by using power spectrum analysis, which allows the identification of underlying frequencies. It has been argued that the higher frequency components in the interbeat interval spectrum (above 0.15 Hz) are related to respiration patterns and may therefore reflect the parasympathetic tone (even though results are sometimes controversial), while the mid-frequency band (0.07-0.15 Hz) may be associated with baroreflex modulation and ortho-sympathetic activity [19-21]. The advantage of using HRV assessment is that it is a non-invasive method that provides a measure of autonomic balance, rather than merely an index of either ortho-sympathetic or parasympathetic activity.

Some studies have shown that relaxation training and hypnosis can influence HRV [22-25].

A review of the literature concerning the relationship among HRV, hypertension and relaxation techniques shows that the use of relaxation approaches may result in decreased blood pressure and increased HRV and parasympathetic activity [25].

De Benedittis et al. [23] found that during hypnosis healthy subjects showed a statistically nonsignificant decrease in LF/HF, compared with the non-hypnotic state, thus indicating dominant activity in the parasympathetic branch or reduced ortho-sympathetic activity. When considering only subjects highly susceptible to hypnosis, as determined by the Stanford Hypnotic Susceptibility Scale [26], De Benedittis et al. found that LF/HF decrease was statistically significant and that subjects showed almost symmetrical activity of the ortho-sympathetic and parasympathetic branches, in contrast to the well-defined dominance of the parasympathetic branch in the more wakeful state. As far as average spectrum frequencies during hypnosis were concerned, results showed that in low susceptibles, LF had a high spectrum power, while HF was weak. Conversely, in high susceptibles the parasympathetic component had a higher peak. The authors argue that:

a. "neutral" hypnosis is associated with a significant LF/HF decrease, determined by a reduction of ortho-sympathetic activity and/or an increase in parasympathetic tone; and

b. there is a positive correlation between high susceptibility to hypnosis and parasympathetic activity.

In another study [24], healthy individuals underwent either relaxation training or were subjected to sham relaxation. A third group of subjects was treated with beta-adrenergic blockade pharmacotherapy, which can reduce resting heart rate even in small doses (thus avoiding the occurrence of undesirable side effects). The relaxation training was structured in weekly group meetings that included theoretical teaching, psychological insight discussion and practical sessions. Subjects were also invited to practice daily for about 30-60 minutes at home. The sham relaxation group received general instructions on behavioral health, and was invited to rest daily for about 30-60 minutes while reading or listening to music. Subjects were tested at baseline and after treatment (four days for the pharmacologically treated group, and three months for both the relaxation training group and the sham relaxation group). Recordings of ECG were performed at rest, during standing and during a mental arithmetic task. Results showed that both beta-adrenergic blockade and relaxation training reduced LF components when individuals where exposed to laboratory stressors, thus showing a reduction in excitatory autonomic responses.

It should be emphasized that the synergistic activity of the ortho-sympathetic and parasympathetic branches of ANS is regulated by automatic mechanisms that work outside conscious and voluntary processes; this activity, however, can also be affected by cerebral integration and by regulation systems located at limbic, cortical and hypothalamic levels [23, 27]. Further research is needed to investigate the neurological mechanisms underlying the relaxation response.

◼ Relaxation Techniques

There is a wide array of self-regulatory techniques by which a relaxation response can be induced. The most commonly applied and clinically established techniques are autogenic training (AT), progressive muscle relaxation (PMR) and meditative techniques [18].

There is considerable evidence of benefit of relaxation techniques in patients with organic diseases. In a meta-analysis of 15 studies evaluating the efficacy of relaxation training in oncologic patients undergoing non-surgical treatment [28], the ability to reduce intervention-related symptoms (such as nausea, pain, blood pressure, heart rate) was examined, together with the ability to improve emotional adaptation (depression, anxiety, hostility and fatigue). Results showed that relaxation techniques resulted in significant benefits in terms of decreasing emotional pressure, as well as levels of depression, anxiety and hostility. Overall, the relaxation training improved general mood in patients undergoing chemotherapy, radiotherapy, hyperthermia and bone marrow transplant.

Other studies have focused on the impact of relaxation techniques on somatic functioning, and report scientifically sound results for the use of relaxation procedures as complements to traditional rehabilitation after surgery [29, 30]. Relaxation training has shown an effect also on immune functioning. Kiecolt-Glaser and colleagues [31] assigned subjects to three different experimental protocols: progressive relaxation, social contact and no treatment. Self-report questionnaires were administered at baseline, after one-month intervention and after one-month followup. Physiological parameters were evaluated through blood exams. Findings showed that only subjects who underwent progressive relaxation experienced a significant increase in NK cells activity, thus indicating improvement in immune system functioning.

The implementation of relaxation therapy has proven to have an important role in helping CHD (coronary heart disease) patients face cardiac rehabilitation challenges. It has been reported that, in five post MI-patients out of six, relaxation training resulted in decreased blood levels of norepinephrine [32]. Cooper and Aygen [33] reported that the daily practice of a relaxation technique (over a period of 11 months) resulted in an 11% reduction of serum cholesterol, compared with 2% in the control group. These results with CHD patients are particularly interesting given that serum cholesterol is an index of sympathetic

activity. According to Italian guidelines for cardiac rehabilitation (task force for activities in cardiac rehabilitation), the main goals of relaxation training are:
1. decreasing psychophysiologic tension;
2. decreasing anxiety levels; and
3. increasing the perception of self-control.

Relaxation techniques can be combined with other intervention procedures intended to foster self-awareness. For example, Type A behavior pattern (TABP) has been classically considered as a constellation of attitudes that typically characterize CHD patients [34, 35]. The most important aspects of TABP are:
- hostility;
- anger;
- mind and body iperactivity; and
- time-urgency [36-38].

Relaxation exercises may help TABP individuals develop an awareness of their behavioral schemes and control the excessive arousal typically associated with TABP.

Moller (in this manual) emphasizes that each patient should be helped to find a relaxation procedure that complies with his/her own specific needs and characteristics. For instance, individuals that are not very introspective may find it easier to learn a simple and repetitive procedure, such as autogenic training and progressive relaxation (ATPR). Other people may prefer meditation or visualization techniques, which usually require more time and effort - along with fairly developed introspective abilities - before desirable results are achieved. Moreover, AT and PR training can occur in the context of a group setting, thus allowing therapists to work with more than one subject at a time, as well as encouraging subjects to motivate each other.

The various relaxation procedures that have been studied have several main features in common, the most important being:
a. Focusing, i.e., the ability to maintain concentration while reducing attention on environmental stimuli;
b. Passivity, or the ability to refrain from goal-oriented activities and analytic thinking; and
c. Receptivity, or the ability to tolerate and accept unusual or paradoxical experiences.

Autogenic Training

Autogenic training has been likened to a mental "gymnastic," due to the fact that it essentially consists of a structured series of mental exercises. The target of the training is to achieve a state of concentration that will eventually automatically and autonomously induce a state of expanded awareness or distension. AT was originally conceived by Schultz [39] as a methodologically sound alternative to externally induced hypnosis, even though AT undeniably has some features in common with hypnosis. One of Schultz's main goals was to reduce the relationship between therapist and client, making the latter completely autonomous in the search for the state of distension [40]. To evaluate the clinical effectiveness of AT, Stetter and Kupper [41] performed a meta-analysis of 60 studies, 35 of which were randomized controlled trials. Results showed medium-to-large effects for pre-post comparisons of disease-specific indications. A previous meta-analysis performed by Linden [42] had shown that AT was associated with medium pre-post effectiveness, ranging from 0.43 for biological outcome measures to 0.58 for psychological and behavioral measures. Both meta-analyses supported the effectiveness of AT in treating a variety of psychological and organic disorders, including, among others, angina pectoris, essential hypertension and recovery from myocardial infarction.

In an investigation of the ECGs and pneumographs of college students, Sakakibara and colleagues [43, 44] found that breathing and heart rate variability during AT showed an increase in parasympathetic tone that was not evidenced during the at-rest control condition.

Despite the fact that AT is supposed to be a tool that clients can use independently, the therapist's role is essential initially in order to learn the technique; thus, AT interventions usually include a preliminary psychoeducational component designed to teach clients how to begin and how to face emerging difficulties. Clients should also receive advice or "hints" on how to proceed when they are not achieving one of the steps of AT; for example, the therapist might suggest that they visualize images such as resting on warm sand in order to start feeling a sense of warmth throughout the body [45]. Practice and motivation help clients learn to independently perform the training in a relatively short time (usually up to eight weeks, but the exact time depends on the number of practice sessions) and finally experience the benefits in terms of both mental and physical relaxation.

Table 1 describes the six steps of AT and the sentences practitioners teach clients to repeat to themselves.

It should be emphasized that AT is not a treatment for a specific disease, but a viable tool for facing various situations that precipitate dysfunctional states of excessive arousal by improving one's ability to obtain a relaxation response.

AT can be included in psychotherapy interventions aimed at improving mental health conditions that have been associated with cardiovascular risk. A longitudinal study showed that psychotherapeutic intervention resulted in a 60% success rate in the treatment of depression, and that, when psychotherapy was associated with AT, the improvement rates increased to 91% [46]. It can be argued that the daily practice of AT may provide a practical way of facing negative reactions to stressors, thus, enhancing an individual's resilience.

Table 1. Autogenic training procedure

Step	Aim	Performance	Summary of procedure
STEP 1	Inducing heaviness	client focuses on the idea of perceiving a heavy body	I am completely calm (once) My right arm is heavy (six times) *(different parts of the body are gradually included: left arm, right leg, left leg and so on)* I am completely calm (once)
STEP 2	Inducing warmth	a warm feeling is thought to spread all over the body	My right arm is warm (six times) *(different parts of body are gradually included: left arm, right leg, left leg and so on)* I am completely calm (once)
STEP 3	The heart practice	attention is focused on heart beats, how fast/slow they are, how they change	My heart beats calmly and regularly (six times) I am completely calm (once)
STEP 4	The breathing practice	client's attention is focused on inhaling and exhaling air	My breathing is calm and regular … it breathes me (six times) I am completely calm (once)
STEP 5	The abdominal practice	a sense of warmth is thought to be spreading from the abdomen toward distal parts of the body	My abdomen is flowingly warm (six times) I am completely calm (once)
STEP 6	The head practice	a sensation of pleasant coolness is perceived n one's forehead	My forehead is pleasantly cool (six times) I am completely calm (once)

■ Biofeedback and Combined Relaxation Procedures

Biofeedback has widely demonstrated its effectiveness in the field of psychological and physical rehabilitation as a result of its ability to increase patients' awareness regarding their (psycho)-physiological processes. The technique requires electronic instrumentation able to provide visual and/or acoustic signals in response to changes in physiological functioning that, usually, are involuntary and not perceived. The aim of biofeedback is to "train" subjects to voluntarily control internal physiological events. Biofeedback is usually used in the treatment of psychosomatic and neurological conditions, different types of headache, and to control heart rate and blood pressure [47]. It is also used to treat hypertension [48]. Biofeedback helps support self-regulating systems that are in charge of homeostasis. Some studies have demonstrated the possibility of even modifying blood pressure [49, 50] and baroreflex [51], thus enabling patients to consciously regulate autonomic responses when stressful events challenge the ability of self-regulating mechanisms that maintain homeostasis. The therapeutic action of biofeedback results from the increase of information flux regarding specific internal events that regulate our body: when specific parameters are out of desirable ranges, the subject receives a visual or audio alert that a rebalancing action has to occur. For example, patients may have to breathe more regularly or relax muscles, usually by using a relaxation technique learned previously or concurrently. Through biofeedback techniques, patients can become skillful in managing symptoms on their own; as a result, the personal involvement of the patient in the learning process becomes a crucial part of the rehabilitation, along with pharmacological therapy and medical intervention). Patients feel less powerless and acquire higher disease-related self-efficacy, which, according to Bandura's theory [52-54], is a predictor of better health outcomes.

Biofeedback is particularly effective when associated with relaxation training. McGrady and colleagues [55, 56] conducted a pilot study to investigate the use of AT and PR in combination with thermal biofeedback in the treatment of neurocardiogenic syncope. Results showed significant differences between treatment and waiting-list control group. Both groups reported a decrease in levels of depression and anxiety, but only the treatment group experienced better outcomes in terms of reduced headache and loss of consciousness.

The combination of biofeedback techniques and relaxation training allows the objective verification of whether a certain relaxation procedure is being effectively implemented. As a matter of fact, the monitoring of physiological parameters provides objective evidence of changes in ortho-sympathetic and parasympathetic branches of ANS. By providing patients with information regarding alterations in heart rate, breathing and muscular tension, a "low arousal modeling" process is implemented [57]. Stoyva [57] proposed an intervention with the association of biofeedback and AT. Initially patients are exposed to a stress-response inducing situation in order to obtain a baseline profile to be used as a comparison when evaluating the psycho-physiological condition obtained after treatment. In the treatment phase, the "heaviness" practice of the AT procedure is performed and the muscular tension of the arms is traced using the electromiograph. Gradually, the whole AT procedure is followed while continuing physiological monitoring.

There may be some disadvantages from the combined use of biofeedback and relaxation training; for example, subjects may learn to rely more on signals coming from the instrumentation than from increased self-awareness of their own physiological functioning.

Biofeedback in CHD Patients' Treatment

The use of biofeedback with cardiac patients requires a preliminary behavioral analysis in order to outline possible risk factors that need to be monitored and eventually modified. Engel and Baile [58, 59] implemented a protocol aimed at learning how to reduce heart rate that included both self-monitoring activities and visits from medical staff. In order to obtain improvements, therapist and patient need to share common assumptions regarding methodology, results and potential problems. Patients should receive comprehensive information and instructions in a clear, non-technical language, and they should be comfortable in sharing with the therapist any doubts they may have regarding the procedure and instruments used.

Some patients may initially find it very difficult to control their state of arousal and become frustrated because of this. It is important that therapists support patients and motivate them to continue with the training, allowing resting periods and respecting their timing. As a rule, whenever a patient experiences a sense of frustration due to the difficulty of training, he or she should be encouraged to go back to an easier step and move forward only after the previous exercise has been fully mastered. Very often, patients are distracted by intrusive thoughts; once again, the therapist should acknowledge patient's needs, allowing him or her to express whatever is going on for a few minutes, and then help redirect the focus back to the relaxation procedure. It is fairly common for patients to engage in a sort of competition with the biofeedback equipment, above all when they present a personality characterized by perfectionism and high competitiveness.

Progressive Muscle Relaxation

Progressive muscle relaxation (PMR) was originally conceived by Jacobson [60, 61], and it is recognized as an effective method for reducing physiological arousal in a mainstream population.

The PMR procedure teaches patients to relax muscles through a two-step process. First, tension is deliberately applied to certain muscle groups, and then patients are instructed to relax. In this manner, the attention is focused on the perception that muscles relax as tension flows away.

Through repetitive practice individuals quickly learn to recognize-and distinguish-the associated feelings of a tensed muscle and a completely relaxed muscle. Based upon this simple learning, physical muscular relaxation can be induced at the first signs of tension that accompany anxiety, thus improving psychological well-being [62]. As a matter of fact, the trophotropic response can be generated by reducing afference of muscular tension inputs to hypothalamic area [23].

In 1973, Bernstein and Borkovec produced a manual for a short version of Jacobson's PR (which may require more than 40 individual sessions)[63]. They specified in a step-by-step procedure for administering relaxation training to clients in about 8-12 sessions. After training, individuals should be able to continue the practice on their own. Table 2 shows the different phases of individual post-training progression, emphasizing specific objectives [64]. A meta-analysis conducted on 29 studies concluded that abbreviated progressive muscle training (APRT) should be viewed as a scientifically sound treatment intervention [65].

In one study, PR was used with the Feldenkrais method in a rehabilitation intervention following myocardial infarction [66]. The aim of the Feldenkrais method is to increase self-awareness of ones bodily schemes so that they can be later modified [67]. The implementation of PR combined with Feldenkrais was compared with standard rehabilitation programs for MI patients. A significant difference was found in the treatment group. Participants reported a better perception of bodily dynamics and an improvement in quality of life, both from a physical and emotional perspective. Authors suggest that PR combined with the Feldenkrais technique can be beneficial in the acute phase of medical treatment, both during in-hospital rehabilitation and at-home care.

Table 2. Individual progression phases after APRT [64]

Phase	Activity	Objective
1	Daily practice of basic technique learned during training sessions	Develop individual mastery of basic procedure
2	Combine original tension-relaxation procedure of 16 muscle groups into seven and eventually four groups	Make induction process less complex and tedious
3	Eliminate the tension cycle of the original procedure	Develop subjects' ability to spontaneously induce the relaxation response
4	Develop skills for differential relaxation of separate muscle groups	Enable subjects to develop the habit of relaxing some muscles while still using others

APRT, abbreviated progressive muscle training

▪ Hypnosis

There is still much controversy over how hypnosis should be defined. It is therefore difficult to specify the psycho- and neuro-biological mechanism underlying hypnotic phenomena.

Early studies demonstrated that the hypnotic state does not produce unique or specific physiological changes [68, 69]. On the contrary, hypnosis may lead to a variety of different physiological patterns, based upon the suggestion given to the subject by the hypnotherapist and on the type of induction procedure used. For instance, it was found that a suggestion of strenuous effort while pedaling at a bicycle ergometer increased pedaling rate, compared with the wakeful state, even though a 20-Watt load was present in both conditions [22]. Hypnosis can also be used to achieve a relaxation response. Some authors refer to this as to a "neutral" state of hypnosis, meaning that suggestions are not aimed at obtaining specific goals, but rather trying to induce a condition of relaxation and well-being. Although there are many different methods for inducing the hypnotic state, the above-mentioned "neutral" state is usually achieved by narrowing subject's attention and reducing environmental stimuli, while simultaneously focusing the attention on inner stimuli. According to Frankel's account of the hypnotic induction technique [10]:

> "The object [of the induction] is to lead the subject, carefully but confidently, to redistribute his attention so as to withdraw it from his general surroundings and focus it on a circumscribed area. Meanwhile, he is encouraged to relax and let happen what will happen... Throughout this [deepening relaxation] procedure the operator fosters [an altered state of consciousness] by offering his comments in a slow, repetitive monotone, exhorting the subject to feel relaxed and calm, or to float and drift."

Today, hypnosis has many clinical applications, chief among which is the relief of pain; hypnosis can also be used as an adjunct to facilitate the effectiveness of specific psychotherapeutic interventions [18]. Its role as modulator in enhancing the immune system response is under investigation as well [31].

Clinical Issues

The existing literature provides basic guidelines for developing a clinically effective treatment protocol using relaxation techniques and/or hypnosis. The main points can be summarized as follows [64]:

A. The basic procedure must be a technique that reliably produces an integrated pattern of physiological changes collectively referred to as "the relaxation response."
B. The program should include instructions from a professional therapist who actively participates in client's training.
C. The procedure should be designed to maximize the client's involvement by requiring home practice and allowing individual rates of progress.
D. The procedure should train clients in the use of both somatic and cognitive relaxation and encourage the generalization of such skills.
E. The program should be cost effective, i.e., available to a large number of individuals without the need for a large number of professional therapists.

In general, techniques aimed at achieving the relaxation response have the advantage of increasing self-awareness of psycho-physiological processes that occur during stressful conditions. The ability to detect states of excessive arousal from a condition of psycho-physiological balance, and eventually to control arousal, results in a significant increase in self-efficacy, which is acknowledged to be a important mediator for behavior change [53].

When trying to elicit a relaxation response in a clinical setting, the therapist may face a significant challenge in helping the patient achieve the basic requirements mentioned above, i.e., passivity and receptivity. Some individuals may find it very difficult to concentrate and not be distracted by environmental stimuli. All this may lead them to feel inadequate and eventually worsen their agitation. Hypnosis offers a viable tool for bypassing such issues. In particular, the work of Milton H. Erickson has provided an innovative approach to hypnosis that tends to incorporate the client's current attitude and behavior into hypnotic induction, rather than trying directly to introduce changes. According to Erickson, hypnotic suggestion has to occur initially as a function of the client's mood and behavior [70]; then, the therapist can shift the client's attention to other stimuli in order for the desired changes to take place. To accomplish this, Erickson used a "naturalistic" approach that involved tracing or imitating the client's state [71], including his/her respiration rate, followed by gradually guiding him/her to a different state through the proper hypnotic suggestions. There is no reason why this procedure couldn't be used to attain a more balanced and functional state of arousal in CHD patients.

As already stated, hypnosis can be used to directly elicit the relaxation response in order to act directly on mechanisms that affect cardiovascular functioning. But therapists can also go further by integrating hypnosis into a psychotherapeutic process aimed at modifying behavioral and personality characteristics that have been associated with cardiac morbidity and mortality. For instance, therapist can give post-hypnotic suggestions that help clients face events that trigger anxiety [72]. Moreover, specific images can be suggested through metaphorical language to reinforce client's self-esteem and self-efficacy [73]. Reinforcing self-esteem may be particularly indicated for CHD patients exhibiting a Type D personality pattern [74], in order to help them cope with negative affectivity and social inhibition. Further research might even explore the moderating role of self-esteem on the association between Type D personality and cardiac morbidity and mortality.

The use of hypnotic psychotherapy may also be beneficial for TABP patients who easily experience anger and hostility toward other people. An emotional and cognitive "restructuring," supported by the use of the hypnotic technique, may help them redefine their "map" of the world, thus lightening their burden and the amount of distress they experience.

As far as therapist's work is concerned, teaching relaxation procedures is fairly easy, compared with inducing a hypnotic state. It is important that therapists receive specialized professional training, and also that they learn different methods of inducing a hypnotic trance.

In conclusion, both relaxation procedures and hypnosis are useful in achieving a specific physiological pattern characterized by decreased arousal of ANS (the relaxation response). Both techniques are also useful in helping clients modify behavioral and personality traits that represent risk factors for CHD onset and recurrence. Further research should clarify the neurobiological mechanisms underlying the relaxed condition. Standardized protocols should be developed and studies should involve larger samples, in order to better understand the effectiveness of the procedures used. Finally, future studies should focus specifically on objective CHD outcomes, since relaxation training and hypnosis may provide viable and less expensive tools for the treatment of chronic CHD patients.

■ References

1. Rozanski A (2005) Integrating psychologic approaches into the behavioral management of cardiac patients. Psychosom Med 67:S67-S73
2. Task force for activities in cardiac rehabilitation (2003) Guidelines for psychological activities in preventive and rehabilitative cardiology. Monaldi Archiv Chest Disease 60:184-234
3. Barr BP, Benson H (1984) The relaxation response and cardiovascular disorders. Behav Med Update 6:28-30
4. Benson H (1977) Systemic hypertension and the relaxation response. N Engl J Med 296:1152-1156
5. Everly GS, Benson H (1989) Disorders of arousal and the relaxation response: speculations on the nature and treatment of stress-related diseases. Intern J Psychosom 36:15-21
6. Stainbrook G, Hoffman JW, Benson H (1983) Behavioral therapies of hypertension: psychotherapy, biofeedback, and relaxation/meditation. Internat App Psychol 32:119-135
8. Meichenbaum D, Henshaw D, Himel N (1982) Coping with stress as a problem-solving process. Series in clinical community psychology: Achiev Stress Anxiety 127-142
8. Sardo A, Goldwurm GF, Sanavio E (1990) Psychosocial intervention with post-myocardial infarction patients: results from a 2-year follow-up. In: Zapotoczky HG, Wenzel T (Eds) The scientific dialogue: from basic research to clinical intervention. Ann Eur Res Behav Ther vol 5. Swets & Zeitlinger Publishers, Lisse, Netherlands pp 229-235
9. Esler M, Kaye D (2000) Sympathetic nervous system activation in essential hypertension, cardiac failure, and psychosomatic heart disease. J Cardiovasc Pharmacol 35:S1-S7
10. Benson H, Arns PA, Hoffman JW (1981) The relaxation response and hypnosis. Internat J Clin Exper Hypnosis 29:259-270
11. Friedman R, Myers P, Krass S, Benson H (1996) The relaxation response: use with cardiac patients. In: Allan R, Scheidt S (Eds) Heart and mind: the practice of cardiac psychology. American Psychological Association, Washington, DC
12. Hoffman JW, Benson H, Arns PA et al (1982) Reduced sympathetic nervous system responsivity associated with the relaxation response. Science 215:190-192
13. Hess WR (1957) Functional organization of the diencephalon. Stratton, New York
14. Cannon WB (1914) The emergency function of the adrenal medulla in pain and the major emotions. Am J Physiol 33:356-372
15. Selye H (1973) The evolution of the stress concept. Am Scient 61:692-699
16. Farrace S, Ferrara M, De Angelis C et al (2003) Reduced sympathetic outflow and adrenal secretory activity during a 40-day stay in the Antarctic. Internat J Psychophysiol 49:17-27
17. Walrath LC, Hamilton DH (1975) Autonomic correlates of meditation and hypnosis. Am J Clin Hypnosis 17:190-197
18. Vaitl D, Birbaumer N, Gruzelier J et al (2005) Psychobiology of altered states of consciousness. Psycholog Bull 131:98-127
19. Akselrod S, Gordon D, Madwed JB et al (1985) Hemodynamic regulation: investigation by spectral analysis. Am J Physiol 241:H887-H875

20. Steptoe A, Johnston D (1991) Clinical applications of cardiovascular assessment. Psychological assessment. J Cons Clin Psychol 3:337-349
21. Task Force of the European Society of Cardiology and the North American Society of Pacing and Electrophysiology (1996) Heart rate variability: standards of measurement, physiological interpretation, and clinical use. Europ Heart J 17:354-381
22. Cigada M, Lucini D, Bernardi L et al (1998) Valutazione della bilancia simpato-vagale durante suggestioni ipnotiche di diverso tipo in soggetti volontari sani. Quaranta anni di ipnosi in Italia: presente e futuro. Atti del XI Congresso Nazionale dell'Associazione Medica Italiana per lo Studio dell'Ipnosi. Edizione AMISI, Milan
23. De Benedittis G, Cigada M, Bianchi A et al (1994) Autonomic changes during hypnosis: a heart rate variability power spectrum analysis as a marker of sympatho-vagal balance. Intern J Clin Exper Hypnosis 42:140-152
24. Lucini D, Covacci G, Miliani R et al (1997) A controlled study of the effects of mental relaxation on autonomic excitatory responses in healthy subjects. Psychosom Med 59:541-552
25. Terathongkum S, Pickler R (2004) Relationship among heart rate variability, hypertension, and relaxation techniques. J Vasc Nursing 22:78-82
26. Weitzenhoffer AM (1962) Estimation of hypnotic susceptibility in a group situation. Am J Clin Hypnosis 5:115-126
27. Benson H, Greenwood MM, Klemchuk H (1975) The relaxation response: psychobiological aspects and clinical applications. Internat J Psychiat Med 6:87-98
28. Luebbert K, Dahme B, Hasenbring M (2001) The effectiveness of relaxation training in reducing treatment-related symptoms and improving emotional adjustment in acute non-surgical cancer treatment: a meta-analytical review. Psycho Oncol 10:490-502
29. Greenleaf M (1992) Clinical implications of hypnotizability: enhancing the care of medical and surgical patients. Psychiatric Med 10:77-85
30. Petry JJ (2000) Surgery and complementary therapies: a review. Altern Ther Med 6:64-74
31. Kiecolt-Glaser JK, Glaser R, Strain EC et al (1986) Modulation of cellular immunity in medical students. J Behav Med 9:311-320
32. Van Dixhoorn J (2000) Implementation of relaxation therapy within a cardiac rehabilitation setting. In: Kenny DT, Carlson JG, McGuigan FJ, Sheppard JL (Eds) Stress and health: research and clinical applications. Harwood Academic Publishers, Amsterdam, Netherlands
33. Cooper MJ, Aygen MM (1979) A relaxation technique in the management of hypercholesterolemia. J Hum Stress 5:24-27
34. Fred HL, Hariharan R (2002) To be b or not to be b-is that the question? Tex Heart Inst J 29:1-2
35. Friedman M, Rosenman RH (1959) Association of specific overt behavior pattern with blood and cardiovascular findings; blood cholesterol level, blood clotting time, incidence of arcus senilis, and clinical coronary artery disease. JAMA 169:1286-1296
36. Dimsdale JE (1988) A perspective on Type A behavior and coronary disease. N Engl J Med 318:110-112
37. Lachar BL (1993) Coronary-prone behavior. Type A behavior revisited. Tex Heart Inst J 20:143-151

38. Lyness SA (1993) Predictors of differences between Type A and B individuals in heart rate and blood pressure reactivity. Psychol Bull 114:266-295
39. Schultz JH, Luthe W (1959) Autogenic training: a psychophysiologic approach to psychotherapy. Grune & Stratton, Oxford, England
40. Wallnöfer H (1993) Anima senza ansia: training autogeno, ipnosi, le vie del rilassamento. Edizioni Universitarie Romane, Rome
41. Stetter F, Kupper S (2002) Autogenic training: a meta-analysis of clinical outcome studies. Appl Psychophysiol Biofeedback 27:45-98
42. Linden W (1994) Autogenic training: a narrative and quantitative review of clinical outcome. Biofeedback Self Reg 19:227-264
43. Sakakibara M, Hayano J (1996) Effect of slowed respiration on cardiac parasympathetic response to threat. Psychosom Med 58:32-37
44. Sakakibara M, Takeuchi S, Hayano J (1994) Effect of relaxation training on cardiac parasympathetic tone. Psychophysiol 31:223-228
45. De Chirico G (1984) Training autogeno. Red Edizioni, Como
46. Krampen G (1999) Long term evaluation of additional autogenic training in the psychotherapy of depressive disorders. Europ Psychol 4:11-18
47. Basmajian JV (1985) Il biofeedback: aspetti teorici ed applicazioni pratiche. Piccin Nuova Libraria, Padova
48. Nakao M, Nomura S, Shimosawa T et al (2000) Blood pressure biofeedback treatment of white-coat hypertension. J Psychosom Res 48:161-169
49. Rau H, Buhrer M, Weitkunat R (2003) Biofeedback of R-wave-to-pulse interval normalizes blood pressure. Appl Psychophysiol Biofeedback 28:37-46
50. Craig A, Lal S (2002) Optimising blood pressure reduction in mild un-medicated hypertensives. In: Shohov, Serge P (Ed) Advances in psychology research, vol. 12. Nova Science Publishers, Inc, Hauppauge, New York pp 199-216
51. Vaschillo E, Lehrer P, Rishe N, Konstantinov M (2002) Heart rate variability biofeedback as a method for assessing baroreflex function: a preliminary study of resonance in the cardiovascular system. Appl Psychophysiol Biofeedback 27:1-27
52. Bandura A (1977) Self-efficacy: toward a unifying theory of behavioral change. Psycholog Rev 84 :191-215
53. Bandura A (1997) Self-efficacy: the exercise of control. Freeman, New York
54. Bandura A (2004) Health promotion by social cognitive means. Health Ed Behav 31:143-164
55. McGrady A (2002) A commentary on "problems inherent in assessing biofeedback efficacy studies". Appl Psychophysiol Biofeedback 27:111-112
56. McGrady AV, Kern-Buell C, Bush E et al (2003) Biofeedback-assisted relaxation therapy in neurocardiogenic syncope: a pilot study. Appl Psychophysiol Biofeedback 28:183-192
57. Stoyva JM (1985) Principi del rilassamento generale: associazione del biofeedback e del training autogeno. In: Basmajian JV (Ed) Il biofeedback: aspetti teorici ed applicazioni pratiche. Piccin Nuova Libraria, Padova
58. Baile WF, Engel BT (1978) A behavioural strategy for promoting treatment compliance following myocardial infarction. Psychosom Med 40:413-419
59. Engel BT, Baile WF (1985) Tecniche comportamentali nel trattamento di pazienti

con disturbi cardiovascolari. In: Basmajian JV (Ed) Il biofeedback: aspetti teorici ed applicazioni pratiche. Piccin Nuova Libraria, Padova

60. Jacobson E (1938) Progressive relaxation. University of Chicago Press, Chicago
61. Jacobson E (1978) You must relax, 5 edn. McGraw-Hill, New York
62. Scogin F, Rickard SK, Wilson J, McElreath L (1992) Progressive and imaginal relaxation training for elderly persons with subjective anxiety. Psychol Aging 7:419-424
63. Bernstein DA, Borkovec TD (1973) Progressive relaxation training: a manual for the helping profession. Research Press, Champaign, IL
64. McReady KF, Berry FM, Kenkel MB (1985) Supervised relaxation training: a model for greater accessibility of behavioral interventions. Professional psychology. Res Pract 16:595-604
65. Carlson CR, Hoyle RH (1993) Efficacy of abbreviated progressive muscle relaxation training: a quantitative review of behavioral medicine research. J Cons Clin Psychol 61:1059-1067
66. Lowe B, Breining K, Wilke S, Wellmann R et al (2002) Quantitative and qualitative effects of Feldenkrais, progressive muscle relaxation, and standard medical treatment in patients after acute myocardial infarction. Psychother Res 12:179-191
67. Dunn PA, Rogers DK (2000) Feldenkrais sensory imagery and forward reach. Perceptual Motor Skills 91:755-757
68. Bauer KE, McCanne TR (1980) Autonomic and central nervous system responding: during hypnosis and simulation of hypnosis. Int J Clin Exp Hypn 28:148-163
69. Case DB, Fogel DH, Pollack AA (1980) Intrahypnotic and long term effects of self-hypnosis on blood pressure in mild hypertension. Int J Clin Exp Hypn 28:27-38
70. Rossi EL (1993) The psychobiology of mind-body healing: new concepts of therapeutic hypnosis (rev. ed) W.W. Norton & Co, Inc., New York
71. Bandler R, Grinder J (1975) Patterns of hypnotic therapy of Milton H. Erickson. Meta Publications, Capitola, CA
72. Purdue V (2003) The use of hypnosis and imagery methods in the treatment of cardiac disorders in women. In: Hornyak, Lynne M, Green JP (Eds) Healing from within: the use of hypnosis in women's health care. Dissociation, trauma, memory, and hypnosis book series. American Psychological Association, Washington, DC pp 65-89
73. Mosconi GP (2001) Ipnosi del 2000: il pensiero di Milton Erickson e dei neo-ericksoniani. Atti del XII Congresso Nazionale dell'Associazione Medica Italiana per lo Studio dell'Ipnosi. Edizione AMISI, Milan
74. Denollet J, Van Heck GL (2001) Psychological risk factors in heart disease: what type D personality is (not) about. J Psychosom Res 51:465-468

Chapter 22

Cardiological and Psychological Mobile Care through Telematic Technologies for Heart Failure Patients: *ICAROS Project*

A. Compare ▪ E. Molinari ▪ L. Bellardita ▪ A. Villani ▪ G. Branzi ▪ G. Malfatto ▪ S. Boarin ▪ M. Cassi ▪ A. Gnisci ▪ G. Parati

Introduction

Currently heart failure is one of the main causes of disability and mortality in western countries. Due to the severity of this illness, as well as the number of clinical interventions necessary (particularly the high frequency of hospitalizations), heart failure comprises a major health expense. Specifically, it accounts for 5% of total hospitalization costs and 1-2% of total healthcare expenses [1]. Better therapies for myocardial infarction (MI) and an increasingly older population will eventually result in even larger numbers of patients with chronic heart failure. Obviously, the increase of patients will necessitate new interventions and support models, including multi-pharmacological prescriptions and close monitoring of clinical conditions over extended periods. Because a patient's psychological condition can influence the course of cardiac disease and therapeutic compliance, the interventions also will need to monitor behavioral and life-style modifications, requiring extensive education efforts, both for the patients themselves and for their families.

Disease management (DM) interventions have been extensively tested and found to be more effective than traditional interventions in improving the prognosis of patients with diabetes, congestive heart failure (CHF) and myocardial infarction (MI). DM consists of a system of coordinated healthcare interventions and patient communication for populations with a high incidence of medical conditions involving patient self-care. A recent meta-analysis that included 102 studies (10 of which were conducted on CHF patients, with a total of 2000 subjects and follow-ups ranging from three months to one year) evaluated the impact of DM as part of a multi-disciplinary approach for treating chronic conditions [2-26]. Results showed that, for the management of CHF, the most common interventions were [2]:
- training patients before dismissal on activities that were to be continued at home (pharmacological therapy, diet, exercise);
- telephone contacts;
- home-based interventions (HBI) involving GP or a trained nurse.

Results confirmed that an integrated management (including multifunction center activities and continuous monitoring) were the most effective interventions. These findings are in marked contrast to the high noncompliance to therapy usually observed in CHF patients after hospital dismissal, a situation that leads to instabilization and a worsening of the clinical condition.

Several studies have focused on the characteristics associated with the likelihood of instabilization. In an Italian sample, for example, it was shown that 46% of CHF and left ventricular dysfunction patients that had been hospitalized for an acute event were re-hospitalized within a year, and that 50% of these re-hospitalizations were due to the lack of adherence to therapy. Moreover, 80% of "unstable" subjects are re-hospitalized within three months from dismissal. Thus, it is clear that patient monitoring during this critical period may have a crucial impact on stability.

New wireless technologies represent a very important resource for managing the complex activities required by DM interventions. There is evidence that some DM programs may reduce disease-associated costs up to 30-40%, mainly in terms of fewer re-hospitalizations, which makes investments in technologically advanced DM interventions extremely worthwhile. New technologies allow easier and better data management. Information can be more easily accessed and distributed, thus improving the productivity-effectiveness relationship. Moreover, the availability of a large amount of data allows advanced statistical analysis (such as Artificial Neural Networks), a capability that, eventually, will lead to better understanding of the variables involved in disease prognosis and even better assistance models.

Up to now, no studies focusing on the integrated management of CHF patients through the use of advanced technologies have been conducted in Italy. The ICAROS (Innovative arChitecture based on wireless and intelligent technology for the cardiological and psychological care of heARt disOrderS)-FIRB project has developed a home-based telecare system for CHD patients, using advanced Internet, as well as emerging wireless and mobile, technologies.

■ The ICAROS - FIRB Project

The ICAROS project was sponsored by the Italian Ministry of University and Scientific Research, with a FIRB (Italian Funds for Base Research) – New Medical Engineering 2001, in co-operation with the following research units:
a) Department of Medicine, Prevention and Applied Biotechnologies of Milano-Bicocca University;
b) Department of Psychology of Università Cattolica del Sacro Cuore, Milan;
c) Istituto Auxologico Italiano.

The technological partner was Mobile Medical Technologies (MMT)[1], a soci-

---

[1] Mobile Medical Technologies s.r.l. (*http://www.m-mt.net*, email *info@m-mt.net*)

ety that offers innovative services in the field of disease management through proprietary Internet and wireless technologies. Not only did MMT provide the technology for wireless clinical monitoring, therapy and acute episode management, they also served as a consultant for developing the project's protocol, implementing the project, and providing the logistic management, training and first-level support needed by the clinical staff.

The project was awarded the CNR (National Research Center) Special Prize for the 6th edition of FORUM P.A. Sanità, issued by the Italian Ministry of Health and other organizations. The FORUM P.A. SANITÀ Prize acknowledges public healthcare organizations who take advantage of information and communication technology (ICT) in creating more efficient healthcare, particularly in terms of managing clinical data as a means of controlling healthcare costs. The CNR special prize was awarded to the ICAROS Project because of its use of ICT in the active prevention of chronic diseases through the administration of complex healthcare programs.

To date, the ICAROS project has been presented at a number of national and international meetings, such as:

- 2nd international e-GOVERNMENT & e-HEALTH conference and exhibition, held in Milan, Italy in July 2005;
- Critical Issues in eHealth Research Conference, held in Washington D.C. (USA) in June 2005;
- Other meetings and exhibits sponsored by the Ministry for Innovation and Technologies.

The project is also a pilot study for a larger investigation, sponsored by a European Commission grant, to be conducted by an international group consisting of researchers from Italian, Spanish and Greek universities and institutions. The larger European project is intended to investigate a universal service for monitoring and managing the cardiac and psychological health of European cardiac patients, and it will include e-Health and advanced mobile services designed to help overcome existing financial and social barriers related to launching such a service at a trans-European level. The project will use trans-European telecommunication network-based applications, exploiting the potential of broadband, advanced mobile networks and multiple platforms in areas of public interest. Its methodology will incorporate the advantages of open standards, interoperability and trusted, secure frameworks. The project will also foster the modernization of related existing public services (eEurope 2005).

As noted by the World Health Organization (WHO), the "…majority of CVDs are preventable and controllable. However, millions are dying in middleage. Activities to prevent this should include strengthening collaborative work with various organizations and community groups involved in this area, promoting the formation of coalitions between key stakeholders, and developing initiatives based on best practices by supporting information exchange among countries." FOR ALL, comprised of groups from several European nations dedicated to enhancing the efforts of present cardiologic disease management and psychosocial support services, is strongly positioned to accomplish this goal. FOR ALL is backed by the existing service from the Istituto Auxologico of Milan, which will be adapted and customized for the market validation phase at the trans -European level, supporting exchange of best practices among European countries. Partners in the project include APIF Moviquity S.A. (Spain); ISTITUTO AUXOLOGICO ITALIANO (Italy); DIANOEMA S.p.a (Italy); ALTEC Information and Communication Systems S.A. (Greece); ATTIKON University Hospital (Greece); and Hospital de Terrassa (CST) (Spain).

The ICAROS study uses a randomized design with parallel groups. Patients are enrolled in the study at three Italian research centers and monitored for one year in order to compare the evolution of clinical and functional conditions between the integrated management (IntM) group (n = 30) and the conventional management (CM) group (n = 30). Upon dismissal from the hospital, patients in the CM group will receive treatment supervised by their GP, and they will undergo clinical check-ups and psychological visits every three months at the HF center. Patients in the IntM group will be monitored daily through a PDA, and they, also, will undergo quarterly visits at the HF center.

The study sample consists of CHF hospitalized systolic dysfunction patients with an ejection fraction lower than 40%, in III-IV NYHA class at hospitalization and with a previous history of HF. In addition, the patients are required to have had one or more hospitalizations during the previous 12 months, or a peripheric edema at dismissal.

The study aims are to:
- Reduce disease progression in terms of clinical events.
- Improve patients' clinical conditions and functional states.
- Monitor psychological state and identify psychological conditions associated with cardiovascular risk in a timely manner.
- Improve CHD patients' quality of life.
- Optimize and personalize therapy, while achieving better cost/benefits efficiency.
- Improve the efficacy and timeliness of interpreting and identifying important clinical signs of acute events that require costly intervention.
- Improve compliance as well as the identification of non-compliant patients.

System Description

The core aspect of the DM model developed for ICAROS-FIRB is therapeutic continuity, i.e., improving the patients' feeling of being cared for by medical staff, while being completely free to move about and go anywhere. Mature internet technologies and emerging multi-channel and wireless technologies allow patients to maintain the interactions and communications established with medical staff during hospitalization.

Overall System Architecture

The service, MMT, provided to the ICAROS-FIRB Project, is headed by the Istituto Auxologico Italiano and Università Cattolica Sacro Cuore, and aimed at improving both the effectiveness and efficiency of chronic disease management. By providing a continuous interaction between patient and doctor, based on new technologies (internet, mobile, wireless), MMT provides continuous monitoring of key medical parameters and psychological conditions using an internet-based software application, which serves as both a medical aid and a psychological care and diagnostic tool.

The front-end designed for the patient provides a portable solution for the day-to-day management of the patient's healthcare needs, while the clinical front-end provides both medical and psychological web-based software designed to facilitate care-related decisions (Fig. 1).

The data repository and the core applications are hosted at a remote server farm. The patient front-end consists of a health organiser resident on the patient's PDA or smartphone. This system is designed to help individuals better manage their lifestyle, medical care and drug intake, to track treatment progress, and to enter information about their therapy by inputting actions performed (e.g., drug intake, exercise, questionnaires). All information collected is automatically report-

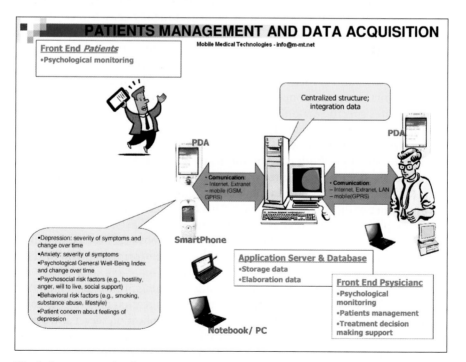

Fig. 1. Remote monitoring system

ed through synchronisation/downloading to their healthcare professional. Each action that the patient performs and enters in the PDA/smartphone is time stamped, which can be viewed by the clinician. Patients are also able to receive printed information regarding their therapies and medical conditions, and to schedule and organise followup visits. Questionnaires are submitted periodically in order to monitor and evaluate psychological conditions. The device used by the patient provides the all information needed for managing the disease, and it allows data input through system prompts. Electronic patient records are available to nurses and/or physicians through a desktop Internet browser. At the initial visit, the physician classifies the patient on the basis of his or her clinical profile and the key variables to be continuously monitored. The physician then initialises the system and loads the key parameters and the therapy into the central repository.

The back end consists of a database and diagnostic software for analysing and comparing data sent by the patient. The collected data will also become the basis for building an integrated, proprietary statistical system that interprets the patient's key clinical symptoms and proposes adjustments to drug intake, exercise and diet. Based on key clinical parameters, the software is designed to be continuously updated with the latest disease-specific information using an evidence-based medical approach and optimal therapeutic targets.

Patient information is entered into the system's medical record database either through synchronisation of the patient's PDA or through a real-time connection with the server. Once the patient has synchronised the device, the doctor receives the information sorted by priority/urgency of each case, and, as appropriate, he or she can update therapy or send messages to the patient (e.g., to schedule visits, warn patients of high-risk behaviors, etc.). Automatic control of adherence to physician instruction (compliance) through analysis of actual data is enabled. Identification by the doctor of out of range parameters/behaviors through automatic data verification will activate an alarm system that facilitates specific action. As soon as the synchronisation takes place, the patient receives new instructions from the system.

The system integrates and stores all clinical data, to provide doctors with a continuous stream of both current and historic information. The objective is to support the doctor in interpreting data and managing the patient. At a given time, for example, the physician may receive a list of priority patients alerting the him or her to the most urgent cases; a list of potential treatment options for a specific patient; charts on key clinical data and forecasts; and information pertaining to patient compliance with respect to diet, physical exercise and drug consumption. Information on when each action was performed, and on medical treatment, safety and tolerability, is also provided.

The ICAROS FIRB Project services – headed by the Istituto Auxologico Italiano – are supplied via a remote software custom application on a remote computer server hosted in a server farm that runs a Java application server and a relational database; the application (an enhanced Electronic Patient Record ERP) is accessible via internet through a standard browser, Java Runtime Environment enabled, in a secure mode (HTTPS).

The overall architecture is protected by a firewall; and the server farm service provides standard features, including SNMP, data back-up, antivirus, uninterruptible power supply, intrusion detection and so on); a service level agreement for maintenance and recovery had been signed.

Help desk operators, nurses, physicians and psychologists are able to interact with the application through Desktop clients; the availability of broadband connections (xDSL/LAN) in the clinical center is required to obtain high performances; the browser uses a Java runtime environment (Java Applet technologies enabled) in order to reach platform independence.

Every desktop client is provided with PDA synchronisation software, making it possible to set up and manage the handheld devices before delivering them to the patients. Mobile devices access the Internet and then go to the application server through a GPRS/EDGE connection supplied by a national Mobile TelCo Operator, as well as by the standard mobile Internet Gateway. The PDA device runs a Windows Mobile 2003 custom application. Data are exchanged between PDAs and the Application Server using a compress XML file format, lowering costs associated with data transmission.

The Electronic Patient Record Application. The system adopted for the ICAROS FIRB project is build upon an existing clinical software layer: an EPR, which is a web-based application developed with Java technologies. This system runs on an Oracle database, in contrast to the mobile application, developed with MSFT Net technologies. The interface between the two layers is managed by a Java servlet and an XML file. Specifically, the ICAROS-FIRB project runs on a customized version of eHealth®.Solutions from GMD mbh (Berlin, Germany), controlled by DN Group (Bologna, Italy); and the custom features consist of proprietary solutions created and owned by MMT.

The current release of eHealth®.Solutions runs on a Microsoft Windows Server platform, and the application server is Tomcat. The reason for adopting an established electronic patient record software framework comes from both the wide diffusion of the software in clinical organizations and the opportunity to rapidly deploy new functionalities for the mobile wireless front end, thanks to the embedded developer tools. Main eHealth® solutions offer further advantages in terms of the high reliability of the EPR, the ability of clinic organizations located in different regions to access the EPR over the Internet, the availability of a document repository for uploading/downloading information, a high degree of usability and data security (involving encryption and authentication, compatibility with both standard HIPAA[2] and stricter Italian privacy laws).

All the EPR and mobile tools the project uses are considered current state-of-the-art technologies.

The application can be run from the ICT department inside the clinical center or from the remote server, without any difference in performance.

---

[2] HIPAA (*http://www.cms.hhs.gov/hipaa/*) **Health Insurance Portability and Accountability Act**

Handheld Device Application. The handheld section of the ICAROS–FIRB project is developed with MSFT Net Windows Mobile 2003 Second Edition, Phone Enabled. The device used by patients:

1. provides all the information necessary for data management (drug intake, diet, exercise, registration parameters, check-up visits); and
2. allows data input when required by the system.

The Windows Mobile devices are equipped with a standard GSM/GPRS Sim Card; some limitation in the functionalities have been activated (only preset telephone numbers are reachable); ICAROS FIRB PDAs could be used also as regular GSM mobile phones and to transmit ECG in acoustic connection thought special purpose devices.

The application serves as a diary for the collection of clinical and vital data, and completed psychological questionnaires. It also serves as a reminder to facilitate adherence to therapy. Collected data can be either locally stored (in the memory of the PDA) or sent to the central repository.

Medical and Psychological Monitoring

Assessment
At intake, physicians classify patients based upon clinical profile, and then they initialise the system with the main variables to be monitored (such as blood pressure) and the pharmacological treatment. This initial phase also includes a psychological assessment, which may occur during either hospitalization or day-hospital rehabilitation. Patients are administered a clinical interview regarding personal history, habits and their social network, and they later complete self-report questionnaires. The psychological assessment process usually occurs over a period of two to three one-hour sessions. The psychological constructs investigated are anxiety, depression, quality of life perception, illness perception and behavior, and anger. Personality traits are investigated as well, with an emphasis on evaluating Type A and D behavior patterns (for further information regarding personality traits, refer to Chapter 11, "Type A, Type D, Anger-Prone Behavior and Risk of Relapse in CHD Patients"). After completing the assessment process, the psychologist at the HF centre compiles a profile, focussed on whether psychological risk factors have emerged.

Patient's Front-End
On a daily basis, patients are required to enter vital parameters on the PDA, including weight, heart rate, diastolic and systolic pressure, liquid intake and diuresis. Patients benefit from an enlarged keyboard that shows up on the PDA display when they need to input numbers or letters. A range-control system prevents the input of improbable data, thus avoiding unnecessary alerts. Figure 2 shows the display for entering vital parameters, as well as the display that serves

as a therapy reminder. PDA screenshots are in Italian, as, thus far, the project has been implemented using an Italian sample.

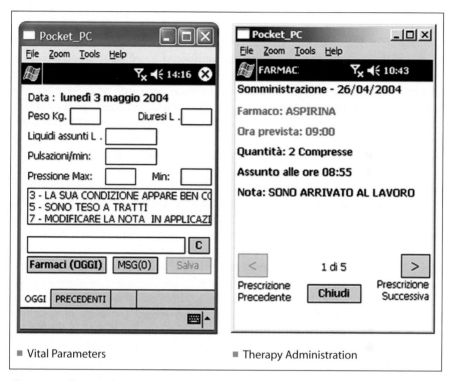

■ Vital Parameters   ■ Therapy Administration

Fig. 2. PDA displays for vital parameters collection and pharmacological therapy administration

Patient's front-end presents, at regular intervals, questionnaires aimed to evaluate depression, anxiety and perception of quality of life. Data synchronization occurs in the same way as it does for medical data. Table 1 lists administered questionnaires, including timing, psychological constructs investigated, and response modality.

Table 1. Psychological constructs and relative assessment instruments

	STAI-short form	PGWB-6	PHQ-9	GENERAL - B
Psychological construct	Anxiety	Quality of life perception	Depression	Psychological general screening
Administration frequency	Weekly	Monthly	Bi-weekly	Weekly
Type of answer	Multiple choice	Multiple choice	Visual analogic scale	Visual analogic scale

Anxiety is measured weekly using a short form of Spielberger's State Trait Anxiety Inventory (STAI -6). Six items were selected by the authors from the state scale, which measures anxiety in terms of feelings of insecurity and powerlessness in front of a perceived threat [27, 28].

Depression is evaluated using the Patient Health Questionnaire (PHQ-9). The PHQ is frequently used to diagnose depressive conditions in medical settings. It consists of nine items for evaluating DSM-IV criteria for major depression. Two studies, one involving 3000 patients with a number of medical problems, and the other, also conducted on 3000 patients at gynecological-obstetric clinics, show the instrument's diagnostic value in relation to measures comprising a larger number of items. Moreover, PHQ-9 not only helps to establish the presence of a depressive condition, but also provides an index of severity of depressive symptomatology [29, 31].

Perception of Quality of Life is measured monthly through PGWB-6, the short form of a standardized self-report instrument developed by Dupuy (Perception of General Well-Being Inventory, or PGWBI) [32-34]. The questionnaire is composed of six sub-scales (anxiety, depression, positivity and well-being, self-control, general health and vitality). The 22-item scale has high internal consistency (Cronbach alpha 0.90-0.94) and has been used in a number of samples varying greatly in terms of socio-demographic variables, health conditions and age. The PGWB-6 has also been used to evaluate changes in subjective well-being after psychotherapy. A study conducted by Università Cattolica of Milan, in cooperation with Bracco, compared the original and the short version, and found a high statistically significant correlation between the two (r = 0.887, p<0.0001). Finally, a multi-trait analysis showed that Cronbach alpha was 0.93 for the standard scale and 0.92 for the short version. Hence, reliability and validity data strongly support the implementation of PGWB-6, which has thus far proved a convenient instrument for monitoring quality of life.

Psychological General Screening B-PGS: Patients also receive a weekly questionnaire used to evaluate psychological well-being (for example, "I feel anxious"). Patients are asked to state what an acceptable condition would be ("Normal/acceptable anxiety for me should be..."). This questionnaire was developed by the group of psychologists involved in the project, and one of the study's aims is to validate it.

Questionnaires can be multiple-choice (an example is shown in Fig. 3), or visual analogic scales (VASs) (an example is shown in Fig. 4). All measures, except for GSB, use normal population indexes as a comparison.

VASs (Fig. 4) provide patients with a response system that is more perceptively immediate, making it easier for them to identify the degree of a particular emotional state. Moreover, numeric data expressed on a continuous scale is without doubt more precise, compared with scales involving the forced choice of a specific number.

Windows Mobile 2003 allows the use of Landscape mode to increase the horizontal scale dimensions and hence questionnaire sensitivity.

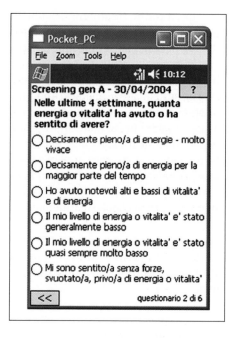

Fig. 3. Display for one of PGWB-6's items

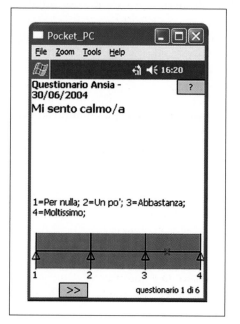

Fig. 4. Visual analogic scale for one of STAI-6's items

Staff Front-End

Medical and psychological visits at the CHF centre are conducted at intake and every three months; physicians may also perform unplanned visits based upon information collected through the system.

Patients are enrolled and randomly assigned to the treatment or control group. When registering the patient into the system, the relevant data are collected and input, including demographic data and information related to mobile devices and SIM card.

As soon as the patient synchronizes the device, the healthcare staff receives information organized by priority/urgency. The system allows medical and psychological staff to identify irregular parameters or behaviors through an automatic verification routine that activates an alert system to facilitate appropriate action. Based upon the information collected, healthcare staff may decide to contact the patient, modify therapy, send the patient a text message or plan a visit. The patient will receive the feedback as soon as he/she performs the next synchronization.

An automatic control system is activated in order to check treatment compliance through analysis of relevant data.

The system holds and integrates all medical and psychological data, and provides health and psychological care staff with a continuous stream of updated and historic information. The aim is to provide an optimal method for interpreting clinical data and managing patients.

Collected data include:
- List of patients with active alerts.
- List of different options for treatment of a specific patient.
- Graphs reporting important data related to clinical picture and development of the condition.
- Information regarding patient compliance, including diet, exercise, drugs intake.
- Information regarding security and tolerance to pharmacological treatment.
- Psychological questionnaire outcomes.

Figure 5 shows the system architecture that allows for the communication of patient information, as well as medical staff-patient exchanges.

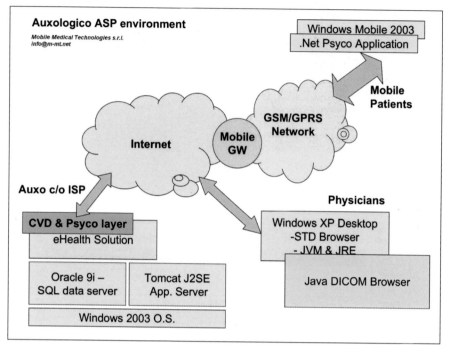

Fig. 5. Communication architecture

Psychologist's Desktop. The answers to self-report questionnaires provided by patients through the PDA are sent directly to the database, along with data regarding vital parameters. The system automatically scores the answers. Total scores for anxiety and depression scales are transformed into percentiles and rated according to clinical significance as follows:
- scores under the 90th percentile are considered normal and reported in a green-coloured cell;
- scores between the 90th and 95th percentile are considered moderate and reported in a yellow-coloured cell; and
- scores corresponding to the 95th percentile or higher are the labeled "High" and reported in a red-coloured cell.

Figures 6 and 7 show displays that track the clinical history of two patients as far as anxiety and depression are concerned. The relevant information was transmitted to the system through PDA questionnaires the patients completed. Data for each questionnaire, including numerical index and qualitative label, are recorded in a dedicated cartel, from most to least recent observation, thus showing the course of patient's condition over time for a specific psychological dimension.

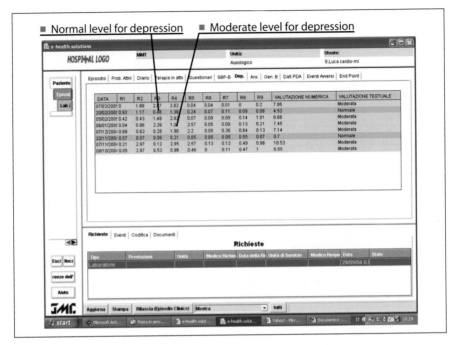

Fig. 6. Database screenshot: depression levels reported by one patient

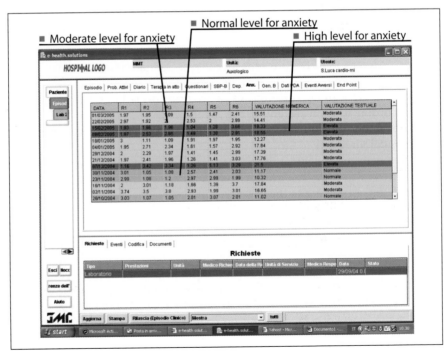

Fig. 7. Database screenshot: anxiety levels reported by one patient

Figure 8 shows the protocol to be followed by the psychologist in charge, based upon alerts regarding the patient's anxiety and depression levels.

Variable	Observation	Action
Anxiety	Normal Level	No action to be performed
	Moderate Level	Verify the presence of two consecutive alerts of moderate level. If trend is confirmed, call patient for psychological inquiry
	High Level	Call patient and plan visit with psychologist. Cardiologist should be alerted as well
Depression	Normal Level	No action to be performed
	Moderate Level	Call patient to verify condition. In case depressive symptomatology is confirmed, plan a visit with psychologist
	High Level	Call patient and plan visit with psychologist. Cardiologist should be alerted as well.

Fig. 8. Psychological reports and types of intervention for anxiety and depressive condition alerts

Medical Staff's Desktop. The visit management part is composed of eight different data files: **Anamnesis, Pharmacological Anamnesis, Objective Examination, Neuro-hormonal, ECG, Chest RX, Ultrasound** and **Ergo Test.** Other visits, including psychological visits, can be stored in a database of electronic documents (text documents, letters, computation sheets, imaging files or scanned documents) as attachments. The visit management section is the same for both treatment and control groups. A separate panel is provided for monitoring each patient in the Integrated Management group. This panel allows access to a number of data files that help control each patient's condition and eventually modify the intervention.

The **Episode** sheet briefly summarizes the information on the registration card for each patient. The **Diary** sheet is a sort of planner that helps staff to register future events, such as visits or telephone calls. The **Active Problems** sheet is extremely important, as it records whether pharmacological prescriptions have been regularly followed and whether vital parameters fall into the acceptable range. From an IT perspective, this sheet is log-file already analyzed from a medical standpoint, reporting information that patients have sent following the PDA-central system synchronization. All clinical data received from the PDA feed appropriate algorithms capable of generating alerts. Figures 9 and 10 show examples of database sheets that report alerts.

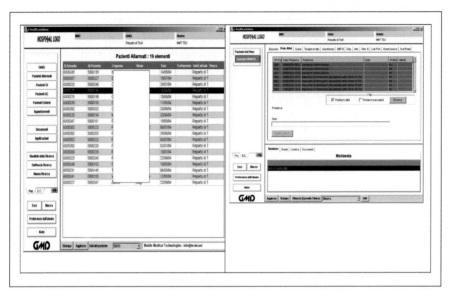

Fig. 9. Patients with alerts   **Fig. 10.** Alerts specification for a specific patient

The **Current Therapy** and **Questionnaires** sheets allow for the management, respectively, of pharmacological therapy and psychological questionnaires, with specific interfaces for administering or modifying therapies and questionnaires as far as parameters such as quantity, timing and so forth, are concerned.

The **SBP-B** (related to PGWB-6 instrument), **Anxiety, Depression and General B** sheets report numerical indices and generate graphical evaluations of responses to individual questionnaires.

The **PDA Data** sheet reports all medical values collected from patients and is referred to for vital parameters details when the Active Problems sheets generate a warning message.

The last two sheets, **Adverse Events** and **End Points,** are used to record cardiac events that occur to patients during the one-year monitoring period.

Final Considerations

Today, electronic patient record technology is widely used in healthcare organizations even if not all the capabilities are exploited. The interest in, and diffusion of, handheld wireless technologies have increased dramatically thanks to technological improvements, especially in terms of and reliability, and to the integration of handheld wireless technology with mobile telephony, Bluetooth and wi-fi. Until now, these technologies were used primarily by sales organizations to automate the operations of their sales forces. The ICAROS Project is solid evidence that the innovation of a complex information system need not result in resistance from staff not trained in information technology methodologies.

In clinical institutions, particularly those that care for elderly CHF patients, the real challenge is the ability to develop very simple systems and devices. Another critical issue involves the training of both system operators and patients. It is essential that this training be provided by qualified professionals, in a step-by-step manner. Although the adoption of a new technology always represents a challenge, we have witnessed the ease with which this process can occur, as demonstrated by the wide diffusion of mobile phones (whose complexity is much greater than that of the ICAROS-provided device).

In the ICAROS project, in-hospital patient training was assigned a key role; sometimes, depending on circumstances, training was also extended to the patient's family. The role of nurses was found to be very important. When they are skilled at information technology (office procedures, data entry) and call-center procedures, nurses are able to solve minor problems in managing the telecare, such as reminding patients to recharge PDA batteries.

The usability of remote monitoring systems obviously involves the ability to simplify data acquisition processes. Technologies capable to acquiring multiple patient inputs through a set of wearable sensors and peripheral special purpose devices located in the patient's home will likely, in the near future, be routine. Also, the continued efforts of computer professionals will result in increased advances in the simplification of the protocol languages used to communicate between computers, computerized devices, and patients and nurses and/or physicians.

At the same time, all the regulations related to more "intrusive" patient management systems will be consolidated to guarantee privacy of the target of care and to improve the confidence in making appropriate use of the increasing amount of data to be analysed.

In a time when population aging is one of most important issues to be solved by welfare systems, it is fundamental to find cost-effective intervention plans. IT systems have proven their usefulness in terms of economic benefits in a number of different fields. Yet, it is not always easy for users to understand related benefits; this becomes even more pronounced for DM interventions, due to their complexity. It is therefore necessary to progressively introduce DM programs, in a process that directly involves patients and clinicians. Ultimately, this will result in a continuity of care not currently provided. For patients, knowing that they are monitored on a daily basis by the clinical center is both comforting and motivating at the same time, thus impacting clinical adherence. It is plausible that using the PDA helps establishing trust between patients and clinical staff. At the same time, patients feel more autonomous in managing their therapy and daily activities, as the PDA also serves as a self-monitoring instrument that increases patient responsibility with respect to pharmacological treatment, subjective psychological well-being and risk factors directly and indirectly related to disease prognosis.

Preliminary information about the ICAROS-FIRB project supports the feasibility of the implementation of DM on a large scale, despite the acknowledged complexity and challenges that are involved.

■ References

1. Cline CM, Israelsson BY, Willenheimer RB et al (1998) Cost effective management programme for heart failure reduces hospitalisation. Heart 80:442-446
2. Weingarten SR, Henning JM, Badamgarav E et al (2002) Interventions used in disease management programmes for patients with chronic illness-which ones work? Meta-analysis of published reports. BMJ:325
3. Gattis WA, Hasselblad V, Whellan DJ, O'Connor M (1999) Reduction in heart failure events by the addition of a clinical pharmacist to the heart failure management team: results of the pharmacist in heart failure assessment recommendation and monitoring (PHARM) study. Arch Intern Med 159:1939-1945
4. Stewart S, Marley JE, Horowitz JD (1999) Effects of a multidisciplinary, home-based intervention on unplanned readmissions and survival among patients with chronic congestive heart failure: a randomised controlled study. Lancet 354:1077-1083
5. Andersson EB, Ehnfors M, Matejka G et al (1998) Feasibility of a nurse-monitored, outpatient-care programme for elderly patients with moderate-to-severe, chronic heart failure. Eur Heart J 19:1254-1260
6. Oddone EZ, Weinberger M, Giobbie-Hurder A et al (1999) Enhanced access to primary care for patients with congestive heart failure. Veterans affairs cooperative study group on primary care and hospital readmission. Eff Clin Pract 2:201-209
7. Rich MW, Beckham V, Wittenberg C et al (1995) A multidisciplinary intervention to prevent the readmission of elderly patients with congestive heart failure. N Engl J Med 333:1190-1195
8. Rich MW, Vinson JM, Sperry JC et al (1993) Prevention of readmission in elderly patients with congestive heart failure: results of a prospective, randomized pilot study. J Gen Intern Med 8:585-590
9. Rich MW (1999) Heart failure disease management: a critical review. J Cardiac Fail 5:64-75
10. Stewart S, Horowitz JJD (2002) Detecting early clinical deterioration in chronic heart failure patients post-acute hospitalisation – a critical component of multidisciplinary, home-based intervention. Eur J Heart Fail 4:345-351

11. Schulman KA, Mark DB, Califf RM (1998) Outcomes and costs within a disease management program for advanced congestive heart failure. Amer Heart J 135:285-292

12. Grady KL, Dracupp K, Kennedy G et al (2000) Team management of patients with heart failure. Circulation 102:2443-2456

13. Shah NB, Der E, Ruggiero C et al (1998) Prevention of hospitalisations fro heart failure with an interactive home monitoring program. Am Hearth J 135:373-378

14. Stewart S, Horowitz JD (2002) Home based intervention in congestive heart failure. Long-term implications on readmission and survival. Detecting early clinical deterioration in chronic heart failure patients post-acute hospitalisation – a critical component of multidisciplinary, home-based intervention. Circulation 105:2861-2866

15. Akosah KO, Shaper AM, Havlik P et al (2002) Improving care for patients with chronic heart failure in the community. The importance of a disease management program. Chest J 122:906-912

16. Whellan DJ, Gaulden L, Gattis WA et al (2001) The benefit of implementing a heart failure disease management program. Arch Intern Med 161:2223-2228

17. Krumholz HM, Parent EG, Tu N et al (1997) Readmission after hospitalisation for congestive heart failure among medicare beneficiaries. Arch Intern Med 157:99-104

18. Cleland JG, Cohen-Solai A, Cosin Aguilar J et al (2002) Management of heart failure in primary care (the IMPROVEMENT of heart failure program): an international survey. Lancet 360:1631-1639

19. Brass-Mynderse NJ (1996) Disease management for chronic congestive heart failure. J Cardiovasc Nurs 11:54-62

20. Naylor MD, Brooten D, Campbell R et al (1999) Comprehensive discharge planning and home follow-up of hospitalised elders. A randomised clinical trial. JAMA 281:613-620

21. Jerant AF, Azari R, Nesbitt TS (2001) Reducing the cost of frequent hospital admissions for congestive hearth failure. A randomised trial of a home telecare intervention. Medical Care 39:1234-1245

22. de Luigan S, Wells S, Johonson P et al (2001) Compliance and effectiveness of 1 year's home telemonitoring. The report of a pilot study of patients with chronic heart failure. Eur J Heart Fail 3:723-730

23. Kornowsky R, Zeeli D, Averbuch M et al (1995) Intensive home-care surveillance prevents hospitalisation and improves morbidity rates among elderly patients with severe congestive heart failure. Am Heart J 129:762-766

24. Gattis WA, Hasselblad V, Whellan DJ, O'Connor CM (1999) Reduction in heart failure events by the addition of a clinical pharmacist to the heart failure management team. Arch Intern Med 159:1939-1945

25. Stewart S, Vandenbroek AJ, Pearson S, Horowitz JD (1999) Prolonged beneficial effects of a home-based intervention on unplanned readmissions and mortality among patients with congestive heart failure. Arch Intern Med 159:257-261

26. Ekman I, Swedberg K (2002) Home-based management of patients with chronic heart failure - focus on content not just form! Eur Heart J 23: 1323-1325

27. Spielberger CD, Sydeman S, Owen AE, Marsh BJ (1999) Measuring anxiety and anger with the State-Trait Anxiety Inventory (STAI) and the State-Trait Anger Expression

Inventory (STAXI). In: Maruish ME (Ed) The use of psychological testing for treatment planning and outcomes assessment 2 edn. Lawrence Erlbaum Associates, Publishers, Mahwah, NJ, US pp 993-1021

28. Spielberger CD, Sydeman S (1994) State-trait anxiety inventory and state-trait anger expression inventory. In: Maruish ME (Ed) The use of psychological testing for treatment planning and outcome assessment. Lawrence Erlbaum Associates, Inc, Hillsdale, NJ, England pp 292-321

29. Kroenke K, Spitzer RL, Williams JB (2001) The PHQ-9: validity of a brief depression severity measure. J Gen Intern Med 16:606-13

30. Kroenke K, SpitzerRL, WilliamsJB (1999) Validation and utility of a self-report version of PRIME-MD: the PHQ primary care study. Primary care evaluation of mental disorders. Patient health questionnaire. JAMA 282:1737-44

31. Lowe B, Kroenke K, Herzog W, Grafe K (2004) Measuring depression outcome with a brief self-report instrument: sensitivity to change of the patient health questionnaire (PHQ-9). J Affect Disord 81:61-66

32. Wool C, Cerutti R, Marquis P et al (2000) Psychometric validation of two Italian quality of life questionnaires in menopausal women. Maturitas 35:129-142

33. Badia X, Gutierrez F, Wiklund I, Alonso J (1996) Validity and reliability of the Spanish version of the psychological general well-being index. Quality of life research: an International Journal of Quality of Life: Aspects of Treatment. Care & Rehabilitation 5:101-108

34. *http://www.bracco.com/Bracco/Internet/Congress/PGWBI+bracco.htm*

Chapter 23

Functioning and Disability in Patients with Cardiovascular Disease within the ICF Classification Framework: Proposals for Using ICF to Classify Functioning and Disability in Patients with Cardiovascular Disease

M. Leonardi ▪ A. Raggi

According to data from the Italian Ministry of Health, cardiovascular disease represents the leading cause of death in Italy, being responsible for 44% of all deaths. More specifically, ischemic heart disease is the first cause (28% of total deaths) and cerebrovascular conditions are the third cause (13% of all deaths). In countries in the European Union, heart disease causes the death of approximately 1.5 million people – this is 42%, or a little less than half, of all deaths - and stroke causes 25% of all deaths [1]. A similar situation is found in the United States, where heart disease accounts for about 930,000 deaths every year, or, 40% of the total deaths [2].

Yet, death is only a part of the picture: people surviving a heart attack often become chronically ill. In Italy, for example, the prevalence of people with a chronic cardiovascular disease is 4.4% - that is, around 250,000 people. Data concerning the European Union [3] report about 2,190,000 hospital discharges following cardiovascular conditions, among which 630,000 are due to coronary heart conditions and about 350,000 to stroke. There is consequently a problem that is linked, not only to the mortality rate due to heart disease, but also to the impact of these conditions on functioning and disability levels in affected people.

Despite the relevance of these epidemiological data, people have scant awareness of the size of the problem. This is apparent if we consider how little they are informed about the main risk factors: smoking, physical inactivity and unhealthy diets.

There are several differences in the clinical and etiological features of heart disease and, although it is quite easy to have a diagnostic classification of different situations and to highlight prognostic factors, it is difficult to achieve a homogeneous and functional classification of the health status in heart patients, especially one that includes the psychosocial correlates that underlie their pathologies.

A psychological approach to the problem - that is, the domain of "psychocardiology" - is able to point out a series of attendant conditions that can be easily, or secondarily, related to heart disease. Furthermore, in some cases psychological features of people affected by heart disease can be considered genuine comorbidities: consider, for example, factors such as anxiety, depression, psychosocial stress and type A-personality behaviors (i.e., behavioral patterns characterized by strong emotional responses, high control and vigilance, and competitiveness and aggressiveness). A multidisciplinary approach to heart disease is essential because, in addition to the effects of the disease *per se*, its related features directly affect patients' functional level. A heart disease patient presenting a high level of anxiety or depression, for example, might have more problems, compared with one who has no comorbidity conditions or milder conditions. Furthermore, the psychological approach plays an important role if we have to address the issue of a patient's adaptation to a lifestyle that, in most cases, is very different from the one the patient had before the heart condition.

From a physical and medical point of view, heart disease, *per se*, is taken care of by cardiologists and heart surgeons by means of drugs or surgery. However, there are a number of issues concerning the way that patients live with their condition and treatment, their emotional correlates and, above all, the impact of disease and rehabilitation on their daily life and work. These disease-related aspects, and their impact on patients, should not be addressed only by physicians, but also by professionals with other skills. Having a heart disease often means experiencing remarkable changes in habits and lifestyle: these changes can often be part of therapeutic prescription.

Referring to changes as therapeutic prescriptions necessarily implies considering the care process in a broader way, due to the fact that a strict distinction between therapeutic and rehabilitative aspects can hardly be endorsed. In the cure and care of cardiopathic patients, therapeutic and rehabilitative aspects become parts of a unified path in which a variety of professional skills play a synergic role.

Psychological support, coupled with the cardiac rehabilitation, should be recommended and considered when planning a rehabilitation program. The program should aim to facilitate those conditions that, in the patient's environment, enable him or her to progress through different stages: from the initial diagnosis, through the rehabilitation process, and to the highest possible level of functioning. This implies not only reducing depression and anxiety, but also improving other areas of functioning - for example, problem solving and the communication and expression of emotions [4].

◼ Heart Disease: Functioning and Disability

Heart disease, like several other clinical conditions, often has a great influence on an individual's practical and daily ability to participate in activities and perform certain tasks. A reduction in everyday activities or ADL (Activities of Daily Living) in individuals affected by heart disease, especially the aged ones, is well documented [5-7]. Restrictions in activities and the need for assistance affect other areas of everyday experience as well - areas related to quality of life, work, etc. Perceived quality of life decreases [8, 9] in each of its components, ranging from the physical to the psychosocial [10]. For individuals with heart disease, the psychological aspects specifically affected are mood profile, anxiety state and psychosocial stress [11-14]. Depressive symptoms are risk factors for myocardial infarction relapse [15, 16], and they are actually the main predictors of decline in quality of life and health status [17]. Depressive disorder is quite common in patients with heart disease: its estimated prevalence is between 15-40% [18], and subclinical depressive conditions are believed to be even more common. Anxiety, also, is common among people with heart disease, both in the acute situation and during rehabilitation [19, 20]. The estimated prevalence of anxiety-related issues is between 70-80% in acute situations, and around 20-25% in chronic situations [19, 21].

Another relevant issue concerns the psychosocial area, particularly work and interpersonal relationships. The latter, especially, is an important factor of protection for patients, both at the onset of disease and during rehabilitation [22-24]. In this connection, a recent contribution [25] highlights how the lack of attentive, thoughtful responses to a patient's needs and symptoms by significant others may actually reinforce the severity of the patient's depressive symptoms and the symptoms associated with heart disease, which, as a consequence, also impacts the patient's level of disability.

Working activity - which exceeds its intrinsic value, affecting domains such as self-esteem and self-efficacy - is also of great importance in terms of quality of life. The importance of getting back to work quickly has been identified as an important health-improving factor; furthermore, rehabilitation training that simulates actual working situations is more effective than focusing only on exercise and effort levels, perhaps because it helps reduce the psychosocial stress associated with the work environment [26, 27].

For the reasons stated above, it is our belief that a successful therapeutic approach cannot do without a broad evaluation of the patient, taking into account clinical features as well as personal and environmental ones, such as marital status, working situation and education level. Such an evaluation cannot be performed without regard to the context of the individual's life, which includes family, professional and social environments, and health practices. So far, all these components have never been systematically addressed, in part due to the fact that different languages are used by different healthcare systems and research centers, and in part due to the fact that the patients themselves can differ radically from one another.

Today, the World Health Organization (WHO) gives us the opportunity to standardize and unify the language used to talk about people's functioning in a multidisciplinary and cross-cultural way [28], enabling us to acquire all the necessary information by means of an ICF (International Classification of Functioning, Disability and Health) [29]. While at a descriptive-diagnostic level, the ICD-10 (International Statistical Classification of Diseases and Related Health Problems) [30], whose 10th edition was released in 1992, is cross-cultural and shareable, there was a need for a classification of health and disability that had the same features. As a matter of fact, the ICIDH-80 (International Classification of Impairments, Disabilities and Handicaps, 1980) had been used since 1980 for research and trials. It is only with ICF, however, that we have made a full transition from a diagnostis classification to another classification, that focused on functioning and disability.

While diagnosis alone can neither explain nor predict what type of health or social service will be needed by a person, evaluating these needs [31] is of utmost importance, especially when the impact of fatal diseases is decreasing and that of chronic diseases is increasing. Capturing health information related to chronic conditions entails changing the type of indicator used to study the population's health, mortality no longer being the most adequate. This epidemiological transition is very evident in the field of cardiology, where advances in medical knowledge and surgical techniques have played a leading role in lowering death rates, while at the same time increasing the number of people with chronic outcomes of heart disease.

The greatest strength of ICF is the fact that it is not tied to a western perspective; on the contrary, it can be applied anywhere in the world, thus allowing cross-cultural comparison at different levels: for example, from the health and social security politicies of different countries to the way they are implemented and the funds each country is willing to invest in the process. Moreover, ICF enables researchers to create world-comparable administrative databases for different health conditions [32]. The ability to make comparisons in this manner will undoubtedly result in improving healthcare services and policies worldwide by identifying as models those countries where disability and mortality rates are lower.

ICF Description

ICF has introduced several cultural changes related to health, functioning and disability issues. For a long time, health concepts coincided with the of absence of disease, a model inspired by the medical perspective, which has now outdated and enriched by other components. Rather than being limited to the absence of disease, health can be better defined as a state of complete physical, psychological and social well being: health is thus strictly related to human functioning at every level. Taking the *environment* into consideration in the concept of health, as in ICF, is of paramount importance: an individual's health has a direct influence on the context of his or her life environment. This is because the state of a person's health can entail substantial changes in his or her habits, work and relationships. Likewise, environmental factors may affect a person's health, either promoting it or serving as a barrier (as in the case of environmental pollution or situational stress).

Functioning, as defined in ICF, goes beyond the old-fashioned concept of "residual ability." It does so by offering a view of the person as a whole in which "functioning" serves as an umbrella term to describe the positive aspects of interaction between healthy individuals and their contextual factors, whether personal or environmental. Functioning is therefore determined both by the patient's health condition (as a result of which, for example, a person with heart disease most likely will not be able to perform strenuous or lengthly physical activities) and by the person's environment (although patients are encouraged to try to reduce stress, a stressful relational context is likely to affect their functioning).

The concept of disability is the most relevant novelty in ICF. *Disability* is viewed as an umbrella term that pinpoints the negative aspects of the interaction between a person and his or her environment. Aspects of disability include physical, structural and functional impairments, as well as, chiefly, restrictions and limitations on the participation and activities that patients have to face in their context, due to a bad fit between their health condition and an environment that hampers them in some ways. Using the term *disability* instead of *handicap* does not represent a semantic modification only. It is a drastic departure from the linear model adopted by ICIDH-80, in which, given a disease, a person was considered impaired and therefore had a handicap. With that classification, the environment was thought of only as a "container" of the expectations and demands related to a role considered "normal" for a specific person.

ICIDH-80 was at first issued for field trials and research only; later on, the great number of comments made by users who, for lack of other official tools, started to use it in a broader way, brought WHO to undertake the revision process from which ICF was developed. ICF does not adopt a linear model (more appropriate for medical understanding) as occurred with ICIDH; it uses a biopsychosocial model that entails a broader and multidimensional vision of functioning and disability. Following the modern theories of complexity, ICF adopts a way of viewing disability that is a result of the mutual interactions between impairments at the structural or functional level, limitations in activity, restrictions in participation and contextual factors (personal as well as environmental).

◾ Structure of ICF Classification

ICF is a classification or a collection of codes used to describe individual health and related conditions by means of a standardized and unified language. There are 1460 alphanumeric codes that are used according to the situation and the specific level needed by the user. These codes are composed of two parts, and each part is divided into two components.

The first part is called "Functioning and Disability," and its two components include: 1) Body Functions and Structures; and 2) Activity and Participation. Body Functions are the physiological functions of body systems, mental function included, whereas Body Structures are the anatomical parts of the body, considered at a recognizable level of detail, without using advanced means and methods of investigation. The second component focuses on Activity, intended as the performance of a task or action by an individual, and on Participation, intended as the involvement of an individual in a life situation. The positive, functioning aspect of "Body Function and Structures" is represented by their functional and structural integrity, while the negative, disability aspect is represented by an impairment, intended as a significant loss or deviation with respect to a set statistical standard. With regard to "Activity and Participation," the positive aspect is represented by the ability to perform tasks and actions and to be involved in life situations, while the negative aspect is represented by activity limitations and participation restrictions. The first definition covers all the difficulties an individual could meet in performing a task, while the second definition covers problems resulting from personal involvement in a life situation.

The second part of ICF is referred to as "Contextual Factors," and these, also, are divided into two components: "Environmental Factors" and "Personal Factors." Personal factors are not classified in ICF at present: given their wide cross-cultural variability, WHO has decided not to classify them, as this would necessarily fall short of achieving a general criteria for universality and cross-cultural comparability.

Environmental factors include all those aspects of the external world that form and determine an individual's life context, as they affect individual functioning. This includes the physical and artificial environment, with its features, relationships, attitudes, policies, systems and services that are available to people (e.g., social, health, and legal services). The presence or absence of these factors can either improve personal functioning, thus reducing disability, or worsen personal functioning, thereby increasing the disability level. In the first case, we talk about Facilitators, and, in the second case, about Barriers. In this manner, by starting from the health condition classified and described according to ICD-10 criteria and referred to as a "body function, structure or both," we can use ICF to describe individual functioning on a global level, not only at the physical components level, but at the environmental level.

As mentioned before, ICF codes are alphanumeric and consist of four letters, corresponding to the ICF domains of Body Functions (b), Body Structures (s), Activity and Participation (d), and Environmental Factors (e). These codes follow the English designation in every country, in order to facilitate cross-cultural comparison. Following each letter are several numbers, depending on the level of the classification to be considered and the needs of the user. The classification is organized in a hierarchical fashion (Table 1) and moves from a first level, which is very generic, to a second, slightly more detailed level, to a third and, finally, a fourth level of detail, as may be seen in this example from Chapter 1, regarding Mental Functions.

Table 1. ICF hierarchical structure

ICF hierarchical structure: mental functions		Level
B1	Mental functions	1
B114	Orientation functions	2
B1142	Orientation to person	3
B11420	Orientation to self	4

As can be seen above, moving down means adding numbers to the starting code. Because ICF is organized in a hierarchical fashion, you can go down in details or do the opposite, i.e., move from a detailed code to a general one (*roll-up* procedure). Each code identifies the item it refers to in an unambiguous and exclusive way, by means of precise and detailed definitions that specify inclusion and exclusions: there are no conceptual overlappings between different codes.

Next to the identification code there is a dot followed by qualifiers, which are used to describe the situation being considered - for example, the severity of the problem. Each code must be followed by one or more qualifiers in order not to lose its intrinsic significance. For the domains of Body Functions, Body Structures, and Activity and Participation, the first qualifier describes the severity of the problem or the extent of the impairment (Table 2). The first qualifier does not represent an assessment or a measure. By "opening up" the code that it refers to, one is able to see the problem and get a rough idea of the extent of the impairment, which, in any case, has to be evaluated by means of a specific assessment.

Table 2. First qualifier, severity scale

First qualifier: severity scale	
0	No problem
1	Mild problem
2	Moderate problem
3	Severe problem
4	Total problem
8	Not specified
9	Not applicable

In the Body Structures classification, two additional qualifiers have to be considered after the first one. The second qualifier is used to describe the nature of the structural change (Table 3), while the third one pinpoints where this structural change, impairment or malformation is located (Table 4).

Table 3. Second qualifier of body structures, nature of change

Second qualifier of body structures: nature of structural change	
0	No structural change
1	Total absence
2	Partial absence
3	A part in excess
4	Abnormal dimensions
5	A discontinous part
6	Deviant position
7	Qualitative change in structure
8	Not specified
9	Not applicable

Table 4. Body structures third qualifier, location of impairment

Third qualifier of body structures: location of impairment	
0	More than one region
1	Right
2	Left
3	Both sides
4	Head on
5	Back
6	Proximal
7	Distal
8	Not specified
9	Not applicable

In classifying Activity and Participation, two qualifiers are used: performance and capacity. They are graduated like the first qualifier and refer to what individuals do in their environment (performance), as well as to the highest possible level of functioning they can reach at a given time, in a standard or uniform environment (capacity). In short, we can say that capacity represents what individuals would be able to do when their environment is neither interfering nor facilitating, and the discrepancy between performance and capacity shows the role of environment.

In classifying Environmental Factors, qualifiers are used to establish whether a factor is a barrier or a facilitator. In the case of barriers, the first qualifier is used according to the standard procedure; however, in the case of facilitators, a plus (+) replaces the decimal point.

As a consequence, each code and its qualifiers are indicative of the body function, structure, activity and participation or environmental factors we are referring to, in a precise and globally shared fashion. This possibility enables us to describe, either at a micro or macro level, which environmental factors are facilitators or barriers and , thus, to assess needs, making it possible to create intervention plans aimed at individuals, the environment or populations.

■ Use of ICF in Cardiological Rehabilitation

Given ICF's descriptive capacity, we may assume that psychological approaches (diagnostic, descriptive and therapeutic) can also follow WHO's biopsychosocial model, which can provide guidelines for planning interventions both for individuals and their environment.

An important step in planning an individual care program using ICF consists in adopting a multidisciplinary approach. Therefore, ICF allows a therapeutic and rehabilitative range of interventions that goes beyond standard psychotherapy or psychological support. Psycho-cardiology as a discipline should encompass different types of interventions, whether strictly therapeutic or designed to enhance the quality, using the contributions, knowledge and resources of many professional domains, not just cardiology and psychology. Only such a methodology can address an array of issues that exceed the domain of psychocardiology, but at the same time can deeply affect it. The use of ICF may serve as a guideline that potentially could encompass the patient's whole care program, from the time a cardiological event occurs, through the rehabilitation program and up to the patient's reintegration into working life.

The most remarkable novelty brought about by ICF in clinical practice is the possibility to making an assessment of needs, both at the individual and population level. Through ICF, we can identify several "access doors" for enhancing an individual's quality of life, apart from clinical situation, by highlighting all functioning and disability items. ICF does not merely point out what is missing, it also underscores what is working and, in patients with the same diagnosis, allows for the identification of different levels of functioning and disability. In this manner, personalized interventions can be planned. ICF clarifies where a person wants to be in terms of his or her disability, and how he/she wants to be treated (transition from compliance to concordance - that is, it provides a shift in perspective from a disease-based approach to one based on the patient as a person).

By identifying environmental factors as essential features in defining disability, it is possible to establish multidisciplinary therapeutic alliances involving many professional skills, which is a very important and useful procedure with cardiopathic patients. A rehabilitative intervention addresses the areas in which an individual is not functioning well, be it physical, psychological or environmental, while making sure that the intervention does not damage functional areas. ICF permits us to classify individuals and their environment. Even in those situations where a patient cannot be cured, ICF - by addressing the individual's needs and the context in which he or she lives - ensures that he or she will be well taken care of.

Once again, we would like to emphasize that ICF is not an assessment tool; its qualifiers are not meant to measure a problem, but, rather, to classify its extent. Every item describing a person's situation should already be associated with a specific assessment; the purpose of ICF is to "translate" the assessment into ICF language through the use qualifiers that, first of all, describe whether a problem exists, and, if so, describe how serious it is.

For psychologists applying ICF in chronic pathologies such as cardiology, this entails focussing their intervention on how the health conditions affect domains such as "Activity and Participation" and "Environmental Factors." These, indeed, are areas that are more likely to be addressed by a psychologist, who, for example, might focus on interventions involving environmental barriers, or, more specifically, those associated with disfunctional relationships and negative attitudes. Here, the psychologist's task is to offer his or her skills to the patient, family and caregivers, in order to help them achieve the most satisfactory psychophysical, social and interpersonal level of functioning possible, while paying special attention to the obstacles or barriers that hinder this optimal level of functioning. This, of course, is a multidisciplinary job, involving not only psychologists and physicians, but also a network of rehabilitation technicians, nursing staff, social workers and legal representatives [33].

Functioning and disability levels in cardiopathic patients may vary according to the specific situation, as well as to the type of medical-rehabilitative intervention needed and the environment, which can serve as either a barrier or facilitator. In some cases, levels of functioning are quite good and therefore rehabilitation will have a modest impact, possibly addressing, for example, ways for improving life habits, such as giving up smoking, eating a healthy diet, or ways of avoiding or dealing with stressful situations. In other cases, such as when the patient's lifestyle itself presents a risk factor, the psychologist may be asked to provide a stronger intervention - for example, helping the patient to work on interpersonal relationships, behavioral patterns, or adaptations to the new condition of disability and its associated stress. It is important to note that limiting an intervention to patients and their lifestyles, and making no changes with respect to the environment, entails ruling out the ICF model in a therapeutic project.

Psychocardiology provides an excellent example of how psychologists, cardiologists and other professionals can pool their skills to develop a cardiological rehabilitation plan if needed, as determined by counseling interviews. At the very least, some psychological counseling is necessary to evaluate whether there is psychological distress associated with the patient's heart disease. If this is the case, then a rehabilitative or psychotherapeutic treatment plan can be devised as necessary, according to the severity of the situation and the capacity of the patient's insight.

Using ICF in a Cardiopathic Patient: Application Example

This is a likely clinical vignette, prepared and simplified for ICF teaching and training purposes.

Man, 50 years old, with dilating cardiomyopathy (ICD-10 code: I42.0); he has to struggle in order to perform ordinary physical activities, during which he has palpitations, tiresome respiratory difficulties and mild pain due to angina pectoris. His motion is limited, especially when lifting and carrying objects (he can handle small, lightweight objects by himself, but he needs help with heavy or large objects. He also needs help walking - he can walk alone for a few meters, or, with the assistance of someone else, for about a hundred metres, provided he changes his position (he has to be supported in order to stand up). Because of the anxiety he suffers as a result of not feeling well, he is not confident enough to use public transportation alone, and he is no longer able to drive a car; therefore, he is unable to travel in town unless somebody goes with him or drives him. He has difficulties in other areas, as well: self care (he needs help to have a bath); social relationships, both formal and informal, which he has cut down; work (he has been forced to retire earlier, in spite of his wish to go on working; however, he is required to perform some tasks compatible with his health status). He regularly takes life-saving drugs, which, however, are not always available at the nearest chemist's; he lives in a house with no architectural barriers and can make use of facilitating tools to perform some of his daily activities. He regularly receives support from his immediate family and friends, which helps him live a less restrictive life. From a psychological point of view, the patient is still unable to accept his new condition that, as he puts it, has caused him only problems. His mood level is very much dysphoric: he sleeps badly and only for a few hours; he reacts to situations in a negative way, especially when he has to be helped in daily activities; and he is unable to cope with the stress associated to his situation, although his difficulties are lessened when his wife is around. He has recently applied for a disability pension; the medical commission granted him 75% invalidity.

This case, simplified in its medical components, was made up to show a possible use of ICF in cardiology; its educational purpose accounts for the lack of details.

By opening up a code we point out a problem. The following codes for Body Functions have been opened up, each of them referring to a single function (for more details regarding the inclusion and exclusion criteria of ICF codes, an ICF online browser is available at www.who.int/classification/icf).

Table 5. Clinical case vignette, body function classification

Body functions		Qualifier (impairment extent)
b134	Sleeping functions	2
b152	Emotional functions	2
b28011	Chest pain	1
b4552	Fatiguability	2
b460	Sensations associated to cardiovascular and respiratory functions	2

We would like to remind the reader briefly that Body Functions qualifiers indicate the extent of an impairment:

0: no problem
1: mild problem
2: moderate problem
3: severe problem

4: total problem
8: not specified
9: not applicable

The same qualifiers used in Body Structures are also used in Activity and Participation. With regard to this case-vignette, Body Structures can be classified as follows:

Table 6. Clinical case vignette, body structure classification

Body structures	First qualifier (impairment extent)	Second qualifier (nature of change)	Third qualifier (impairment location)
s4100 Heart structure	3	4	8

In the domain of Body Structures, the second qualifier indicates the nature of change in anatomical structures, while the third one shows the location of a structural change or impairment.

EXTENT	NATURE	LOCATION
0: no problem	0: no structural change	0: more than one region
1: mild problem	1: total absence	1: right
2: moderate problem	2: partial absence	2: left
3: severe problem	3: a part in excess	3: both sides
4: total problem	4: abnormal dimensions	4: head on
8: not specified	5: a discontinuous part	5: back
9: not applicable	6: deviant position	6: proximal
	7: qualitative change in structure	7: distal
	8: not specified	8: not specified
	9: not applicable	9: not applicable

With respect to Body Structures, it is evident that the qualifiers used to classify and describe the situation in our case-vignette indicate a status of severe, due to an abnormality in heart dimensions, whose location is not better specified for lack of specific information from the case-vignette.

In the Activity and Participation domain, a performance qualifier shows what the patient is actually able to do in his environment, and it takes into account both factors that help and those that hinder the patient's functioning. The Capacity qualifier identifies the highest possible level of the patient's ability to function with no facilitators (e.g., people, helping tools, drugs, etc.) and no barriers. With regard to our case-vignette and according to the available description of the subject, the following Activity and Participation codes may be opened, using these qualifiers for performance and capacity.

Table 7. Clinical case vignette, activity and participation classification

Activity and participation	First qualifier (performance)	Second qualifier (capacity)
d420 Handling stress	1	3
d430 Lifting and carrying objects	1	3
d450 Walking	2	3
d470 Using means of transportation	0	2
d475 Driving	4	4
d510 Bathing	1	3
d740 Formal relationships	2	2
d750 Informal relationships	0	1
d850 Paid work	4	4

It is important to remember that, in the domain of Environmental Factors, a plus (+) is added to a qualifier to indicate the presence of a facilitator, while the standard decimal point is used in the case of a barrier.

Table 8. Clinical case vignette, environmental factors classification

Environmental factors	qualifier (barrier or facilitator)
e1101 Drugs	+4
e115 Products and technologies for personal use in daily life	+3
e155 Design, construction and building products and technology of building for public use	+3
e310 Immediate family	+4
e320 Friends	+4
e410 Individual attitudes of immediate family members	+4
e420 Individual attitudes of friends	+4
e570 Social security services, systems and policies	+3
e590 Labour and employment services, systems and policies	2

ICF makes it possible to take a picture of an individual's functioning, and of the interactions between health status and the environment. In this case-vignette, we can see the important facilitating and protecting role of the environment for this person. In the domain of Activity and Participation, each performance qualifier is less severe than, or equal to, its corresponding capacity qualifier, meaning that environment has a positive effect on the life of this person. Likewise, in Environmental Factors, all codes except one are classified as facilitators: the only barrier is found in the field of labour system and policies, because the company he used to work for was not able or willing to alter his job responsibilities or offer him another job position, forcing this man to retire before due time.

In view of the above information and ICF structure, it would seem important - in addition to managing the cardiological situation – to consider a counseling program or psychotherapy, particularly with respect to helping the patient as far as mood and psychosocial stress management are concerned. Beyond this, we might also consider a home support program for some basic activities, particularly those related to self-care. Although at the present time, this intervention does not seem necessary, in the future it could become urgent, both in view of possible clinical worsening and in the event of a change in family relationships.

As already mentioned, ICF is not an assessment tool. Given a certain health condition at a specific moment, it classifies and describes a person's level of functioning; therefore, it cannot be used to describe the probable course of a disease. Nevertheless, by using the classification at different times, it is possible to get *different* pictures of the person's functioning. This enables professionals to identify needs and plan targeted interventions, the length of which depends on the nature of the situation. Just as health conditions and environmental factors change over the time, the same thing happens for functioning levels. Such a change may be due to the worsening or improving of a health condition, or to a modification of the life context. Remember that disability, according to ICF, is determined by health condition in a disadvantaged environment; as a result, modifications in a person's current environment may inadvertently create other barriers, resulting in further functional limitations and, consequently, a higher level of disability. Using ICF, it is possible to monitor these functional levels over the time, and to see which codes are opened, which qualifiers are used, and the differences between capacity and performance, on the one hand, and the presence of environmental barriers or facilitators, on the other hand. In general, the more pictures are taken over time, the better equipped we are to modulate different interventions and identify the best program of individualized cure and care.

■ References

1. Rayner M, Petersen S (2000) European cardiovascular disease statistics. British Heart Foundation, London
2. U.S. Department for Disease Control and Prevention (2004) Preventing heart disease and stroke. Addressing the Nation's Leading Killers
3. Peterson S, Rayner M (2002) Coronary heart disease statistics 2002 edition. British Heart Foundation, Health Promotion Research Group, Department of Public Health, Oxford
4. Weissman MM, Markowitz JC, Klerman GL (2000) Comprehensive guide to interpersonal psychotherapy. Basic Books, New York
5. Mendes de Leon CF, Guralnik JM, Bandeen-Roche K (2002) Short-term change in physical function and disability: the women's health and aging study. J Gerentol B Psychol Sci 57:S355-S365
6. Reynolds SL, Silverstein M (2003) Observing the onset of disability in older adults. Soc Sci Med 57:1875-1889
7. Brach JS, VanSwearingen JM, Newman AB, Kriska AM (2002) Identifying early decline of physical function in community-dwelling older women: performance-based and self-report measures. Physical Ther 82:320-328
8. Simko LC, McGinnis KA (2003) Quality of life experienced by adults with congenital heart disease. AACN Clinical Issues 14:42-53
9. Huo N, Chui MA, Eckert GJ et al (2004) Relationship of age and sex to health-related quality of life in patients with heart failure. Am J Critical Care 13:153-161
10. Berry C, McMurray J (1999) A review of quality of life evaluations inpatients with congestive heart failure. PharmacoEconomics 16:247-71
11. Carels RA (2004) The association between disease severity, functional status, depression and daily quality of life in congestive heart failure patients. Quality of life research 13:63-72

12. Martensson J, Dracup K, Canary C, Fridlud B (2003) Living with heart failure: depression and quality of life in patients and spouses. J Heart Lung Transplant 22:460-467

13. Kim P, Warren S, Madill H, Hadley M (1999) Quality of life of stroke survivors. Quality of Life Research 8:293-301

14. Havranek EP, Masoudi F, Westfall K et al (2002) Spectrum of hearth failure in older patients: results from the natural heart failure project. Am Heart J 143:412-417

15. Bush D, Ziegelstein R, Tayback M et al (2001) Even minimal symptoms of depression increase mortality risk after acute myocardial infarction. Arch Int Med 158:2469-2475

16. Ferketich A, Schwartzbaum J, Frid D, Moeschberger M (2000) Depression as an antecedent to heart disease among women and men in the NHANES I atudy. Arch Int Med 160:1261-1268

17. Rumsfeld JS, Havranek EP, Masoudi F et al (2003) Depressive symptoms are the strongest correlate of short-term declines in health status in patients with heart failure. J Am Coll Cardiol 146:646-652

18. Lesperance F, Frasure-Smith N (2000) Depression in patients with cardiac disease: a practical review. J Psychosom Res 48:379-391

19. Moser DK, McKinley S, Riegel B et al (2002) Perceived control reduces in-hospital complications associated with anxiety in acute myocardial infarction. Circulation 106(Suppl II):369

20. Sirois BC, Burg MM (2003) Negative emotion and coronary heart disease. A review. Behav Mod 27:83-102

21. Januzzi JL, Stern TA, Pasternak RC, DeSanctis RW (2000) The influence of anxiety and depression on outcomes of patients with coronary artery disease. Arch Int Med 160:1913-1921

22. Jaracz K, Kozubski W (2003) Quality of life in stroke patients. Acta Neurologica Scandinavica 107:324-329

23. Westlake C, Dracup K, Creaser J et al (2002) Correlates of health-related quality of life in patients with heart failure. J Critical Care Heart Lung 31:85-93

24. Bennett SJ, Perkins SM, Lane KA et al (2001) Social support and health related quality of life in chronic heart failure patients. Quality of life research 10:671-682

25. Itkowitz NI, Kerns RD, Otis JD (2003) Support and coronary heart disease: the importance of significant other responses. J Behav Med 26:19-30

26. Mital A, Shrey DE, Govindaraju M et al (2000) Accelerating the return to work (RTW) chances of coronary heart disease (CHD) patients: part 1 - development and validation of a training programme. Dis Rehab 22:604-620

27. Shrey DE, Mital A (2000) Accelerating the return to work (RTW) chances of coronary heart disease (CHD) patients: part 2 - development and validation of a vocational rehabilitation programme. Dis Rehab 22:621-626

28. Üstün TB, Chatterji S, Kostansjek N, Bickenbach J (2003) WHO's ICF and functional status information in health records. Health Care Financing Review 24:77-88

29. Organizzazione Mondiale della Sanità (2001) Classificazione internazionale del funzionamento, della disabilità e della salute. Ginevra

30. Organizzazione Mondiale della Sanità (1992) Classificazione statistica internazionale delle malattie e dei problemi sanitari correlati, decima revisione. Ginevra

31. Leonardi M (2003) ICF: la classificazione internazionale del funzionamento, della disabilità e della salute dell'Organizzazione Mondiale della Sanità. Proposte di lavoro e di discussione per l'Italia. Giornale Italiano di Medicina Riabilitativa, vol. 17 N.1
32. Iezzoni LI, Greenberg MS (2003) Capturing and classifying functional status information in administrative databases. Health Care Financing Review 24:61-76
33. Scherer MJ, Blair KL, Banks ME et al (2004) Rehabilitation psychology. In: Craighead WE, Nemeroff CB (Eds) The concise Corsini encyclopedia of psychology and behavioral science, 3rd edition (pp 801-802). John Wiley & Sons, Inc., Hoboken, NJ

Chapter 24

Coherence-Building Techniques and Heart Rhythm Coherence Feedback: New Tools for Stress Reduction, Disease Prevention and Rehabilitation

R. McCraty ▪ D. Tomasino

Ms. C, a very active professional woman who enjoyed skiing, scuba diving and sky-diving, was diagnosed with a cardiac arrhythmia and mitral valve prolapse in 1989. By 1993, she was experiencing 700 extra heartbeats per hour and was told that she was at risk for sudden death. She was prescribed beta-blockers, Valium and aspirin, the side effects of which were stomach-aches, headaches and hair loss. In July 1994, Ms. C suffered a near-fatal episode of ventricular tachycardia and underwent radio frequency catheter ablations. Ms. C's ventricular tachycardia events continued to recur throughout the following nine months, during which time she had surgery four times. In April 1995, she was told that another catheter ablation might perforate her heart, causing death. Feeling like an invalid, depressed, and afraid to live, Ms. C was forced to take an extended medical leave from her high-level job at a global technology company. Ms. C describes herself during the period that preceded her illness as follows: "I was the type of person who was trying to be the perfect mother, the perfect wife, the perfect employee. I used to sleep four hours a night because there was so much to do. I thrived on it. I was so used to that adrenaline rush that I didn't know what it was like not to have it".

In the fall of 1995, Ms. C's cardiologist referred her to a seminar where she learned the HeartMath coherence-building techniques to help her manage her stress and improve her health. When Ms. C returned to work after the training, a coworker remarked that, "the difference in her was like night and day". She immediately began practicing the techniques on a regular basis and diligently applied them at work whenever she felt her stress level rising. She notes, "After my weekend at HeartMath, whenever that adrenaline would start to rush again, I could stop the trigger. Now I can pull myself back into balance at will".

The change was impressive to Ms. C's colleagues, who observed that she exhibited far less stress, anxiety and tension, and more calmness and ease, even during a particularly hectic work period. Ms. C's physicians were similarly impressed with the change in her physical health. With daily practice of the

HeartMath tools, within several weeks after the seminar Ms. C was taken off Valium; within six months her beta-blocker (Sotalol) dosage was cut in half, and later further reduced. A 24-hour ECG recording the following fall (1996) found not a single irregular heartbeat. Furthermore, 24-hour heart rate variability analysis showed marked improvements in autonomic nervous system (ANS) function. While Ms. C's heart rate variability was abnormally low for her age before she began practicing the HeartMath techniques, it increased to normal values within two months after she began using the techniques.

Over four years later, there have been no further episodes of ventricular tachycardia and no further need for surgery. Feeling she has regained her health and her life, Ms. C declares, "I feel absolutely incredible". As she made no dietary, exercise, or other lifestyle changes during this time, Ms. C attributes her recovery to the HeartMath interventions.

The relationship between psychological stress and heart disease has been well documented. There is growing evidence that stress, sourcing from a wide array of emotional and psychosocial factors, significantly affects virtually all stages of the disease process-genesis, progression and recovery (reviewed in [1,2]). Furthermore, patients with heart disease frequently suffer considerable emotional distress, such as anger, anxiety, fear and depression, in the process of learning to live with and manage their illness. Increasingly, the medical community recognizes the need for effective stress reduction interventions in order to improve the emotional health of heart disease patients and assist in their physiological rehabilitation, as well as to prevent disease in those at risk. The HeartMath system, which employs heart-based emotion refocusing and restructuring techniques and heart rhythm feedback technology, has proven effective in significantly reducing emotional stress and improving patient outcomes. In some cases, such as Ms. C's above, this intervention has facilitated profoundly transformative changes in patient health and overall quality of life. HeartMath techniques and technology have been shown to promote the maintenance of a highly efficient and regenerative psychophysiological state, characterized by improved sympathovagal balance and increased synchronization and harmony in system-wide functioning. The resulting state, termed *psychophysiological coherence*, is conducive to healing and rehabilitation, emotional stability and optimal performance.

In this chapter, we provide an overview of the Institute of HeartMath's research on the physiological correlates of positive emotions, which led to the characterization of the psychophysiological coherence mode. We describe the positive emotion-focused techniques of the HeartMath system and introduce the Freeze-Framer heart rhythm coherence feedback system. The scientific basis of the effectiveness of the HeartMath interventions is examined from a psychophysiological perspective. This discussion builds on a conceptual framework that emphasizes the emotional component of the experience of stress and further maintains that in order to truly transform stress an intervention at the emotional level is required. To understand how stress is generated and processed in the brain and body, we present a model of emotion based on Karl Pribram's theory, in which the brain functions as a complex pattern-matching system.

This perspective holds that the heart is a key component of the emotional system, with the patterns of its extensive inputs to the brain making an important contribution to emotional experience. Through the use of tools and technologies that foster positive emotions and psychophysiological coherence, individuals can effectively initiate a *repatterning* process, whereby habitual emotional and physiological patterns underlying stress and disease are replaced with new, healthier patterns that establish increased emotional stability, mental acuity and physiological efficiency as a new familiar baseline or norm. The latter part of the chapter discusses applications of the HeartMath coherence-building tools and heart rhythm coherence feedback in the prevention and treatment of cardiac disease.

The Emotional Basis of Stress

The term "stress" has become one of the most widely exercised words in everyday vernacular. People describe themselves as "stressed" when stuck in traffic and also when experiencing the dissolution of a long-term relationship. Preparing for an examination, having difficulty communicating with a coworker, dealing with serious illness, and adjusting to new living or working conditions can all be "stressful". But what is the common thread that unites these diverse experiences, making them worthy of a common descriptor? What defines the essence of the experience of "stress"?

A widely accepted model of stress involves the perception and appraisal of a stimulus as threatening, and the consequent activation of set of physiological reactions characterized as the "stress response". Thus, stress research has traditionally been oriented towards studies examining the cognitive processes that influence the perception of stress (a cognitive perspective) or the body's response to stress (a physiological perspective). Surprisingly, however, comparatively little attention has been given to the role of the emotional system in the stress process. From a psychophysiological perspective, emotions are central to the experience of stress; indeed, it is *emotions* – such as anger, anxiety, irritation, frustration, helplessness or hopelessness – that are truly what we are experiencing when we describe ourselves as "stressed". All of the above examples of "stressors"- whether minor inconveniences or major life changes – are experienced as "stressful" to the extent that they trigger emotions such as these.

While mental processes clearly play a role in stress, it is most often unmanaged emotions that provide fuel for their sustenance. It is well recognized that thoughts carrying an "emotional charge" are those that tend to perpetuate in consciousness. It is also emotions – more than thoughts alone – that activate the physiological changes comprising the "stress response". A purely mental activity, such as cognitively recalling a past situation that provoked anger, does not produce nearly as profound an impact on physiological processes as actually engaging the emotion associated with that memory – actually re-experiencing the *feeling* of anger. It is the emotion that activates the ANS and hypothalamic-pituitary-adrenal axis, leading to changes in the activity and function of the body's systems and organs. Thus, many of the deleterious effects of "stress" on the brain and body are in fact physiological repercussions of negative emotions.

In essence, stress is conceptualized here as *emotional unease* – the experience of which ranges from low-grade feelings of emotional unrest to intense emotional upset. It is further contended that stress arises not only in direct response to external situations or events, but also, to a large extent, involves the ongoing internal emotional processes and attitudes that individuals perpetuate even in the absence of any identifiable extrinsic stimulus. Recurring feelings of agitation, worry, anxiety, anger, judgmentalness and resentment, discontentment and unhappiness, as well as insecurity and self-doubt, often consume a large part of our emotional energy and disrupt our "feeling world," even as we engage in the flow of everyday life, not necessarily confronted with a specific, current "stressor". Indeed, many people do not realize the extent to which these internalized, habitual emotional patterns dominate their internal landscape, diluting and limiting positive emotional experience, and eventually becoming so familiar that "stress" essentially becomes a defining part of their sense of self-identity [3, 4]. Over the long term, such recurring emotional patterns can contribute to the genesis of cardiac disease, intensify symptoms, or impede recovery.

■ Breaking the Stress Cycle: The Power of Positive Emotions

Although most stress has an emotional source, *most of the widely used stress management interventions do not directly focus on emotions*. For example, relaxation has long been seen as the ultimate remedy for stress; many individuals believe that if they could just learn to relax, then they would be healthier and happier. Relaxation is a helpful and beneficial process in that it temporarily draws attention away from distressing feelings and reduces physiological arousal, thereby promoting regeneration of the body. However, relaxation techniques generally do not address the unmanaged emotions that are the root cause of stress – nor do they seek to transform the deeper, recurring emotional patterns that give rise to stress-producing feelings. Without these more fundamental changes at the emotional level, any relief from stress that is experienced is likely to be short-lived.

Other techniques commonly used to manage stress are derived from cognitive-behavioral psychotherapy. The cognitive-behavioral model operates from the theory that maladaptive thoughts drive unhealthy behaviors and that these thoughts should therefore be the focus of therapeutic intervention. Cognitive-behavioral therapy by definition excludes emotions as a primary focus for attention, and although emotions may be explored, they are seen as a consequence of maladaptive thoughts. According to the cognitive model, all emotions follow a cognitive assessment of sensory input, which then leads to a behavioral response. The basic theoretical framework is that if emotions always follow thought, then one can gain control over one's emotions by changing one's thoughts.

In the last decade, however, research in the neurosciences has made it quite clear that emotional processes operate at a much higher speed than thoughts, frequently bypassing the mind's linear reasoning process entirely [5]. Further, although emotions can be induced by thoughts, they may also arise from unconscious associations triggered by external or internal events. In other words, not all emotions follow thoughts: emotions often occur independently of the cognitive system and, moreover, can significantly bias or color the output of cognitive processes [5, 6]. For this reason, a therapeutic focus on thought processes alone often fails to identify the fundamental cause of an emotional disturbance. In some cases, try as one may to rectify one's thinking, one can fall short of achieving emotional relief simply because the underlying maladaptive emotional pattern is driven largely by unconscious triggers that operate independently of the intellect.

Current research in the neurosciences confirms that emotion and cognition can best be thought of as interacting but separate functions and systems, which communicate via bidirectional neural connections between the neocortex and emotional centers such as the amygdala. These connections allow emotion-related input to modulate cortical activity, and cognitive input from the cortex to modulate emotional processing. However, research indicates that the neural connections that transmit information from the emotional centers to the cognitive centers in the brain are stronger and more numerous than those that convey information from the cognitive to the emotional centers [5]. This fundamental asymmetry accounts for the powerful influence of input from the emotional system on cognitive functions such as attention, perception and memory, as well as on higher-order thought processes. Conversely, the comparatively limited influence of input from the cognitive system on emotional processing helps to explain why it is generally so difficult to willfully modulate our emotions through thought alone.

This is why strategies that encourage "positive thinking" – *without also engaging positive feelings* – may frequently provide only temporary, if any, relief from emotional distress. While the individual may make a conceptual shift (which is important), the fundamental source of stress and driver of unhealthy behavior – the underlying maladaptive emotional pattern – remains largely intact. Understanding of how the cognitive and emotional systems interact has significant implications for emotion regulation interventions: it suggests that *intervening at the level of the emotional system itself* is a more direct, efficient and powerful way to override and transform the maladaptive patterns underlying unhealthy psychological, behavioral and physiological stress responses.

Specifically, the *activation of positive emotions* can play a critical role in breaking the stress cycle by effectively transforming stress at its source. The transformative power of positive emotions is far from a new concept, having been noted for centuries by religious scholars, artists, scientists, medical practitioners and lay authors alike. However, it is only recently that positive emotions have begun to be systematically examined in a scientific light (e.g., see [7]). Hardly surprisingly, a growing body of research is now beginning to provide objective evidence of the centrality of positive emotions to optimal functioning in nearly all spheres of human experience. Positive emotions have been linked to improved health and increased longevity [8, 9]. They have also been shown to affect the way we think and address challenges – increasing cognitive flexibility, creativity, receptivity and innovative problem solving, and enhancing psychological resilience in the face of adversity. Positive emotions further shape our behavior, promoting helpfulness, generosity and cooperation. In short, it is suggested that positive emotions are critical to our effective adaptation to life's challenges, and to our growth and development as human beings [3, 10, 11].

Intriguingly, research is now beginning to reveal some of the underlying physiological processes that may help explain *how* positive emotions improve health, enhance cognitive function and promote constructive behavior. As described in detail below, we have found that positive emotions are associated with a specific physiological state characterized by increased system-wide coherence, which in turn is associated with improved physiological functioning, emotional stability and cognitive performance.

The Physiology of Positive Emotions

In the early stages of research at the Institute of HeartMath, we focused on how psychophysiological patterns change during stress and various emotional states, and we sought to determine which physiological variables were most sensitive and responsive to changes in emotion. In analyzing many different physiological measures, we discovered that the rhythmic beating patterns of the heart were consistently the most reflective of changes in emotional states, in that they covaried with emotions in real time.

Specifically, we examined the natural fluctuations in heart rate, known as *heart rate variability* (HRV) or *heart rhythms*, which are a product of the dynamic interplay of many of the body's systems. Short-term (beat-to-beat) changes in heart rate are largely generated by the interaction between the heart and brain via the neural signals flowing through the efferent and afferent pathways of the sympathetic and parasympathetic branches of the ANS. HRV is thus considered a measure of neurocardiac function that reflects heart-brain interactions and ANS dynamics.

Utilizing HRV analysis, we have demonstrated that distinct heart rhythm patterns characterize different emotional states [12-14]. In general, emotional stress – created by emotions such as anger, frustration and anxiety – leads to heart rhythm patterns that appear *incoherent* – erratic, disordered and jagged (Fig. 1). Overall, compared to a neutral baseline state, this indicates less synchronization in the reciprocal action of the parasympathetic and sympathetic branches of the ANS. This desynchronization in the ANS, if sustained, taxes the nervous system and bodily organs, impeding the efficient synchronization and flow of information throughout the psychophysiological systems.

In contrast, sustained positive emotions, such as appreciation, care, compassion and love, generate a smooth, ordered, sine wave-like pattern in the heart's rhythms. Relative to a neutral baseline, this reflects increased synchronization between the two branches of the ANS and a general shift in autonomic balance towards increased parasympathetic activity. As is visually evident (Fig. 1) and also demonstrable by quantitative methods [12-14], heart rhythms associated with positive emotions such as appreciation are clearly more *coherent* than those generated during a negative emotional experience such as frustration.

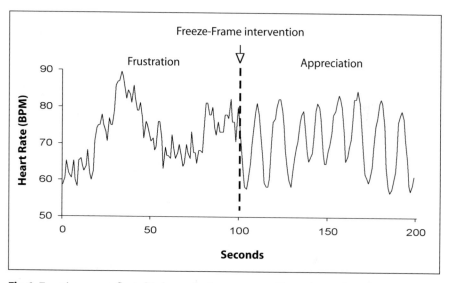

Fig. 1. Emotions are reflected in heart rhythm patterns. The real-time heart rate variability (heart rhythm) pattern is shown for an individual making an intentional shift from a self-induced state of frustration to a genuine feeling of appreciation by using HeartMath's "Freeze-Frame" positive emotion refocusing technique (at the dotted line). It is of note that when the recording is analyzed statistically, the *amount* of heart rate variability is found to remain virtually the same during the two different emotional states; however, the *pattern* of the heart rhythm changes distinctly. Note the immediate shift from an erratic, disordered (incoherent) heart rhythm pattern associated with frustration to a smooth, harmonious, sine wave-like (coherent) pattern as the individual uses the positive emotion refocusing technique and self-generates a heartfelt feeling of appreciation

We observed that these associations held true in studies conducted in both laboratory and natural settings, and for both spontaneous emotions and intentionally generated feelings. It is important to emphasize that – although heart *rate* and the *amount* of HRV can also covary with emotional changes – our findings showed that it is the larger-scale *pattern* of the heart's rhythmic activity that is most directly related to emotional dynamics [14].

Taking this research further, we also observed that when positive emotional states are intentionally maintained, coherent heart rhythm patterns can be sustained for longer periods, which also leads to increased synchronization and entrainment between the heart's rhythm and the activity of multiple bodily systems. To describe the distinctive set of physiological and psychological correlates consistently observed in such states across diverse subject populations, we have introduced the term *psychophysiological coherence* [14].

Psychophysiological Coherence

At the physiological level, the psychophysiological coherence mode is characterized by increased order, efficiency and harmony in the activity and interactions of the body's systems, encompassing phenomena such as autocoherence, entrainment, synchronization and resonance [3, 14]. As described above, this mode is associated with increased coherence in the heart's rhythmic activity (autocoherence), which manifests as a sine wave-like pattern oscillating at a frequency of approximately 0.1 Hz. In this mode, the HRV power spectrum is dominated by a narrow-band, high-amplitude peak near the center of the low frequency range (Fig. 2).

Furthermore, during the psychophysiological coherence mode, there is increased cross-coherence or entrainment among the rhythmic patterns of activity generated by different physiological oscillatory systems. Because the heart is the body's most powerful rhythmic oscillator and generates the strongest rhythmic wave pattern, as the heart's rhythm becomes more coherent it pulls other oscillatory systems into entrainment with it. Typically, entrainment is observed between heart rhythms, respiratory rhythms and blood pressure oscillations; however, other biological oscillators, including very low frequency brain rhythms, craniosacral rhythms, and electrical potentials measured across the skin, can also become entrained [14].

Finally, psychophysiological coherence is characterized by increased synchronization between the activity of the heart and brain. Specifically, we have found that the brain's alpha rhythms exhibit increased synchronization with the cardiac cycle during this mode [3, 14].

In terms of physiological functioning, the coherence mode confers a number of benefits to the system. These include: (i) improved sympathovagal balance and ANS synchronization; (ii) resetting of baroreceptor sensitivity, which is related to improved short-term blood pressure control and increased respiratory efficiency; (iii) increased vagal afferent traffic, which is involved in the inhibition of pain signals and sympathetic outflow; (iv) increased cardiac output, in conjunction with increased efficiency in fluid exchange, filtration and absorption between the capillaries and tissues; (v) increased ability of the cardiovascular system to adapt to circulatory requirements; and (vi) increased temporal synchronization of cells throughout the body. This results in increased system-wide energy efficiency and conservation of metabolic energy [3, 14]. These observations support a link between positive emotions and increased physiological efficiency, which may partially explain the growing number of documented correlations between positive emotions, improved health and increased longevity. We have also shown that practicing techniques that increase psy-

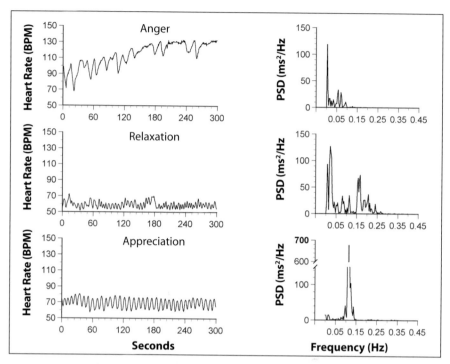

Fig. 2. Heart rhythm patterns during different psychophysiological states. The graphs to the left are heart rate tachograms, which show beat-to-beat changes in heart rate. The graphs to the right show the heart rate variability power spectral density plots of the tachograms at left. Anger is characterized by a lower frequency, disordered heart rhythm pattern and increasing heart rate. As can be seen in the corresponding power spectrum to the right, the rhythm during anger is primarily in the very low frequency band, which is associated with sympathetic nervous system activity. Relaxation produces a higher frequency, lower-amplitude heart rhythm, which indicates reduced autonomic outflow. In this case, increased power in the high frequency band of the power spectrum is observed, reflecting increased parasympathetic activity (the relaxation response). In contrast, sustained positive emotions such as appreciation are associated with a highly ordered, smooth, sine wave-like heart rhythm pattern, indicative of the psychophysiological coherence mode. As can be seen in the corresponding power spectrum, the coherence mode is associated with an unusually high-amplitude peak (note the scale difference) in the low frequency band, centered around 0.1 Hz. This indicates system-wide resonance, increased synchronization between the sympathetic and parasympathetic branches of the nervous system, and entrainment between the heart rhythm pattern, respiration and blood pressure rhythms. The psychophysiological coherence mode is also associated with increased parasympathetic activity, thus encompassing a key element of the relaxation response, yet it is physiologically distinct from relaxation because the system is oscillating at its natural resonant frequency (~0.1 Hz) and there is increased harmony and synchronization in nervous system and heart-brain dynamics. In addition, the coherence mode does not necessarily involve a change in heart rate *per se* or in the *amount* of heart rate variability, rather, it involves a change in heart rhythm *pattern*

chophysiological coherence is associated with both short-term and long-term improvement in several objective health-related measures, including enhanced humoral immunity [15, 16] and an increased DHEA/cortisol ratio [17].

Psychophysiological coherence is similarly associated with beneficial psychological correlates, including reduced perception of stress, sustained positive affect and a high degree of mental clarity and emotional stability. Studies have also shown that the coherence mode is associated with significant improvement in cognitive performance [14].

It is important to note that the psychophysiological coherence mode is both physiologically (as shown in Fig. 2) and psychologically distinct from a state of relaxation. At the physiological level, relaxation is characterized by an overall reduction in ANS outflow and a shift in ANS balance towards increased parasympathetic activity. The coherence mode is also associated with an increase in parasympathetic activity, thus encompassing a key element of the relaxation response, but it is physiologically distinct from relaxation because the system is oscillating at its natural resonant frequency and there is increased harmony and synchronization in nervous system and heart-brain dynamics. Further, unlike relaxation, the coherence mode does not necessarily involve a lowering of heart rate, *per se*, or a change in the *amount* of HRV, but rather a change in heart rhythm *pattern* [14].

Not only are there fundamental differences in the physiological correlates of relaxation and coherence, the associated psychological states are also quite different. Relaxation is generally a dissociative state, conducive to rest or sleep, in which attention is primarily drawn away from cognitive and emotional processes. In contrast, coherence generally involves the active experience of positive emotions. This mode promotes a calm, balanced, yet alert and responsive state, conducive to everyday functioning, including problem-solving, decision-making, and the performance of tasks requiring mental acuity, focus, coordination and discrimination [3, 14].

◼ Positive Emotion-Focused Tools and Techniques

The research described above has informed the development of the HeartMath system, a set of positive emotion-focused techniques that enable people to reliably self-generate and sustain psychophysiological coherence and its associated benefits. Studies conducted across diverse populations in laboratory, organizational, educational and clinical settings have demonstrated that HeartMath coherence-building techniques are effective in producing both immediate and sustained reductions in stress, together with improvements in many dimensions of psychosocial well being. Moreover, these interventions have also resulted in significant improvements in key health and performance-related measures (summarized in [3, 18]). Collectively, results indicate that such techniques are easily learned and used, produce rapid improvements, have a high rate of compliance, and are readily adaptable to a wide range of demographic groups.

HeartMath positive emotion refocusing techniques are designed to enable individuals to intervene *in the moment* that stress is experienced, in order to reduce or prevent the psychophysiological stress response. Briefly, these interventions combine a shift in the focus of attention to the physical area around the heart (where many people subjectively feel positive emotions) with the intentional self-induction of a sincere positive emotional state, such as appreciation. This prevents or interrupts the body's normal stress response and initiates a shift toward increased psychophysiological coherence. As result of this shift, higher cognitive faculties and emotion-regulation abilities, which are normally compromised during stress and negative emotional states, are activated. This quick and simple process enables one to temporarily disengage from the distressing thoughts or emotions and often facilitates a perceptual shift, which allows the original stressor to be assessed and addressed from a broader, more emotionally balanced perspective. By enabling individuals to intercede in the moment that stress is experienced – rather than recuperate "after the fact" – the techniques can help save tremendous amounts of energy that otherwise would be drained, thereby preventing (often hours) of emotionally-induced wear and tear on the body and psyche.

As well as helping people modify their responses to stressful events in the external environment, the HeartMath tools also help individuals identify and modify more subtle internal stressors (i.e., persistent self-defeating and energy-depleting thought patterns and feelings, such as anxiety, fear, hurt, anger, resentment, criticalness, perfectionism, and projections about the future). As individuals practice the techniques when feeling inner emotional unrest, they gain increased awareness of the habitual mental and emotional processes underlying their stress, and they become better at noticing onset of these feelings and patterns, thus diminishing their influence.

In addition to its positive emotion refocusing techniques, which are generally used to address stress in the moment, the Institute of HeartMath has developed several emotional restructuring techniques. These help individuals hold a positive emotional focus and maintain a state of psychophysiological coherence for longer periods (5-15 minutes at time, or longer if desired). The process is typically accompanied by feelings of deep peacefulness and a sense of inner harmony. These emotional restructuring techniques can be an effective means of diffusing accumulated stress and negative feelings and facilitating physical, mental and emotional regeneration. This process also quiets the normal stream of mental dialogue. As a result, many users report the spontaneous emergence of increased intuitive clarity and insight relative to problems or troublesome issues.

Consistent use of coherence-building techniques over longer periods helps people develop the capacity to sustain positive emotions and the benefits of the psychophysiological coherence state. This effectively facilitates a repatterning process, whereby the synchronous, harmonious patterns of psychophysiological activity associated with the coherent state become increasingly familiar to the brain and nervous system. Once this is accomplished, the system attempts to maintain this state automatically, thereby establishing a new, healthier psychophysiological baseline or norm.

◼ The Generation of Emotions: A Pattern-Matching Process

Recent years have seen the emergence of a new understanding of how the brain functions, as well as of the brain-body dynamics involved in emotional processing. Rather than assembling thoughts and feelings from bits of data like a digital computer, the brain is an analog processor that relates whole concepts or *patterns* to one another and looks for similarities, differences and relationships between them. This new way of understanding brain processes has challenged long-held views of how emotions are generated. Psychologists once maintained that emotions were purely mental expressions generated by the brain alone. We now know that emotions have as much to do with the body as they do with the brain. The emergence of an emotional experience results from the ongoing interaction between the brain, the body and the external environment.

Our research findings support a systems model of emotion that includes the heart, brain, and the nervous and hormonal systems as fundamental components of a dynamic, interactive network underlying the emergence of emotional experience [19]. This model is based on the theory of emotion first proposed by Pribram [20], in which the brain functions as a complex pattern-identification and matching system. In this model, past experiences build a set of familiar patterns, which are instantiated in the neural architecture. Inputs to the brain from both the external and internal environments contribute to the maintenance of these patterns via a feedback process. Within the body, the patterns of activity of many processes provide constant rhythmic inputs with which the brain becomes familiar. These include the heart's rhythmic activity; digestive, respiratory, and hormonal rhythms; and muscular tension activation patterns, particularly facial expressions. These inputs are continuously monitored by the brain and help organize sensory perception, cognition, feelings and behavior.

Recurring input patterns from prior experience form a stable backdrop, or *reference pattern*, against which the input patterns from present experience are compared. According to this model, current patterns that match the reference pattern are processed and experienced as "familiar," and therefore do not produce a change in emotional arousal or experience. However, when an input pattern in the present is sufficiently different from the reference pattern, a discontinuity or *"mismatch"* occurs. This mismatch, or *departure from the familiar pattern*, is what generates feelings and emotions.

In order to maintain the stability of an established reference pattern, the neural systems attempt to preserve a match between the reference pattern, current inputs and future behaviors. When the input to the brain does not match the existing reference pattern, an adjustment must be made to achieve control and return the system to stability. One way to reestablish stability is by executing an outward action. We are motivated to eat if we feel hungry, run away or fight if threatened, do something to draw attention to ourselves if feeling ignored, etc. Alternatively, we can gain control and reestablish stability by making an internal adjustment (without any overt action). For example, a confrontation at work may lead to feelings of anger, which can prompt inappropriate behavior (e.g., outward actions such as shouting, fighting, etc.). However, through intentional internal adjustments, we can *self-manage* our feelings in order to inhibit these responses, reestablish stability, and maintain our job. Ultimately, when we achieve stability through our efforts, the results are feelings of satisfaction and gratification. In contrast, when there is a failure to assert control to reestablish psychophysiological stability, feelings such as anxiety, panic, annoyance, apprehension, hopelessness or depression result.

In short, since our psychophysiological systems are designed to maintain stability, returning to the familiar reference pattern gives us a feeling of security, while remaining in unfamiliar territory causes unrest. Importantly, this is true even if the established reference pattern is one of chaos and confusion: *if the reference pattern becomes maladapted, the system will still strive to maintain a match to that pattern, even though it may be dysfunctional.*

In addition to processes that monitor the inputs and controls for maintaining stability (pattern matching) in the here-and-now, there are also matching processes that appraise the degree of congruity or incongruity between the past and the here-and-now and between the here-and-now and the projected future. Inputs to the neural systems are appraised and compared to memories of past outcomes associated with similar inputs or situations. These prospective appraisals can be either optimistic or pessimistic. If the historical outcomes of similar situations are positive (resulting in the ability to maintain control and reestablish stability), an optimistic affect (e.g., interest, confidence or hope) will result.

Conversely, if the appraisal does not result in a projected ability to return to stability, the current inputs are accompanied by pessimistic feelings about the future (e.g., annoyance, apprehension, hopelessness or depression). A pessimistic appraisal can be due to the expectation of failure to achieve stability based on the outcomes of past similar situations, or based on a lack of experience in the projected future situation. However, as we encounter novel situations, experience new inputs, and learn new strategies to reestablish and maintain stability, we expand our repertoire of successful outcomes. The more repertoires available, the more likely a novel input will be appraised optimistically, with a high probability of success in maintaining stability. Once we learn how to handle new challenges effectively and maintain stability, the strategies (complex patterns) for dealing with the challenges also become familiar and part of our repertoire. It is through this process that we mature, increasing our internal self-control and management of emotions, as well as our ability to respond effectively to external situations.

Importantly, this model provides a psychophysiological basis for understanding why chronic stress can be so difficult to change. Through repeated experiences of stress, the brain learns to recognize the patterns of psychophysiological activity associated with "stress" as familiar, and therefore "comfortable". To the extent that these patterns of activity become part of our baseline reference, the system then automatically strives to maintain a match with these habitual psychophysiological patterns through a feedback process, despite their detrimental impact on health, emotional well being and behavior. As a result, without effective intervention, stress tends to become self-perpetuating and reinforcing.

Because the system is in a dynamic relationship with its environment, however, this model also incorporates the means for change and development. Through a *feed-forward* process, like resetting a thermostat, as new input patterns are consistently experienced and thus reinforced in the neural architecture, they become familiar to the system, and the reference pattern is thus modified and fed forward to a new stability. Once the new reference pattern is stabilized, the system strives to maintain a match with inputs that characterize this new baseline.

Usually this process occurs automatically and unconsciously. *However, such a feed-forward, repatterning process can also be intentionally initiated.* This occurs as a pattern-matching operation in which the individual deliberately holds and projects a new emotional or behavioral pattern into the future as a target of achievement, to use Pribram's terms [21]. Holding the new pattern as a target in this way causes the psychophysiological systems to feed forward as new patterns of input are experienced and processed. Essentially, the system makes continual adjustments in its patterns of activity until a match is achieved between the target and the current pattern of system activity. Eventually, if this process is sustained, a new baseline is created in which the new pattern is instantiated in the system as the reference pattern. It is on this principle that the HeartMath technology is based. To further understand the technology, it is necessary to examine the key role of the heart in this model.

More Than a Pump: The Heart's Key Role

Our model of emotion involves the critical function of afferent (ascending) input from the bodily organs to the brain in contributing to the input patterns that ultimately determine emotional experience [19, 20]. Although complex patterns of activity originating from many different bodily organs and systems are involved in this process, it has become clear that the heart plays a particularly important role. The heart is the primary and most consistent source of the body's dynamic rhythmic pattern. The afferent networks connecting the heart and cardiovascular system with the brain are far more extensive than the afferent systems associated with other major organs [22]. Furthermore, it is now established that the heart is a sophisticated information encoding and processing center, with an intrinsic nervous system sufficiently sophisticated to qualify as "little brain" in its own right. Its circuitry enables it to learn, remember and make functional decisions independent of the cranial brain, and its rhythmic input to the brain reflects these processes [23].

The heart also functions as a sensory organ, and is particularly sensitive and responsive to changes in a number of psychophysiological systems. For example, heart rhythm patterns are continually modulated by changes in the activity of either branch of the ANS, and the heart's extensive intrinsic network of sensory neurons also enables it to detect and respond to variations in hormonal rhythms and patterns [23]. Finally, the heart is itself an endocrine gland that manufactures and secretes multiple hormones and neurotransmitters [14].

Thus, with each beat, the heart not only pumps blood, but also continually transmits dynamic patterns of neurological, hormonal, pressure and electro-magnetic information to the brain and throughout the body [14]. An extensive body of research has shown that cardiac afferent input not only exerts homeo-static effects on cardiovascular regulatory centers in the brain, but also influ-ences the activity and function of higher brain centers involved in perceptual, cognitive and emotional processing (reviewed in [14, 19]). The multiple and continuous inputs from the heart and cardiovascular system to the brain, are, therefore, a major contributor in establishing the familiar reference pattern against which the current input of the "here-and-now" is compared. It follows, also, from this model that *changes* in the heart's pattern of activity can have an immediate and profound impact on emotional perception and experience.

Given this connection between heart rhythm patterns and emotion, it is rea-sonable that interventions that enable individuals to *intentionally* change the pattern of the heart's rhythmic activity might modify one's emotional state. In fact, people commonly use just such an intervention when feeling stress – by taking several slow, deep breaths to alter their breathing rhythm. It is not gen-erally realized, however, that an important reason breathing techniques are effec-tive in helping to shift one's emotional state is because *changing one's breathing rhythm modulates the heart's rhythmic activity*. The modulation of the heart's rhythm by respiratory activity is referred to as respiratory sinus arrhythmia.

While it can provide short-term relief from stress, cognitively directed, paced breathing is difficult for most people to maintain for more than about a minute. We have found, however, that characteristic shifts in the heart's rhythmic activ-ity can be generated naturally and more easily sustained through the inten-tional self-induction of positive emotions.

▨ Revisiting the HeartMath Techniques: A Repatterning Process

Now that we understand the psychophysiological processes involved in the gen-eration of emotion, the key role of the heart in the emotional system, and the dis-tinctive physiological changes accompanying positive emotions, we are in a position to more fully understand how the HeartMath techniques work, as well as their larger implications for health and well-being.

The HeartMath tools offer a systematic and reliable means by which one can intentionally feed forward out of a state of emotional unease or stress into a "new" positive state of emotional calm and stability. This occurs as a result of a process in which the individual intentionally creates a new positive emotional state as the system's future target and activates changes in patterns of psychophysiological activity that enable the system to achieve and maintain that new state.

Intervening at the level of the emotional system, HeartMath techniques uti-lize the heart as a point of entry into the psychophysiological networks underly-ing emotional experience. The model of emotion we have just discussed eluci-dates the brain's role as a pattern-identification and matching system, and under-scores the importance of afferent bodily input in establishing the familiar patterns that are critical in determining emotional experience. As a principal and consistent source of rhythmic information patterns that impact the physiological, cognitive and emotional systems, the heart provides an access point from which system-wide dynamics can be quickly and profoundly affected [14, 19].

We have found that the process of coupling an intentional shift in attention to the physical area of the heart with the self-induction of a sincere heartfelt positive emotional *feeling* appears to excite the system at its resonant frequency, thus facilitating the natural emergence of the psychophysiological coherence mode (Fig. 1). This shift to coherence, in turn, results in a change in the pattern of afferent cardiac signals sent to the brain, which is of significance for several reasons. First, at the physiological level, this shift serves to interrupt or prevent the triggering of the body's normal stress response. Second, at the emotional level, the movement to a more organized pattern of cardiac afferent input that accompanies a coherent heart rhythm pattern is one that the brain associates with feelings of security and well-being, resulting in a "pattern match" with positive emotional experience. This shift in the pattern of the heart's input to the brain thus serves to *reinforce* the self-generated positive emotional shift, making it easier to sustain. Through consistent use of the HeartMath tools, the coupling between the psychophysiological coherence mode and positive emotion is further reinforced. This subsequently strengthens the ability of a positive feeling shift to initiate a beneficial physiological shift towards increased coherence, and a physiological shift to facilitate the experience of a positive emotion.

A further outcome of the shift to a state of psychophysiological coherence manifests at the cognitive level, as a result of the change in the pattern of cardiac afferent information reaching the brain's higher cognitive centers. Research has shown that changes in input to the brain from the cardiovascular system can modify the brain's electrophysiological activity and lead to significant changes in perceptual and cognitive processing (reviewed in [14]). Specifically, evidence suggests that the self-induction of positive emotions and the coherence mode can increase mental clarity and facilitate higher cognitive functions [14]. The activation of this state thus often results in a change in perception or attitude about a given stressor, and the ability to address it from a more objective, discerning and resourceful perspective.

The process of activating the psychophysiological coherence mode not only leads to immediate benefits by helping to reduce stress in the moment it is experienced, it can also contribute to long-term improvements in emotion regulation abilities and emotional well-being, which, ultimately, may affect many aspects of one's life. This is because each time an individual intentionally arrests and overrides the psychophysiological and behavioral patterns associated with stress by self-generating a positive emotion and activating a state of psychophysiological coherence, the "new" coherent patterns – and "new" repertoires for responding to challenge – are reinforced in the neural architecture. With consistent practice, the patterns are further reinforced and become increasingly familiar to the brain, eventually becoming established as a new baseline or reference pattern, which the system then strives to maintain.

It is in this way that the HeartMath tools facilitate a repatterning process. The maladaptive patterns that underlie the experience of stress are progressively replaced by healthier physiological, emotional, cognitive and behavioral patterns as the "automatic" or familiar way of being. Our research supports the efficacy of this process in establishing emotional stability, mental acuity and physiological efficiency as a new familiar baseline, and thereby diminishing the future likelihood of experiencing prolonged stress. Even when stress or emotional instability is subsequently experienced, the familiar, coherent state is readily accessible, enabling a quicker and more enduring emotional shift.

The occurrence of such a repatterning process is supported by both physiological and psychological data. At the electrophysiological level, ambulatory recordings demonstrate a greater frequency of *spontaneous* (without conscious practice of the tools) periods of coherence in the heart rhythm patterns of individuals practiced in the HeartMath techniques, compared with the general population. There are also data linking the practice of HeartMath tools to favorable changes in hormonal patterns. Specifically, a significant increase in the DHEA/cortisol ratio was demonstrated in individuals who consistently used the HeartMath tools for 30 days. This finding, which has recently been independently replicated, provides evidence that a repatterning process occurs at a fundamental level, given that there is normally little physiological variability in the levels of these hormones from month to month [17].

The physiological changes observed with the use of the interventions typically occur in conjunction with significant changes in psychological patterns. Reductions in measures of emotional distress, including anxiety, depression, anger, hostility, guilt, and burnout, have been consistently observed in many different populations with practice of the HeartMath tools (summarized in [3, 18]. These observations suggest that the interventions are effective in helping to modify the habitual emotional patterns that are a major source of stress.

Heart Rhythm Coherence Feedback Training: Facilitating Coherence

The learning and effective use of HeartMath positive emotion-focused tools can be significantly facilitated by heart rhythm coherence feedback training. This technology provides real-time physiological feedback and objective validation in the process of learning to self-generate increased psychophysiological coherence [24].

An HRV feedback and coherence-building system known as the FreezeFramer® (Quantum Intech, Boulder Creek, California) incorporates a patented technology that enables heart rhythm coherence, the key physiological marker of the psychophysiological coherence mode, to be objectively monitored and quantified. Using a noninvasive fingertip or earlobe plethysmographic sensor to record the pulse wave, this interactive hardware/software system plots changes in heart rate on a beat-to-beat basis. The software also includes a tutorial that provides instruction in the HeartMath coherence-building techniques. As users practice the techniques, they can readily see and experience the changes in their heart rhythm patterns – which generally become more ordered, smoother, and more like a sine wave – as they experience positive emotions. This process enables individuals to easily develop an association between a shift to a more healthful and beneficial mode of physiological functioning and the positive emotional feeling experience that induces such a shift. The software also analyzes the heart rhythm patterns for their coherence level, and this is fed back to the user either as an accumulated score or as "success" in playing one of three interactive games designed to reinforce the emotion refocusing skills. Finally, the system includes a multi-user database to store results and track client progress. This heart rhythm coherence feedback technology is available on two platforms: a personal computer-based version and a newly developed handheld version.[1]

Because this technology uses a pulse wave sensor and involves no electrode hook-up, it is extremely versatile, time-efficient and easy to use in clinical settings, as well as at home, in the workplace, in schools, etc. Heart rhythm coherence feedback training and positive emotion-focused coherence-building techniques have been successfully used in diverse contexts by mental health professionals, physicians, law enforcement personnel, educators, athletes and corporate executives. Applications include stress and anger management; decreasing anxiety, depression, and fatigue; promoting improved academic, work, and sports performance; reducing physical and psychological health risk factors; and facilitating improvements in health and quality of life in patients with numerous clinical disorders [3, 18, 24].

■ Clinical Applications

Because coherence-building interventions reduce stress-induced autonomic and hormonal activation, improve sympathovagal and neuroendocrine balance, and promote increased efficiency and synchronization in the functioning of physiological systems, these tools can be a powerful aid in facilitating healing and rehabilitation. Health professionals have found the HeartMath techniques and the Freeze-Framer heart rhythm coherence feedback technology to be an effective addition to treatment programs for patients with a wide variety of conditions that are associated with or exacerbated by emotional stress.

---

[1] For additional information on the Freeze-Framer® technology, see: *www.heartmath.com/freezeframer*. Newly updated versions of this technology, in both personal computer-based and handheld formats, will be released in 2006 under the name emWave™. For additional information on this technology, see: *www.emwave.com*

Hypertension

HeartMath techniques and heart rhythm coherence feedback have been shown to be effective in reducing blood pressure in individuals with hypertension. In a recent workplace study, hypertensive employees were trained in the Heart-Math techniques and provided with the Freeze-Framer system for use in the workplace as well as at home. Trained employees demonstrated a mean adjusted reduction of 10.6 mm Hg in systolic blood pressure and 6.3 mm Hg in diastolic blood pressure three months after the completion of the training program. These changes were evident over and above the effects of antihypertensive medication. Several of the participants were also able to reduce their medication usage, with their physician's approval, during the study period, and one was permitted to discontinue medication usage entirely following completion of the study. Concurrent with these changes, study participants also exhibited significant improvements in emotional health, including reductions in stress symptoms, depression, and global psychological distress, and increases in peacefulness and positive outlook [25].

Congestive Heart Failure

A study conducted at Stanford University tested the efficacy of the HeartMath techniques in a population of elderly patients with congestive heart failure. The intervention emphasized guided and regular home practice of two core Heart-Math techniques over a 10-week period. Post-intervention, the treatment group exhibited significant reductions in perceived stress, depression, and emotional status relative to an untrained control group. Positive trends were noted for measures of anxiety, optimism, perceived physical fitness and health-related quality of life. Finally, on a measure of functional capacity, the six-minute walk, a significant improvement was observed. Treatment group members walked, on average, 175 feet further at post-test than at pre-test, indicating significantly increased functional capacity, while the control group showed a slight decline over this period. Compliance was excellent, and in post-test interviews patients expressed singular appreciation for the program, reporting the experience to be both enjoyable and valuable [26].

Cardiac Arrhythmia

HeartMath interventions have been used with great success by patients with cardiac arrhythmias. Patients often report being able to stop or attenuate arrhythmic episodes by using a HeartMath technique in the moment that symptoms are experienced. Furthermore, many patients experience significant long-term improvements in symptomatology, medication requirements and overall quality of life. The case of Ms. C, with which we opened this chapter, provides a noteworthy example of the types of changes patients see after learning and practicing the techniques. In this case, a patient with ventricular tachycardia was able to effect a dramatic improvement in her symptoms and general well being.

The HeartMath techniques have also proven particularly effective in helping individuals with atrial fibrillation – in some cases leading to profound and lasting improvements in symptoms even after a range of invasive procedures and aggressive pharmacological interventions failed. The Pacemaker Clinic for Kaiser Hospitals in Orange County, California, conducted an internal study on the use of HeartMath interventions in patients suffering from atrial fibrillation. Seventy-five patients were randomly selected to receive a home-study program as an educational aid for learning and practicing the HeartMath tools. (This program included the book *Freeze-Frame*, the facilitative music *Heart Zones*, and a workbook that provides step-by-step instruction and practice guidelines for the Freeze-Frame and Heart Lock-In techniques.) The patients were asked to work with the program for three months, during which time they also received coaching in the use of the techniques by the Pacemaker Clinic Coordinator. At the end of the three-month period, the patients were individually interviewed to assess what benefits they had derived from their practice. Seventy-one of the 75 patients reported substantial improvements in their physical and emotional health. Fifty-six patients were able to better control their paroxysmal atrial fibrillation and hypertension to the extent that they were able to reduce their antiarrhythmic and antihypertensive medications, with their physician's approval. Fourteen were able to discontinue their antiarrhythmic medications altogether.

In examining the cost benefits, a number of the patients were taking Amiodarone, Sotolol, or mixes of both, to help control their atrial fibrillation. They were also taking beta-blockers and nitrates for their hypertension. The coordinator of the Pacemaker Clinic reported that the reduction in pharmacy costs to the health maintenance organization (HMO) as a result of the improvements in patients' health were in the thousands of dollars per month. She concluded: "The overall benefits to the patients were significant, life-changing and priceless".

Cardiac Risk Reduction

Another promising application of HeartMath coherence-building techniques and heart rhythm coherence feedback technology is in patient populations who are at risk of developing heart disease. Individuals suffering from autonomic exhaustion ensuing from maladaptation to high stress levels typically manifest abnormally low HRV. Chronically, low HRV connotes reduced flexibility of the cardiovascular system, and has been found to be predictive of increased risk of heart disease and premature mortality [27-29]. The HeartMath interventions have proven highly effective in facilitating the recovery of individuals suffering from stress-induced autonomic exhaustion. Notably, increases in HRV, from low to normal values, have been measured in as little as six weeks' time in individuals who regularly practiced the techniques.

A recent organizational study investigated the efficacy of a HeartMath intervention program in reducing physiological and psychological health risks in correctional peace officers. An analysis of baseline data revealed that officers in this study were under greater stress and at greater health risk, compared with a reference sample of working adults. A within-group analysis of pre-post changes showed that three months after the intervention program, HeartMath-trained employees demonstrated significant reductions in stress and health risk factors. Physiological changes in the experimental group included significant reductions in total cholesterol, LDL cholesterol levels, the total cholesterol/HDL ratio, fasting glucose levels, mean heart rate, and systolic and diastolic blood pressure. Psychological changes included significant reductions in overall psychological distress, anger, fatigue, hostility, interpersonal sensitivity, speed and impatience, and global Type A behavior, and increases in gratitude and positive outlook. There were also improvements in key organizationally relevant measures in the experimental group after the program, including increased productivity, motivation, goal clarity and perceived manager support. Projections for cost savings (in healthcare and absentee costs) were approximately $700 per employee [30].

Conclusions and Implications

Heart-based techniques that enable the self-activation of positive emotions show promise as a simple and powerful means of modifying engrained emotional patterns that contribute to the experience of stress and its debilitating effects on health and well being. We have shown that the use of such techniques creates psychophysiological coherence, a highly efficient and regenerative functional mode that appears to have wide-ranging benefits. By virtue of the brain's pattern-matching function, the intentional generation of positive emotions and psychophysiological coherence enables individuals to activate a feed-forward process whereby stress-producing psychophysiological and behavioral patterns engrained through past experience are progressively replaced by new, healthier patterns of activity. Thus, through the establishment of a new reference pattern, individuals effectively create an *internal environment* that is conducive to the maintenance of physiological efficiency, mental clarity and emotional stability – one that is both resilient and adaptive to life's inevitable challenges. The occurrence of such a "repatterning" process is consistent with the experience of many practitioners of positive emotion-focused techniques, who have reported that the use of these tools has led to lasting positive changes in their health, emotions and attitudes, social relationships, and sense of personal empowerment and fulfillment.

The use of positive emotion-based interventions and heart rhythm coherence feedback has been shown to be an effective addition to treatment programs for individuals with heart disease and cardiovascular disorders. By providing patients with tools for reducing stress and its deleterious repercussions, the interventions not only reduce symptomatology, they also promote physical rehabilitation and significantly enhance emotional well being, as well as overall quality of life. Another promising application for these tools is cardiac disease prevention and health risk reduction. Data indicate that they can facilitate significant reductions in major cardiac risk factors over a relatively brief period of time. In sum, positive emotion-focused, coherence-building tools and technologies provide a practical, versatile and cost-effective intervention that has broad-based applications in disease prevention, rehabilitation and the enhancement of long-term health and well being.

Acknowledgments

HeartMath, Freeze-Frame, and Heart Lock-In are registered trademarks of the Institute of HeartMath. Freeze-Framer is a registered trademark and emWave is a trademark of Quantum Intech, Inc.

■ References

1. Rozanski A, Blumenthal JA, Davidson KW et al (2005) The epidemiology, pathophysiology, and management of psychosocial risk factors in cardiac practice: the emerging field of behavioral cardiology. J Am Coll Cardiol 45:637-651
2. Rozanski A, Blumenthal JA, Kaplan J (1999) Impact of psychological factors on the pathogenesis of cardiovascular disease and implications for therapy. Circulation 99:2192-2217
3. McCraty R, Childre D (2004) The grateful heart: the psychophysiology of appreciation. In: Emmons RA, McCullough ME (Eds) The psychology of gratitude. Oxford University Press, New York, pp 230-255
4. Childre D, Rozman D (2005) Transforming stress: the HeartMath solution to relieving worry, fatigue, and tension. New Harbinger Publications, Oakland, CA
5. LeDoux J (1996) The emotional brain: the mysterious underpinnings of emotional life. Simon and Schuster, New York
6. Niedenthal P, Kitayama S (1994) The heart's eye: emotional influences in perception and attention. Academic Press, San Diego
7. Snyder CR, Lopez SJ (2002) Handbook of positive psychology. Oxford University Press, New York
8. Ostir GV, Markides KS, Black SA, Goodwin JS (2000) Emotional well-being predicts subsequent functional independence and survival. J Am Geriatr Soc 48:473-478
9. Danner DD, Snowdon DA, Friesen WV (2001) Positive emotions in early life and longevity: findings from the nun study. J Pers Soc Psychol 80:804-813
10. Isen AM (1999) Positive affect. In: Dalgleish T, Power M (Eds) Handbook of cognition and emotion. John Wiley & Sons, New York, pp 522-539
11. Fredrickson BL (2001) The role of positive emotions in positive psychology: the broaden-and-build theory of positive emotions. Am Psychol 56:218-226
12. McCraty R, Atkinson M, Tiller WA et al (1995) The effects of emotions on short-term power spectrum analysis of heart rate variability. Am J Cardiol 76:1089-1093
13. Tiller WA, McCraty R, Atkinson M (1996) Cardiac coherence: a new, noninvasive measure of autonomic nervous system order. Altern Ther Health Med 2:52-65
14. McCraty R, Atkinson M, Tomasino D, Bradley RT (2006) The coherent heart: heart-brain interactions, psychophysiological coherence, and the emergence of system-

wide order. HeartMath Research Center, Institute of HeartMath, Boulder Creek, CA, Publication No. 06-022

15. Rein G, Atkinson M, McCraty R (1995) The physiological and psychological effects of compassion and anger. J Advancement Med 8:87-105

16. McCraty R, Atkinson M, Rein G, Watkins AD (1996) Music enhances the effect of positive emotional states on salivary IgA. Stress Med 12:167-175

17. McCraty R, Barrios-Choplin B, Rozman D et al (1998) The impact of a new emotional self-management program on stress, emotions, heart rate variability, DHEA and cortisol. Integr Physiol Behav Sci 33:151-170

18. McCraty R, Atkinson M, Tomasino D (2001) Science of the heart: exploring the role of the heart in human performance. HeartMath Research Center, Institute of Heart-Math, Boulder Creek, CA, Publication No. 01-001

19. McCraty R (2003) Heart–brain neurodynamics: the making of emotions. HeartMath Research Center, Institute of HeartMath, Boulder Creek, CA, Publication No. 03-015

20. Pribram KH, Melges FT (1969) Psychophysiological basis of emotion. In: Vinken PJ, Bruyn GW (Eds) Handbook of clinical neurology. North-Holland Publishing Company, Amsterdam, pp 316-341

21. Pribram KH (1991) Brain and perception: holonomy and structure in figural processing. Lawrence Erlbaum Associates, Hillsdale, NJ

22. Cameron OG (2002) Visceral sensory neuroscience: interoception. Oxford University Press, New York

23. Armour JA, Kember GC (2004) Cardiac sensory neurons. In: Armour JA, Ardell JL (Eds) Basic and clinical neurocardiology. Oxford University Press, New York, pp 79-117

24. McCraty R, Tomasino D (2004) Heart rhythm coherence feedback: a new tool for stress reduction, rehabilitation, and performance enhancement. In: proceedings of the first baltic forum on neuronal regulation and biofeedback, Riga, Latvia (Also available at *http://wwwheartmathorg/research/research-papers/HRV_Biofeedback2pdf*)

25. McCraty R, Atkinson M, Tomasino D (2003) Impact of a workplace stress reduction program on blood pressure and emotional health in hypertensive employees. J Altern Complement Med 9:355-369

26. Luskin F, Reitz M, Newell K et al (2002) A controlled pilot study of stress management training of elderly patients with congestive heart failure. Prev Cardiol 5:168-172

27. Tsuji H, Larson MG, Venditti FJ et al (1996) Impact of reduced heart rate variability on risk for cardiac events. The Framingham Heart Study. Circulation 94:2850-2855

28. Tsuji H, Venditti FJ Jr., Manders ES et al (1994) Reduced heart rate variability and mortality risk in an elderly cohort. The Framingham Heart Study. Circulation 90:878-883

29. Dekker JM, Schouten EG, Klootwijk P et al (1997) Heart rate variability from short electrocardiographic recordings predicts mortality from all causes in middle-aged and elderly men. The Zutphen Study. Am J Epidemiol 145:899-908

30. McCraty R, Atkinson M, Lipsenthal L, Arguelles L (2003) Impact of the power to change performance program on stress and health risks in correctional officers. Boulder Creek, CA: HeartMath Research Center, Institute of HeartMath, Report No. 03-014, November

Subject Index

Activities of daily living 102, 251, 472
Activity 12, 26-29, 39, 51-54, 72, 73, 75, 89,
    90, 93, 99, 111, 122, 135, 136, 172, 175,
    195, 200, 217, 221, 225, 228, 281, 282, 286,
    289, 312, 319, 324, 341, 370, 393, 394, 415,
    421, 436-439, 444, 473, 475-479, 481-483,
    489-491, 493-502, 507
Acute myocardial infarction 1, 55, 100,
    122-125, 128, 131, 133, 274, 393, 414
Adherence 2, 6, 10, 12, 13, 86, 90, 93, 111,
    122, 173, 174, 180, 382, 425, 452, 456,
    458, 468
Affiliation 235-237, 245-247, 249
Anger 25, 36, 54, 73-76, 80, 113, 136,
    166-168, 174, 175, 177, 179, 187, 189-195,
    198, 200-210, 217-219, 222, 227, 249, 288,
    341, 342, 354, 365, 372, 375, 384, 400, 401,
    414, 421-423, 426, 427, 439, 446, 458,
    488-490, 492, 495, 497, 498, 503, 504, 507
Angina pectoris 71, 85, 154, 196, 274,
    440, 480
Angiography 25, 138, 218
Antidepressant 29, 94, 105, 159, 370, 373,
    375, 378, 385
Anxiety 1-3, 9, 14, 26, 29, 30, 51, 55, 87, 90,
    110, 112, 115, 121-140, 149, 150, 152, 154,
    156, 158, 168, 179, 203, 204, 207, 208, 219,
    221, 227, 282, 287, 288, 291-293, 296,
    311-313, 320, 363, 393, 395-397, 424, 435,
    438, 439, 442, 443, 446, 458-460, etc.
Approach-avoidance conflict 217, 224, 227
Artificial neural network 282, 310

Autogenic training 422, 438, 439, 441
Autonomic nervous system 56, 89, 93, 135,
    136, 157, 225, 227, 436, 488

Baroreflex 56, 135, 437, 441
Biofeedback 176, 441-443
Biopsychosocial model 6, 15, 21, 168, 177,
    311, 370, 475, 478
Blood pressure 1, 2, 7, 22, 24, 25, 28, 29,
    35-61, 72, 89, 103, 128, 135-137, 139,
    165-180, 189, 198-200, 209, 217-219,
    221, 223, 225, 226, 244, 245, 247, 249,
    254, 287-289, 313, 378, 392, 395, 419,
    436-438, 441, 458, 494, 495, 505, 507

Cardiac
    arrhythmia 487, 505
    risk reduction 506
Cardiological rehabilitation 478, 480
Cardiovascular
    diseases 35, 52, 99, 219
    reactivity 35-37, 39-42, 51, 56, 58-61,
        135, 167, 173-176, 180, 184, 198, 221,
        224-226, 244, 395
Central nervous complication 158
CHD 21-30, 85-91, 93, 94, 121, 122, 130-132,
    134, 135, 138, 157, 187-190, 196-199,
    203-206, 209, 210, 217-221, 223-225, 244,
    275, 281, 391-398, 400, 402, 413-415, 418,
    420, 421, 429, 435, 438, 439, 442, 445, 446,
    452, 454, 458
Chronic heart failure 99, 155, 451

Clinical
  interview 11, 12, 112, 458
  psychology 5-7, 11, 13, 15, 349
Cognitive
  behavioural therapy 13, 14, 115
  restructuring 420, 422-425, 446
Coherence 328, 487-489, 492, 494-497,
    502-507
Coherence-building techniques 487, 496,
    497, 504, 506
Compliance 9, 10, 12, 113, 158, 184, 312,
    369, 381, 395, 451, 454, 456, 462, 479,
    496, 505
Congestive heart failure 26, 105, 106, 369,
    451, 505
Cook-Medley hostility scale 202
Coronary
  artery disease 12, 29, 35, 36, 51, 53-55, 58,
    60, 61, 71, 85, 99, 105, 109-112, 114,
    136, 137, 154, 157, 166, 174, 188, 218,
    282, 369, 374, 382, 383, 385, 436
  disease 52, 93, 111, 113, 197, 202, 273,
    274, 276
  flow reserve 77, 138
  heart disease 1-3, 21, 60, 85, 91, 102, 115,
    121, 131, 155, 157, 188, 190, 217, 220,
    244, 281, 369, 374-376, 386, 391-393,
    395, 413, 414, 438
Couple therapy 395, 397, 399, 402, 408

Data mining 281, 305
Defensive hostility 168, 217, 220, 221
Depression 1-3, 8, 9, 14, 22, 25, 26, 29, 30,
    51, 55, 57, 72, 85-94, 99-106, 109-116,
    122, 130, 138, 151, 153-157, 168, 171,
    174, 179, 204, 206-208, 247, 276, 282,
    287, 288, 291-293, 297, 311, 313, 320,
    322, 341, 354, 369-386, 392, 393, 395,
    402, 438, 440, etc.
  major 86-88, 90, 100, 101, 104, 105, 110,
    112, 114, 115, 154, 369, 370, 373, 375,
    376, 379, 383-386, 460
  treatment 91
Depressive symptoms 2, 57, 87-91, 100-103,
    105, 106, 110, 111, 113, 114, 149-151, 153,
    154, 157, 159, 226, 250, 251, 274, 276, 291,
    369-373, 375, 383, 392, 473
Diabetes 2, 22, 57, 58, 100, 102, 125, 134, 189,
    220, 226, 274, 275, 379, 414, 451

Disability 6, 9, 121, 122, 225, 319, 323,
    324, 329, 331, 334, 369, 451, 417-476,
    479-481, 484
Discrimination 254, 496
Disease management 13, 451, 453-455
Dominance 235-238, 242-245, 437

E-health 453
Emotional restructuring techniques 497
Emotionally focused therapy 391, 398, 408
Endothelial function 57, 78
ENRICHD 91-94, 105, 115, 116
Environmental factors 1, 223, 234, 474, 476,
    478, 479, 483, 484
Evaluation 9, 11, 30, 112, 116, 149, 151, 154,
    158, 172, 192, 193, 195, 197, 199, 200, 202,
    204, 208, 290, 308, 322, 365, 375, 376, 381,
    383, 423, 473
Evolutionary algorithm 294, 309
Exhaustion 8, 22, 25, 30, 89, 110-116, 153,
    168, 206, 207, 226, 421, 506

Family context 10, 349
FIM 331, 333, 334
Freeze-framer 488, 504, 505, 508
Functioning 7, 9, 11, 14, 56, 88, 155, 187,
    188, 220, 226-228, 243, 244, 250, 283, 289,
    307, 319, 371, 373-375, 377, 379, 392, 395,
    396, 400, 435, 436, 438, 441, 442, 446,
    471-476, 478-480, 482-484, 488, 492, 494,
    496, 504

Gender differences 128, 129, 236, 273, 313
Guidelines 10-13, 166, 173, 178, 286, 290,
    370, 376, 439, 445, 478, 506

Health behaviours 408
Heart
  disease 1-3, 21-23, 29, 30, 35, 60, 72, 80,
    85, 91, 100, 102, 105, 115, 121, 131, 136-
    138, 155, 157, 188-190, 198, 206, 209,
    210, 217-220, 226, 227, 244, 274, 281-
    283, 286, 291, 369, 374-376, 386, 391-
    393, 395, 413, 414, 436, 438, 471-475,
    480, 488, etc.
  failure 26, 99-106, 110, 139, 149, 154, 155,
    159, 325, 369, 436, 451, 505
  rate 24-26, 28, 29, 35-45, 47-49, 51-56, 60,
    72, 89, 135-137, 139, 174, 199, 200, 221,

222, 244, 281, 287-292, 296, 308, 313,
370, 419, 436-438, 440-442, 458, 488,
492, 493, 495, 496, 503, 507
  recovery 281, 287, 290-292, 296, 308
  variability (*see also* HRV, heart
    rhythm) 24, 26, 28, 29, 55, 89, 135,
    136, 370, 436, 440, 488, 492, 493, 495
  rhythm (*see also* heart rate variability,
    HRV) 89, 492, 493, 495, 496, 500-504
    coherence feedback 487-489, 503-507
    transplantation 26, 149, 152, 154-157
Heart-based techniques 507
HeartMath 487-489, 492, 493, 496, 497,
  500-508
High blood pressure 1, 7, 22, 25, 166, 167,
  171, 189, 209, 217, 218, 226
Hostility 8, 14, 25, 29, 30, 55, 73, 74, 113,
  167, 168, 171, 172, 174, 175, 179, 190-195,
  198-205, 209, 210, 217-223, 226, 227, 235,
  244, 246, 248, 249, 251, 254, 288, 312,
  375, 413-417, 421-424, 426, 438, 439, 446,
  503, 507
HRV (*see also* heart rate variability, heart
  rhythm) 55, 56, 89, 90, 436, 437, 492-494,
  496, 503, 506
Hypertension 7, 22, 35, 36, 41, 51-54, 56-61,
  86, 89, 99-101, 103, 109, 113, 125, 165-181,
  184, 189, 197, 202, 217, 220, 223, 225-227,
  247, 255, 282, 283, 286, 374, 376, 383, 395,
  414, 436, 437, 440, 441, 505, 506
Hypnosis 422, 435-437, 440, 444-446

ICF, International Classification
  of Functioning, Disability and Health
  471-481, 483, 484
Illness behavior 9
Inflammation 2, 30, 57, 86, 88, 111, 113,
  136, 157, 226, 227
In-hospital complications 123, 132
Interpersonal
  circumplex 235
  conflict 7, 217, 220, 243, 244, 375
  psychotherapy 369-371, 374
Ischemic heart disease 23, 60, 72, 80, 100,
  105, 282, 283, 286, 291, 413, 414, 471

Left ventricular function 91
Listening 10, 248, 251, 343, 344, 349-355, 359,
  360, 363, 365, 366, 428, 437

Longitudinal 38, 51, 60, 102, 168, 171, 175,
  179, 180, 223, 224, 241, 249, 250, 252, 295,
  369, 440

Marital satisfaction 10
Marlowe-Crowne social desirability
  scale 219
Measure 49, 55, 60, 74, 89, 91, 123, 167, 170,
  171, 174, 193, 195, 202, 207, 219, 221, 282,
  288, 289, 291, 320, 321, 323, 324, 326, 328,
  330, 331, 333, 364, 420, 436, 437, 477, 479,
  492, 505
Mechanisms 8, 14, 15, 21, 23-25, 28, 35, 36,
  39, 45, 51, 53, 55, 72, 75, 76, 78-80, 85, 88,
  89, 93, 94, 102-104, 109, 116, 134, 135,
  139, 140, 157, 165, 167-169, 172, 179-181,
  184, 198, 205, 208, 225, 227, 239, 241, 243,
  245, 253, 282, 284, 313, 324, 369, 371, etc.
Mental stress 25-27, 38, 53-57, 72, 76-80,
  113, 135-139, 167, 169, 175, 223
  ischemia 71-73, 76, 78, 80
Metabolic equivalent 287, 292, 296
Mobile care 451
Multidisciplinary approach 472, 478
Myocardial
  blood flow 73, 76, 77, 80
  infarction 1, 23, 45, 55, 60, 78, 85, 91, 100,
    103, 105, 110, 114, 115, 122-125, 128,
    131, 133, 157, 197, 207, 250, 274, 324,
    369, 391, 393, 395, 414, 419, 440, 451, 473

Narrative 165, 171, 176, 355-358, 365
Noncompliance 25, 157, 452
Non-linear
  clustering 301
  mapping 293
Non-linearity 283-285, 293, 301

Ortho-sympathetic 436-438, 442
Outcome(s) 12, 15, 51, 56, 79, 80, 86, 92, 94,
  100, 101, 104, 105, 109, 110, 113, 114, 116,
  130-132, 134, 139, 155, 157, 168, 171-176,
  178-180, 188, 192, 208, 210, 243, 250, 254,
  282, 283, 289-291, 296, 298, 299, 305-308,
  310, 311, 313, 319-321, 323, 324, 329, etc.

Parasympathetic 55, 89, 109, 135, 157,
  198-200, 436-438, 440, 442, 492, 493,
  495, 496

Pathophysiology 71, 72, 76, 78, 79, 88, 134, 217, 225
Personality 1, 8, 104, 113, 150, 168, 187-192, 201, 202, 206-210, 217, 234, 238-242, 250, 251, 282, 287, 288, 292, 293, 296, 298, 305, 311-313, 357, 361, 371, 372, 385, 443, 446, 458, 472
Person-metric 320-325
Positive emotion refocusing technique(s) 493, 497
Positive emotion-focused techniques 488, 496, 507
Positive emotions 206, 488-497, 501, 502, 504, 507
Post-traumatic stress disorder 26
Predictor variable 22
Prevalence 27, 29, 57, 85-87, 90, 93, 99-102, 105, 106, 109, 110, 121-123, 152, 154, 158, 166, 174, 322, 471, 473
Prognosis 1, 11, 12, 25, 28, 30, 71, 78, 79, 85-88, 90-93, 130, 138, 188, 207, 208, 250, 276, 341, 374, 451, 452, 468
Psycho-cardiology 6-8, 10, 11, 13, 14, 311, 313, 339, 478
Psychological
    distress 9, 26, 111, 150, 154, 166, 206, 391, 393, 394, 396, 435, 480, 505, 507
    factors 9, 15, 25, 29, 36, 73, 134, 136, 155, 165, 167, 168, 170, 171, 173, 174, 176, 178-181, 184, 192, 218, 234, 282, 340, 342
    pain 349, 350, 356, 364, 365
    risk profile 282
    stress 9, 26, 36, 55, 56, 58, 59, 137, 150, 173, 174, 188, 273, 343, 488
    well-being 11, 443, 460, 468
Psycho-metric 321
Psychophysiological coherence 488, 489, 494-497, 502, 503, 507
Psychosocial 1-3, 11, 21, 22, 25, 27, 30, 35, 58, 60, 73, 92, 113, 116, 122, 123, 149, 150, 152, 155, 157, 158, 165, 175, 176, 179, 180, 187, 196, 206, 210, 217, 218, 220, 221, 223, 228, 234, 235, 238, 240, 249, 252, 253, 256, 274, 282, 311, 369, 373, 378, 394, 397, etc.
    predictors 155
    risk factors 3, 22, 30, 51, 116, 234, 242, 250, 311

stress 1, 3, 51, 54, 61, 167, 174, 175, 436, 472, 473, 483
support 3, 153, 154, 158, 454
vulnerability 73
Psychotherapy 10, 91, 92, 369, 370, 372, 374, 378, 386, 397, 440, 446, 460, 478, 483, 490

Quality of life 11, 13, 14, 29, 92, 102, 104, 106, 110, 122, 127, 149, 152, 153, 159, 166, 173, 178, 179, 250, 393, 443, 454, 458-460, 472, 473, 479, 488, 504, 505, 507

Rasch
    analysis 319, 328, 331
    model 325-330
Rational-emotive behavior therapy 424
Rehabilitation 3, 7, 10-13, 87, 92, 114, 122, 151, 173, 281, 282, 286, 291, 305, 307, 308, 310, 311, 313, 319, 320, 323-325, 333, 353, 376, 379, 381, 385, 386, 395, 397, 435, 438, 439, 441-444, 458, 472, 473, 478-480, 487, 488, 504, 507, 508
Relaxation 2, 13, 92, 115, 158, 176, 180, 421, 422, 435-446, 490, 495, 496
    response 436, 438, 440, 444-446, 495, 496
Repatterning 489, 497, 500, 501, 503, 507
Reproducibility 39, 40, 72, 76, 326
Review 25, 26, 35, 71, 80, 85, 100, 104, 116, 126, 127, 136-138, 150, 165, 168, 169, 218, 224, 225, 234, 237, 246, 252, 376, 377, 379, 381-386, 399, 414, 415, 420, 437
Risk factor 2, 21, 22, 25, 26, 55, 60, 100, 113, 115, 158, 170, 174, 175, 180, 189, 196, 197, 201-203, 206, 208, 218, 234, 244, 245, 256, 274, 282, 284, 311, 374, 392, 395, 413-415, 480

Screening 3, 22, 103-105, 112, 116, 459, 460
Self 7, 8, 11, 13, 14, 51, 87, 88, 91, 100, 104, 105, 110, 112, 122, 131, 132, 159, 167, 170, 175, 188, 192, 193, 195, 196, 202, 204, 219, 220, 222, 226-228, 235, 237, 239, 248, 274, 307, 309, 312, 320, 326, 331, 344, 351, 352, 355, 358, 361, 371, 376, 382, 385, 386, etc.
Self-efficacy 6, 12, 14, 158, 394, 395, 423, 442, 445, 446, 473
Self-organising maps 301
Semantic 355-357, 365, 475
    polarities 357

Serotonin reuptake inhibitors 2, 29, 114
Silence 350, 352-354
Social
  defensiveness 217, 219-221, 223
  support 3, 10, 12, 51, 92, 115, 152, 154,
    155, 158, 168, 175, 180, 220, 234, 236,
    239, 243, 246-248, 251, 312, 382, 393,
    417
SSRI 29, 93, 105, 114, 115, 159
Stress 1-3, 8, 9, 12, 14, 21, 23-28, 30, 35-39,
  44, 44, 45, 51-61, 72, 76-80, 86, 90, 92, 113,
  123, 124, 135-139, 155, 167-169, 174-178,
  180, 187-189, 209, 218, 220-223, 225-228,
  239, 243, 244, 246-249, 251, 253, 255,
  273-276, 289, 290, 340, 343, 379, 380, etc.
Structured interviews 112
Syndrome X 28, 226
Systemic therapy 5, 6, 10, 14, 36, 57, 73, 77,
  78, 137, 399, 400

Temporal
  breakdown 362-364
  dimension 349, 350, 360-365
Training 3, 5, 7, 12-14, 79, 92, 112, 281,

282, 302, 303, 305, 307-310, 352, 370,
  422, 435, 437-446, 451, 453, 467, 473,
  480, 487, 503-505
Trait 73, 152, 153, 190, 201, 203, 204, 207,
  210, 219, 236, 239, 245, 287, 291, 292,
  296, 311, 313, 460
Transactional 188, 192, 235, 237-240, 242,
  245, 253, 254, 418
Trauma 12, 93, 391, 395, 396, 398, 401,
  402, 408
Treatment 2, 7, 10, 15, 29, 54, 71, 78-80, 85,
  91-94, 99, 102, 103, 105, 106, 109-111,
  114-116, 121, 125, 138, 140, 149, 151,
  157, 165, 166, 169, 172-174, 176-181,
  184, 198, 283, 284, 312, 324, 339, 343,
  344, 358-360, 363, 370-378, 380-382,
  384-387, 391, etc.
  of the Type A behavior 418
Type A behavior pattern 8, 25, 29, 74, 168,
  188-191, 209, 218, 413-415, 439
Type D personality 8, 190, 206-210, 446

World Health Organization 1, 85, 319,
  453, 473